AF680833

Jesse E. Edwards

His Legacy to Cardiovascular Medicine

Edited by:

Brooks S. Edwards
James H. Moller

Science International Corp.

Science International, Corp.
31 Sunset Court
Stamford, CT 06903
www.ScienceInternational.org

Copyright information available upon request.

Library of Congress Control Number: 2011932842

ISBN 13: 978-0-9788169-1-9

Cover and Interior Design: J. L. Saloff
Typography: Garamond Premier Pro.

Published in the United States of America on acid-free paper.
First Edition: v. 1.0

Portions of the text are Copyright ©2011 by Brooks Edwards, rights reserved. No part of this work may be reproduced or transmitted in any form by any means, electronic or mechanical, including photocopying and recording, or by any information storage or retrieval system, except as may be expressly permitted by the 1976 Copyright Act or in writing by the publisher.

To Marjorie Helen Brooks Edwards for her love
and caring for Jesse, their children, Ellen and Brooks,
and grandchildren, and for her profound interest in
Jesse's work, his colleagues and friends.

All proceeds from the sale of this book will be provided to the Jesse E. Edwards Registry of Cardiovascular Diseases to support its mission of education and research.

Contents

Commentary Contributors x

Preface 1

Jesse E. Edwards Curriculum Vitae 3

Jesse E. Edwards Profile 7

Congenital Heart Disease

1. Anomalies of the Derivatives of the Aortic Arch System
Jesse E. Edwards, M.D. 11
Reprinted from Medical Clinics of North America 1948
Commentary by: Paul Julsrud, M.D.; Nandan Anavekar. M.B., B.Ch. 36

2. The Collateral Circulation in Coarctation of the Aorta
Jesse E. Edwards, M.D., O. Theron Clagett, M.D., M.S., Russell L. Drake, Norman A. Christensen, M.D. 38
Reprinted from Mayo Clinic Proceedings 1948
Commentary by: Dave Hunter, M.D. 45

3. The Lewis A. Conner Memorial Lecture: Functional Pathology of the Pulmonary Vascular Tree in Congenital Cardiac Disease
Jesse E. Edwards, M.D. 47
Reprinted from Circulation 1957

The Pathology of Hypertensive Pulmonary Vascular Disease: A Description of Six Grades of Structural Changes in the Pulmonary Arteries with Special Reference to Congenital Cardiac Septal Defects
Donald Heath, M.D. and Jesse E. Edwards, M.D. 80
Reprinted from Circulation 1958
Commentary by: Marc Pritzker, M.D. 95

4. The Developmental Complex of "Parachute Mitral Valve," Supravalvular Ring of Left Atrium, Subaortic Stenosis, and Coarctation of Aorta
John D. Shone, M.B., Robert Sellers, M.D., Ray C. Anderson, M.D., Paul Adams, Jr., M.D., C. Walton Lillehei, M.D., F.A.C.C., Jesse E. Edwards, M.D. 97
Reprinted from American Journal of Cardiology 1963
Commentary by: Kenneth Jue, M.D. 109

5. Termination of Left Superior Vena Cava in Left Atrium, Atrial Septal Defect, and Absence of Coronary Sinus: A Developmental Complex
Gunay Raghib, M.D., Herbert D. Ruttenberg, M.D., Ray C. Anderson, M.D., Kurt Amplatz, M.D., Paul Adams, Jr., M.D., Jesse E. Edwards, M.D., ... 111
Reprinted from Circulation 1965
Commentary by: Robert Anderson, BSc, M.D., FRCPath 124

6. Persistent Truncus Arteriosus: A Classification According to Anatomic Types
Robert W. Collett, M.D. and Jesse E. Edwards, M.D. 126
Reprinted from Surgical Clinics of North America 1949
Commentary by: Mary Ella Pierpont, M.D. 152
Commentary by: Anton Becker, M.D. 154

7. Origin of Both Great Vessels from the Right Ventricle: I. Without Pulmonary Stenosis
Henry N. Neufeld, M.D., James W. DuShane, M.D., Earl H. Wood, M.D., John W. Kirklin, M.D., Jesse E. Edwards, M.D. 156
Reprinted from Circulation 1961

Origin of Both Great Vessels from the Right Ventricle: II. With Pulmonary Stenosis
Henry N. Neufeld, M.D., James W. DuShane, M.D., Jesse E. Edwards, M.D. 170
Reprinted from Circulation 1961
Commentary by: Richard Van Praagh, M.D. 180

8. Coronary Arterial Patterns in Transposition Complexes: Anatomic and Angiographic Studies
Larry P. Elliott, M.D., Kurt Amplatz, M.D., Jesse E. Edwards, M.D. 183
Reprinted from American Journal of Cardiology 1966
Commentary by: Julien Hoffman, M.D. 200

9. Congenital Cardiac Disease Associated with Polysplenia: A Developmental Complex of Bilateral "Left-Sidedness"
James H. Moller, M.D., Ahmad Nakib, M.D., Ray C. Anderson, M.D., Ph.D., Jesse E. Edwards, M.D. 202
Reprinted from Circulation 1967
Commentary by: James Moller, M.D. 213

10. A Classification of Total Anomalous Pulmonary Venous Connection Based on Developmental Considerations

Jesse E. Edwards, M.D. and H. Fred Helmholz, Jr., M.D. 214
Reprinted from Mayo Clinic Proceedings 1956
Commentary by: Fouad Butto, M.D. 224

11. Lesions of the Atrioventricular Conduction System after Repair of Ventricular Septal Defect: Relation to Heart Block

Jack L. Titus, M.D., Guy W. Daugherty, M.D., John W. Kirklin, M.D.,
Jesse E. Edwards, M.D. 226
Reprinted from Circulation 1963

Anatomy of the Atrioventricular Conduction System in Ventricular Septal Defect

Jack L. Titus, M.D., Guy W. Daugherty, M.D., Jesse E. Edwards, M.D. 233
Reprinted from Circulation 1963
Commentary by: James Kirklin, M.D. 242

12. Pathologic Spectrum of Dysplasia of the Tricuspid Valve: Features in Common with Ebstein's Malformation

Anton E. Becker, M.D., Mies J. Becker, M.D., Jesse E. Edwards, M.D. 244
Reprinted from Archives of Pathology 1971
Commentary by: Joseph Dearani, M. D. 256

13. Diagrammatic Portrayal of Variations in Cardiac Structure: Reference to Transposition, Dextrocardia and the Concept of Four Normal Hearts

Paul Stanger, M.D., Robert C. Benassi, M.S., Michael E. Korns, M.D., Kenneth L. Jue, M.D.,
Jesse E. Edwards, M.D. 257
Reprinted from Circulation 1968
Commentary by: William Edwards, M.D. 283

14. Dissecting Aneurysm Complicating Marfan's Syndrome (Arachnodactyly) in a Mother and Son

Claude M. Grondin, M.D., Charles L. Steinberg, M.D., Jesse E. Edwards, M.D. 284
Reprinted from American Heart Journal 1969
Commentary by: Heidi Connolly, M.D. 290

15. Sudden Death in Patients with Hypertrophic Cardiomyopathy: Characterization of 26 Patients Without Functional Limitation

Barry J. Maron, M.D., William C. Roberts, M.D., F.A.C.C., Jesse E. Edwards, M.D., F.A.C.C.,
Hugh A. McAllister, Jr. M.D., F.A.C.C., Daniel D. Foley, M.D., Stephen E. Epstein, M.D.,
F.A.C.C. 292
Reprinted from American Journal of Cardiology 1978
Commentary by: Barry Maron, M.D. 300

Acquired Diseases of the Heart

16. Pathologic Anatomy of Mitral Insufficiency
Jesse E. Edwards, M.D. and Howard B. Burchell, M.D. 303
Reprinted from Mayo Clinic Proceedings 1958
Commentary by: Maurice Enriquez-Sarano, M.D., FACC, FAHA 316

17. The Myxomatous Mitral Valve and Sudden Death
Elliot Chesler, M.D., Richard A. King, M.D., Jesse E. Edwards, M.D.. 318
Reprinted from Circulation 1983
Commentary by: Paul Friedman, M.D. 326

18. Pathologic Changes in Aortic-Coronary Arterial Saphenous Vein Grafts
Zeev Vlodaver, M.D. and Jesse E. Edwards, M.D. 328
Reprinted from Circulation 1971
Commentary by: Zeev Vlodaver, M.D. 338

19. Ventricular Septal Rupture Complicating Acute Myocardial Infarction: Identification of Simple and Complex Types in 53 Autopsied Hearts
Brooks S. Edwards, M.D., William D. Edwards, M.D., Jesse E. Edwards, M.D. 340
Reprinted from American Journal of Cardiology 1985
Commentary by: Robert Wilson, M.D. 345

20. The Congenital Bicuspid Aortic Valve
Jesse E. Edwards, M.D. 347
Reprinted from Circulation 1961
Commentary by: William C. Roberts, M.D. 351

21. Atherosclerosis: An Impossible Mission?
Jesse E. Edwards, M.D. 352
Reprinted from Circulation 1969
Commentary by: Brooks Edwards, M.D. 356

22. The Mechanism of Balloon Angioplasty
Wilfrido R. Castaneda-Zuniga, M.D., Augustin Formanek, M.D., Murthy Tadavarthy, M.D., Zeev Vlodaver, M.D., Jesse E. Edwards, M.D., Christoph Zollikofer, M.D., Kurt Amplatz, M.D. 385
Reprinted from Radiology 1980
Commentary by: John Bass, M.D. 365

Perspectives

23. The Autopsy: Do We Still Need It?
Jesse E. Edwards, M.D. 369
Reprinted from Mayo Clinic Proceedings 1981
Commentary by: Michael Ackerman, M.D., Ph.D. 371

24. Epilogue: The Pathologist
Jesse E. Edwards, M.D. 372
Reprinted from American Journal of Cardiology 1982
Commentary by: Brooks Edwards, M.D. 375

Final Thoughts 377
Brooks Edwards, M.D.

Permissions 379

Commentary Contributors

Michael J. Ackerman, M.D., Ph.D.
Professor of Medicine, Pediatrics, and Pharmacology
Consultant in Cardiovascular Diseases and Pediatric Cardiology
Director of the Long QT Syndrome Clinic and
the Windland Smith Rice Sudden Death Genomics Laboratory
Mayo Clinic
Rochester, Minnesota

Nandan S. Anavekar, M.B., B.Ch.
Assistant Professor of Medicine
Resident in Cardiology & Echocardiography
Mayo Clinic
Rochester, Minnesota

Robert H. Anderson BSc, M.D., FRCPath
Visiting Professor at Newcastle University
Emeritus Professor at University College, London
Emeritus Visiting Professor at Manchester University
Visiting Professor at Medical University of South Carolina

John L. Bass, M.D.
Associate Professor of Pediatrics
University of Minnesota
Minneapolis, Minnesota

Anton E. Becker, M.D.
Emeritus Professor of Cardiovascular Pathology
Academic Medical Center
University of Amsterdam
The Netherlands

Fouad Butto, M.D.
Director of Pediatric Cardiology
Toledo Children's Hospital
Associate Professor of Pediatrics
University of Toledo
Toledo, Ohio

Heidi M. Connolly, M.D.
Professor of Medicine, Mayo Clinic College of Medicine
Vice Chair for Education, Division of Cardiovascular Diseases
Director of the Marfan and Thoracic Aortic Clinic and Congenital Heart Center
Mayo Clinic
Rochester, Minnesota

Joseph A. Dearani, M.D.
Chair, Division of Cardiovascular Surgery
Professor of Surgery
Mayo Clinic
Rochester, Minnesota

Brooks S. Edwards, M.D.
Professor of Medicine, Mayo Clinic College of Medicine
Consultant, Division of Cardiovascular Medicine
Director, William J. von Liebig Transplant Center
Mayo Clinic
Rochester, Minnesota

William D. Edwards, M.D.
Professor of Pathology
Department of Laboratory Medicine and Pathology
Mayo Clinic
Rochester, Minnesota

Paul A. Friedman, M.D.
Professor of Medicine
Mayo Clinic
Rochester, Minnesota

Julien I.E. Hoffman, M.D.
Emeritus Professor of Pediatrics
University of California San Francisco
San Francisco, California

David W. Hunter, M.D.
Professor of Radiology
University of Minnesota
Minneapolis, Minnesota

Kenneth L. Jue, M.D.
Pediatric Cardiologist, Children's Hospital Central California
Madera, California
Professor of Pediatrics, University of California Los Angeles
Los Angeles, California

Paul R. Julsrud, M.D.
Professor of Radiology
Supplemental Consultant
Division of Cardiac Radiology
Mayo Clinic
Rochester, Minnesota

James K. Kirklin, M.D.
Professor and Director
Division of Cardiothoracic Surgery
University of Alabama at Birmingham
Birmingham, Alabama

Barry J. Maron, M.D.
Director, Hypertrophic Cardiomyopathy Center
Minneapolis Heart Institute Foundation
Minneapolis, Minnesota

James H. Moller, M.D.
Adjunct Professor of Medicine
Professor (retired) and former Head of Pediatrics
University of Minnesota
Minneapolis, Minnesota

Mary Ella Peirpont, M.D., Ph.D.
Associate Professor of Pediatrics and Ophthalmology
University of Minnesota
Pediatric Cardiologist and Geneticist
Children's Hospitals and Clinics of Minnesota
Minneapolis, Minnesota

Marc Pritzker, M.D.
Professor of Medicine
University of Minnesota
Minneapolis, Minnesota

William C. Roberts, M.D.
Executive Director, Baylor Heart and Vascular Institute
Dean, A. Webb Roberts Department of Continuing Medical Education
Baylor University Medical Center
Editor in Chief, American Journal of Cardiology and the Baylor University Medical Center Proceedings
Dallas, Texas

Maurice Enriquez-Sarano, M.D., FACC, FAHA
Professor of Medicine, Mayo Clinic College of Medicine
Director, Valvular Heart Disease Clinic
Consultant, Cardiovascular Diseases and Internal Medicine
Mayo Clinic
Rochester, Minnesota

Richard Van Praagh, M.D.
Emeritus Professor of Pathology
Harvard Medical School
Boston, Massachusetts

Zeev Vlodaver, M.D.
Former Senior Research Associate in Cardiovascular Pathology
Jesse E. Edwards Registry, United Hospital
St. Paul, Minnesota
Former director, Non-invasive Cardiology, Unity Hospital
Fridley, Minnesota

Robert F. Wilson, M.D.
Professor, Cardiovascular Division
University of Minnesota
Minneapolis, Minnesota

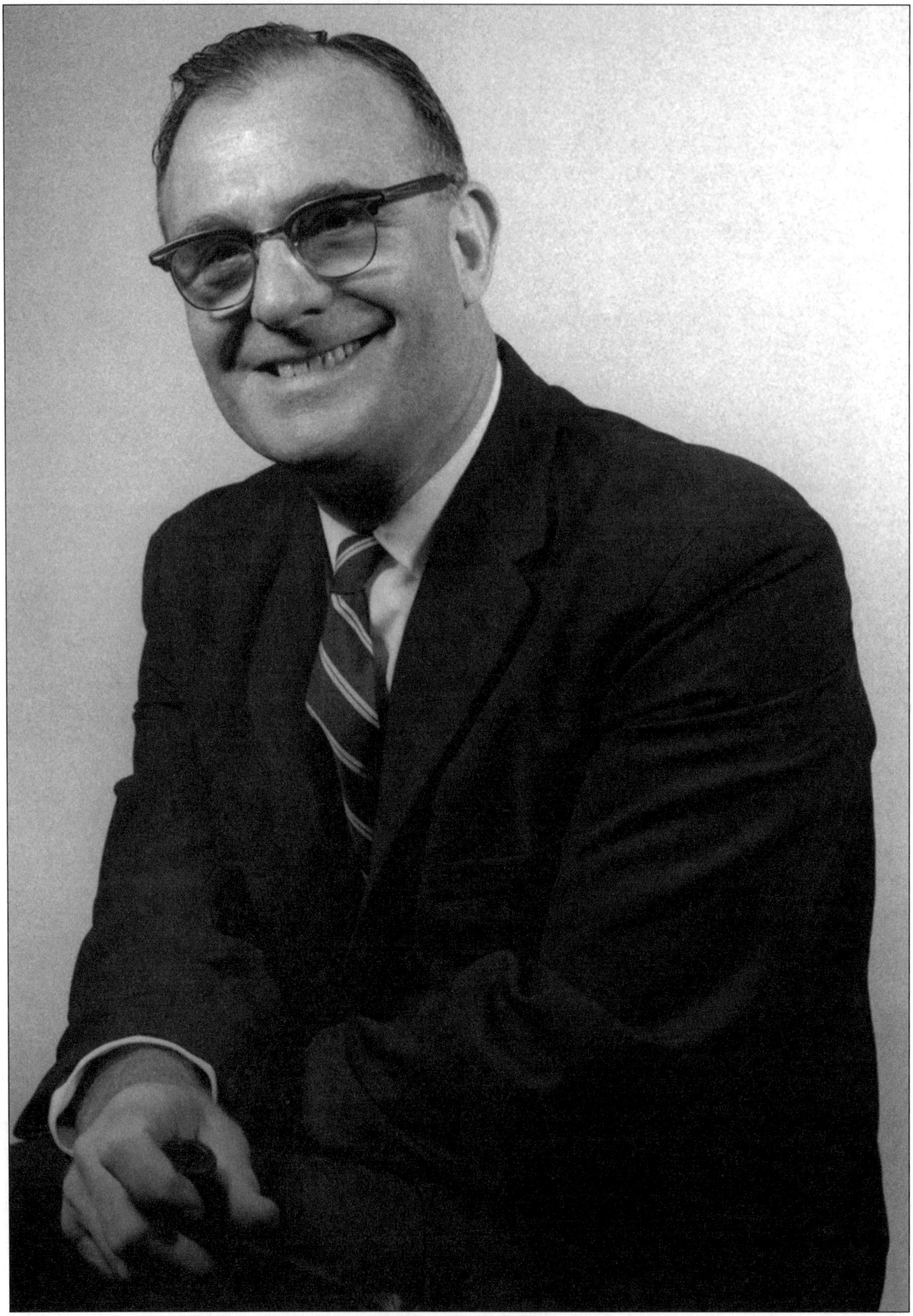

Jesse E. Edwards, M.D.

Preface

July 14, 2011, is the 100th anniversary of the birth of Jesse E. Edwards. This book honors his life and contributions to cardiology through the study and clinical application of pathology. His major influence was describing the structure of malformed or diseased hearts through the clarity of his writing and effective teaching of learners at all levels from medical students to professors. He strove to provide a framework for conditions of the cardiovascular system.

In this book are reprinted 27 of the 725 papers he wrote in collaboration with others, often with those beginning their careers in cardiology, pathology or cardiac surgery. The papers reflect a range of topics and about 2/3 relate to congenital heart disease and 1/3 to acquired conditions affecting the heart. This division mirrors the overall distribution of his articles. This probably reflects that fact that he was a key contributor at two institutions in Minnesota, the Mayo Clinic and the University of Minnesota, which were the first centers to perform open heart operations for congenital heart disease.

Each of the reprinted articles is accompanied by a commentary from an internationally recognized authority, a colleague or a trainee. These individuals were asked to discuss the importance of the original article with a view to its influence on current management of patients and our understating of the condition.

The articles were selected by a group of cardiologists or cardiac pathologists associated with the Jesse E. Edwards Cardiovascular Registry at the United Hospital in St. Paul, Minnesota. They were: Brooks Edwards MD, Michael Garr MD, Shannon Mackey-Bojack MD, James H. Moller MD, Victor Tschida MD and Zeev Vladovar MD. Appreciation is given to Daniel Foley MD, Vice President of Medical Affairs at United Hospital, St. Paul, Minnesota for his ongoing support and interest in our project and in the Cardiovascular Registry, itself. Jesse's daughter, Ellen Villa, contributed her editorial skills to help shape this work. Judy Anderson and Krista Barsness of the Jesse Edwards Registry of Cardiovascular Pathology provided exemplary secretarial help in gathering articles and preparing the materials. Michelle Ward, Brooks Edwards' secretary, was a joy to work with on this project. She compiled the material to send to the publisher and doggedly pursued copyright approvals and the reprinting of a number of the papers.

Shannon Mackey-Bojack, MD, is the current director of the Jesse E. Edwards Cardiovascular Registry and interestingly as an undergraduate student worked there preparing cardiac specimens and assisting the students, residents and fellows. She maintains the spirit of Jesse by demonstrating cardiac specimens at hospitals, holding teaching sessions around a table, contributing to the literature, being available for "curb-side" consultation and exploring new areas of cardiology. A couple of these relate to the histology of the conduction system as it is affected by disease and the effects of interventional procedures on the heart and great vessels. A continued focus of the Registry is the study and prevention of sudden death. The Registry is fortunate to have the support of the United Hospital Foundation. Their efforts for this unique and valuable resource continue to benefit the field of cardiovascular disease. The ultimate beneficiaries of the Registry are the children and adults afflicted by a cardiac condition and their families.

The success of any book depends on the publisher. Steven Korn has guided us through the preparation of this book. His specific questions and suggestions have helped us define our purpose and shape the book into a fitting tribute to Jesse. His dedication to this project was out of deep affection for Dr. Edwards and his family. To him we owe our thanks.

The editors thank the publishers of the following journals: American Heart Journal, American Journal of Cardiology, Archives of Pathology, Circulation, Medical Clinics of North America, Proceedings of the Mayo Clinic, Radiology and Surgical Clinics of North America for their permission to reprint these articles which appeared in their respective journals.

Jesse E. Edwards, M.D.
Condensed Curriculum Vitae

I. BIRTH: Hyde Park, Massachusetts, July 14, 1911

II. MARITAL STATUS: Married (Marjorie Helen Brooks)

Children (Ellen {Mrs. John K. Villa} and Brooks Sayre)

Grandchildren (Kate Villa, John Jesse Villa, Jeremy Edwards, Max Edwards, Jessica Edwards)

III. EDUCATION:

Tufts College, BS 1932
Tufts College Medical School, MD 1935

IV. TRAINING:

1935–36, Resident in Pathology, Mallory Institute of Pathology, Boston
1936–37, Mixed Clinical Internship, Albany Hospital, Albany, NY
1937–40, Assistant to the Pathologist, Mallory Institute of Pathology, Boston City Hospital, Boston
1940–42, Research Fellow, National Cancer Institute, US Public Health Service, Bethesda, Maryland

V. HOSPITAL AND CLINIC AFFILIATIONS:

United Hospital (Formerly The Charles T. Miller Hospital)

A. Program of research and training in Cardiovascular Pathology (Currently, The Jesse E. Edwards Registry of Cardiovascular Disease),

Senior Consultant, 1987–2008

Director, 1960–1987

B. Department of Pathology, United Hospital

Senior Consultant in Anatomic Pathology, 1978–1987

Directory of Laboratories, 1960–1978

Other

A. Minneapolis Children's Medical Center, Minneapolis, MN
Honorary Staff Member - 1980–1998

B. St Paul-Ramsey Medical Center, St Paul, MN
Consultant, Department Of Pathology, 1968–1998

C. VA Medical Center, Minneapolis, MN
Consultant, Department of Pathology, 1966–1998

D. Hennepin County Medical Center, Minneapolis, MN
Consultant, Department of Pathology, 1966–1998

E. Mayo Clinic, Rochester, MN
Consultant, Sect. Of Pathology Anatomy, 1946–1960

VI. ACADEMIC AFFILIATIONS:

University of Minnesota

A. Professor of Pathology, Graduate School, 1960–2008

B. Clinical Professor, Pathology, School of Medicine, 1960–2008

C. Assistant Professor (1946–51); Associate Professor (1951–54); And Professor (1954–60) of Pathology Mayo Foundation, Graduate School

Other

A. Instructor in Pathology, Bacteriology and Surgery
Tufts College Medical School, 1939–40

B. Instructor in Pathology
Boston University School of Medicine, 1938

VII. PUBLICATIONS:

A. Papers - 725 (majority in the field of cardiovascular disease)

B. Books - 14

C. Chapters - 70

VIII. EXTRACURRICULAR PROFESSIONAL EXPERIENCES:

A. Editorial Boards

1. American Journal of Cardiovascular Pathology
2. Laboratory Investigation
3. Circulation
4. American Journal of Cardiology
5. American Heart Journal
6. Geriatrics
7. Pediatric Cardiology

B. Societies:

1. Member, Path. Study Section, US Public Health Service 1957–62
2. President, Minnesota Heart Association, 1962– 63
3. President, International Academy of Pathology, 1955–56
4. President, American Heart Association, 1967–68
5. President, World Congress of Pediatric Cardiology, 1980
6. Review Committee: Member, Mortality Review Committee, Multicenter Diltiazem Postinfarction Trial (MDPIT), University of Rochester, NY
7. Chairman, Mortality Review Committee, Program on the Surgical Control of Hyperlipidemias, University of Minnesota, Minneapolis
8. Member, End Point Event Subcommittee, Multicenter Study of Silent Myocardial Ischemia, University of Rochester, NY

IX. MILITARY EXPERIENCE: 1942–46 progressively Capt., Major, Lt. Col.,

US Army Medical Corps

A. Active Service:

1. Chief, General Hospital Laboratories in US and European Theater, 1942–45
2. Pathologist, War Crimes Investigating Team, European Theater, US Army, 1945
3. Commanding Officer, Central Laboratory for US Army in Europe and concurrently Laboratory Consultant to the Chief Surgeon, European Theater, 1945–46

B. Col., Medical Corps, US Army Reserve, ret.

C. Civilian Consultant to Surgeon General, US Army, 1947–1967

X. CERTIFICATION AND LICENSURE:

A. Diplomat of National Board of Medical examiners, 1936

B. Certified by American Board of Pathology (Pathologic Anatomy), 1940

C. Licensed to practice medicine in Minnesota,

XI. SCIENTIFIC HONORS:

A. Alpha Omega Alpha

B. Gifted Teacher Award, American College of Cardiology

C. Gold Heart Award, American Heart Association

D. Research Achievement Award, American Heart Association

E. Distinguished Teacher Award, American Heart Association

F. Honorary Member, American College of Chest Physicians

G. Honorary Member, Council on Clinical Cardiology, AHA

H. Doctor of Science (Honorary), Georgetown University, 1990

I. University of Minnesota Medical School Teacher of the Year

J. Harold S. Diehl Award, Minnesota Medical Foundation 1998

K. Mayo Clinic Distinguished Alumni Award 1987

XII. BIOGRAPHIC REFERENCES:

A. Who's Who in the World

B. Who's Who in America

C. American Men of Science

D. Directory of Medical Specialists

Profile of Jesse E. Edwards

James H. Moller, M.D.

Who inspires you? A question I was asked recently for a hospital publication. My first thought was Jesse Edwards. While gone for nearly four years now he remains an inspiration to me and many others who came into his presence. Yes, he inspired us to work hard learning about the heart and its conditions, and to be dedicated to cardiology and contribute to its advancement. His life and attitudes inspired us. He was a thoughtful teacher, an attentive listener, and concerned about each of us as individuals. One day, a rather assertive fellow was pontificating on a subject at our daily heart review session. Jesse sat patiently listening until the individual had finished and then continued the session. Later when asked how he could put up with the interruption, he replied, "He might have had something important to say."

Our lives at the University of Minnesota changed immensely in the summer of 1960 when Jesse moved from the Mayo Clinic, where he had been for over a decade, to the Charles T. Miller Hospital in St Paul, Minnesota. He quickly became an invaluable resource for us in pediatric cardiology and cardiac surgery at the University of Minnesota and the various teaching hospitals in our metropolitan area. He was an active participant in conferences, taught about the structure of malformed hearts and provided opportunities to study cardiac pathology in the "Miller Basement"- a suite of offices, laboratory space and conference room on the lower floor of the hospital. Often a half dozen or so pediatric or cardiac surgical residents or fellows or medical students worked, reviewed cardiac specimens and wrote reports or papers about them. With Jesse's warm and encompassing personality we developed a sharing attitude by teaching each other, reviewing cardiac specimens together and exchanging knowledge from our own specialties. Undergraduate premedical students were employed as assistants and many of whom became medical students and some ultimately cardiologists, cardiac surgeons or pathologists. This experience was possible because he embraced us and valued our presence. In his low-key, quiet manner he encouraged and was an example to us.

Open-heart surgery for congenital heart disease in children began in 1954 and 55 at two sites 80 miles apart both in Minnesota – The Mayo Clinic and the University of Minnesota. Jesse played a major collaborating role at both institutions in those pioneering days. The cardiologists, cardiac surgeons, physiologists and radiologists appreciated his collaboration for he understood their challenges and questions of surgeons and was able to provide clear answers based on his knowledge of cardiac anatomy and pathology. Furthermore, he developed frameworks and classifications, which organized the diverse types of cardiac malformations, making our knowledge more orderly. Many of the papers reprinted here reflect his working relationships with specialists in other disciplines of medicine. The striking ability to develop collegial relations with a broad range of specialists reflected the respect they felt for him as a trustworthy individual with much to share.

Around academic institutions we often hear the word "mentor". The term is loosely applied to relationships between teacher and student. That relationship may be advisor-advisee, supervisor-staff member, division head-division member. But true mentorship is something much greater and has a broad meaning.

Mentors are individuals with advanced knowledge and experience who take a personal interest in helping the careers and advancement of their protégés. They may not be in the same discipline as their protégé, but a close friendship develops that becomes one of the most important relationships in the protégées life. The relationship is informal and develops on the basis of mutual identification and the fulfillment of career needs. Thus, it cannot be assigned, it is chosen

Mentoring is from the Greek word meaning enduring and is defined as a sustained relationship between a youth and an older person.

Mentorship is a long-term relationship, one that even if people are apart for a period of time when they meet again their relationship is strong. They often share other interests in common besides the focus of their mutual activity. Through continued involvement the adult offers support, guidance and assistance as the younger person goes through a difficult period, faces new challenges. Jesse was my mentor in every sense of the word.

I never had another teacher like Jesse. And my associates would say the same. He spent more individual time with me in a teacher – student relationship (and subsequently mentor-mentee) than anyone else ever has. That teaching was often done at a ledge-like counter along one wall of his office. There was a window above the counter and the afternoon sun streamed in, which was so welcome on wintery days. We sat side-by-side and worked on manuscripts. The discussion about the manuscript involved anatomy, clinical correlations, surgical approaches, developmental relationships and writing skills. On the counter were his tools - unlined punched yellow paper, scissors with long blades and Elmer's glue. This was cut and paste before it became a computer command. He explained that over my lifespan I would save a year's time by this technique. So we worked cutting and rearranging sentences and paragraphs, interspersed with new sentences. All this to be retyped by his secretary of many years - Jane Jungbauer. But most importantly he discussed why he was making the changes to the manuscript you had so carefully prepared. I cherish those afternoon sessions with him. They taught me so much about the obvious - cardiology and writing and about the not so obvious - those more subtle lessons of attitudes-patience, concern for others, respect and the responsibility to help younger people – students, residents, fellows develop their careers.

As I was in the last phase of my pediatric cardiology fellowship, I did not have a position to go to. Jesse offered me my first "job" and that as a senior research fellow in cardiac pathology - a bit different from what I had been trained to do as a pediatric cardiologist. As we discussed my responsibilities, I said I would probably be spending part of some Saturdays in the pathology laboratory. He asked, "What about your family?" This question emphasized the importance of family as it was so evident in the lives of Jess and his wife, Marge. In the hallway of their home were photographs of their children, Ellen and Brooks and their grandchildren, Jeremy, Max and Jessie Edwards and Kate and Johnny Villa. Each summer, the three families went to northern Minnesota to celebrate Jess' birthday on July 14th, an annual event which usually included fishing. After Jess's death his daughter, Ellen, prepared a beautiful booklet about Jesse and his family. Each grandchild wrote a very touching remembrance of their grandfather, known as Gaga. He was an outstanding role model showing the importance of family and friends for completeness in life.

I visited Jess and Marge shortly before he passed. I gave him a copy of a small book I had written for medical students. I inscribed it "to the best English teacher I have ever had". But he was so much more to me and to all of us who were privileged to work with him in the "Miller basement."

Congenital Heart Disease

ANOMALIES OF THE DERIVATIVES OF THE AORTIC ARCH SYSTEM

JESSE E. EDWARDS

IT is known that certain vascular anomalies resulting from maldevelopment of the derivatives of the aortic arch system may be responsible for symptoms resulting from compression of either the trachea or the esophagus. The symptoms, physical signs, roentgenographic features and surgical therapy have been the subjects of many articles. The symptoms vary considerably. In some instances no symptoms may be present during a full lifetime.[3,11,23,36,42,44] In other instances symptoms may be noticed at birth or shortly thereafter.[10,16,20,26,28,41,45,51] When they appear at this early time of life, manifestations of respiratory involvement usually overshadow those of esophageal malfunction, although the reverse may be true.[21] In the newborn, symptoms include cough, inspiratory and expiratory stridor, intercostal and suprasternal retraction with inspiration and attacks of cyanosis which may be precipitated by ingestion of food. Regurgitation may follow ingestion of food, and drinking may be associated with apparent discomfort. There is a tendency toward pulmonary infection. The symptoms cited are sometimes attributed to an enlarged thymus and since roentgenographic examination of the thorax may reveal a widened mediastinal shadow, consistent with an enlarged thymus, the initial impression may be that an enlarged thymus is the basis for the infant's difficulties. So strongly may the diagnosis of enlarged thymus be entertained that it is not uncommon for radiation to be applied in an effort to shrink the thymus. This proves of no avail. Unless surgical measures are employed to correct those vascular anomalies causing pronounced symptoms, it is common for the infant to die of pulmonary infection.

The clinical impression that some sort of vascular anomaly is responsible for the symptoms may be gained from bronchoscopic examination which may reveal a zone of tracheal narrowing. It is usually simpler and more advisable to administer a small amount of barium and to visualize the esophagus roentgenographically. A zone of constriction of the

Medical Clinics of North America, July 1948

esophagus in the upper thoracic region will usually be readily evident and will lead the physician to the correct interpretation as to the basis for the symptoms. If no symptoms occur during infancy, the patient may never suffer as a result of his vascular abnormality. On the other hand, symptoms may first become evident later in life.[6,8,27,29,40,43] As a result of aging changes which cause dilatation of the aorta and its branches, anomalies which produced no symptoms during infancy or childhood may become troublesome during adult life, especially during advancing age. When symptoms first appear in adult life they are usually in the form of persistent cough, dysphagia and rarely, hoarseness.

The exact anatomic nature of the vascular anomaly can frequently be ascertained by the application of several roentgenographic technics and criteria. These have been described.[3,4,6,17,18,20,29,33,34,40,42,43,45] It is not the purpose of this communication to consider these to any extent.

Knowledge concerning the configuration of the various anomalies of the aortic arch derivatives is important to the clinician, to the roentgenologist and to the surgeon who treat patients who have symptoms attributable to these anomalies. To the clinician and roentgenologist, this knowledge may be used to advantage in evaluating the findings in cases in which symptoms may result from the presence of vascular anomalies. To the surgeon, realization of the possible vascular configurations which may interfere with the function of either the esophagus or the trachea will serve as a guide, while exploring the region of the aortic arch, in determining the exact nature of the anomaly in a given case. This determination will serve to guide the surgeon to perform those procedures most suitable for the correction of the condition or for the relief of symptoms resulting from it.

The primary purpose of this communication is to describe and to illustrate* those anomalies of the derivatives of the

---

* I am indebted to Mr. Russell L. Drake for the preparation of the illustrations. It is to be emphasized that these are diagrammatic representations. At times it was necessary to make minor modifications of relations in order that the salient features of a given condition could be brought out in one illustration. For the preparation of the illustrations of those anomalies which have been reported, use has been made of the author's personal experience and of illus-

aortic arch system which may interfere with the function of either the esophagus or the trachea. The subjects of persistent patent ductus arteriosus and coarctation of the aorta are not included. The majority of the anomalous configurations to be presented have been described. To these will be added several configurations which, as far as the author knows, have not been reported. Yet these stand out as distinct possibilities. Consequently, they will be included as hypothetical forms. This is done with the hope that when they are encountered, they will be understood and not be viewed with undue surprise. Furthermore, it is hoped that whosoever observes these hypothetical possibilities will be stimulated to place them on record in order that the literature may contain a more comprehensive accumulation of this group of anomalies.

In discussions such as this it is customary to employ the standard Rathke diagram of the six aortic arches in explaining the developmental basis for the various aortic arch anomalies and in relating the various types to each other. While this approach is perfectly logical and correct, the reader, nevertheless, is likely to be somewhat confused. The reason for this is explained by several factors. Not only do a number of structures of the primitive aortic arch system disappear, but there are important alterations in the shape of the aortic arch pattern. This results from the fact that while some portions of the primitive arterial pattern grow in equal proportion to the growth of the body, other portions grow relatively little with respect to the growth of the body as a whole. This produces distortions of the basic diagram of six arches. Moreover, there are important shifts in the relative situation of the subclavian arteries to that of the six aortic arches (ducti arteriosi). Thus in the basic diagram of the six aortic arches, which is customarily employed, the subclavian arteries lie caudad to the sixth arches. Yet, by the time of birth, important differences in the rates of growth of the portions of the aortic arch system result in the presence of the subclavian arteries in a cephalad position with respect to the sixth aortic arches.

I feel that a better understanding of the relationship of

---

trations in such works as those of Bayford, Quain, Turner, Abbott, Thomson,[4] Holzapfel, Kopsch, Poynter, Arkin, Wolman, Gross[22] and others.

the aortic arch anomalies, from a developmental point of view and with respect to each other, can be had by an approach other than the employment of the basic primitive and diagrammatic six arch pattern. It seems best to employ, as the basic pattern, an anomaly which, while it contains the essential features of the primitive aortic arch pattern, has as well gone through the growth adjustments that take place in all persons.

For this reason, the anomaly known as the functioning double aortic arch is chosen as the basic pattern. To fulfill completely the line of reasoning, this anomaly should contain right and left ducti arteriosi but usually only one ductus arteriosus is present. The one adjustment that the reader must make is to realize that the functioning double aortic arch represents with one exception the primitive aortic arch pattern, in which growth adjustments have taken place. The one exception is that one of the sixth aortic arches has largely disappeared.

In my opinion, malformations of the aortic arch derivatives may be divided into two groups depending upon whether the ductus arteriosus* takes its origin from the left pulmonary artery or from the right pulmonary artery. Arbitrarily, in cases in which the ductus arteriosus arises from the left pulmonary artery the anomalies are classified under Group I while in cases in which the ductus arteriosus takes its origin from the right pulmonary artery the anomalies are placed in Group II. Group I is by far the larger of the two. Although exceptions to the rule occur, the upper portion of the descending aorta lies on that side of the body on which the ductus arteriosus is found.

In those cases in which the upper portion of the descending aorta lies on the right side, the lower portion of the descending aorta crosses to the left at about the level of the body of the eighth or ninth thoracic vertebra to leave the thorax through the aortic hiatus.

* The term "ductus arteriosus" will be used interchangeably with the term "ligamentum arteriosum." Patency of the ductus arteriosus is not an essential part of the anomalies to be considered although it may be encountered, additionally.

GROUP I. LEFT-SIDED DUCTUS ARTERIOSUS AND LEFT-SIDED DESCENDING AORTA

A. Functioning Double Aortic Arch.—The double aortic arch has the following characteristics. The ascending aorta arises normally from the left ventricle and then divides into two arches, a left and a right. The left or so-called anterior arch follows closely the course of the normal aortic arch. It passes in front of the trachea and over the left major bronchus to join the descending aorta, which lies on the left side of the body. The right or so-called posterior arch passes over the right major bronchus and then turns rather abruptly to the left behind the esophagus and in front of the vertebral column. It joins the left arch either to the left of or behind the esophagus at the point at which the latter arch joins the descending aorta. The branches of the aortic arches are symmetrically arranged. The right common carotid and the subclavian arteries arise independently in that order, from before backward, from the right aortic arch. Similarly, the left common carotid and subclavian arteries arise from the left arch. The ductus arteriosus is inserted into the left arch between the origin of the left subclavian artery, in front and the junction of the left and right arches, behind. The lower attachment of the ductus arteriosus is to the left pulmonary artery (fig. 130*a*).

It is evident that in the case of functioning double aortic arch the trachea and esophagus are encircled by a vascular ring composed of the bifurcation of the ascending aorta in front, the right and the left aortic arches laterally, and either the posterior limb of the right aortic arch alone or the junction of the two arches, behind. If the vascular ring is sufficiently tight to compress the two tubes which it encircles, the trachea is usually compressed at each side and is thus converted into a triangular-shaped tube at the level of the arches. The esophagus is compressed from behind forward. The connections of the ductus arteriosus are such as to hold the bifurcation of the pulmonary trunk tightly against the front of the trachea, which increases the pressure of vessels against this tube.

This appears to be particularly true if the posterior junc-

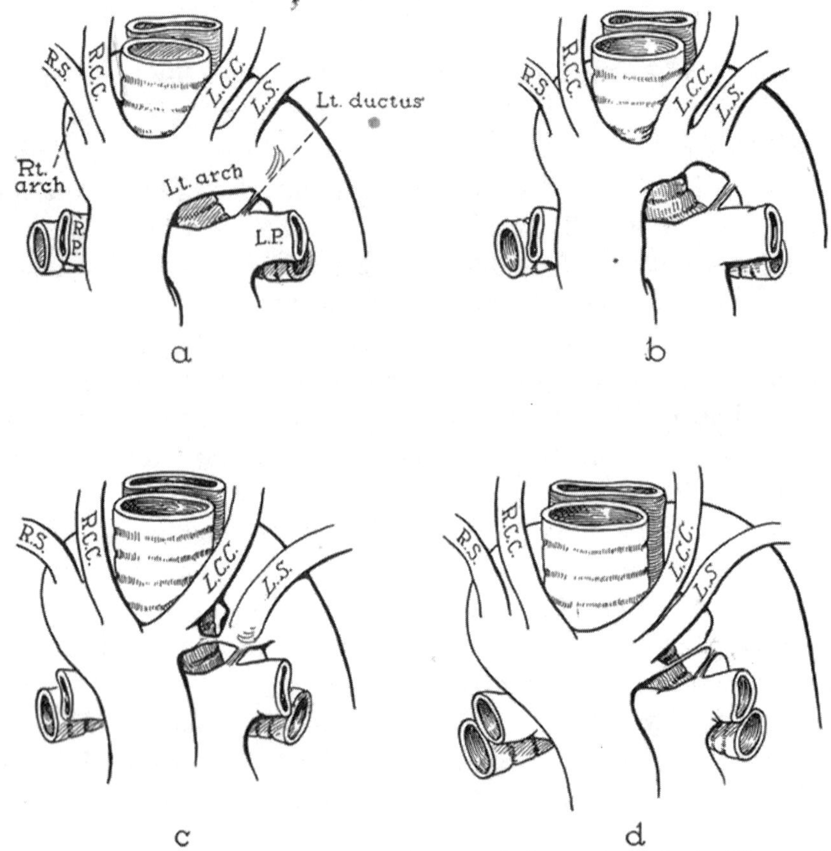

Fig. 130.—*Left-Sided Ductus Arteriosus and Descending Aorta* (Group I). *a. Functioning Double Aortic Arch.* This is the basic pattern from which all the anomalies of Group I, shown in figures 130 and 131, are derived. In functioning double aortic arch, two arches are derived from the ascending aorta. The left pursues a course similar to that of the normal aortic arch. The right arch, after crossing over the right major bronchus, deviates to the left, behind the esophagus, to join the left arch and descending aorta to the left of the midline. Occasionally, this junction may be behind the esophagus. The trachea and esophagus are encircled by the aortic structures. The left-sided ductus arteriosus holds the left pulmonary artery and the bifurcation of the pulmonary trunk against the anterior surface of the trachea. The right and left arches are of approximately equal caliber.

b. Functioning Double Aortic Arch. The vascular pattern is identical to that in figure 130*a*. This is a more common form of functioning double arch. In it the left arch is the more narrow of the two.

c. Partial Atresia of Double Aortic Arch. In this anomaly the basic pattern shown in figure 130*a* is altered in such a way that there is a zone of atresia of the left aortic arch between the origin of the left common carotid artery and that of the left subclavian artery. Although there is no longer a functioning double arch, there is still a vascular ring about the esophagus and trachea, as in the functioning double aortic arch. This anomaly is hypothetical.

d. Partial Atresia of Double Aortic Arch. In contrast with figure 130*c*, the zone of atresia of the left aortic arch lies between the origin of the left subclavian artery and the aortic insertion of the ductus arteriosus.

ANOMALIES OF DERIVATIVES OF AORTIC ARCH 931

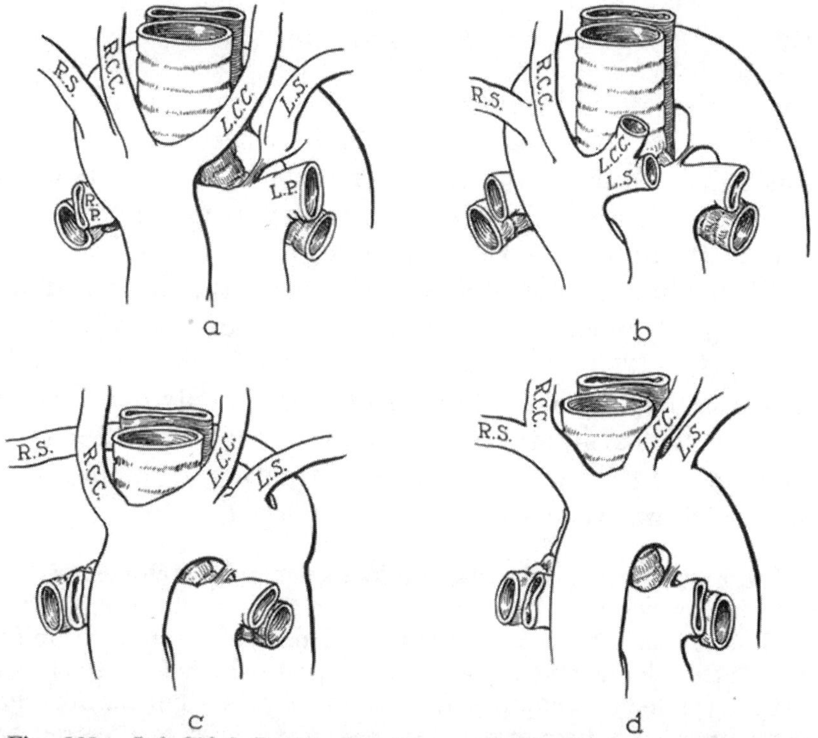

Fig. 131.—*Left-Sided Ductus Arteriosus and Left-Sided Descending Aorta* (Group II). *a. Right-Sided Aortic Arch with Retro-Esophageal Segment and Left-Sided Descending Aorta; Left Subclavian Artery Originating from Aortic Diverticulum.* In figure 130*c* there was illustrated a zone of atresia in the left portion of a double aortic arch. The zone lay between the origins of the left common carotid and subclavian arteries. In that type of anomaly the atresia would be expected to occur late in fetal life or after birth; therefore, the atretic segment would be still recognizable. If the atresia occurs in the same situation in early intra-uterine life, the anomaly illustrated in this figure occurs. There is a right-sided aortic arch with a retro-esophageal segment which joins the left-sided, upper portion of the descending aorta. The left subclavian artery arises as the fourth branch of the aorta from a diverticulum to which the ductus arteriosus also is attached. The diverticulum represents the pervious, most posterior part of a left aortic arch. There is a vascular ring about the trachea and esophagus; this ring is composed of the right aortic arch, on the right, the retro-esophageal segment of the right aortic arch, behind, the aortic diverticulum and the ductus arteriosus on the left, and the bifurcation of the pulmonary trunk in front.

b. Right-Sided Aortic Arch with Retro-Esophageal Segment and Left-Sided Descending Aorta; Left Subclavian Artery Originating from Left Innominate Artery. This anomaly varies from that shown in figure 131*a* only in that the gap in the left aortic arch lies between the origin of the left subclavian artery and the aortic insertion of the ductus arteriosus. Consequently, the left subclavian artery arises from a left-sided innominate artery. The ductus arteriosus is inserted into a remnant of the posterior portion of the left arch which usually appears in the form of an aortic diverticulum. As the anomaly shown in figure 131*a* is comparable with the one shown in figure 130*c*, this anomaly is com-tion of the left and right aortic arches is behind rather than to the left of the esophagus. In such instances there is greater tension upon the ductus arteriosus, which, in turn, tends to pull the bifurcation of the pulmonary trunk more firmly against the anterior surface of the trachea.

When a functioning double aortic arch exists the two arches are often of unequal diameter; the right one usually is the wider[8] (fig. 130*b*). Occasionally, the two arches may be of approximately equal caliber.[10] I have personally observed an example of this. In still other instances, the left arch may be the larger of the two. This was the situation in the following case which was reported by Gordon (case 4).

The patient was a boy, five weeks of age, whose clinical history was characterized by noisy breathing which was intensified when the infant was lying down or was fed. Roentgenographic examination of the thorax revealed a wide mediastinal shadow which was first interpreted as a manifestation of an enlarged thymus. Bronchoscopy revealed a high-grade compression stenosis of the trachea, at the carina, and similar compression of both main bronchi. Roentgenologic examination of the esophagus with barium revealed esophageal compression. It was believed that a vascular malformation was responsible for the clinical features described. A left thoracotomy disclosed a left-sided ligamentum arteriosum. The aorta seemed to show a normal configuration; the left arch was of normal size and blended in a normal manner with the descending aorta, which was on the left side. A sudden attack of cyanosis occurred three days after the operation and the child died. Necropsy revealed a double aortic arch. The left arch was of normal size but the right arch was smaller.

---

parable with the one shown in 130*d*.

c. Left-Sided Aortic Arch and Left-Sided Descending Aorta; Right Subclavian Artery Arising from the Distal Arch or from the Upper Portion of the Descending Aorta. If the right portion of the double arch shown in figure 130*a* disappears between the points of origin of the right common carotid and right subclavian arteries, the pattern shown in this figure occurs. The right subclavian artery arises as the fourth branch of an otherwise normal aorta. The right subclavian artery passes in close relation to the esophagus as it proceeds to the right side of the body and may compress that tube. The artery usually passes behind the esophagus.

d. Left-Sided Aortic Arch and Left-Sided Descending Aorta (Normal Pattern). If that portion of the double arch illustrated in figure 130*a* disappears posterior to the origin of the right subclavian artery, the right subclavian artery arises from the innominate artery. A normal vascular pattern is then produced.

In cases of double aortic arch, the left arch usually is the smaller of the two but the case reported by Gordon proves that this does not always hold true. The two arches may be of equal size or the right arch may be the smaller of the two.

B. **Partial Atresia of One Aortic Arch.**—An accentuation of the inequality of the two aortic arches leads to anomalies in which part of one of the arches is atretic and resembles a fibrous cord. As a rule, the atresia is situated in the left arch but it is a hypothetical possibility that portions of the right arch, instead, may be atretic. In general, three anatomic forms may represent this subgroup, depending upon the site of the atretic segment of the left arch. Hypothetically, the atresia may involve that part of the left aortic arch which lies between the origins of the left common carotid artery and the left subclavian artery (fig. 130*c*); it usually lies between the origin of the left subclavian artery and the aortic insertion of the ductus arteriosus[3,7,9,15,47] (fig. 130*d*); or it may involve the most distal part of the left arch, between the aortic insertion of the ductus arteriosus and the region of the posterior junction of the left and right aortic arches.[50] In any of the varieties of partial atresia of a double aortic arch the trachea and esophagus are encircled by a vascular ring, partly atretic, and, if the ring is sufficiently narrow, compression effects upon these structures are identical to those produced by a narrow vascular collar caused by a double aortic arch in which the two arches are pervious.

C. **Right-Sided Aortic Arch with Retro-esophageal Segment and Left-Sided Descending Aorta.**—In cases of double aortic arch in which a portion of one arch is atretic but recognizable, it is evident that the atresia occurred rather late during fetal life or after birth. Should the process of obliteration of a portion of a double aortic arch occur relatively early in fetal life, it is possible that the atretic segment would no longer be present as an identifiable structure at the time of birth. The double arch would cease to exist as a continuous structure. Such variants of the double aortic arch are included in the next subgroups.

1. *Right-Sided Aortic Arch with Retro-esophageal Segment and Left-Sided Descending Aorta; Left Subclavian Artery Origi-*

nating from Aortic Diverticulum.—If that segment of the left aortic arch between the origin of the left common carotid artery and left subclavian artery disappears, the following aortic arch pattern is achieved (fig. 131*a*). There is but one complete aortic arch, the right, which after passing over the right bronchus, turns to the left, at about the level of the body of the third or fourth thoracic vertebra, between the esophagus in front and the spinal column behind. Either directly behind the esophagus or to its left, the aortic arch joins the descending aorta, which usually lies to the left of the midline. The first three branches of the aortic arch are the left common carotid, the right common carotid and the right subclavian arteries in that order from before backward. The left subclavian artery arises as a fourth branch of the aorta from a diverticulum-like outpouching that lies at the left upper angle of the junction of the right aortic arch with the descending aorta. The diverticulum usually lies against the left side of the esophagus and into its lower anterior aspect is inserted the upper portion of the ductus arteriosus. The lower attachment of the ductus arteriosus is to the left pulmonary artery.[7,15,27,36,38,39,47,49]

This condition is comparable with that illustrated in figure 130*c*, in which there was predicted atresia of that segment of the left aortic arch between the origins of the left common carotid and left subclavian arteries. In that condition, the atretic segment would be identifiable as a fibrous-like cord. In the condition under this heading, the atretic segment is no longer identifiable; therefore, on casual examination, one might not identify the anomaly as a variant of the double aortic arch which, however, it should be considered to be. The aortic diverticulum which gives rise to the left subclavian artery and which is a point of attachment for the ductus arteriosus should be interpreted as a patent posterior portion of a left aortic arch. The segment of the left aortic arch between the origin of the left subclavian and common carotid arteries has disappeared during early embryonic life and is not identifiable.

In certain instances, the aortic diverticulum has approximately the same diameter as the subclavian artery to which it gives origin. Under such conditions, the diverticulum appears as the proximal part of the left subclavian artery, and the ductus arteriosus which actually is attached to the diverticulum appears to be attached to the beginning of the left subclavian artery.[2,24] Such variations in gross appearance do not alter the basic concepts concerning the significance of the vascular pattern. Rather they represent minor variations in relative rates of growth.

While there is absence of the symmetrically constricting effects of a continuous double aortic arch, there is, nevertheless, a vascular ring about the trachea in anomalies of this subgroup. The ring is formed by the right aortic arch on the right, the retro-esophageal segment of the right aortic arch, behind, the aortic diverticulum and the ductus arteriosus on the left, and the bifurcation of the pulmonary trunk in front. The subclavian artery plays no role in forming the vascular ring. In such instances a break in the continuity of the vascular ring may be accomplished by the division of the ductus arteriosus, which allows left lateral expansion of the trachea and the esophagus. The procedure also allows the bifurcation of the pulmonary trunk to sag away from the front of the trachea with relief of pressure against that tube. In addition, Gross in discussing this type of anomaly, stressed the possibility of compression of the trachea by the left common carotid artery which arises to the right of the midline and crosses in front of the trachea to achieve its usual position on the left side of the superior mediastinum. He recommended dislocating this vessel from its close association with the trachea if it compresses the air passage unduly.[22]

2. *Right-Sided Aortic Arch with Retro-esophageal Segment and Left-Sided Descending Aorta; Left Subclavian Artery Originating from Left Innominate Artery.*—Referring to the double aortic arch (fig. 130*a*), it is evident that if the portion of the left aortic arch between the origin of the left subclavian artery and the insertion of the ductus arteriosus disappears, the aortic arch pattern appears as follows (fig. 131*b*). There is one aortic arch, the right. This passes over the right major bronchus after which it turns to the left, passes between the esophagus and the spinal column, as in the other anomalies

previously described. Behind, or to the left of the esophagus, it joins the left-sided descending aorta. As in Group C-1 there is a diverticulum at the junction of the aortic arch and descending aorta.[3,24] The ductus arteriosus is inserted into this diverticulum. The left subclavian artery does not arise from the diverticulum but instead arises from a left-sided innominate artery in common with the left common carotid artery. The left innominate artery is the first branch of the aortic arch, the second and third branches being the right common carotid and right subclavian arteries, respectively.

As in Group C-1, there is a constricting vascular ring about the trachea and the esophagus. It is to be remembered that the aortic insertion of the ductus arteriosus is actually to a remnant of the most posterior portion of the left aortic arch and that this diverticulum is shorter than it is in the comparable anomaly in which the left subclavian artery arises from an aortic diverticulum. Consequently, in the type of anomaly described in this section, the diverticulum is expected to be small and it often is. Moreover, on the basis of molding of vessels with growth, it is possible for a diverticulum not to be immediately apparent. It is to be remembered, however, that the aortic insertion of the ductus arteriosus is to tissue which must be considered tissue of the left aortic arch.

D. Left-Sided Aortic Arch and Left-Sided Descending Aorta.—The types of anomalies that have been considered thus far were characterized not only by the presence of the ductus arteriosus on the left side but also by the presence of a right-sided aortic arch either alone or associated with a left-sided aortic arch. Since the upper part of the descending aorta lay either in the midline or to the left of the midline, the posterior portion of the right aortic arch possessed a horizontal segment, behind the esophagus, which was directed toward the descending aorta. In the remaining two types of vascular patterns to be considered in Group I, the left aortic arch is the only one that is present as a continuous functioning vessel. Portions of the right arch have disappeared.

1. *Left-Sided Aortic Arch and Left-Sided Descending Aorta; Right Subclavian Artery Arising from Distal Portion of Aortic Arch or from the Descending Aorta.*—This aortic arch pattern

is characterized by the disappearance of the segment of the right portion of the double aortic arch between the origins of the right common carotid and the right subclavian arteries. Consequently, the first branch of an otherwise normal left-sided aortic arch is the right common carotid artery rather than the innominate artery. The second and third branches of the arch are the left common carotid and the left subclavian arteries, respectively. The right subclavian artery arises as the fourth branch of the aorta from either the aortic arch or the upper part of the descending aorta (fig. 131*c*). The origin of this artery is frequently wider than the rest of the intrathoracic portion of the vessel, a feature that is not surprising since the origin of the right subclavian artery in this anomaly represents the most posterior portion of a right-sided aortic arch. From its origin on the left side of the midline, the right subclavian artery proceeds upward and to the right in an oblique direction. It crosses the midline usually by passing between the esophagus, in front, and the spinal column, behind. Less often, the artery lies between the esophagus and the trachea as it passes from the left side of the body to the right side, and even less commonly does it cross in front of the trachea.[13,19,30,37,48] This type of anomaly of the aortic arch is the one most frequently observed, and, as a rule, it does not give rise to symptoms. When the right subclavian artery arises as the fourth branch of the aortic arch and is responsible for symptoms, the symptoms usually result from esophageal compression and appear in the form of dysphagia.

2. *Left-Sided Aortic Arch and Left-Sided Descending Aorta; Normal Arch and Branches.*—It seems logical to include the features of the normal aorta at this point in the consideration since it too can be visualized as a modification of the double aortic arch. If one assumes that the double aortic arch is modified in such a way that there is loss of the right arch between the origin of the right subclavian artery and the descending aorta, one arrives at the structure of the normal aorta (fig. 131*d*).

Under these circumstances, the first branch of the aortic arch is the innominate artery, which soon divides into the right common carotid and right subclavian arteries. The second branch is the left common carotid artery and the third is the left subclavian artery. The descending aorta lies on the left side and no undue compression upon the trachea or the esophagus is caused by the aortic arch or its branches. The ductus arteriosus extends from the left pulmonary artery to the aorta at a point beyond the origin of the left subclavian artery.

GROUP II. RIGHT-SIDED DUCTUS ARTERIOSUS WITH UPPER PORTION OF DESCENDING AORTA ON THE RIGHT SIDE

The second group of anomalies of the derivatives of the aortic arch system is characterized by the ductus arteriosus being a right-sided structure and extending from the right pulmonary artery, below, to the aorta, above.

The upper portion of the descending aorta lies in the right side of the thorax, to the right of the esophagus. In the lower part of the thorax, usually at the level of either the body of the eighth or ninth thoracic vertebra, the aorta crosses to the left behind the esophagus and then emerges from the thorax through the aortic hiatus of the diaphragm.

In this group, the anomalies of the aortic arch, its branches and the upper portion of the descending aorta are essentially mirror images of the various anomalies of the first group. Anomalies of Group II are encountered less frequently than those of Group I but the counterparts of all the types in the first group have either been observed or exist as hypothetical possibilities in Group II.

A. **Functioning Double Aortic Arch.**—As far as I have been able to determine, there is no case on record which fulfills all the criteria of the functioning double arch of Group II, yet this anomaly must be considered as a hypothetical possibility. Reference will be made, after the description, to two reported cases in which some of the features conform to those of the vascular structure which will be described.

In this type, the aortic arch divides into two arches, a right and a left. The right arch passes in front of the trachea and over the right major bronchus to join the descending aorta, which is on the right side of the body. The left arch passes over the left major bronchus and then passes behind the esophagus to the right to join the right arch at the point at which it becomes continuous with the descending aorta (fig. 132*a*). The upper portion of the descending aorta lies to the right of the midline. As in its counterpart of Group I, the branches of the double arch of this group, the common carotid and subclavian arteries arise in that order from before backward from the arch of the respective side. The ductus arteriosus arises from the right pulmonary artery and is inserted into the right aortic arch between the origin of the right subclavian artery and the posterior junction of the two aortic arches.

The second case in the report of Sweet, Findlay and Reyersbach fulfills the aortic arch pattern of this anomaly but the matter of the site of the ductus arteriosus is problematic. The case history is interesting and instructive, not only from the diagnostic but also from the surgical points of view.

The patient, a boy aged 4 years, had a cough that was associated with wheezing shortly after birth. There were numerous attacks of pulmonary infection and dysphagia. At the age of 4 years, he was able to eat only liquids or strained foods and vomited these. There was evidence of esophageal and tracheal obstruction on roentgenographic examination. A left-sided thoracotomy was performed. At operation it was observed that the left arch assumed an unusual course. Instead of remaining on the left side of the body, as it does in the double aortic arch of Group I, the left arch, after crossing over the left major bronchus, deviated to the right and crossed the midline behind the esophagus. The opening in the left side of the thorax was closed and a right thoracotomy was performed about three weeks later. This procedure revealed that the right arch, which had a diameter an eighth as large as that of the left arch, passed over the right main bronchus, which it compressed, and then became continuous with the descending aorta, the upper portion of which was on the right side. The left arch, after passing behind the esophagus, reached the right side of the body and joined the right arch at the point at which the latter joined the descending aorta. The descending aorta remained on the right side of the body until it reached the lower portion of the thorax, where it deviated toward the midline. Division of the right arch resulted in disappearance of symptoms. The features of the aortic arch conformed to that illustrated in figure 132*b*.

One major problem in this case, however, is the matter of the ductus arteriosus. The authors said that at the operations they made a search for a ductus arteriosus on the left and the right sides but found none. They concluded, therefore, that none was present and assumed that in the absence of a ductus arteriosus, the fetal circulation was balanced by either a defect in the atrial or ventricular septum and that such a defect closed shortly after birth, which explained the absence of clinical signs of a septal defect. It is doubtful that such an assumption is correct. It is more reasonable to assume that a ductus arteriosus was in fact present but was not discovered at the time of operation. When one considers the rather intricate dissection necessary to find a closed right-sided ductus arteriosus, when present under ideal conditions at necropsy, it is understandable that one might be overlooked, even after a search was made for it, at operation. If one assumes that a right-sided ductus arteriosus were present in this case, the essential features of the double aortic arch of Group II would be fulfilled. Since proof of the existence of a right-sided ductus arteriosus is lacking in the case cited the functioning double aortic arch of Group II must remain, for the time being, as a hypothetical anomaly. It is interesting to contrast the aortic arch configuration in this case with the findings in the fourth case in the report of Gordon, to which reference has herein been made. In each case there was a double aortic arch and the right arch was more narrow than the left. In Gordon's case the anomaly definitely belongs to Group I since it was the right arch that passed behind the esophagus to join a left-sided descending aorta and the ductus arteriosus lay on the left side. In the second case in the report by Sweet, Findlay and Reyersbach, the presence of the upper descending aorta on the right side coupled with the fact that the left arch was the one that crossed the midline behind the esophagus created

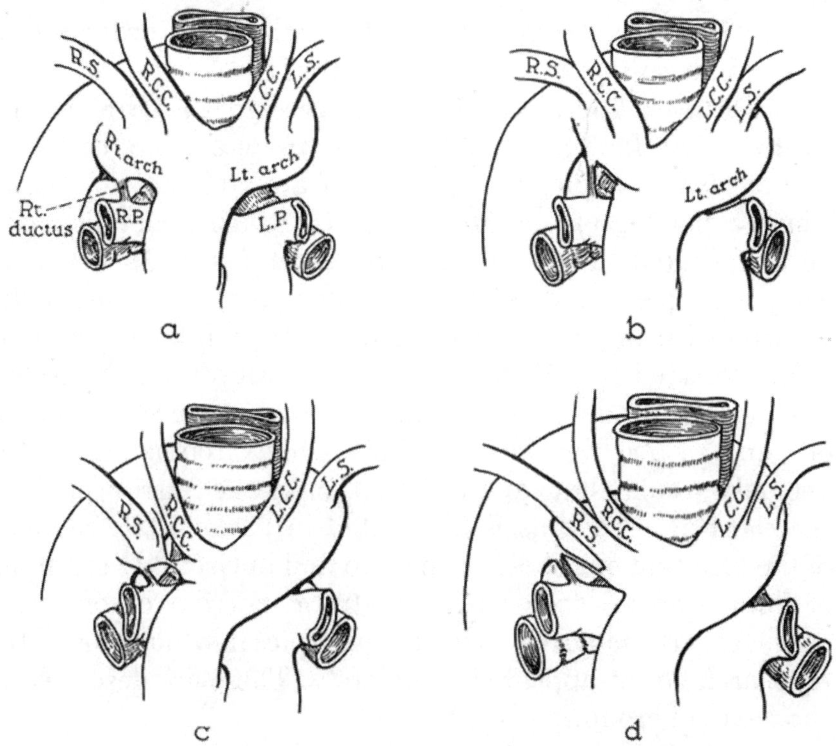

Fig. 132.—*Right-Sided Ductus Arteriosus with Upper Portion of Descending Aorta on the Right Side* (Group II). The aortic arches, the ductus arteriosus and upper part of the descending aorta, in the anomalies of Group II, illustrated in figures 132 and 133, are mirror images of the vascular patterns of Group I which are illustrated in corresponding portions of figures 130 and 131.

a. Functioning Double Aortic Arch. The difference from the pattern illustrated in figure 130*a* lies in the fact that it is the left arch that passes behind the esophagus in this anomaly; the ductus arteriosus and the upper portion of the descending aorta lie on the right side. As the anomaly shown in figure 130*a* is the basic type of Group I, the one here illustrated is the basic pattern for Group II. This is as yet a hypothetical anomaly.

b. Functioning Double Aortic Arch. In Group I, the left arch is usually the more narrow of the two. In this pattern, which to date is a hypothetical one, the right arch is expected to be the more narrow of the two.

c. Partial Atresia of Double Aortic Arch. To fulfill the mirror image of the anomaly illustrated in figure 130*c*, the atretic segment lies in the right arch between the origins of the right common carotid and right subclavian arteries. This is a hypothetical form.

d. Partial Atresia of Double Aortic Arch. The mirror image of the pattern shown in figure 130*d* is illustrated. The atretic segment lies in that portion of the right arch between the origin of the right subclavian artery and the aortic insertion of the ductus arteriosus. This form is hypothetical.

an aortic arch pattern different from that in Gordon's case and similar to the anomalies of Group II.

B. **Double Aortic Arch with Atresia of One of the Arches.**—As far as I have been able to determine, there are no reported examples in Group II of a double aortic arch in which a portion of one arch is atretic. Such anomalies may be anticipated. They are illustrated in figure 132*c* and *d*. They are represented as the mirror images of those anomalies of Group I in which a portion of the left arch is atretic. It is to be expected that if examples of the group under consideration are found the atretic segment will have a greater chance of lying in the right arch. Under such circumstances, the anomaly would show an accentuation of the narrow state of the right arch such as is illustrated in figure 132*b*. Support of the idea that one should expect to find in Group II examples of double aortic arch with an atretic portion of one arch exists from the fact that there are examples in which part of the right arch has disappeared completely. These are described in the next subgroup.

C. **Left-Sided Aortic Arch with Retro-Esophageal Segment and Upper Portion of the Descending Aorta on the Right Side.**—1. *Right Subclavian Artery Originating from Aortic Diverticulum.*—This aortic arch pattern (fig. 133*a*) is the mirror image of that member of Group I illustrated in figure 131*a*. This anomaly is rare but I recently reported a case in which it was present.[14] When this type of anomaly is present, the appearance of the aortic arch system is as follows. There is only one complete aortic arch; that is, the left. After passing over the left major bronchus the arch turns to the right to cross the midline behind the esophagus. After it reaches the right side of the thorax it joins the descending aorta, the upper portion of which is also on the right side. At the right upper angle of the junction of the arch and descending aorta there is a diverticulum which lies along the right side of the esophagus. The right-sided ductus arteriosus is inserted into the lower anterior aspect of the diverticulum. The right subclavian artery is the fourth branch of the aortic arch arising from the upper aspect of the aortic diverticulum. The first three branches of the aorta are the right common

ANOMALIES OF DERIVATIVES OF AORTIC ARCH 943

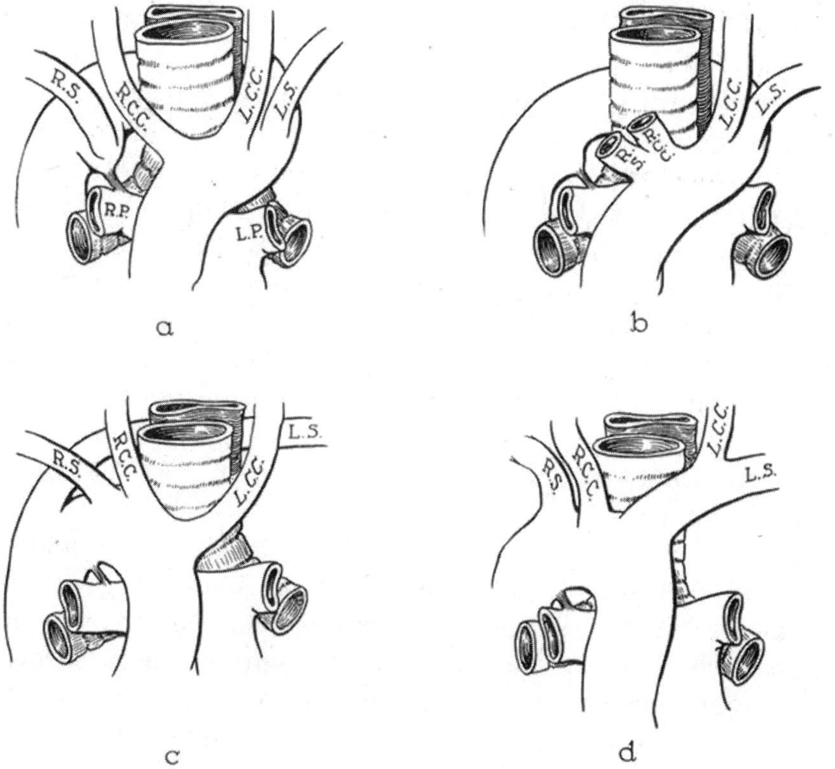

Fig. 133.—*Right-Sided Ductus Arteriosus with Upper Portion of Descending Aorta on the Right Side* (Group II). *a. Left-Sided Aortic Arch with Retro-Esophageal Segment and Upper Portion of Descending Aorta on the Right Side; Right Subclavian Artery Originating from Aortic Diverticulum.* If that portion of the double aortic arch of Group II which is illustrated in figure 132*a* disappears between the points of origin of the right common carotid and right subclavian arteries, this anomaly occurs. There is a vascular ring about the trachea and the esophagus which is formed by the aortic arch on the left, by the retro-esophageal portion of the aortic arch behind, by the aortic diverticulum and the ductus arteriosus on the right, and by the bifurcation of the pulmonary trunk in front. The aortic diverticulum represents the patent posterior portion of the right arch. The form illustrated is the mirror image of the anomaly illustrated in figure 131*a*.

b. Left-Sided Aortic Arch with Retro-Esophageal Segment and Upper Portion of Descending Aorta on the Right Side; Right Subclavian Artery Originating from the Right Innominate Artery. This form varies from that shown in figure 133*a* only in that the portion of the right arch between the origin of the right subclavian artery and the aortic insertion of the ductus arteriosus has disappeared. This form is a mirror image of that illustrated in figure 131*b*.

c. Right-Sided Aortic Arch with Upper Part of Descending Aorta on the Right Side; Left Subclavian Artery Originating from the Aortic Arch or from the Descending Aorta. This form may result from modification of the double aortic arch (illustrated in figure 132*a*) in such a way that that portion of the left arch between the origins of the left common carotid and left subclavian arteries carotid, the left common carotid and the left subclavian arteries in that order from before backward. As in its counterpart in Group I, this pattern is characterized by a vascular ring surrounding the trachea and the esophagus. Should symptoms result from this ring, division of the ductus arteriosus by means of a right thoracotomy would be indicated. It is of interest that the right common carotid artery arises to the left of the midline and crosses this line to get to its definitive position. In its course the artery may compress the trachea, and should symptoms result from this factor, dislocation of the artery might be helpful. Gross has advocated this procedure for the left common carotid artery in the condition which is the mirror image of the one under consideration.[22]

The configuration of this type of anomaly may be understood if one studies the illustration of functioning double aortic arch in figure 132*a*. If one assumes that that part of the right arch between the origin of the right common carotid and right subclavian arteries disappears, one immediately recognizes the anomaly which is shown in figure 133*a*. The diverticulum to which the ductus arteriosus is attached and from which the right subclavian artery arises represents the patent posterior extremity of the right arch.

2. *Left-Sided Aortic Arch with Retro-Esophageal Segment and Upper Portion of Descending Aorta on the Right Side; Right Subclavian Artery Originating from a Right-Sided Innominate Artery.*—If one assumes that a double aortic arch of Group II is altered in such a way that that segment of the right arch between the origin of the right subclavian artery and the right-sided ductus arteriosus disappears, the arterial configuration representative of this anomaly is obtained (fig. 133*b*).

---

disappears. The end result is a mirror image of the anomaly illustrated in figure 131*c*.

d. Right-Sided Aortic Arch with Upper Portion of Descending Aorta on the Right Side; Branches Forming a Mirror Image of the Normal Branches. If that portion of the left aortic arch illustrated in figure 132*a* disappears posterior to the point of origin of the left subclavian artery, the latter vessel arises in common with the left common carotid artery from a left-sided innominate artery. The pattern is a mirror image of the normal, which is illustrated in figure 131*d*.

It varies from the type illustrated in figure 133*a* only in the mode of origin of the right subclavian artery. In the type already described, the subclavian artery arose as the fourth branch of the aorta from a diverticulum thereof. Inasmuch as the right arch is interrupted posterior to the subclavian artery in the anomaly now being considered, the right subclavian artery arises in common with the right common carotid artery from the innominate artery. The ductus arteriosus is attached to an aortic diverticulum. This pattern is a mirror image of that member of Group I illustrated in figure 131*b*. At one time, the anomaly under consideration remained as a hypothetical possibility but recently Paul has reported two cases in which the roentgenographic and surgical findings indicated the presence of an anomaly of this type. The configuration of the great vessels in these cases was identical with that described in this article but the site of the ductus arteriosus was not identified at operation for congenital cardiac disease. Since the aortic configuration in these cases was the same as it is in Group II-C-1, except for minor difference in the origin of the subclavian arteries, it is reasonable to postulate that the ductus arteriosus was situated on the right side.

D. **Right-Sided Aortic Arch and Upper Portion of the Descending Aorta on the Right Side.**—1. *Left Subclavian Artery Originating from the Aortic Arch or from the Descending Aorta.*—If one studies the double aortic arch of Group II (fig. 132*a*) and assumes that that portion of the left arch between the origin of the left common carotid artery and that of the left subclavian artery disappears, he will have a clear understanding of the anomaly illustrated in figure 133*c*. It is characterized by the presence of only one arch, that is, the right. This passes over the right major bronchus and blends with the descending aorta, the upper portion of which lies in the right side of the thorax. The branches of the aorta from before backward are the left common carotid, the right common carotid, the right subclavian and the left subclavian arteries.[12,25,31,32] Figures 132*a* and 133*c* illustrate that the very first part of the left subclavian artery is actually the remaining posterior extremity of a left aortic arch. The configuration of this anomaly is essentially a mirror image of that illustrated in figure 131*c*; that is, it is a mirror image of the common anomaly in which the right subclavian artery arises as a fourth branch of an otherwise normal aorta. As is true in cases of that configuration, the aorta does not interfere with either the esophagus or the trachea but the subclavian artery, which crosses the midline, usually behind the esophagus, may compress that tube and cause dysphagia.

2. *Right-Sided Aortic Arch and Upper Portion of the Descending Aorta on the Right Side. Left Subclavian Artery Originating from Left-Sided Innominate Artery.*—This is the most common type of anomaly in Group II. The pattern of the aortic arch and of its branches is a mirror image of that of the normal aorta. The aortic arch passes over the right major bronchus and blends with the descending aorta, the upper portion of which lies to the right of the esophagus and to the right of the midline. In the lower part of the thorax the descending aorta crosses to the left and enters the abdomen through the aortic hiatus of the diaphragm. Figures 132*a* and 133*d* reveal that this anomaly is a modification of the double aortic arch of Group II in the following respects. That portion of the left arch posterior to the origin of the subclavian artery disappears; the left subclavian artery arises, therefore, in common with the left common carotid artery from a left-sided innominate artery. The left-sided innominate artery is the first branch of the aortic arch; the right common carotid and right subclavian arteries are the second and third branches, respectively.[15,39,44] Since the aortic arch, its branches, and the upper part of the descending aorta are mirror images of the structures of the normal aorta, they do not encroach upon the trachea or the esophagus and symptoms relative to interference with the function of either of these tubes by the vascular anomaly are not ordinarily encountered. It is of interest that the anomaly being considered is frequently associated with congenital cardiac disease, particularly with the tetralogy of Fallot. According to Taussig, about 20 to 25 per cent of patients with the tetralogy of Fallot have this aortic configuration.[46] The other types of malformations de-

rived from the aortic arch derivatives may be associated with congenital cardiac disease but that is not the rule.

TREATMENT

If a patient suffers from symptoms resulting from an anomaly of the derivatives of the aortic arch system, certain rules concerning surgical therapy can usually be followed. Relief may be obtained by division of the smaller of the two aortic arches, by division of that part of the arch which is atretic, by division of the ductus arteriosus, by dislocation of a common carotid artery, or by division of a subclavian artery. Usually, the structure or structures which must be treated surgically are either the ductus arteriosus or some structure which lies in the same side of the body as the ductus; therefore, it is advantageous for the surgeon to know, preoperatively, on which side the ductus arteriosus lies in order that he may perform the thoracotomy on that side. Since the roentgenologist is not able to visualize the ductus arteriosus directly, he must rely on indirect evidence in predicting its situation. The following rule, although not infallible, will be helpful. The ductus arteriosus usually lies on the same side of the thorax as does the upper portion of the descending aorta. By visualizing the site of the latter structure, the roentgenologist may predict, with reasonable accuracy, the situation of the ductus arteriosus and guide the surgeon as to the proper side on which to perform the thoracotomy.

REFERENCES

1. Abbott, F. C.: Specimen of left aortic arch with abnormal arrangement of the branches. J. Anat. & Physiol. (Proc. Anat. Soc. Gr. Brit. & Ireland). *26*:xiii–xv, 1892.
2. Annan, J. L.: Case of an abnormal sinuous aorta. J. Anat. & Physiol. *44*:241–243 (Apr.) 1910.
3. Arkin, Aaron: Double aortic arch with total persistence of the right and isthmus stenosis of the left arch: a new clinical and x-ray picture; report of six cases in adults. Am. Heart. J. *11*:444–474 (Apr.) 1936.
4. Assmann, Herbert: Die klinische Röntgendiagnostik der inneren Erkrankungen. Leipzig, F. C. W. Vogel, 1924, p. 103.
5. Bayford, David: Singular case of obstructed deglutition. Mem. M. Soc. Lond. (Ed. 2). *2*:275–286, 1794.
6. Bedford, D. E. and Parkinson, John: Right-sided aortic arch (situs inversus arcus aortae). Brit. J. Radiol. n.s. *9*:776–798 (Dec.) 1936.

7. Biedermann, F.: Der rechtsseitige Aortenbogen in Röntgenbild. Fortschr. a. d. Geb. d. Röntgenstrahlen. *43:*168–187 (Feb.) 1931.
8. Blincoe, Homer, Lowance, M. I. and Venable, John: A double aortic arch in man. Anat. Rec. *66:*505–517 (Nov.) 1936.
9. Brigham, R. O.: A right aortic arch. Ohio State M. J. *18:*484–486 (July) 1922.
10. Crystal, D. K., Edmonds, H. W. and Betzold, P. F.: Symmetrical double aortic arch; report of a case. West. J. Surg. *55:*389–392 (July) 1947.
11. Curnow, John: Double aortic arch enclosing trachea and oesophagus. Tr. Path. Soc. London. *26:*33–37, 1875.
12. Dittrich, P.: Quoted by Renander, Axel.
13. Dolgopol, Vera B.: Anomalous origin of right subclavian artery from the descending arch of aorta. J. Tech. Methods. *13:*112–118 (Mar.) 1934.
14. Edwards, J. E.: Retro-esophageal segment of the left aortic arch, right ligamentum arteriosum and right descending aorta causing a congenital vascular ring about the trachea and esophagus. Proc. Staff Meet., Mayo Clin. *23:*108–116 (Mar. 3) 1948.
15. Ewald, Wilhelm: Einige Fälle von Arcus Aortae dexter. Frankfurt. Ztschr. f. Path. *34:*87–97, 1926.
16. Faber, H. K., Hope, J. W. and Robinson, F. L.: Chronic stridor in early life due to persistent right aortic arch; report of two cases. J. Pediat. *26:*128–137 (Feb.) 1945.
17. Fray, W. W.: Right aortic arch. Radiology. *26:*27–36 (Jan.) 1936.
18. Garland, L. H.: Persistent right-sided aortic arch. Am. J. Roentgenol. *39:*713–719 (May) 1938.
19. Goldbloom, A. A.: The anomalous right subclavian artery and its possible clinical significance. Surg., Gynec. & Obst. *34:*378–384 (Mar.) 1922.
20. Gordon, Susanna: Double aortic arch. J. Pediat. *30:*428–437 (Apr.) 1947.
21. Gross, R. E.: Surgical treatment for dysphagia lusoria. Ann. Surg. *124:*532–534 (Sept.) 1946.
22. Gross, R. E.: Surgical treatment for abnormalities of the heart and great vessels. Springfield, Illinois, Charles C Thomas, 1947, pp. 39–47.
23. Gross, R. E. and Ware, P. F.: The surgical significance of aortic arch anomalies. Surg., Gynec. & Obst. *83:*435–448 (Oct.) 1946.
24. Gruber, G. B.: Zwei Fälle von Dextropositio des Aortenbogens. Frankfurt. Ztschr. f. Path. *10:*375–382, 1912.
25. Hammer, G.: Situs inversus arcus aortae (Hohe Rechtslage der Aorta). Fortschr. a. d. Geb. d. Röntgenstrahlen. *34:*517–523, 1926.
26. Herbut, P. A. and Smith, T. T.: Constricting double aortic arch; report of a case. Arch. Otolaryng. *37:*558–562 (Apr.) 1943.
27. Herringham, W. P.: Right aorta with persistent left aortic root giving origin to the left subclavian. J. Anat. & Physiol. (Proc. Anat. Soc. Gr. Brit. & Ireland). *25:*vi–vii, 1891.
28. Herrmann, W. W.: Double aortic arch. Arch. Path. *6:*418–425 (Sept.) 1928.
29. Herzog, F. and Firnbacher, E.: Beitrag zu den Anomalien der Aorta und des Ösophagus. Fortschr. a. d. Geb. d. Röntgenstrahlen. *35:*1236–1243, 1927.
30. Holzapfel, Gotthold: Ungewöhnlicher Ursprung und Verlauf der Arteria subclavia dextra. Anat. Hefte (Abt. 1). *12:*369–523, 1899.

31. Kopsch, F.: Rauber's Lehrbuch der Anatomie des Menschen. Leipzig, Georg Thieme, 1914, vol. 3, p. 277.
32. Lockwood, C. B.: Right aortic arch. Tr. Path. Soc. London. *35:*132, 1884.
33. Mohr, R.: Zur Diagnostik der kongenitalen Herzfehler. Deutsche Ztschr. f. Nervenh. *47–48:*371–387, 1913.
34. Neuhauser, E. B. D.: The roentgen diagnosis of double aortic arch and other anomalies of the great vessels. Am. J. Roentgenol. *56:*1–12 (July) 1946.
35. Paul, R. N.: A new anomaly of the aorta; left aortic arch with right descending aorta. J. Pediat. *32:*19–29 (Jan.) 1948.
36. Pense, Gertrud: Ein Fall von rechtsseitigem Aortenbogen und seine entwicklungsgeschichtliche Deutung. Anat. Anz. *70:*257–274 (Sept.) 1930.
37. Poynter, C. W. M.: Arterial anomalies pertaining to the aortic arches and the branches arising from them. Lincoln, Nebraska, University Studies of the University of Nebraska. *16:*229–345 (Oct.) 1916.
38. Quain, Richard: The anatomy of the arteries of the human body with its applications to pathology and operative surgery, with a series of lithographic drawings. London, Taylor & Walton, 1844, 550 pp.
39. Reid, D. G.: Three examples of a right aortic arch. J. Anat. & Physiol. *48:*174–181 (Jan.) 1914.
40. Renander, Axel: Roentgen-diagnosed anomaly of oesophagus and arcus aortae. Dysphagia lusoria. Acta radiol. *7:*298–308, 1926.
41. Schall, L. A. and Johnson, L. G.: Dyspnea due to congenital anomaly of aorta. Ann. Otol., Rhin. & Laryng. *49:*1055–1060 (Dec.) 1940.
42. Spencer, Jack and Dresser, Richard: Right-sided aorta. Am. J. Roentgenol. *36:*183–187 (Aug.) 1936.
43. Sprague, H. B., Ernlund, C. H. and Albright, Fuller: Clinical aspects of persistent right aortic root. New England J. Med. *209:*679–686 (Oct. 5) 1933.
44. Sprong, D. H., Jr. and Cutler, N. L.: A case of human right aorta. Anat. Rec. *45:*365–375 (May) 1930.
45. Sweet, R. H., Findlay, C. W., Jr. and Reyersbach, Gertrud C.: The diagnosis and treatment of tracheal and esophageal obstruction due to congenital vascular ring. J. Pediat. *30:*1–17 (Jan.) 1947.
46. Taussig, Helen B.: Congenital malformations of the heart. New York, The Commonwealth Fund, 1947, chaps. 5 and 21, pp. 109–149; 442–463.
47. Thomson, Allen: Quoted by Turner, William.
48. Thomson, Arthur: Question III. Variation in the arrangement of the branches arising from the arch of the aorta. J. Anat. & Physiol. *27:*189–192 (Jan.) 1893.
49. Turner, William: On irregularities of the pulmonary artery, arch of the aorta, and the primary branches of the arch, with an attempt to illustrate their mode of origin by a reference to development. Brit. & For. M. Rev. *30:*173–189 (July); 461–482 (Oct.) 1862.
50. Watson, M.: Notes of a case of double aortic arch. J. Anat. & Physiol. *11:*229–234 (Jan.) 1877.
51. Wolman, I. J.: Syndrome of constricting double aortic arch in infancy; report of case. J. Pediat. *14:*527–533 (Apr.) 1939.

Anomalies of the Derivatives of the Aortic Arch System

Paul R. Julsrud, M.D.,
Anavekar S. Nandon M.B. B.Ch.

As a practicing cardiac radiologist, I am constantly reminded of Dr. Jesse Edwards' enormous contribution to our current understanding of cardiovascular malformations. His landmark paper, *Anomalies of the Derivatives of the Aortic Arch System*, still provides the basis for recognizing and properly classifying vascular rings and related entities. With the advent of advanced imaging techniques, such as computed tomography and magnetic resonance imaging, we are now able to noninvasively clearly demonstrate the anatomic features he described in such elegant detail. (Figure 1 and 2) Furthermore, we are only able to take full advantage of these recent imaging advances due to his comprehensive understanding of these complex anomalies.

Those of us who were privileged to know Jesse were continually amazed at his uncanny ability to make sense of complicated cardiovascular anomalies. His paper categorizing aortic arch anomalies is a prime example of this ability. In this paper, he masterfully unravels the myriad malformations encompassing vascular rings and associated aortic arch anomalies using an innovative system that employed his now famous "functional double arch with bilateral ducti (ligamentum) arteriosi." This ingenious system, using a developmental perspective, was recognized from the outset as a medical breakthrough providing an intelligible, clinically useful approach to this confounding subject. None other than the most preeminent pediatric radiologist of his time, Dr. Edward B.D. Neuhauser, commenting on the atlas that was the direct extension of the paper under consideration, states that Jesse's work on this subject was "concise, logical, and beautifully written and should prove to be the classic treatise on anomalies of the aortic arch system." Since this system continues to inform us regarding the proper diagnosis and treatment of these anomalies, I can attest that more than 60 years later these words are still true.

In further considering this paper, it should be noted that Jesse emphasized that the key to the accurate diagnosis and proper treatment of these anomalies was the location of the ligamentum arteriosum. In vintage Edwards' style, he concludes the paper with a section titled "Treatment," in which he reiterates the relevance of the ligamentum arteriosum position to his proposed classification, as well as the consequent surgical implications. In addition, he comments that "since the roentgenologist is not able to visualize the ligamentum arteriosum directly, he must rely on indirect evidence in predicting its situation." One can only imagine his delight if he were with us now to see this important structure demonstrated so clearly with modern cardiac computed tomography.

Another amazing attribute of this paper was that the proposed system not only explained known conditions, but also hypothesized arch anomalies not previously described. Since this paper was published in 1948, many of the predicted anomalies have been reported, confirming Jesse's predictions, and once again testifying to his wizard-like abilities.

A personal anecdote provides yet another example of Jesse's abiding interest in the subject under discussion. One morning, in the early '90s, his son Brooks brought him by to visit me (PRJ) at work. I had just finished reviewing a magnetic resonance scan of a young boy that clearly demonstrated a left-sided ipsilateral duplicated arch, which is thought to represent a persistence of the left 5th aortic arch. Jessie was obviously moved as he saw for the first time an arch anomaly that had been one of the hypothetical variants. To see this anomaly so accurately defined noninvasively seemed to stir his imagination regarding the possibilities his earlier work had facilitated.

Although Dr. Jesse Edwards' contributions to the medical literature are legendary, what I remember most about him was his prowess as a gifted, insightful and gracious teacher and mentor. His anatomic explanations always stressed the imaging correlations and surgical implications. He consistently emphasized the fact that accurate knowledge of anatomy, either by pathological inspection or careful attention to imaging, was crucial to the clinical understanding of the patient's problem. His gentle manner was always combined with a persistent drive to make sure his work was relevant to patient care. This, in part, accounts for the fact that his work currently remains so useful and certainly will for years to come. Because of this, I am in the habit of instructing my trainees to first "Google" Jesse Edwards on the subject when they encounter a congenital or acquired cardiac abnormality with which they are not familiar.

In closing, even though other contributors to this book commemorating Jesse may also want to use this famous quotation, we would be remiss if we neglected to invoke Sir Isaac Newton's famous words which so aptly apply to Jesse. It is only by *".....standing on the shoulders of giants"* that ensuing generations are able to "see so far."

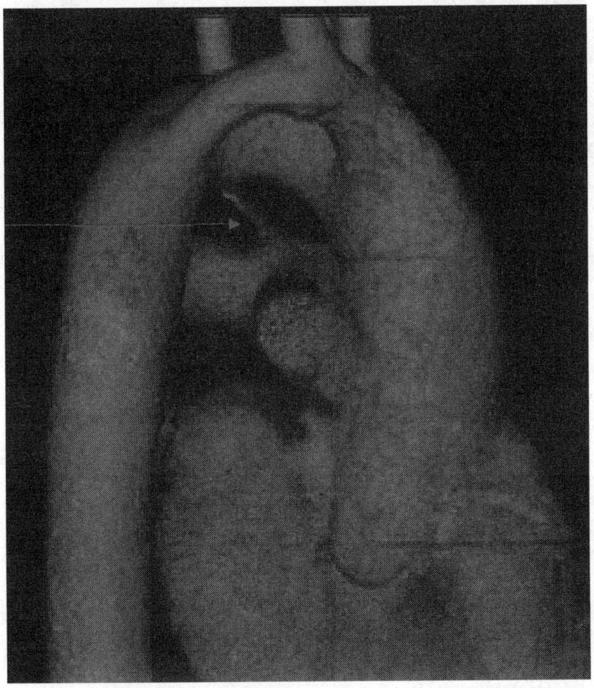

Figure 1

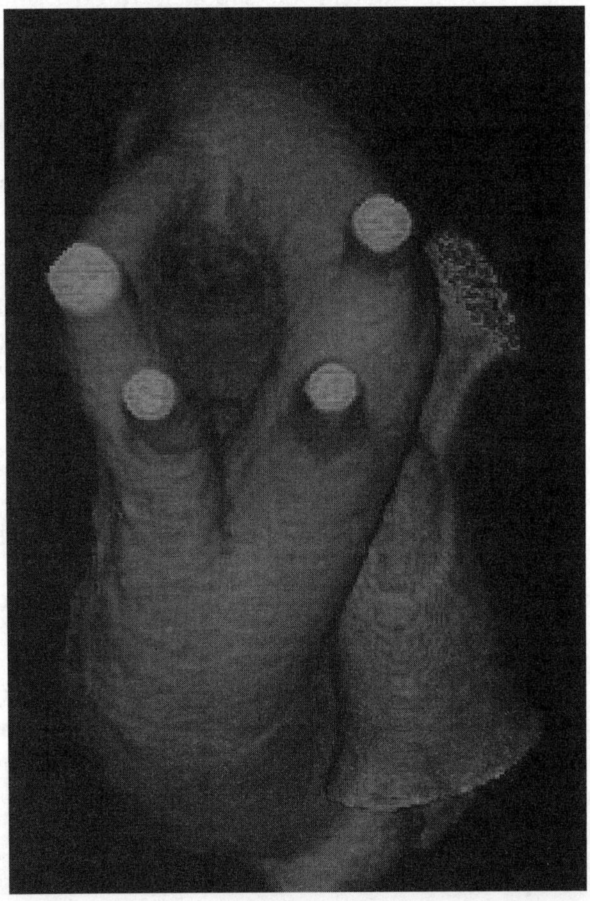

Figure 2

THE COLLATERAL CIRCULATION IN COARCTATION OF THE AORTA

Jesse E. Edwards, M. D., Section on Pathologic Anatomy, O. Theron Clagett, M. D., M. S. in Surgery, Division of Surgery, Russell L. Drake, Head of the Medical Art Studio, and Norman A. Christensen, M. D., Division of Medicine: In 1827 Meckel[1] reported on the existence of a prominent system of collateral arteries in coarctation of the aorta. In the century that followed, more data were added. These facts were reviewed by King[2] Blackford,[3] and Abbott[4] and important additional contributions have been made by others since the time of these reviews.[5-8] Rösler[5] and Railsback and Dock[6] reported that the defects of the ribs caused by the enlarged intercostal arteries could be demonstrated roentgenographically and that these changes could be used in establishing the clinical diagnosis of coarctation. Substantial evidence concerning the anatomy of the collateral arterial system was supplied by Love and Holms[9] and Bramwell and Jones.[8]

Using the facts supplied by published accounts [1, 4, 8-12] and those gained by our own experience, we have prepared a diagram (fig. 1) of the collateral circulation in the usual type of coarctation of the aorta in which the ductus arteriosus is closed.

In figure 1 the details shown on the left side include the arteries that are essentially part of the thoracic cage, as well as the circulation to the left side of the abdominal wall and to the left lower extremity, while the details on the right side represent the vessels concerned with the circulation of the scapula and adjacent tissues. The details for the left side are applicable to the right as well, and vice versa. The diagram shows that in the type of aortic coarctation represented, the

1. Meckel, A.: Verschliessung der Aorta am vierten Brustwirbel. Arch. f. Anat. u. Physiol. 1827, pp. 345-354.
2. King, J. T., Jr.: Stenosis of the Isthmus (Coarctation) of the Aorta and Its Diagnosis During Life: Report of Four Cases. Arch. Int. Med. *38*:69-95 (July) 1926.
3. Blackford, L. M.: Coarctation of the Aorta. Arch. Int. Med. *41*:702-735 (May) 1928.
4. Abbott, Maude E.: Coarctation of the Aorta of the Adult Type. II. A Statistical Study and Historical Retrospect of 200 Recorded Cases, with Autopsy, of Stenosis or Obliteration of the Descending Arch in Subjects above the Age of Two Years. Am. Heart J. *3*:392-421 (Apr.) 1928.
5. Rösler, H.: Beiträge zur Lehre von den angeborenen Herzfehlern. IV. Untersuchungen an zwei Fällen von Isthmusstenose der Aorta. Wien. Arch. f. inn. Med. *15*:521-538, 1928.
6. Railsback, O. C. and Dock, William: Erosion of the Ribs due to Stenosis of the Isthmus (Coarctation) of the Aorta. Radiology *12*:58-61 (Jan.) 1929.
7. Fray, W. W.: The Roentgenologic Diagnosis of Coarctation of the Aorta (Adult Type). Am. J. Roentgenol. *24*:349-362 (Oct.) 1930.
8. Bramwell, Crighton and Jones, A. M.: Coarctation of the Aorta: the Collateral Circulation. Brit. Heart J. *3*:205-227, 1941.
9. Love, W. S., Jr. and Holms, J. H.: Coarctation of the Aorta with Associated Stenosis of the Right Subclavian Artery. Am. Heart J. *17*:628-631 (May) 1939.
10. Walshe, W. H.: A Practical Treatise on the Diseases of the Heart and Great Vessels, Including the Principles of Their Physical Diagnosis. Ed. 4, London, Smith, Elder & Co., 1873, pp. 533-542.
11. Lewis, Thomas: Material Relating to Coarctation of the Aorta of the Adult Type. Heart *16*:205-261 (June 14) 1933.
12. Wolke, Knut: Two Cases of Coarctation (Stenosis of the Isthmus) of the Aorta. Acta radiol. *18*:319-329, 1937.

subclavian arteries, through the communications of their branches, play the paramount role in carrying blood from that part of the aorta above the coarctation to that part below. The common carotid arteries are of minor importance in the collateral circulation in coarctation of the aorta.

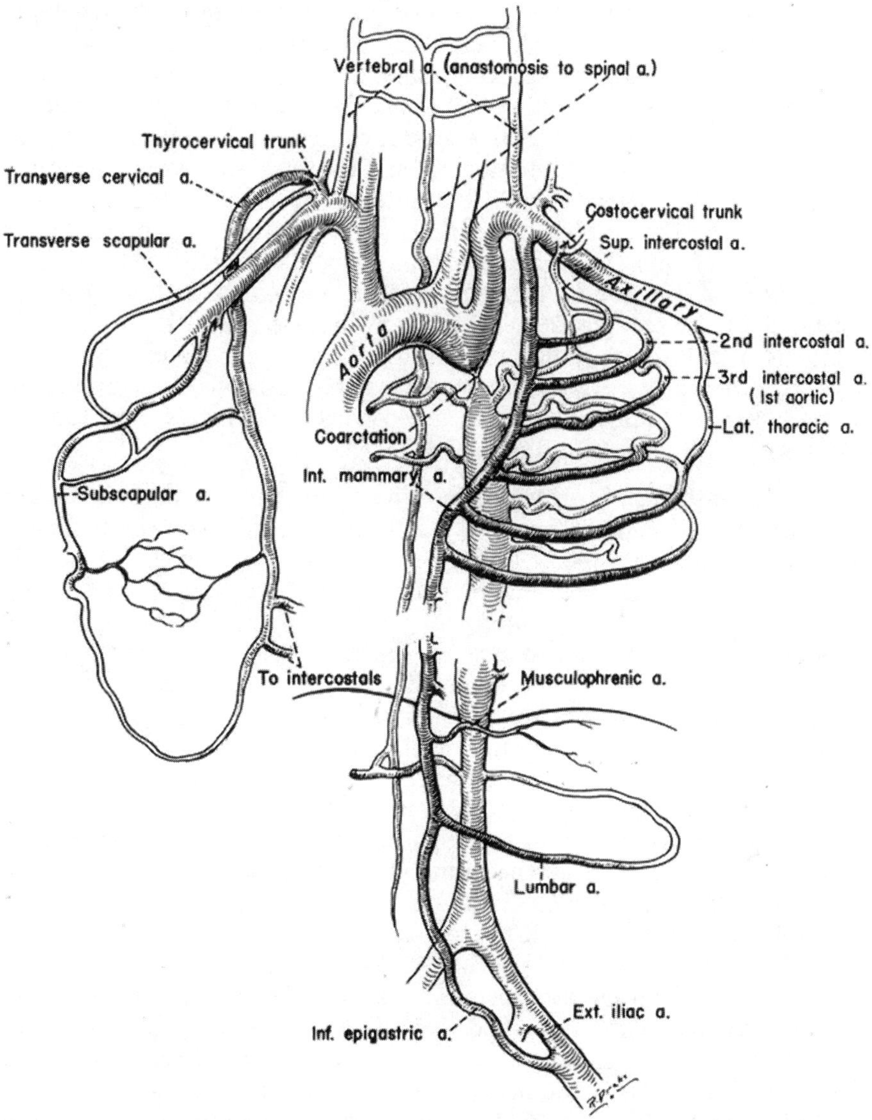

Fig. 1. The major collateral channels in coarctation of the aorta.

The intercostal arteries, with the exception of the first two of each side, are most important anastomotic bridges because of their communication with the aorta below the level of the coarctation on the one hand and with the internal mammary, musculophrenic, superior epigastric, anterior spinal and lateral thoracic arteries and the descending branch of the transverse cervical artery on the other. In this way the intercostal arteries carry blood which is ultimately derived from the aorta above the level of the coarctation to that portion of the aorta which lies below the coarctation. It is undoubtedly true that the vessels about the scapula, which communicate directly or indirectly with the intercostal arteries, contribute materially to the function of the collateral system portrayed. Bramwell and Jones indicated that these communications by far overshadow those of the intercostal arteries with the internal mammary artery and its terminal branches. The illustrations from the case they presented are in support of this view. Railsback and Dock, on the other hand, while cognizant of the communications of the intercostal arteries with the arteries of the scapula, stated that in their case the anterior communications of the intercostal arteries with the internal mammary arteries seemed to represent the important avenues of collateral circulation. The internal mammary arteries are consistently dilated and tortuous in coarctation (fig. 2*a* and *b*).

The intercostal arteries, by virtue of their function, become greatly dilated and tortuous. Posteriorly in particular, the tortuosity produces pressure atrophy of the adjacent ribs. At times this atrophy takes the form of mere enlargement of the costal grooves of the ribs. At other times, at the points of greatest tortuosity, there is gross focal erosion of the substance of the rib[12] (fig. 2*c* and *d*). When this feature occurs, it represents an important roentgenologic diagnostic feature in coarctation of the aorta since the notches are readily recognized on roentgenograms of the thorax. It is of interest that while it is commonly stated that the lower margin of the rib is notched in coarctation, such is usually not the case. On the contrary, the notching occurs on the inferior and anterior aspect of the main body of the rib at the point at which it joins that part of the rib which forms the wall of the costal groove (fig. 2*c* and *d*). This pathologic feature was illustrated by Ernstene and Robins[13] in 1931 and has been observed by Hodges.[14] Since the inferior portion of the rib which forms the posterior wall of the costal groove is thin in comparison to the upper portion of the rib, it may be sufficiently penetrated by roentgen rays as to become invisible in the roentgenogram.[15] Under such conditions, the notching appears to involve the inferior margin of the rib. This picture, however, is an illusion produced by roentgen-ray penetration of the lower portion of the rib.

13. Ernstene, A. C. and Robins, S. A.: The Roentgenologic Diagnosis of Stenosis of the Descending Arch (Coarctation) of the Aorta. Am. J. Roentgenol. 25:243-246 (Feb.) 1931.
14. Hodges, F. J.: Personal communication to the authors.
15. Crafoord, C., Ejrup, B. and Gladnikoff, H.: Coarctation of the Aorta. Thorax 2:121-147 (Sept.) 1947.

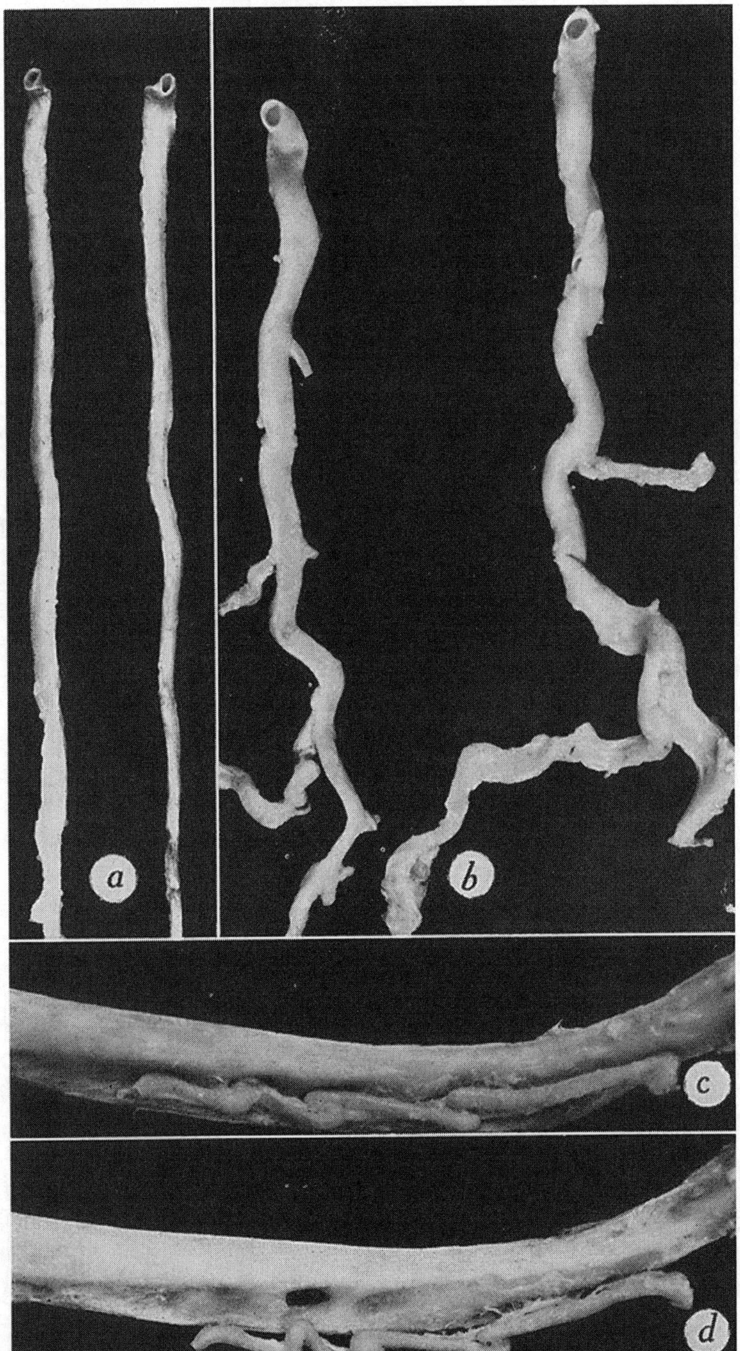

Fig. 2. Legend appears on facing page.

Pugh[16] has demonstrated that when roentgenograms of the thorax in patients with coarctation of the aorta are examined carefully, one frequently can demonstrate a portion of the rib inferior to that which is notched, thus visualizing roentgenographically the changes which are shown to be present pathologically.

The reason that the first two intercostal arteries do not play a great role in the collateral system lies in the fact that they usually do not communicate with the aorta posteriorly, as the other intercostal arteries do. Posteriorly, the first two intercostal arteries communicate with the superior intercostal artery, which in turn is in communication, either directly or through the costocervical trunk, with the subclavian artery of the same side. The superior intercostal artery may, however, play a bridging function by its anastomosis with the third intercostal artery at a point anterior to the site at which the latter vessel arises from the aorta as the first aortic intercostal artery.

The communication of the two terminal branches of the internal mammary, the musculophrenic and the superior epigastric arteries with the lower intercostal arteries, which occurs anteriorly, has already been mentioned. A prominent and additional communication of the superior epigastric artery is that with the upper portion of the inferior epigastric artery. Through this channel a substantial amount of blood may be carried from the subclavian artery above to the external iliac and femoral arteries below (figs. 1, *3a* and *b*).

Anastomoses between the inferior epigastric and the lumbar arteries serve as additional channels through which blood enters the lower part of the aorta.

The position and the communications of the anterior spinal artery are represented in figure 1. This artery may serve as a collateral channel in coarctation of the aorta since it lies along the entire length of the spinal cord and, so, forms a continuous channel past the level of the aortic narrowing. By receiving communications from the vertebral arteries in the cervical region, it receives blood derived from the subclavian arteries, which ultimately comes from the aorta above the level of stenosis. Furthermore, by its communications with the intercostal and lumbar arteries in the thoracic and lumbar regions, respectively, the anterior spinal artery may carry blood flowing into it from the vertebral arteries, above, toward the aorta below.

16. Pugh, D. G.: Value of Roentgenologic Diagnosis in Coarctation of the Aorta. Proc. Staff Meet., Mayo Clin. 23:343-347 (July 21) 1948.

Fig. *2a*. A pair of normal internal mammary arteries for comparison with those in figure *2b*; *b*, internal mammary arteries from a case of coarctation of the aorta in a male 18 years of age. The vessels are dilated and tortuous; *c*, a rib and intercostal artery from a case of aortic coarctation; the internal mammary arteries in this case are illustrated in figure *2b*. The intercostal artery is dilated and tortuous. At the points of greatest tortuosity of the artery there is notching of the rib; *d*, the same specimen as illustrated in figure *2c*. The intercostal artery has been retracted exposing the notches in the rib. The notches do not lie at the lower margin of the rib. Rather, they lie at the junction of the main body of the rib and that portion of the bone forming the posterior wall of the costal groove.

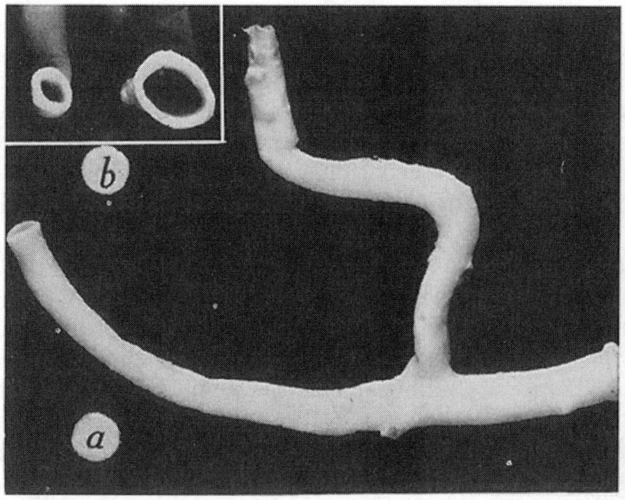

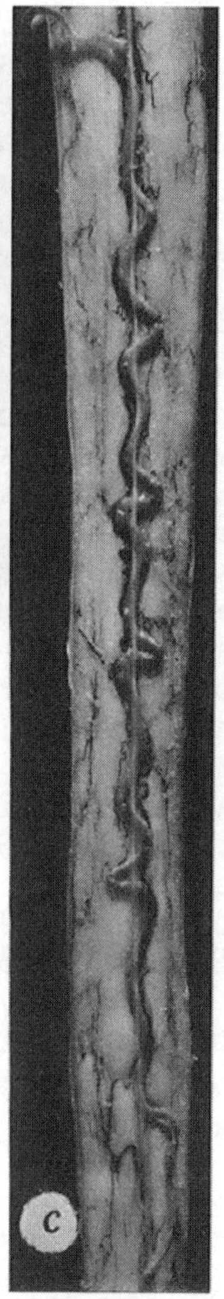

Fig. 3*a*. External iliac artery and inferior epigastric artery from a case of aortic coarctation in a boy 13 years of age. The external iliac artery runs more or less horizontally. Its proximal portion is to the left, its distal to the right. The inferior epigastric artery runs vertically. The latter artery is wide and tortuous. The iliac artery widens below the entrance of the inferior epigastric artery; *b*, the proximal and distal ends of the external iliac artery illustrated in figure 3*a*. The distal end, below the entrance of the inferior epigastric artery, is considerably wider than the proximal. This feature gives morphologic evidence of the function of the inferior epigastric artery in carrying blood to the lower extremity; *c*, anterior view of the lower cervical and upper thoracic portions of the spinal cord in a man 28 years of age with coarctation of the aorta. The anterior spinal artery is dilated and tortuous.

The role of the anterior spinal artery as a collateral channel has received relatively little attention in the past, although, in our experience, it is often dilated and tortuous in cases of aortic coarctation, particularly in the cervical and thoracic regions (fig. 3*c*). Evidently, symptoms resulting from the dilated state of the anterior spinal artery are not common. One exception is the case of Haberer, quoted by Herxheimer[17] and by Abbott, in which a transverse myelitis resulted from dilated spinal collaterals associated with coarctation.

17. Herxheimer, Gotthold: Missbildungen des Herzens und der grossen Gefässe. In Schwalbe, Ernst: Die Morphologie der Missbildungen des Menschen und der Tiere. Vienna, Gustav Fischer, 1910, vol. 3. Lieferung III, Abteilung 2, ch. 4, pp. 339-504.

It is to be emphasized that the relative size of the collateral channels may vary from case to case, and in a given case they may vary from side to side. The disproportion in size of the collaterals on one side as compared with the other may be remarkable, especially in atypical forms of coarctation. For example, when the site of aortic narrowing lies between the origins of the left common carotid and left subclavian arteries, the chief load of collateral function falls upon the right subclavian artery and its branches.[18] The left side of the body receives blood from the right side by means of midline anastomoses and from the lower part of the aorta after blood to it has come from right subclavian sources. Conversely, in those unusual cases in which aortic coarctation occurring near the ligamentum arteriosum is associated with stenosis of the origin of the right subclavian artery,[9] the major collateral function falls upon the left subclavian artery and its branches and upon the vessels which anastomose with them.

Major disproportion between the size of the collateral channels on one side as compared with the size of those of the other may be used as an aid in establishing the diagnosis of unusual types of coarctation.

SUMMARY

The anatomy of the collateral system of arteries in coarctation of the aorta is discussed and illustrated by a diagram and by photographs. It is emphasized that the notching of the ribs in coarctation does not usually involve the anatomic lower margin of these bones. Rather, it occurs at the junction of the main body of the rib and that portion which forms the wall of the costal groove. The role of the anterior spinal artery as a collateral channel is discussed.

CLINICAL FEATURES IN COARCTATION OF THE AORTA: A REVIEW OF 96 CASES*

Norman A. Christensen, M. D. and Edgar A. Hines, Jr., M. D., M. S. in Medicine, Division of Medicine: From 1925 to 1947, 119 Clinic patients were diagnosed as having coarctation of the aorta. This group forms the basis for this study. Important features in the diagnosis of coarctation of the aorta are (1) characteristic differences in the arterial pulsations and in indirect blood pressure in the upper and lower extremities, (2) the presence of one or more cardiac or cardiovascular murmurs, (3) the presence of a well-developed collateral arterial system that by-passes the coarctation, (4) characteristic

18. Parker, R. L. and Dry, T. J.: Coarctation of the Aorta at an Unusual Site, Associated with a Congenitally Bicuspid Aortic Valve: Report of Case. Am. Heart J. 15:739-745 (June) 1938.

*Abridgment of a portion of the thesis submitted by Dr. Christensen to the Faculty of the Graduate School of the University of Minnesota in partial fulfillment of the requirements for the degree of Master of Science in Medicine.

The Collateral Circulation in Coarctation of the Aorta

David W. Hunter, M.D.

This article by Jesse Edwards was written in 1948, one year after I was born. It is always humbling to find out how much about medicine was known before you were born, and particularly long before the work that you and your contemporaries did to further medical knowledge. In this seminal article on the anatomy of the collateral circulation associated with coarctation, Dr. Edwards summarizes the work of anatomists who came before him and manages to put all of their work and his extensive observations into a wonderful brief perspective accompanied with his usual fabulous illustrations.

His two colleagues on this paper reflect his lifelong dedication to working closely with clinicians who both contributed to his work and benefited from it immensely. Dr. O. Theron (Jim) Clagett (1908-1990) of the Mayo Clinic was one of the most prominent thoracic surgeons of his time, and Dr. Norman A. Christensen (1915-2008) was an equally renowned Mayo Clinic internist with a broad range of interests including vascular problems that led him to produce two papers in 1948 and 1949 with Dr. Edwards on the circulation disturbances associated with coarctation. The clarity and thoroughness of detail in this article gave surgeons of the era the anatomic understanding that allowed them to develop the currently practiced surgical repair techniques. From the subclavian flap technique, which was developed soon after the first report by Clarence Crafoord of Stockholm, Sweden, of coarctation surgery in 1944 using a resection and end-to end anastomosis technique, surgeons throughout the years have owed a great debt to Jesse Edwards. More recently, the modern imaging techniques of CTA and MRA are able to give us pictures, which are astonishingly much like Dr Edwards' beautiful anatomic drawings, and confirm all of the observations that he made so long ago. In this article, Dr Edwards reveals his most valuable asset as a clinical researcher, and that was his incredible powers of observation. As you read this article, you begin to appreciate his unbelievable attention to detail down to the exact position of the intercostal artery indentations of bone and exactly what they meant for the radiographic images that were being used at the time to make the diagnosis. You also note how Dr. Edwards always had something innovative to say. In my brief experience working with him, I tried to write a paper based on findings associated with complex septal defects. He reviewed my first attempt and smiled, commenting only "If you can find something novel to say about the issue let's go forward. If not, let's look for another topic."

In the last two decades, there has been a significant debate about whether coarctation will be best treated with endovascular or surgical techniques. Although surgery still seems to have the upper hand for coarctation repair in infancy, the question as to which technique has more long-term successes and complications when applied to older children and adults is slowly evolving to favor the endovascular route. It has been a little more than 60 years since the publication of this article, and yet today we are just beginning to come to grips with the genetic, vascular and multisystem problems for which coarctation is simply a signpost. It is astonishing and refreshing how complex the human organism can be and how, no matter when you live, there is always more work to be done, peeling away one layer at a time we finally find ourselves coming closer to the center of this wonderfully complex onion of life.

The Lewis A. Conner Memorial Lecture

Functional Pathology of the Pulmonary Vascular Tree in Congenital Cardiac Disease

By JESSE E. EDWARDS, M.D.

While there are many anatomic varieties of congenital malformations of the heart and great vessels, most may be divided, from a functional point of view, into 3 types: (1) communication between the ventricles or between the aorta and pulmonary arteries, (2) anomalous drainage of pulmonary venous blood into the right atrium, and (3) obstruction to pulmonary venous flow. In each of these categories the responses of the pulmonary vascular tree have to be considered in understanding the altered dynamics. Depending on the type and degree of response in the pulmonary vascular bed, there may be a varying functional picture among patients having the same anatomic or functionally comparable malformation.

*"A teacher affects eternity; he can never tell where his influence stops."**

A PHYSICIAN with great vision and energy, Dr. Lewis A. Conner, was a leader in medical education and in preventive medicine. It is clear both from his writings and from conversations with one of his former interns, my good friend, Dr. Norman Keith, that Dr. Conner also had keen insight into the specific problems of the individual patient. He was a pioneer more than 40 years ago in emphasizing facts which then were controversial and which we accept today as commonplace. His interests in the pulmonary complications of the patient with typhoid fever led to a clear appreciation of the relationship of peripheral venous thrombosis to pulmonary embolism.

He indicated that peripheral venous thrombosis might be clinically latent and yet be responsible for pulmonary embolism.[1, 2] The pulmonary embolism might be recurrent and not necessarily fatal. In stressing these facts, he brought out the concept that in a patient with a disease seemingly unrelated to the lungs, there might be pulmonary manifestations that were, in fact, somehow related to the basic nonpulmonary disease.

Read at the meeting of the American Heart Association, Cincinnati, Ohio, October 26 to 31, 1956.

From the Mayo Clinic and the Mayo Foundation. The Mayo Foundation is a part of the Graduate School of the University of Minnesota.

Abstracted, Circulation **14:** 903, 1956.

* The Education of Henry Adams (Henry Brooks Adams). Chap. 20. 1907.

With this background of the man for whom this lecture is named, and with my own personal interest in congenital cardiac disease, when invited to give this lecture I chose a subject that dealt with the interrelationship of the heart and the lungs. I believe this choice to be appropriate for this particular lecture, since, as we shall see, the pulmonary vessels play significant roles in many patients with congenital cardiac disease; patients in whom the primary difficulty is not pulmonary but rather is in another organ, as in this instance, the heart.

Historically, congenital cardiac disease may be divided into two periods separated in time and thought by two nearly simultaneous major developments. These were the reintroduction of cardiac catheterization by Cournand and Ranges[3] in 1941 and the devising of the anastomotic operation for pulmonary stenosis by Blalock and Taussig[4] in 1945. While there is some overlapping in approach between these two periods, they are, in general, rather sharply separated.

The earlier period began with anatomic description of the various malformations, a sphere in which Rokitansky made notable contributions and to which Sir Arthur Keith and Lev added materially.

The natural consequences of the establishment of various malformations anatomically were the attempts at clinicopathologic correlation. In this regard we readily think of Peacock,

Fallot, the Gibsons, Roger and Brown. Coming from this era the clinicopathologic correlations of Maude Abbott, a pathologist, were classic and served to keep the light of congenital cardiac disease, however dim the flicker, from being extinguished. One cannot help realizing the personal satisfaction that had come to this devoted worker when, during the final years of her career, she witnessed a road to definite therapy. First came the attempted closure of a patent ductus arteriosus by Graybiel, Strieder, and Boyer[5] and finally the report in 1939 of success in such attempts by Gross and Hubbard.[6]

In the earlier of the 2 historical periods in congenital cardiac disease there was a strong tendency to attribute specific functional derangement to specific anatomic cardiac malformations. The outstanding exception to this was Abbott's teaching of the occurrence of *cyanose tardive*;[7] that is, patients with certain malformations might not be cyanotic for a period of time and then develop cyanosis. The basis for this change in function for a given patient was not clearly defined. Although some reference was made to a role that pulmonary vessels might play in such a change, no specific correlations between the changing clinical manifestations and functional or anatomic changes in the pulmonary vessels were forthcoming. In 1927, however, Moschcowitz[8] suggested that cyanosis in congenital cardiac disease might result from pulmonary hypertension.

The arrival of the second period in congenital cardiac disease was marked by a secure background regarding the anatomic nature of the various malformations but almost a complete void regarding the interrelationships between the pulmonary vessels on one hand and the function of the heart with the anatomic defect on the other.

That the pulmonary vessels might play a significant role in determining the behavior of the cardiovascular system in a given patient rapidly became apparent as some cyanotic patients on whom an anastomotic operation was to be done were found to have severe pulmonary hypertension, a condition that would not allow an increased pulmonary flow were the procedure done. Also, early in this period Bing's group[9, 10] and Dexter's group[11, 12] by the use of cardiac catheterization, studying patients with the same anatomic defect, found some to have normal pulmonary arterial pressures while in others the pulmonary pressure was as high as the systemic arterial pressure.

Such observations raised many questions: Is pulmonary hypertension a complication of certain types of congenital cardiac disease? Is it an integral part of the disease? Is the elevated pressure simply a product of altered function without changes in structure? Are there structural changes that accompany the elevated pulmonary resistance and pressure? If anatomic changes are present in the pulmonary vessels, are they the same in all cases with pulmonary hypertension? If differences in structure exist, are any of the changes potentially reversible with correction of the defect? Are any permanent?

Early attempts at answers to these questions were inhibited by inadequate material. What was needed was both histologic and physiologic data on a sufficient number of cases of any particular condition to reveal the entire story for that condition. By studying individual cases, even with pathologic and physiologic data at hand, one did not know just where he was with regard to the over-all manifestations of the condition. With the passage of time such accumulations have been made, notably by Dammann and his associates[13–15] and by the English workers Heath and Whitaker.[16]

From such organized studies, an orderly process becomes evident, so that now a number of the foregoing questions may be answered with confidence although mechanisms involved for certain phenomena are still lacking. Some of the questions still require conditional answers, but the stage is set for comprehensive understanding of the problem of the interrelationships between the pulmonary circulation and the heart which has one or another malformation. This leads us to appreciate that among a group of patients with the same anatomic diagnosis regarding the cardiac malformation, the physiologic and clinical behavior may be so diverse, depending on pulmonary vascular response, that superficially some patients could hardly seem to be harboring the same malformation as others.[17–22]

One of our early experiences with the interrelationship of the pulmonary vessels and cardiac malformations concerned a 7-year-old girl who was observed in 1947. Dr. Howard B. Burchell, who had studied the patient clinically, thought that she had coarctation of the aorta proximal to a patent ductus arteriosus, and that the right ventricle was supplying blood to the descending aorta. The predicted anatomic arrangement was found at operation. The patient was one of the early cases of coarctation on whom operation was performed. Unfortunately, she died of hemothorax from separation of the aortic suture line on the thirteenth postoperative day.

Before the lungs were examined histologically, Dr. Burchell indicated that in view of his postulate that the right ventricle was supplying blood to the descending aorta, the pulmonary arterial pressure would have had to be equal to or in excess of aortic pressure. Was the high pulmonary vascular resistance necessary to maintain such a high pressure associated with structural change in the pulmonary vessels?

Histologic examination of the lungs revealed arteries that were so thick-walled they suggested the structure of peripheral systemic arteries. Our first reaction to describe these was the term "peripheralization" of the pulmonary vessels. After reflecting further on this, we recognized that the connections of the ductus and postulated direction of flow in this case after birth were like those in the normal fetus. This led us to postulate that the pulmonary vessels had not acquired a systemic arterial structure but that the changes were a carry-over into postnatal life of features normal in the fetus. Parenthetically, this case was one of four of coarctation and patent ductus arteriosus of which the pulmonary vessels were reported before this society at the 1948 meeting.[23]

I have derived much pleasure, encouragement, and guidance from the continuous interest that Dr. Burchell has evidenced in co-ordinating our pathologic findings with those of the clinician, physiologist, and surgeon. Much gratitude is due him for having been a major factor in making the story as organized in my mind as it now is.

However, should the audience judge that it is not organized, I must personally take the responsibility, not he.

Definition of Terms

There are 3 terms that are frequently used in a discussion of the dynamics of the pulmonary circulation: (1) pressure, (2) flow, and (3) resistance.

The first 2, pressure and flow, are real and measurable, while resistance is an abstract value derived from knowing the other 2. Yet the 3 are closely interrelated.

The level of pulmonary arterial pressure depends on the volume rate of pulmonary flow and the resistance to that flow. For a constant flow the pressure will vary directly with the resistance: the higher the resistance, the higher the pressure, and vice versa. For a constant resistance the pressure will vary with the flow: the higher the flow, the higher the pressure, and vice versa.

Pulmonary arterial hypertension refers to elevated pressure. A value of about 25 mm. of mercury, or about one fifth the systemic arterial pressure, is normal for pulmonary arterial systolic pressure. The dividing line between normal and abnormal values is not clear-cut. In many patients who have elevated pulmonary arterial pressure, however, the level of pressure is so high that the pulmonary arterial systolic pressure is about the same as the systemic arterial systolic pressure. At such equal levels the pulmonary arterial and systemic pressures are sometimes referred to as representing equivalent pressures.

A measured fall in pulmonary pressure without knowledge of the volume rate of flow does not tell us whether the observed phenomenon in pressure change is due to a lowering in flow, to a fall in resistance or both.

Certain Features of Normal Pulmonary Circulation

We are not concerned here with acquired cardiac disease, and so our discussion regarding the interrelationship between cardiac disease and the pulmonary vessels cannot logically start with a normal postnatal pulmonary vascular tree.

We are, on the contrary, concerned with congenital diseases of the heart. These diseases are present both before and after birth and their relationship to the pulmonary vessels must therefore include a consideration of the responses of the pulmonary vascular tree in these various types of diseases during fetal life, at birth and in the postnatal state. To avoid consideration of events at the time of birth deprives us of an important link in the story.

With this background it is pertinent first to consider some of the features of the normal fetal circulation and the changes that take place at the time of birth and later.

Fetal Circulation

Blood returns to the heart by way of the 2 venae cavae (fig. 1*a*). Most of the superior caval blood flows through the tricuspid valve to the right ventricle.[24] The inferior caval stream splits at atrial level, some flowing through the foramen ovale into the left atrium, where it is joined by what blood returns through the pulmonary veins from the lungs. The mixture enters and leaves the left ventricle. Most of this blood is distributed to the branches of the aortic arch.

That part of the inferior caval blood that does not flow through the foramen ovale joins the superior caval blood, enters the right ventricle, then flows into the pulmonary trunk.

The principles concerned with distribution of the blood leaving the pulmonary trunk of the normal fetus are worthy of particular attention, since they are also applicable to those anomalies in which an abnormal communication exists between the lesser and the greater circulation.

In the fetus the pulmonary arterial bed is in free communication with the descending aorta by way of the ductus arteriosus. In view of this free communication the pressures in the pulmonary arteries and aorta and in the 2 ventricles are of the same magnitude.[25-27] Of the blood that leaves the right ventricle only a small proportion enters the pulmonary vascular

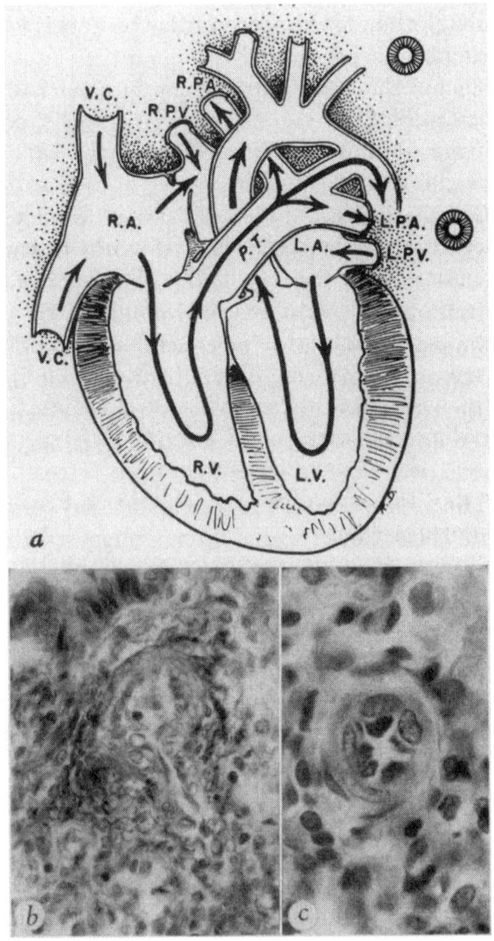

FIG. 1. *a*. Diagrammatic representation of the intracardiac circulation in the fetus. The circles beside the left pulmonary artery and the left subclavian artery indicate relative resistances to flow in the 2 systems. Here they are assumed to be equal. *b*. A small pulmonary muscular artery and arteriolar branch of a control stillborn full-term fetus. Characteristically the muscle of the mediae is thick and the lumina are narrow [ELVG (This abbreviation here and in subsequent illustrations indicates Verhoeff's elastic-tissue stain counterstained with van Gieson's connective-tissue stain.); reduced from × 500]. *c*. High-power view of pulmonary arteriole of a stillborn full-term fetus. The media is composed of thick muscle and the lumen is narrow (hematoxylin and eosin; reduced from × 900).

bed. The major part of it is propelled through the ductus arteriosus into the descending aorta and on to the placenta. In order for the flow through the ductus arteriosus to be possible, there must exist a high resistance to flow through the pulmonary vascular bed. This high resistance is at one and the same time responsible for the pulmonary hypertension that is characteristic of the fetus and for right ventricular blood to be driven into the descending aorta.

The basis for the high resistance to pulmonary flow may in part be caused by the features associated with the collapsed lung,[27] and it may in part be brought about by action of the pulmonary arteriolar and arterial bed. The latter possibility is supported by the fact that in the normal fetus the pulmonary arteries and arterioles have thick muscular medial layers and narrow lumina[28] (fig. 1*b* and *c*).

The appearance of these small arterial vessels with their thick medial layers suggests that they are capable of significant degrees of vascular constriction, and the fact that their lumina are narrow suggests further that in the fetus the small pulmonary arterial vessels are in fact in a vasoconstricted state.

Changes at Birth

After birth the ductus arteriosus closes, at first functionally and later anatomically, thus eliminating the free communication between the 2 circuits at arterial level.[26, 29] Closure of the foramen ovale occurs almost simultaneously.[29, 30]

With these 2 fetal channels closed, there is complete partitioning of the 2 circulations, a circumstance that allows each to have its own resistance and pressure without affecting the flow through the other.

Early after birth the pulmonary pressure becomes lower than the systemic pressure and, since the same volume of blood flows through each circuit, the postnatal fall in pulmonary pressure has to be a consequence of a fall in pulmonary vascular resistance.[26]

While there is an abrupt fall in pulmonary vascular resistance at birth, the development of the fully established adult relationship between pulmonary and systemic resistance, wherein the pulmonary resistance is about one-fifth of the systemic resistance, is in part a gradual process. The latter opinion, until such time as direct observations are made, must rest on indirect, but presumably reliable evidence.

In the normal fetus the 2 ventricles are of about the same thickness. Usually by the end of the third postnatal month the adult disproportion between the thickness of the 2 ventricles is established both by anatomic and by electrocardiographic evidence (fig. 2*a* and *b*). The other supporting factor is that the thick pulmonary arteries and arterioles of the fetus gradually are transformed into the thin vessels of the adult (fig. 2*c*). The latter process is usually complete by about the age of 3 months but certainly by 6 months.[14, 28]

Adult Pulmonary Vascular Tree

We shall now consider the structure of the pulmonary vascular bed in the adult, both to contrast it with the fetus and also to have it serve as another point of reference in the consideration of the pulmonary vascular tree in the various congenital cardiac diseases.

There are 3 major categories of arterial vessels in the lungs as follows: (1) the elastic arteries, (2) the muscular arteries, and (3) the arterioles.

The elastic arteries are characterized by having numerous layers of elastic tissue arranged in a concentric manner identical with that in the aorta. Included as elastic pulmonary arteries are the pulmonary trunk and the various branches that accompany the cartilaginous bronchi. The smallest ones measure about 1 mm. in diameter. As in the aorta, there are collagenous fibers and smooth muscle cells between the elastic layers. The intima is a thin connective-tissue layer covered by endothelium. The adventitia is composed of dense collagen.

From the review of Burton[31] on the functional significance of the structural elements in walls of blood vessels, it is proper to consider that the elastic fibers of the elastic pulmonary arteries impart to this class of vessel a high degree of resistance to distention, while the relatively small amount of muscle would indicate that the elastic arteries have very little capability of actively constricting.

Arising from the elastic arteries is the next class of vessel, the muscular arteries. These vessels branch into lower orders of the same class of vessel. The muscular arteries are associated with the bronchioles, the respiratory bronchioles, and the alveolar ducts. The char-

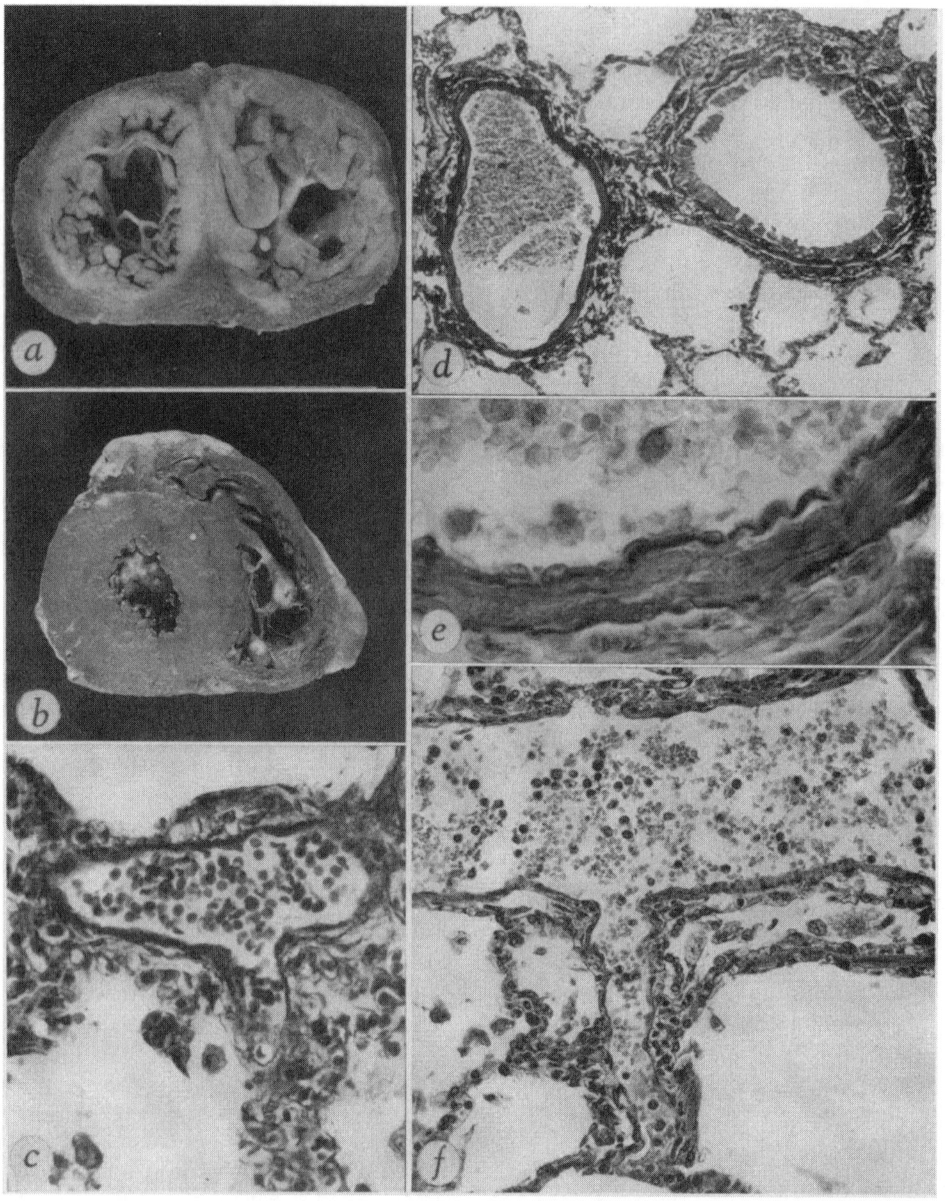

FIG. 2. *a*. Cross section of ventricles viewed from above in a control newborn infant. The 2 ventricles are of about the same thickness. *b*. Cross section of the ventricles in a control adult heart, showing the characteristic disproportion in thickness between the left ventricle and the right. This contrasts with the fetal state shown in *a*. *c*. A small pulmonary muscular artery and an arteriolar branch from a control 6-week-old infant. The thick media characteristic of similar vessels in the fetus has disappeared, leaving the adult type of change in which the walls are thin and the lumina are wide (ELVG; × 330). *d*, *e*, and *f*. From a control male patient aged 23 years. *d*. Large muscular artery and a bronchiole (ELVG; × 70). The arterial wall is thin and its lumen is wide. *e*. A segment of the artery illustrated in *d* (ELVG; × 570). *f*. An arteriole arising from a small muscular artery, each with characteristically thin walls and wide lumina. At the origin of the arteriole a small amount of muscle is present in the media (hematoxylin and eosin; × 200).

acteristic media of the elastic arteries changes fairly abruptly with the origin of the muscular branches. Two sheaths of elastic tissue from the elastic arteries enter a muscular artery to be the internal and external elastic laminae of that vessel. In that class of muscular arteries arising from the elastic arteries there may be additional laminae of elastic fibers, but these

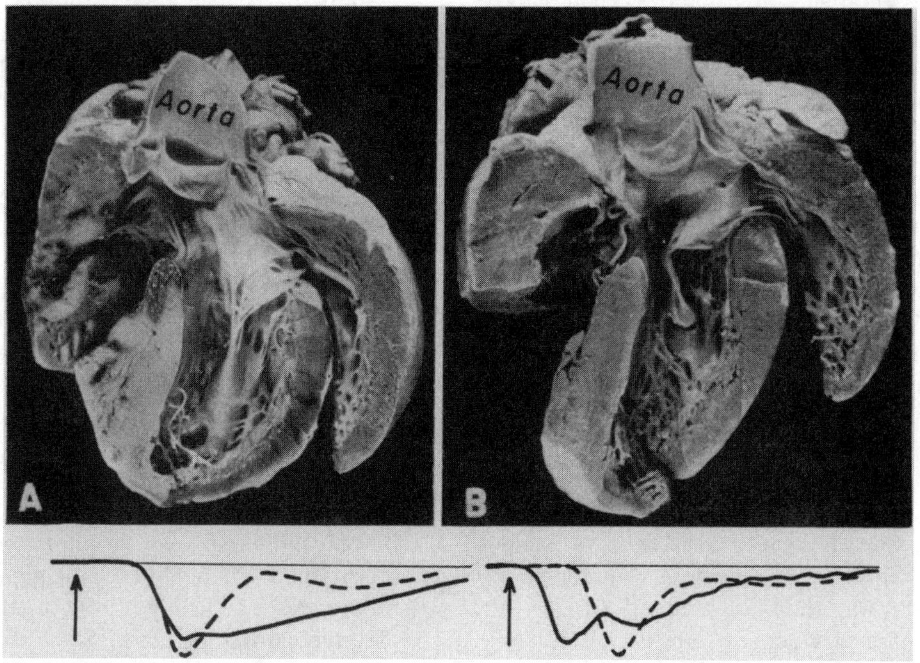

FIG. 3. Gross specimens and dye-dilution curves in 2 cases of ventricular septal defect, showing different hemodynamic features while the structure of the heart is essentially the same (solid curves for particular cases; dotted curves for anticipated normal). Total pulmonary resistance (dynes sec. cm.$^{-5}$) *A*. 305, *B*. 3197; systemic resistance (dynes sec. cm.$^{-5}$) *A*. 2500, *B*. 1886; pulmonary artery pressure (mm. Hg) *A*. 79/55, *B*. 135/83; radial artery pressure (mm. Hg) *A*. 93/62, *B*. 135/84.

are normally lost after further branching. In all classes of muscular arteries the major element of the artery lies between the internal and the external elastic membrane. This is a layer of the circularly oriented smooth muscle. There are a thin intima and a relatively thin adventitial layer of collagen. In the normal adult the wall of a pulmonary muscular artery is thin while the lumen is wide (fig. 3). The anatomic structure suggests a low resistance to flow; yet the presence of muscle suggests that a vasoconstrictive function may be found in the muscular arteries.

Arising from those muscular arteries which are related to the respiratory bronchioles are the muscular arterial branches which accompany the alveolar ducts. As the latter arteries are traced distally, they give off branches that arise about at right angles. The latter vessels are termed "arterioles." Beyond the origin of the arterioles the artery accompanying the alveolar duct loses its identifiable muscular media.

Here the vessel wall is composed of an endothelial layer lying on a thin layer of connective tissue that contains a single elastic layer. Beyond this level the arterial vessel communicates with the capillaries related to the air spaces.

The branches that are termed "arterioles" are small replicas of the arteries from which they arise (fig. 2*d*, *e*, and *f*). At their origins they have a media that has a circularly oriented thin layer of muscle. Shortly beyond their origins the arterioles lose identifiable muscle. Here they are composed of an endothelial lining, a small amount of supporting collagen, a single elastic layer, and a thin collagenous adventitia.

Our anatomic classification of the arterial vessels is similar to that of Brenner[32] with but one exception. By classifying vessels according to their caliber, segments which we would consider the proximal portions of arterioles would be classified as small arteries by Brenner's criterion, which indicates that the dividing line between small muscular arteries and arterioles is 100 microns. We have observed the proximal part of vessels arising from arteries accompanying alveolar ducts to have diameters more than this in the normal, whereas the same class of vessel may have a considerably narrower diameter under abnormal conditions. Were one to apply a classification based on diameter, the same class of vessel would be called an artery in the normal and an arteriole in the abnormal. Furthermore, there are circumstances wherein an arteriole has a diameter less than 100 microns in the normal and in excess of this under certain abnormal conditions. From the foregoing it is apparent that there is in the lung a small class of vessel, which we call the arteriole. This has a muscular media at its origin and none in its remaining portion. Even at its thickest and muscular portion the normal arteriole of the adult has a very thin wall compared to the size of its lumen. A common ratio of lumen-to-wall thickness is about 8:1.

The pulmonary arteries and arterioles accompany and branch with the bronchial system, while the veins, as indicated by Miller,[33] are as far removed from the bronchial system as is possible within the anatomic confines of the respiratory units. On one side of the capillaries lie the arterioles, while on the opposite side lie the venules. The latter then proceed away from the bronchiole of their respiratory units toward the interlobular septum, where they join the venous trunks. Knowledge of this is particularly helpful, especially in studying single sections, since a thin-walled structure near an alveolar duct may suggest a venous structure, yet from its position the vessel must be of arterial or arteriolar nature.

If we were to judge functional potential from structural characteristics of the normal adult pulmonary arterial tree, with its thin walls and wide lumina, we could conclude that it is a low-resistance system. Functional observations in the normal indicate that this is the case.[34–38]

At the same time it is well to recognize that even in the normal the arterial side of the pulmonary circulation is more than a passive series of communications from the right ventricle to capillaries. Responses in the normal of increased resistance to flow when breathing gas mixtures low in oxygen suggest the possibility of a vasoconstrictive response.[39–43]

Vasodilatory effect may be observed in the normal pulmonary arteriolar bed, as judged by the fact that a significant increase in flow may not be associated with any appreciable rise in pressure. This can be accounted for only by a decrease in vascular resistance.[44, 45]

The same class of pulmonary vessel has so remarkably a different appearance from one patient to another that by study of individual sections one may not be certain that he is in fact comparing the same class of vessel. By serial sections, given classes of vessels may be identified by their origins and terminations and by their relations to the respiratory system.

While such studies are laborious, the assurance obtained when identifying a given class of vessel more than justifies the effort involved.

In our pathologic collection of congenital malformations of the heart and great vessels there are about 500 cases. In 96 of these, comprehensive cardiac catheterization studies had been done during life under the direction of Dr. E. H. Wood. In many of these the functional studies included obtaining multiple dye-dilution curves.[46–48]

I am indebted to Drs. Earl H. Wood, F. H. Helmholz, Jr., H. J. C. Swan, P. S. Hetzel, and I. J. Fox for making readily available to me the results of these various studies and for their helpfulness in reviewing these with me. In addition to reference to this specific material I have had free interchange of ideas with Dr. Wood and his group for some years, a fact which has given me a clearer insight into cardiovascular physiology than I would otherwise have had.

The major part of the presentation to follow is based on the cases in which functional studies had been done. In 50 of these, serial sections of pulmonary tissue were examined. Also, in a smaller number of cases that had not had physiologic studies similar sections were studied.

Functional Classification of Congenital Cardiac Disease

While there are many different anatomic types of cardiac anomalies, in most of these there is 1 of 2 anatomic derangements that place functional responsibility on the pul-

TABLE 1.—*Classification of Congenital Malformations of the Heart*

Functional category	Representative anatomic types
Communication between ventricles or systemic and pulmonary arteries	Ventricular septal defect, "tetralogy of Fallot," single functioning ventricle, patent ductus arteriosus
Pulmonary venous drainage into right atrium	Atrial septal defect, anomalous pulmonary venous connection
Pulmonary venous obstruction	Mitral stenosis, chronic left ventricular failure

monary vascular tree. One of the 2 anatomic derangements is an abnormal opening between the lesser and the greater circulation; the other is an abnormal obstruction somewhere in the circulatory system.

The abnormal opening may be at the level of the atrial septum, at the ventricular septum, or between the aorta and the pulmonary arterial system.

The important sites of obstruction may be anatomically located in the pulmonary arterial tract or in the mitral valve. More commonly there are defects other than mitral stenosis that produce essentially the same effect as though an anatomic site of obstruction had in fact been at the mitral valve. If the majority of congenital malformations of the heart are defined in a functional manner they fall into 3 major categories as shown in table 1.

VENTRICULAR SEPTAL DEFECT

I shall begin with a discussion of ventricular septal defect, realizing that what I say about this condition pertains in many ways also to patent ductus arteriosus.

When a ventricular septal defect exists, it is convenient to view this functionally as a communication not only between the ventricles but also between the left ventricle and the pulmonary arteries. It is proper at the outset to distinguish those cases of ventricular septal defect without gross pulmonary stenosis from those in which the defect is associated with pulmonary stenosis.

Ventricular Septal Defect without Pulmonary Stenosis

Three features of ventricular septal defect without pulmonary stenosis have occupied the minds of many in attempting to determine why the behavior in some cases differs significantly from that in others.

These features are (1) the relation of the aortic valve to the defect; (2) the size of the defect; (3) the pulmonary vascular changes.

1. Relation of the Aortic Valve to the Defect. Earlier teaching emphasized that the relation of the aortic valve to the defect represented an essential basic factor in difference of behavior among patients with ventricular defect. There is now sufficient evidence to indicate that these conclusions were based on insufficient examination of varied material, and are not valid.

The older concept stems principally from a review that Maude Abbott[49] made of a report by Eisenmenger.[50] The earlier author had reported the case of a cyanotic patient who at necropsy had a large ventricular septal defect and communication of the aorta, above the defect, with both ventricles. Abbott reasoned that the continuity of the right ventricle with the aorta would make a right-to-left shunt obligatory and named the combination of biventricular origin of the aorta above a ventricular septal defect without pulmonary stenosis and with cyanosis as the Eisenmenger complex. This name is in general use today for this combination of circumstances. In 7 of 8 cases with this anatomic arrangement she observed cyanosis. What Abbott failed to point out was that among many patients with the same anatomic arrangement between the aorta and the heart a right-to-left shunt does not occur. This negates the thesis that communication of the aorta above a ventricular septal defect with the right ventricle makes a right-to-left shunt obligatory.

Support for the present view is to be had from 2 representative cases illustrated in figure 3. In each, the anatomic relation of the aorta to the heart above a large ventricular septal defect was identical, showing free communication between the right ventricle and the aorta.

In each case the pulmonary arterial systolic pressure was essentially equivalent to that in the systemic arteries. Yet in one case there was a large left-to-right shunt and no right-to-left shunt. In the other case a significant right-to-left shunt was present, possibly associated with a small left-to-right shunt. Since the anatomic arrangements are the same in the 2 cases, the reason for different behavior must be sought elsewhere than in the anatomic features of the malformation. This difference is found in the response of the pulmonary vascular tree, as suggested by Selzer and Laquer[51] and by Dexter and associates[11] and later by Dammann and associates[13, 15] and Blount and co-workers[22] among others.

In the first case the pulmonary vascular resistance, although mildly elevated, was significantly less than the systemic vascular resistance. In the second case the pulmonary vascular resistance was very high, being greater than systemic level.

We may therefore conclude that in ventricular septal defect the relation of the aorta to the right ventricle is not the primary factor in determining the direction of the shunt. Rather, the determining factor is the height of the pulmonary vascular resistance as compared to the resistance in the systemic circulation.

It is of interest to point out that Eisenmenger[52] himself, in a paper subsequent to the original one referred to by Abbott, indicated that in any case with defect of the ventricular septum lying near the aortic valve, the aorta is in communication with the right ventricle. He demonstrated that this situation could be reproduced even in a normal heart by artificially creating a defect near the aortic valve. This has been confirmed.[51, 53]

Simply by virtue of the fact that most ventricular septal defects are in close relationship with the aortic valve, it is likely that, in a random case of ventricular septal defect with a right-to-left shunt, the aorta will be found communicating with the right ventricle. However, if a defect is distant from the aortic orifice, as in a case described by Heath and associates,[54] the same dynamics may apply as when the defect is near the aorta. We have had similar experience.

The foregoing leads to the dilemma as to what to do about the term, "the Eisenmenger complex." Two avenues are open.

We may retain the term for those cases of ventricular septal defect with cyanosis, or we may discard it and indicate for such a case the descriptive designation, "ventricular septal defect with right-to-left shunt."

To do the latter would better convey the thought that the occurrence of a right-to-left shunt in a case of ventricular septal defect is simply one manifestation in the wide spectrum of functional behavior in ventricular septal defect and is not causally related to a specific anatomic type of ventricular septal defect.

2. Size of Defect. In each of the cases in the foregoing discussion the defect was large, and hence what influence the size of the defect had in one case was equally applicable to the other.

Small Defects. During fetal life, it is normal for the pressure in the 2 ventricles to be equal. At this time a ventricular septal defect, regardless of its size, is of little functional significance, there probably being very little flow through the abnormal opening.

After birth, when the tendency for pulmonary vascular resistance to fall is manifest, the size of the defect takes on paramount importance. A small defect, though an opening, is one that presents a high degree of resistance to flow through it (fig. 4*a*). It represents an obstruction between the left ventricle on one hand and the right ventricle and the pulmonary arteries on the other. In view of this obstruction the left ventricle obviously is not in free communication with the lesser circulation. It is possible for a differential in pressure to be built up between the 2 compartments. This happens[55, 56] as the pulmonary vascular resistance falls toward normal postnatal levels and a normal postnatal evolution of the pulmonary arteries and arterioles is manifest. The small defect is a controlling factor in preventing large volumes of blood from shunting from the left ventricle to the lesser circulation. The pulmonary and right ventricular pressures are normal.

Large Defects. Defects that have about the same diameter as the aorta are said to be large.[56] Allowing free communication between the left ventricle and the right ventricle and pulmonary arteries, they lack the obstructive character of the small defect (fig. 4*b* and *c*).

It is at this point important to recognize a principle of interrelationship between the 2 circulations when there is free communication between them. Burchell and Wood[57] and Hamilton and associates[58] have clearly demonstrated that the direction and volume of flow through such a communication depend principally on

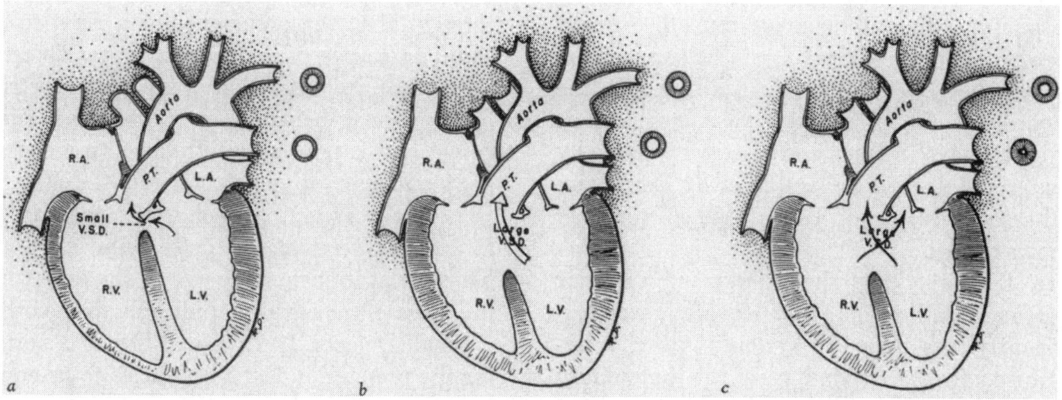

FIG. 4. Diagrammatic representation of hemodynamics in small (*a*) and large (*b* and *c*) ventricular septal defects. In the small defect the pulmonary resistance is significantly less than the systemic; the defect itself represents an obstruction. In the large defects, when the pulmonary resistance is less than the systemic a left-to-right shunt occurs. When the pulmonary resistance exceeds the systemic a right-to-left shunt appears.

relative resistances to flow in the pulmonary as compared to the systemic circulation. The blood flows into the system with the lower resistance.

The size of the defect determines whether it itself is an effective barrier between the left ventricle and the pulmonary arteries. When the defect is large, significant changes, both functional and structural, are evident in the pulmonary vascular tree.

3. Pulmonary Vascular Changes. After birth, without obstruction at the defect, and with pulmonary vascular resistance falling, there would be a tendency for a large runoff of left ventricular blood into the pulmonary circulation. If the pulmonary vascular resistance fell to normal adult levels, 2 possible lethal consequences of such a runoff might exist. In the presence of a defect so large that it exerts no obstruction between the ventricles, the systolic pressures in the 2 ventricles and in the systemic and pulmonary arteries approach identity.[59, 60] With left ventricular blood diverted to the pulmonary circulation and assuming that the systemic vascular resistance did not change, the resulting lowered flow to the systemic circulation would lead to a fall in systemic pressure. This might be so low as to result in inadequate perfusion of the tissues. The other possibility assumes that, though the systemic pressure would fall, it might still be high enough to perfuse the tissues adequately. However, the large volume shunted through the pulmonary circuit and back to the left ventricle might be responsible for left ventricular failure.

In acquired diseases such phenomena may occur. One or the other of these mechanisms may perhaps be the basis for early death in adult patients with myocardial infarction who suffer a large rupture of the ventricular septum. Likewise these factors may operate to cause early death in experimental animals in which ventricular septal defects beyond a certain size are created.[61] In each of the examples of acquired defects cited the pulmonary vessels are assumed to be of normal type with little muscle in the small arteries and arterioles.

With the sudden stimulus these pulmonary vessels are not structurally prepared to meet the sudden demand on them. Because of the lack of sufficient muscle for effective vasoconstriction they cannot produce a "protective" resistance.

Quite a different situation exists in the patient born with a large ventricular septal defect. At this time the pulmonary vessels are equipped with thick muscular coats and are capable of significant vasoconstriction and so of maintaining a higher-than-normal resistance to pulmonary flow. By this means the pulmonary vessels usually prevent a left-to-right shunt of such magnitude as would be lethal. At the same time it is recognized that even in the presence of a low pulmonary resistance a fall in systemic resistance would tend to reduce the magnitude of the left-to-right shunt.

Dammann and Ferencz[15] have traced the behavior of the vascular system in patients of varying ages with large ventricular septal defects. In the early postnatal months there seems to be an inherent tendency for the resistance to fall toward normal. After this the pulmonary vascular resistance tends to become stabilized at a level less than systemic resistance, but greater than normal pulmonary resistance. In time there may be a progressive rise in pulmonary vascular resistance. Divertie and Swan[62] in our physiology laboratory have made similar observations.

Since the direction and volume of flow through the large defect depend on relative resistances to flow through the pulmonary and systemic circulation, the early postnatal months when the resistance falls are particularly critical.[63] It is in this period that patients are particularly susceptible to death from left ventricular failure as a result of the large shunt. In later years when the pulmonary vascular resistance rises, the left-to-right shunt falls off in volume and may be superseded by or associated with a right-to-left shunt.

In cases with small ventricular septal defects the pulmonary vessels cannot be distinguished from the normal (fig. 5*a*). This correlates well with observations that with a small defect functional studies yield essentially normal values for resistance. In all cases with large defects that we have studied the pulmonary vessels are abnormal, although there are different kinds and degrees of change. In a given case 1 of 3 anatomic types of pulmonary vascular beds is encountered which may be called (1) high resistance-high reserve, (2) high resistance-low reserve, or (3) a form transitional between the first two.

The type of vascular bed termed "high resistance-high reserve" is essentially like that of the normal fetus. It has the following characteristics (fig. 5*b* and *c*).

The muscular arteries of all sizes show prominently thick muscular mediae associated with thick elastic laminae. At times there is increased thickness of the adventitia by dense collagen. The arterioles show prominently thick muscular medial layers and often well-defined elastic layers as well as suggestions of thickened adventitiae. The thickening of the medial muscular layer extends for varying distances down the length of the arterioles, but consistently the origins of the arterioles are the most strikingly involved by the medial thickening and luminal narrowing. At times the muscle fibers of the thickened arterioles have a vacuolated character.

Intimal fibrous lesions are usually absent or, if present, are few and restricted to small arteries or arterioles.

The reason why this type of vascular bed is characterized as a "high resistance-high reserve" system is that when measurements are available patients who have this type of bed as a group show resistances above normal adult levels. The basis for this seems to lie in vasoconstriction. The constricted vessels seem to have a potential for vasodilatation, thereby potentially decreasing the total pulmonary resistance or, stated otherwise, increasing the capacity of the bed.

Judging from the similarity in structure between the high resistance-high reserve pulmonary vascular bed in large ventricular septal defect on one hand and the bed of the normal fetus on the other, it seems probable that a decrease in pulmonary vascular resistance could occur after the abnormal communication between the 2 circulations is obliterated. The type of vascular bed that I have designated as having a high resistance-low reserve characteristic has a remarkably different appearance from that in the foregoing type. Here the large muscular arteries show characteristic obliterative intimal lesions (fig. 5*d*, *e* and *f* and fig. 6). The small muscular arteries and arterioles may show similar lesions, but the majority are thin-walled and dilated. The intimal lesions involve arteries as large as 300 microns in diameter. These lesions frequently show a plexiform arrangement in individual cross section. In serial sections, the involved segment of artery shows irregularly deposited collections of young connective tissue, creating a markedly narrowed lumen with irregular configuration. Older lesions are acellular and hyalinized. The irregular spaces in the lumen of the artery with intimal thickening may yield a picture suggesting organized thrombus.

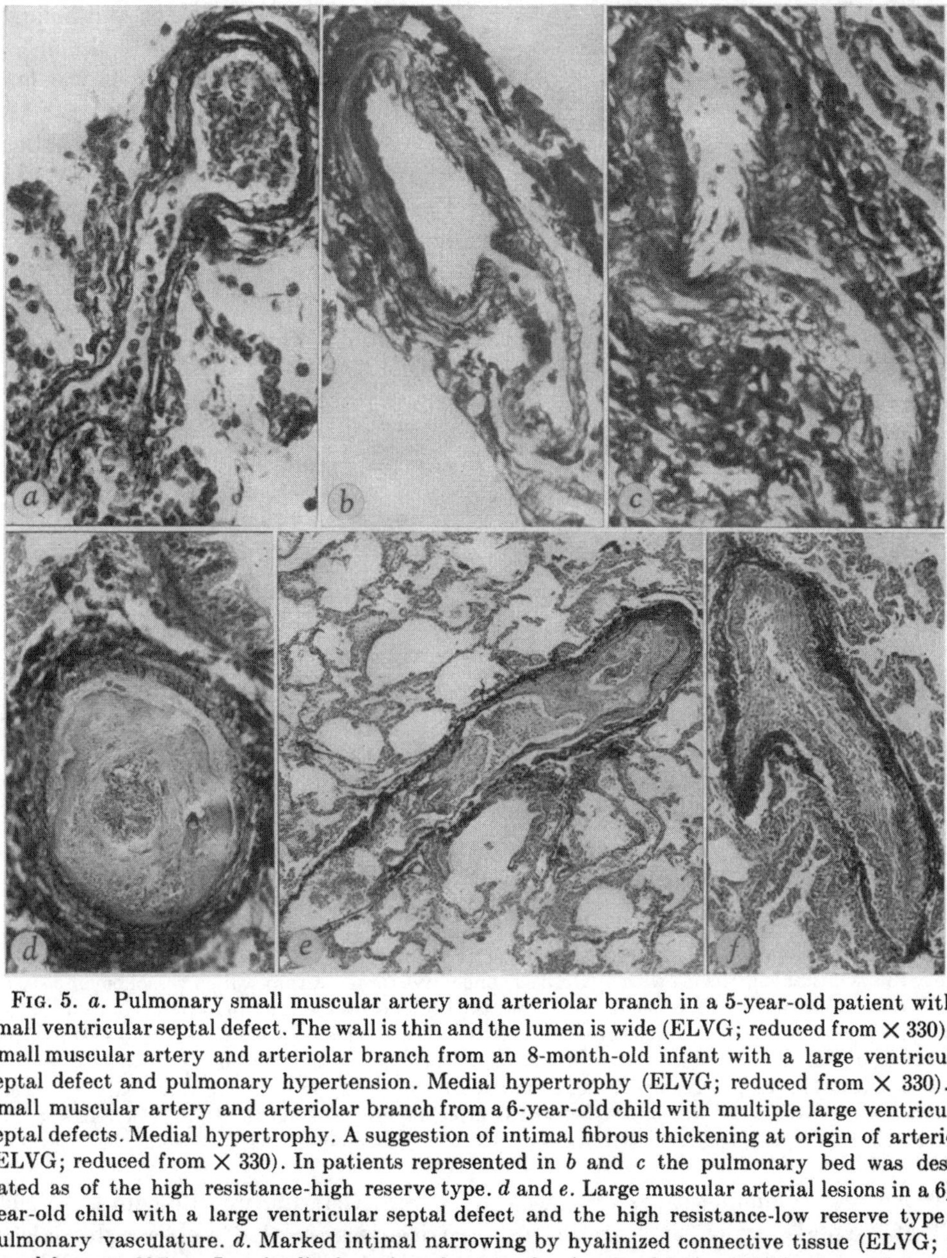

FIG. 5. *a*. Pulmonary small muscular artery and arteriolar branch in a 5-year-old patient with a small ventricular septal defect. The wall is thin and the lumen is wide (ELVG; reduced from × 330). *b*. Small muscular artery and arteriolar branch from an 8-month-old infant with a large ventricular septal defect and pulmonary hypertension. Medial hypertrophy (ELVG; reduced from × 330). *c*. Small muscular artery and arteriolar branch from a 6-year-old child with multiple large ventricular septal defects. Medial hypertrophy. A suggestion of intimal fibrous thickening at origin of arteriole (ELVG; reduced from × 330). In patients represented in *b* and *c* the pulmonary bed was designated as of the high resistance-high reserve type. *d* and *e*. Large muscular arterial lesions in a 6½-year-old child with a large ventricular septal defect and the high resistance-low reserve type of pulmonary vasculature. *d*. Marked intimal narrowing by hyalinized connective tissue (ELVG; reduced from × 200). *e*. Longitudinal section of artery showing focal intimal thickening with hyalinized and cellular connective tissue yielding a narrow and irregular lumen. There is thinning of the arterial wall distal to the intimal lesions (ELVG; reduced from × 50). *f*. A small muscular artery from a 6½-year-old child with a large ventricular septal defect and patent ductus arteriosus; a high resistance-low reserve pulmonary tree. Intimal fibrous thickening (ELVG; reduced from × 100).

The characteristic lesion is not an organized thrombus in our opinion, although in the same case organized thrombosis may also exist. The intimal arterial lesions which may be seen in ventricular septal defect are also observed in some cases of patent ductus arteriosus, atrial septal defect and so-called primary pulmonary hypertension. These lesions have been the subject of considerable interest in the literature.[64] Some have claimed them to be glomuslike congenital malformations.

Others have suggested that these lesions

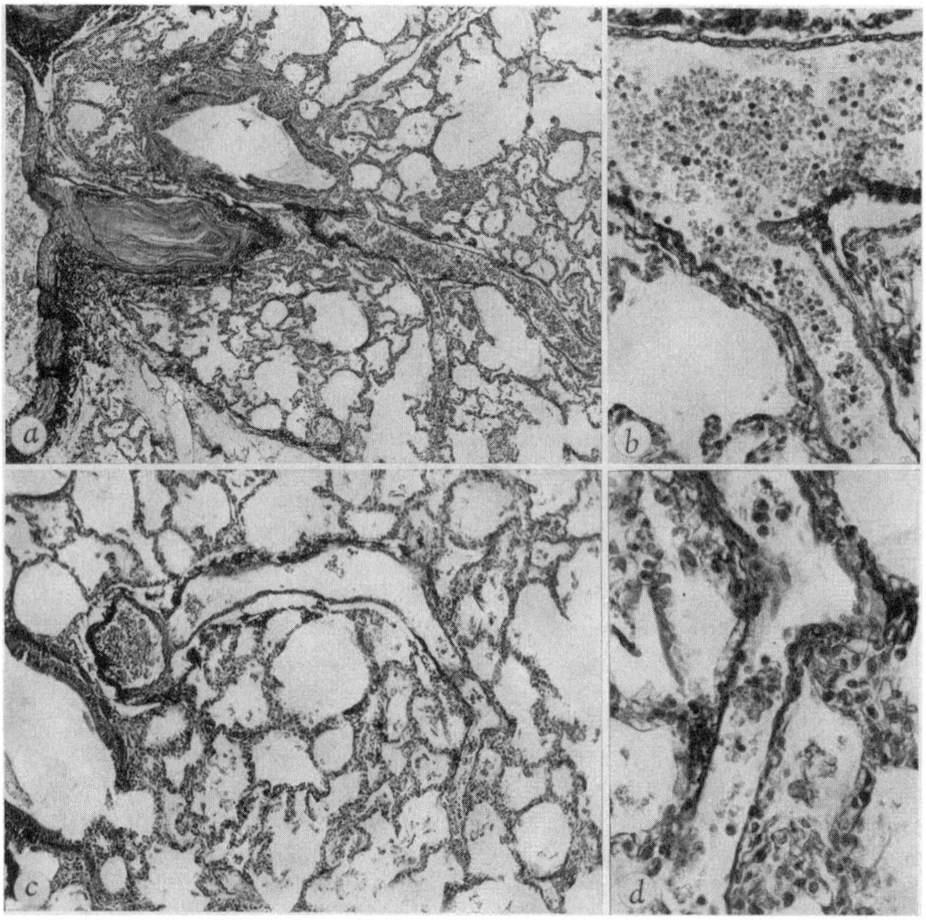

FIG. 6. From the case illustrated in figure 5*d* and *e* of a 6½-year-old child with a large ventricular septal defect and a high resistance-low reserve type of pulmonary vasculature. *a*. A large muscular artery shows intimal narrowing with hyalinized connective tissue. A thin-walled vessel beyond (to the right) was shown on serial section to arise from the occluded vessel (ELVG; reduced from × 45). *b*. High-power view of an arteriole arising from the thin-walled segment of artery illustrated in *a* (hematoxylin and eosin; reduced from × 200). *c*. An artery and an arteriole not associated with intimal occlusion of the parent artery. The lumina are wide and the walls are thin (ELVG; reduced from × 90). *d*. High-power magnification of the arteriole arising from the thin-walled artery illustrated in *c* (ELVG; reduced from × 330).

are arteriovenous communications.[65-67] This implies that cyanosis, which may appear in ventricular septal defect, is a consequence of a shunt through these hypothesized channels. Neither of these claims can be supported, since the lesions may readily be demonstrated by serial sections to be confined to arteries.[54, 64, 68-72] Additional support comes from physiologic studies in patients with ventricular septal defect who have such arterial lesions. When dye-dilution curves are compared following injection of dye into the right ventricle and into the pulmonary trunk, it becomes readily apparent that the injection into the right ventricle is associated with a right-to-left shunt, while the injection into the pulmonary trunk shows no evidence of a right-to-left shunt. This evidence therefore does not support the presence of an arteriovenous shunt in the lung, nor does it support any other claim that the cyanosis in patients with ventricular septal defect is of pulmonary origin. The evidence, as well as the observation of fully saturated blood in the left atrium,[73] establishes that the desaturation of the systemic arterial blood is derived from a shunt through the ventricular septal defect rather than pulmonary vessels.

The lung that has the anatomic characteristic that I have called "high resistance-low reserve" has a remarkable difference at the level of the small arteries and arterioles when compared to the lung classified as "high resistance-high reserve" (fig. 6). Whereas in the latter the arteries and arterioles show medial hypertrophy with correspondingly narrow lumina, most of the small vessels of the high resistance-low reserve lung show wide lumina and thin walls. The thinning and dilatation of the vessel wall are universal, occurring both beyond obstructed arteries and in areas where arteries are not obstructed.

In some cases, the dilatation of the small arteries and of the arterioles may reach extreme proportions with aneurysmlike formation. Where these dilated vessels lie near the air spaces, they may herniate into them. Rupture may perhaps be the basis for hemoptysis, which occurs in patients with this type of pulmonary vascular bed.[54, 74]

Brewer[71] has indicated that some of these dilated vessels represent collateral channels arising from pulmonary arteries above the sites of obstructed lumina to the vascular bed beyond. Heath[74] has suggested that some are collateral channels from the bronchial arterial system. The majority of the dilated vessels have normal sites of origin and termination.

The location of the intimal occlusive lesions in relatively large arteries correlates well with observations in postmortem angiographic studies, where the arteries show a blunted configuration.[75, 76] This has been called a "pruning" effect by Evans.[68] In addition to the intimal lesions of large muscular arteries, necrosis and thrombosis may be observed in similar vessels.[77-82]

The pulmonary vascular bed with occlusive intimal arterial lesions always displays a high resistance to flow. What then is the explanation for the apparent paradox of a high resistance to flow in the presence of dilated small arteries and arterioles?

The occluded arteries are large ones, often being 0.3 mm. or wider in diameter, and therefore are the channel for the blood supply to a relatively large area of pulmonary tissue. With multiple lesions of this type, a considerable amount of the pulmonary vascular bed is eliminated from the effective perfusion channel of the lesser circulation, even allowing for some collateral circulation to this area from the pulmonary arteries. As far as the functional capacity of the pulmonary vascular bed is concerned, it is as though portions of the lung had been extirpated (fig. 7*a*). Ferguson and Varco[83] have removed portions of the lung and produced pulmonary hypertension by reducing the total capacity of the vascular bed and additionally by increasing the flow to the remaining pulmonary tissue.

The atrophy and dilatation of the vessels beyond areas of obstruction are a feature which is similar to that in small vessels in cases with obstruction at the major pulmonary pathway. The atrophy and dilatation in the vessels not associated with obstructed arteries seem to be a response on the part of the effective portion of the pulmonary circuit to accommodate as much blood as is possible in this remaining functional area.

It is of significance that in spite of this compensatory mechanism, however it is brought about, the total capacity of the effective pulmonary bed is so limited that a high pulmonary vascular resistance exists. This type of pulmonary vascular bed may be said to have reached the limits of its capacity to receive blood from the right ventricle, even though the vessels participating individually are widelumened and thin-walled.

The intimal lesions of large muscular arteries, in our opinion, are specific for pulmonary hypertension of a severe degree and of chronic nature. We have not observed them in other circumstances.

In addition to the 2 clear-cut types of pulmonary vascular beds that are usually encountered among patients with ventricular septal defect (fig. 7*a*), there is an occasional case that presents a transitional type of pattern (fig. 7*b* and *c*). In this, a few small arteries, usually about 100 microns or less in diameter, are occluded by intimal fibrous tissue. The unoccluded small arteries and the arterioles show a wall-thickness that is either normal or slightly greater than normal, while the lumina are of

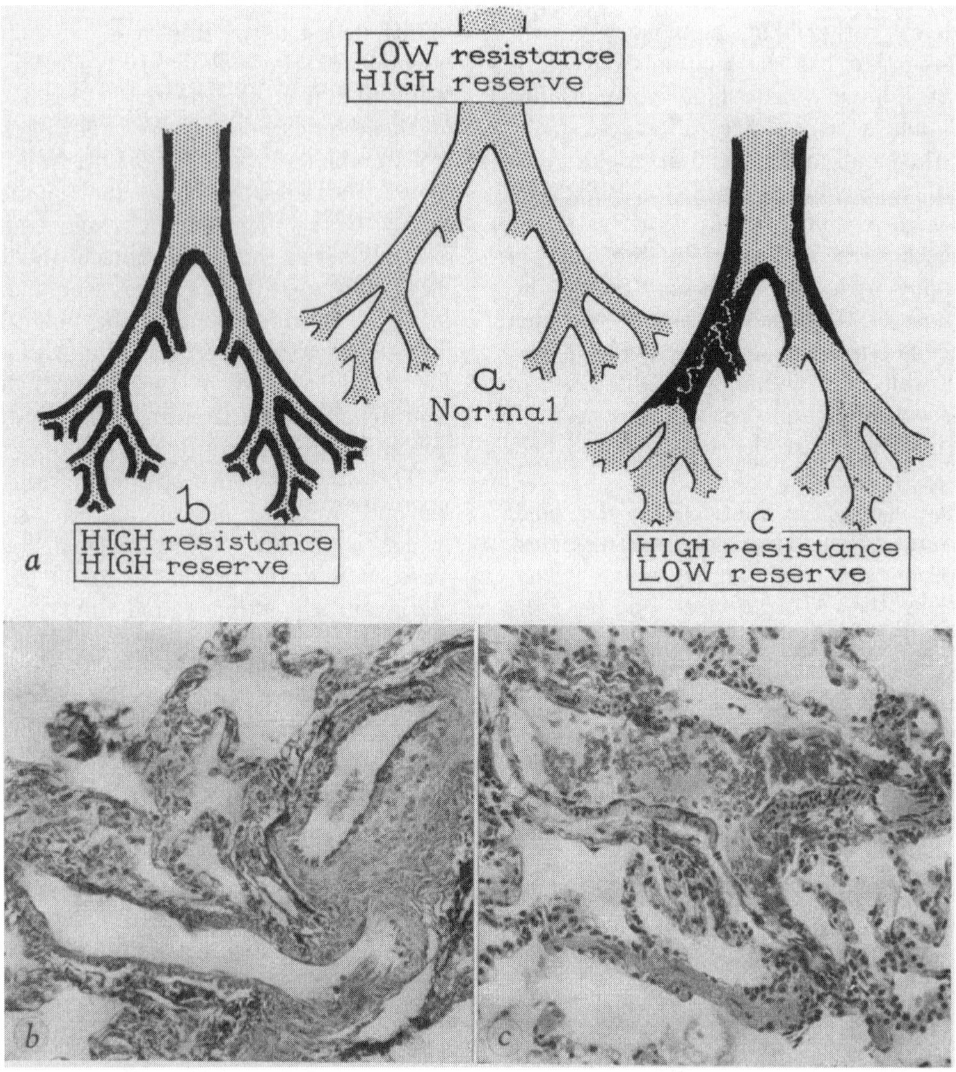

FIG. 7. *a.* Diagrammatic representation of the normal pulmonary arterial system and that in the 2 basic types with a free communication between the ventricles or great arteries. *b* and *c.* Photomicrographs of pulmonary vessels from a 6-year-old girl patient with a patent ductus arteriosus and pulmonary hypertension, showing a transitional type of pulmonary vascular tree. *b.* The 2 vascular channels were shown by serial section to communicate through a zone of intimal narrowing at the origin of the small arterial branch (ELVG; reduced from × 200). *c.* An artery and an arteriolar branch not related to intimal fibrous thickening, showing essentially a normal structure (hematoxylin and eosin; reduced from × 200).

normal width. There is lacking the element of excessive width of small vessels seen in cases with intimal occlusion of larger arteries. In the transitional forms the large muscular arteries have medial layers thicker than normal.

Correlation of Functional Features with Structural Changes in the Pulmonary Vascular Bed. That there are 2 basic types of pulmonary vascular patterns in patients with ventricular septal defect is of very great importance for practical reasons. In one type closure of the defect may yield essentially normal pulmonary pressure, while in the other type closure of the defect is associated with retention of pulmonary hypertension. In fact, with the defect closed, the pulmonary arterial pressure may even rise above aortic pressure.

Cases known to have the high resistance-

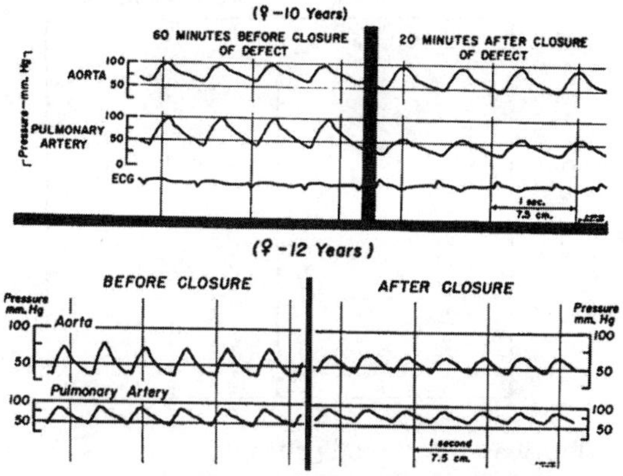

FIG. 8. Preoperative and postoperative pressure studies in 2 patients with ventricular septal defect. In the 10-year-old girl the pulmonary vascular pattern was of the high resistance-high reserve type. The heart and preoperative dye-dilution curves of this patient are illustrated in the left-hand column of figure 3. In the 12-year-old girl the pulmonary vascular pattern was of the high resistance-low reserve type. Illustrations of the pulmonary vessels from this case appear in figure 5*d* and *e* and in figure 6. The defects were closed by Dr. J. W. Kirklin.

high reserve type of pulmonary vascular bed show a lowering of pulmonary pressure after closure of the defect (fig. 8). This may simply reflect the reduction in pulmonary flow without change in resistance. It does not necessarily mean that the fall in pulmonary pressure is an expression of fall of pulmonary resistance. While it is expected that such would occur in this type of patient after the defect is closed, the pulmonary resistance need not be expected to fall immediately with the surgically created change in circulation. From the demonstration of a gradual rather than abrupt fall in pulmonary vascular resistance after surgical relief of mitral stenosis one would expect that in ventricular septal defect a postoperative fall in pulmonary resistance would also be gradual. The demonstration of a fall in pulmonary vascular resistance after closure of the defect is yet to be accomplished and will require cases in which complete physiologic studies preoperatively and postoperatively have been done.

Among cases known to have the high resistance-low reserve type of pulmonary vascular bed the pulmonary pressure may rise or remain constant after closure of the defect. When it rises, the reason is probably best explained as follows. Before closure of the defect and in the face of a very high pulmonary vascular resistance, the defect operated as an "escape valve" allowing a right-to-left shunt of that volume of blood in excess of that which caused pulmonary pressure to be at systemic levels. With closure of the escape valve, no shunt is possible and all the right ventricular blood is ejected into the pulmonary vascular bed. The volume of pulmonary flow is now greater than when a right-to-left shunt existed. In the presence of a fixed pulmonary vascular resistance the increased pulmonary flow yields increased pulmonary arterial and right ventricular pressures. If this becomes sufficiently high the right ventricle may fail abruptly in the postoperative period.

With this difference in behavior among cases it is important to predict, if possible, which type of vascular tree is present before surgical treatment is recommended. For this reason it was pertinent to see whether functional studies could indicate the anatomic type of vascular bed present.

In 15 cases having large ventricular septal defect, a single ventricle without stenosis or patent ductus arteriosus with pulmonary hypertension in which serial sections of lungs had been examined there were available physiologic studies that yielded figures for pulmonary and systemic flows when the patients breathed air and 100 per cent oxygen. From these figures, values for total systemic and total pulmonary resistance could be calculated under these 2 conditions. Dr. H. F. Helmholz, Jr., reviewed the physiologic data independently of the observations on structural changes and then the two were correlated[84] in an attempt to see whether the structural type of pulmonary vascular tree could be predicted from the hemodynamic characteristics.

The most reliable basis for prediction, as judged by this material, is to know the ratio of total pulmonary resistance to total systemic resistance when the patient breathed air and when he breathed 100 per cent oxygen.

In a flexible pulmonary vascular bed total pulmonary resistance falls when the inspired gas has a greater oxygen content than air. This is true not only in the normal but also in certain patients with congenital cardiac disease.[85]

The cases were divided according to the 3

structural types of pulmonary vascular bed already described.

The results are illustrated in figure 9.

The high resistance-high reserve and transitional types of vascular beds were associated with varying ratios of total pulmonary and total systemic resistance when the patient breathed air but in no case was the ratio more than 0.7:1. That is, though the pulmonary resistance might be elevated, it did not exceed total systemic resistance. In each of these 2 types of vascular beds with breathing of 100 per cent oxygen there was a significant fall in pulmonary resistance compared to systemic, so that in no case was the ratio greater than 0.4:1 under these circumstances.

In contrast, when the patients with the high resistance-low reserve type of pulmonary vascular bed breathed air the total pulmonary resistance approached, equaled or exceeded the systemic resistance.

When 100 per cent oxygen was administered to this group, there was usually a slight fall in pulmonary resistance compared to systemic, but in no case that we observed did it fall below a ratio of 0.6:1. In some cases the ratio did not differ much from 1:1.

These observations indicate that from hemodynamic data there is possible a rough separation between the cases having the high resistance-high reserve or transitional types of pulmonary vascular beds on one hand and the high resistance-low reserve bed on the other, even when the patient breathes air. The distinction becomes much more evident when 100 per cent oxygen is administered.

It is probable that biopsy of a chance section of the lung might yield a high degree of accuracy as to the structural type of pattern. The type with only medial changes is simple to identify. In the types with intimal arterial lesions there is no certainty that a biopsy would necessarily yield a characteristically occluded vessel. The finding of prominently dilated small vessels in a patient with known high resistance to pulmonary flow would be strong evidence favoring the presence of intimal arterial lesions even if these were not present in the particular piece of tissue.

The question naturally arises as to the relationship between the 3 types of vascular trees.

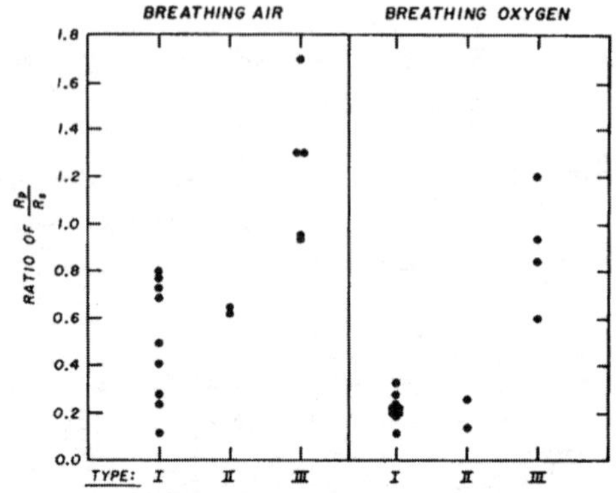

FIG. 9. Ratios of total pulmonary to total systemic vascular resistance among 15 patients with a free communication between the ventricles or great arteries. A sixteenth case with a ratio of 0.9:1 on air did not have studies on oxygen. Type I refers to a high resistance-high reserve pulmonary vascular bed, type II to a transitional form, and type III to a high resistance-low reserve pulmonary vascular tree.

Our opinion is that the high resistance-high reserve type of bed is essentially an integral part of the anatomicofunctional complex of a congenital unobstructed communication between the ventricles without pulmonary stenosis. We believe this to be the type of lung with which such patients are born. The medial hypertrophy does not represent a malformation, but rather we believe that it represents a persistence of a fetal type of pulmonary vessel, just as in the over-all function of the heart with the defect there is carried over from the fetal into the postnatal state a free communication between the 2 circulations.

The transitional and high resistance-low reserve types of vascular tree, in our opinion, are complications of long-standing pulmonary hypertension in which the pulmonary systolic pressure equals or approaches systemic systolic pressure. That one type gives way to the other is supported by different age patterns between the cases without intimal arterial lesions on one hand and those with such lesions on the other. Among patients with a free communication between the ventricles or great arteries we have observed only the high resistance-high reserve type of bed among patients less than 2 years of age. This type of pattern persists for varying lengths of time. We have observed it in patients aged 10 and 37 years respectively, but the last case is most unusual. In general, the older the patient, the more likely he is to have 1 of the other 2 types of pattern. While occasional patients as young as 2 years may show the transitional or the high resistance-low reserve type, the high resistance-low reserve pattern is usually present in patients who have carried a defect of the type under discussion for 20 or more years. It is only the exceptional patient who does not.

Ventricular Septal Defect with Pulmonary Stenosis

We have just completed the description of ventricular septal defect without pulmonary stenosis. In this discussion it was brought out that while the aortic ostium is in free communication with both ventricles, the nature and direction of shunts depend principally on relative resistances to the flow of blood through the 2 circulations. When a high resistance to pulmonary flow exists, the basis for this resides in changes within the pulmonary arterioles and arteries. In some instances of ventricular septal defect without pulmonary stenosis, the resistance to pulmonary flow may be greater than the resistance to systemic flow. This results in a right-to-left shunt. The same functional derangements as in ventricular septal defect without pulmonary stenosis may occur in a condition that in the past has been considered quite a separate one from ventricular septal defect without pulmonary stenosis. This is the so-called tetralogy of Fallot, characterized anatomically by biventricular origin of the aorta above a large ventricular septal defect, right ventricular hypertrophy, and stenosis of the major pulmonary pathway. In the past, it was thought that this condition was always associated with a significant right-to-left shunt and with cyanosis. Recent experiences have shown that among patients with basically the same anatomic complex of malformations, there is a spectrum of functional changes essentially identical with that in ventricular septal defect without stenosis.[86-88] The reason for the similarity in spectra between the 2 conditions resides in the fact that in the so-called tetralogy of Fallot, there are varying degrees of pulmonary stenosis.

The range in behavior among patients having anatomically the tetralogy of Fallot is well illustrated by 3 cases with varying degrees of pulmonary stenosis shown in figure 10. In the first instance, the degree of pulmonary stenosis was mild. The pulmonary arterial pressure, though lower than the right ventricular pressure, was still elevated above normal. There was only a left-to-right shunt and no right-to-left shunt.

Histologically, the pulmonary vessels showed medial hypertrophy of the arteries and arterioles indistinguishable from that seen in cases of large ventricular septal defect without pulmonary stenosis.

We may recall the concept that, when a ventricular septal defect is present, the left ventricle is functionally in communication with the pulmonary arteries. The pulmonary stenosis represents an obstruction in that communication. In the case with the mild pulmonary stenosis, the obstruction was so mild that it did not represent an effective barrier between the left ventricle and the pulmonary vessels, as evidenced by the elevated pulmonary arterial pressure. This mild obstruction represented 1 focus of increased resistance to pulmonary flow, but was ineffective in controlling the amount of blood flowing through the lungs. A second zone of increased resistance to pulmonary flow lay in the small vessels of the lung, just as in large ventricular septal defect without pulmonary stenosis.

In the second case, the pulmonary stenosis was of moderate degree, and the pulmonary arterial pressure was essentially normal. Functionally, a small right-to-left shunt and a larger left-to-right shunt were demonstrated. Histologically, the pulmonary vessels were normal. Here, the pulmonary stenosis was an effective barrier between the left ventricle and the pulmonary arteries, and it was the main controlling factor in the volume of flow to the lungs. The small pulmonary vessels are thus relieved of the responsibility of being a governing factor controlling blood flow to the lungs.

Realizing the fact that this patient had a large ventricular septal defect, the pulmonary stenosis here was of a degree that might be termed ideal. While allowing sufficient pulmo-

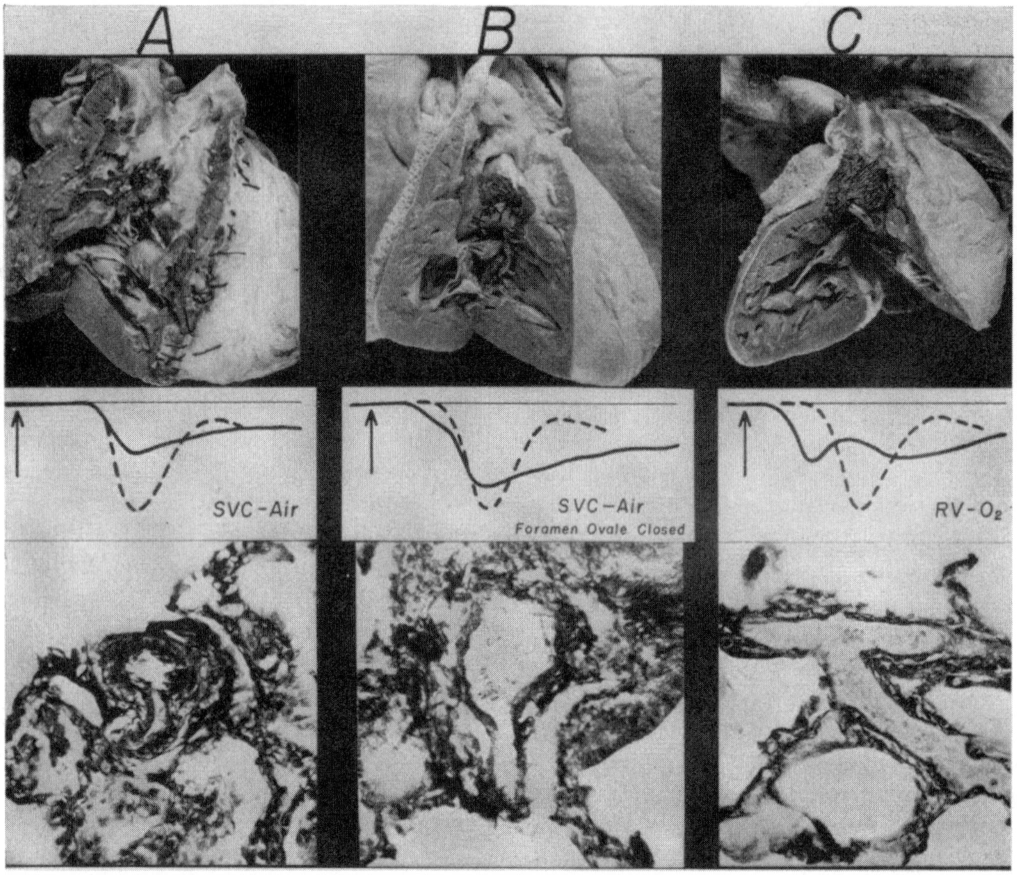

FIG. 10. The outflow tract of the right ventricle, preoperative dye-dilution curves (solid curves for particular cases; dotted curves for anticipated normal) and the small arteries with arteriolar branches in three cases of ventricular septal defect with infundibular stenosis of varying degrees. In each case the ventricular septal defect had been closed and infundibular resection had been performed at operation (see text for contrasting features among the cases).

nary flow it removed from the small pulmonary vessels the responsibility of governing volume of pulmonary flow and did not allow them to be subjected to high levels of pressure, with the attendant complications. At the same time, while the pulmonary vessels were effectively protected from the ventricular pressure, the right-to-left shunt caused by the pulmonary stenosis still was only of minor magnitude. Such an ideal arrangement is the one sought in the procedure of creating pulmonary stenosis in patients with ventricular septal defect in whom closure of the ventricular septal defect is not attempted.[13]

In the third case, the pulmonary stenosis was so severe that a large right-to-left shunt resulted, making the patient cyanotic. Here we have the traditional picture of the tetralogy of Fallot with so high a degree of resistance to pulmonary flow at the right ventricular outflow tract as to exceed systemic resistance. Here then, the shunt was predominantly right-to-left. The pulmonary vessels were normal or thinner than normal. Thus while in the first case the pulmonary vessels were insufficiently protected, in the third case the pulmonary vessels were effectively protected from ventricular pressure but only at the expense of a right-to-left shunt.

I have indicated that the term "Eisenmenger complex" might with advantage be replaced by a descriptive term indicating the characteristics of the hemodynamic derangement. Likewise, it is evident that the term "tetralogy of Fallot" might also be conveniently abandoned.

Because the functional derangement of patients with basically the same anatomic defect is so varied, it seems more appropriate to identify cases by such functionally descriptive terms as, for example, "ventricular septal defect with mild pulmonary stenosis and left-to-right shunt," "ventricular septal defect with moderate pulmonary stenosis and bidirectional shunts" or "ventricular septal defect with severe pulmonary stenosis and right-to-left shunt."

If we recall that in a ventricular septal defect there is functionally a communication between the left ventricle and the pulmonary arteries, then we recognize certain similarities in the behavior of this communication among patients with small ventricular septal defect without pulmonary stenosis, on the one hand, and patients with large ventricular septal defects and significant degrees of pulmonary stenosis, on the other hand. In each instance, there is a barrier between the left ventricle and the pulmonary arteries, and the pulmonary vascular bed is normal. In the case of the small ventricular septal defect without pulmonary stenosis, the barrier in the communication lies at the small obstructing ventricular septal defect. In the case of large ventricular septal defect with severe pulmonary stenosis, the obstruction between the left ventricle and the pulmonary arteries is at the site of pulmonary stenosis.

Functional Single Ventricle

In cases of single ventricle, whether this represents a single ventricle anatomically or only functionally, the basic dynamics are essentially like those in ventricular septal defect. Two major subgroups exist, namely, single functioning ventricle without pulmonary stenosis and single functioning ventricle with pulmonary stenosis. In the cases of single functioning ventricle without pulmonary stenosis, the pulmonary and systemic pressures are essentially equal and the regulation of distribution of blood flow to the systemic circulation, on one hand, and to the pulmonary circulation, on the other, is dependent on relative resistances in the two circulations.

Assuming that the systemic resistances are at normal levels, which is usually the case, the variable factor is the pulmonary resistance, exactly as in large ventricular septal defect. Cases with functional single ventricle without pulmonary stenosis show the same range of vascular changes in the lung as in large ventricular septal defect.[74, 80] While theoretically there is a tendency for free mixing of blood in the same ventricle, this has not proved to be the case, at least in regard to the anatomic single ventricle. Here there is a tendency for the blood entering through the tricuspid valve to stream toward the pulmonary trunk, while the blood entering through the mitral valve streams toward the aorta. Under these circumstances, the pulmonary arterial oxygen saturation is lower than that of the systemic arterial circulation. Even with functional studies, it may be impossible to distinguish the single ventricle without pulmonary stenosis from a large ventricular septal defect.[89]

Just as the single ventricle without pulmonary stenosis may be difficult to distinguish from ventricular septal defect without pulmonary stenosis, so the single ventricle with pulmonary stenosis may not be readily distinguished from ventricular septal defect with pulmonary stenosis.

In cases in which the single ventricle is associated with pulmonary stenosis, the governing factor in distribution of blood is the zone of obstruction leading to the pulmonary trunk. Usually, the resistance to flow through this is so high that the greater proportion of blood leaving the common ventricle enters the aorta and there is therefore a significant right-to-left shunt.

When the common ventricle is associated with significant pulmonary stenosis, the pulmonary vessels are in the range of normal structurally.

Patent Ductus Arteriosus

The dynamics in patent ductus arteriosus are very closely related to those in ventricular septal defect. Were there significant resistance to flow through the ductus arteriosus during fetal life, the right ventricular pressure would have to exceed the left ventricular pressure in order for blood to enter the descending aorta through the ductus.

We know that the pressure in the 2 ventricles is essentially equal, and we must therefore conclude that in the fetus the ductus arteriosus does not constitute an obstructed channel. It may be said therefore to allow free communication between the aorta and the pulmonary arteries.

In the patient who is destined to postnatal persistent patency of the ductus arteriosus, it is not known whether at birth the functional occlusion of the ductus thought to be present in the normal is also present here. It is possible that, in the patient who is to have persistent patency of the ductus, the ductus does act normally at the time of birth. Subsequent to birth, however, persistent patency of the ductus arteriosus results from failure of growth of the structural elements of the media and intima of the ductus which normally close the ductus. The persistently patent ductus seems simply to have maintained the same structure that it had in the normal before birth.

Recognizing that during fetal life the ductus is a nonobstructing channel of all individuals, one may assume that it is a similar channel in the neonatal period of individuals who are to maintain patency of the ductus. This means that the arterial sides of the lesser and greater circulations are in free communication at this time. From this we may imply that in all patients with persistent patency of the ductus arteriosus, there is a phase of pulmonary hypertension in which the pulmonary and systemic arterial pressures are about equal. The absence of a continuous murmur in most infants with patent ductus arteriosus may thus be due to equivalent pressures in both circulations.[90, 91] In later life, patients with patent ductus arteriosus can readily be separated into 2 major groups, comparable to patients with small and with large ventricular septal defects. The majority of patients with patent ductus arteriosus have an arrangement which is like that of patients with small ventricular septal defects in that the ductus represents an obstructing communication between the left ventricle and the pulmonary arteries. A differential in pressure exists between the left ventricle and aorta on one hand, and the pulmonary arteries on the other. In cases of this type, the pulmonary vascular bed is protected from the pressure in the left ventricle and systemic circulation by the obstructive type of ductus arteriosus. The small pulmonary vessels are normal.[16]

The second type is the one in which the ductus arteriosus is so short and wide that there is no significant pressure difference across it. These cases may therefore be compared with the large ventricular septal defect. In them, the systemic and pulmonary arterial pressures are in the same general range. The regulation of the volume and direction of shunt depend primarily on the relation of the systemic to the pulmonary resistances. The pulmonary resistance is usually higher than normal.

The pulmonary vascular changes are like those in large ventricular septal defect. One may be termed the high resistance-high reserve type of vascular tree; the other, the high resistance-low reserve vascular tree. As in ventricular septal defect, transitional forms between the two exist.

Let us return to the fact that in children and adults 2 types of ductus arteriosus are present, while in the neonatal period it is hypothesized that all patients with patent ductus arteriosus have pulmonary hypertension. What is the basis for persistence of pulmonary hypertension in one group and its disappearance in the other? The basis for this seems to lie in a different type of resistance to flow through the ductus, high in one and low in the other.

In the patient who develops a high resistance to flow through the ductus, a possible explanation is that, as the patient grows, there is a differential quality to the growth. That is, the aorta and the pulmonary artery may grow in diameter out of proportion to that of the patent ductus. The relatively narrow state of the ductus constitutes an obstruction to flow and permits a pressure differential to exist across the ductus, a feature which is characteristic of the so-called classic patent ductus arteriosus.

In the second group, the orifice of the ductus

arteriosus seems to grow in concert with the diameters of the aorta and pulmonary trunk. This short and wide type of ductus represents a nonobstructive opening allowing equivalent pressures in the aorta and the pulmonary arteries.[92]

ATRIAL SEPTAL DEFECT

For purposes of discussion, patients with atrial septal defect may be divided into 2 age groups, (1) infants and children, and (2) adults. Adults may be further subdivided into those with low pulmonary vascular resistance and normal pulmonary pressures and those with elevated pulmonary vascular resistance and pressures.

The story as regards infants and children still has many unsettled points. In adults the situation is clearer. We shall first discuss the adult with atrial septal defect.

Adult Patients

Low Pulmonary Vascular Resistance and Normal Pulmonary Pressure. In atrial septal defect with low pulmonary vascular resistance and normal pressure and high pulmonary flow as determined by functional studies, the structural nature of the pulmonary vascular tree is that of a low-pressure system. Throughout the arterial system, including the arterioles, the lumina are wide and the walls thin (fig. 11*a* and *b*). Anatomically, the system cannot be distinguished with certainty from normal, but the tortuosity of the arteries not seen in the normal suggests a high flow.

Elevated Pulmonary Vascular Resistance and Pressure. There is a tendency for patients with ordinary atrial septal defect to develop, gradually, an increasing pulmonary vascular resistance and pulmonary hypertension while retaining for a time, at least, a high pulmonary flow. This tendency is apparent in patients reaching the fourth decade of life, although there are exceptions both ways: younger adult patients may manifest pulmonary hypertension while some older patients delay or never show, within the period of study, a tendency for elevating pulmonary vascular resistance and pressure.

Adult patients who have an increased pulmonary vascular resistance and increased pulmonary arterial pressure may conveniently be divided into 2 groups. In the first group the pulmonary pressures are below those in the systemic arteries. Among these patients, pulmonary arterial systolic pressures from 40 to 80 mm. of mercury are frequently encountered. This group may be said to have moderate pulmonary hypertension. In the second group the pulmonary arterial pressures are in the range of aortic pressures, although not necessarily identical. The pulmonary pressure may even exceed the aortic. This group may be said to have severe pulmonary hypertension.

The foregoing 2 groups of patients with elevated pulmonary arterial pressures are separated, not because they are basically different, but because 1 group, the first, seems to represent an earlier and lesser degree of a complication of atrial septal defect than the latter.

There are different anatomic pictures in the pulmonary vascular tree in these 2 groups of patients with elevated pulmonary arterial pressures, the 2 anatomic types functionally representing different degrees of elevated pulmonary vascular resistance.

Moderate Pulmonary Hypertension. The patients with moderate pulmonary hypertension show a widely varying pattern in the small muscular arteries and arterioles, ranging from completely occluded vessels to very thin-walled, abnormally wide ones (fig. 11*c*, *d*, *e*, and *f*).

The large muscular pulmonary arteries show medial hypertrophy, a feature that closely reflects the degree of pulmonary arterial and right ventricular pressures.

Significant occlusive lesions in the form of cellular fibrous intimal thickening are seen in the small arteries and at the beginnings of arterioles. With serial sections, it is readily demonstrated that these lesions are focal.

For example, as one traces an occluded arteriole distally, the lumen eventually opens up and the vessel is wide. It is obvious that, were the distal unobstructed part of such a vessel examined in a chance single section, one would falsely gain the impression that it was

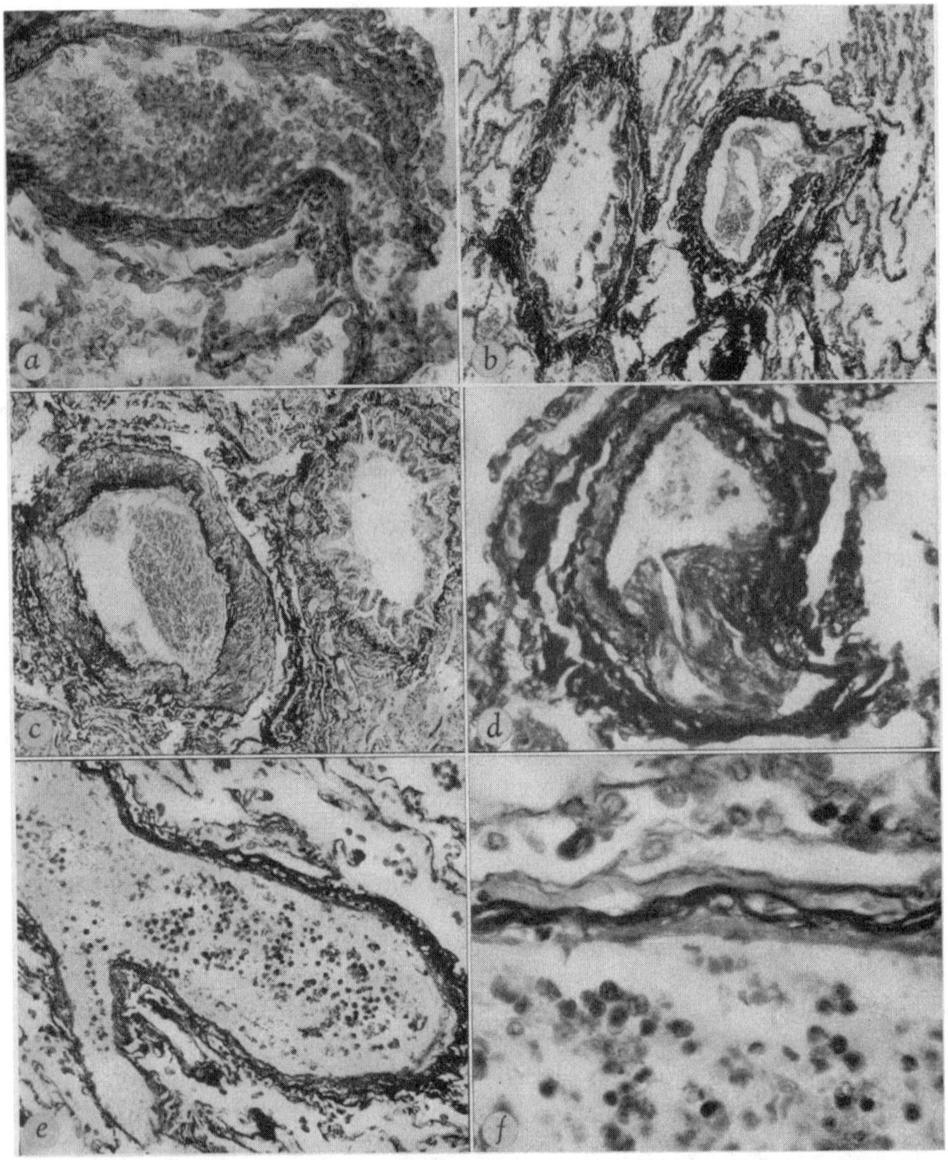

FIG. 11. Photomicrographs of pulmonary vessels in adult patients with atrial septal defect. *a* and *b*. From a 41-year-old woman with high pulmonary flow and normal pulmonary arterial pressures. *a*. Small muscular artery and arteriolar branch, showing thin walls and wide lumina (ELVG; reduced from × 330). *b*. A large muscular artery and a bronchiole. The arterial wall is thin and the lumen is wide, features not distinguishable from the normal (ELVG; reduced from × 70). *c*. From a 46-year-old patient with left-to-right shunt and moderate pulmonary hypertension (pulmonary arterial pressure 89/20 to 100/37). Medial hypertrophy of the large muscular artery, which lies beside a bronchiole (ELVG; reduced from × 70). *d*, *e*, and *f*. From a 34-year-old patient with moderate pulmonary hypertension. *d*. A small muscular artery and an arteriolar branch. Medial hypertrophy of the artery, intimal occlusion by fibrous tissue of the arteriolar origin (ELVG; reduced from × 330). *e*. A small muscular artery and an arteriolar branch not related to occlusive intimal lesions, showing exceedingly wide lumina (reduced from × 200). The wall of the artery is atrophic, as illustrated in *f*. *f*. Detail of wall in dilated artery shown in *e*. The medial muscle is almost entirely absent, the wall now being represented by the condensation of the 2 elastic laminae and fibrous thickening of the intima and adventitia (ELVG; reduced from × 570).

an unobstructed vessel, when in reality it is completely closed more proximally. When the complication of intimal small arterial and arteriolar occlusion develops, the extensiveness of its distribution can therefore never be fully appreciated from individual histologic sections, regardless of how many sections are taken.

The intimal lesions at arteriolar level lie in thin-walled vessels. Some small arteries with intimal occlusive lesions show thin media, while in some this layer is hypertrophied. Why is there this difference? The answer may perhaps be found in the large muscular arteries. These vessels in patients having atrial septal defect and no pulmonary hypertension are thin, in the range of normal. Yet when pulmonary hypertension develops, they become thickly muscular. They accompany the myocardium with regard to hypertrophy and in their hypertrophy the large muscular arteries reflect the level of pressure within them. With regard to the varying picture in the media of the small arteries that have intimal occlusive lesions, it may be postulated that in the thick ones obstruction existed more peripherally and that elevation of arterial pressure existed before the small artery itself developed intimal lesions. By the same reasoning, those arteries with thin mediae and occluding intimal lesions developed the intimal lesions early, before significant elevation of pressure had occurred.

This leads us to a consideration of the nonobstructed small arteries and arterioles among the patients with moderate pulmonary hypertension.

These show unusually wide lumina and often atrophic mediae. The arterial walls may no longer have identifiable muscle, being composed principally of the elastic membranes and varying amounts of collagen. Frequently, there is a thick, uniformly deposited layer of acellular collagen in the intima. The latter type of change may be seen in normal control patients of comparable age, but the number of vessels involved in the normal is far less than in patients with atrial septal defect.

What is the functional significance of the structural changes encountered in the patients with moderate pulmonary hypertension and elevated pulmonary vascular resistance?

While the development of medial hypertrophy of the larger muscular arteries may be a contributing factor to elevated resistance, the intimal lesions of the small arteries and arterioles are most peripherally located and seem to be the initiating factor in elevating the pulmonary vascular resistance. Recognizing that the intimal lesions of the smallest arterial vessels are characteristic of the patients with moderate or only slightly elevated levels of arteriolar resistance, they cannot be charged to elevated pressure. These intimal lesions seem properly to be credited to the factor of high flow. The turbulence and abnormal vibrations that are probably set up in these small vessels as great volumes of blood flow through them may represent mechanical irritation. The intimal cellular fibrous response may be in the category of a reparative reaction.

Although elevation of total pulmonary resistance results from the occlusion of many small arteries and arterioles, a high flow characteristically continues through the lungs and with this combination of circumstances there is an elevation of pulmonary arterial pressure. This factor is probably responsible for distention of the unoccluded small vessels—being the ones through which the pulmonary blood must inevitably flow. Whether such a process of distention causes simply atrophy or causes disruption in the normal attachments of the medial smooth muscle fibers, and secondarily atrophy, is not known. What is known, as has been indicated, is that many of the unobstructed small arterial vessels are devoid of distinct muscle layers. The connective tissue, including the elastic tissue of the vessel, represents the only remaining significant element that maintains the integrity of the vessel. It is realized, however, that a vessel so altered may offer little, if any, active constriction, now being simply a passive structure with a wide lumen and a connective-tissue wall.

It is demonstrable, however, that in a patient with such elements in the pulmonary vascular tree, there still remains a vasoconstrictive function. Perhaps this is brought about by action of the hypertrophied media of the large muscular arteries, for structurally,

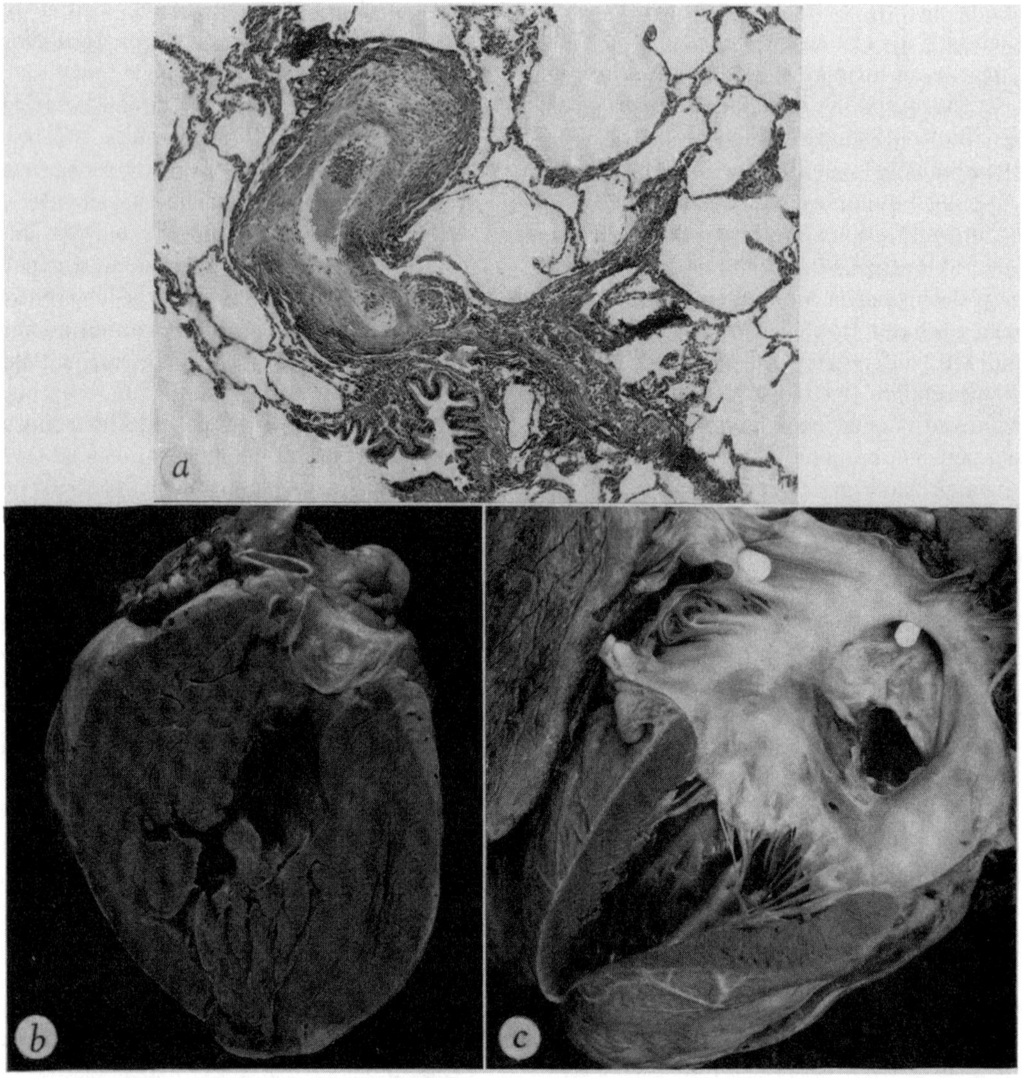

FIG. 12. From a 24-year-old man with atrial septal defect, severe pulmonary hypertension and only a right-to-left shunt. *a*. Photomicrograph of a large muscular artery showing intimal fibrous occlusion (hematoxylin and eosin; reduced from × 135). Such lesions were widely distributed and in addition many foci of arterial necrosis were present in the lung. *b*. The right ventricle. Marked hypertrophy. *c*. The left atrium and ventricle. The atrial septal defect is shown. Probes are present in the right and left upper pulmonary veins. The left ventricle, being of normal thickness, is thinner than the markedly hypertrophied right ventricle illustrated in *b*.

at least, these are so equipped as to suggest that they may have a vasoconstrictive action.

Severe Pulmonary Hypertension. In patients with atrial septal defect who have pulmonary arterial pressures at the levels of systemic arterial pressures, occlusive intimal lesions are present in the large arteries (fig. 12). Vessels involved frequently have diameters in the range of 300 microns. The lesions may be plexiform in nature and identical to those in ventricular septal defect. At this stage the pulmonary vascular bed is difficult to distinguish from that of the high resistance-low reserve type of vascular bed seen in patients with ventricular septal defect.

Necrotizing arterial lesions may occur in the arteries and be associated with thrombosis, which further reduces the capacity of the vascular bed. Both the intimal fibrous and the necrotizing arterial lesions are considered to be complications of long-standing severe pulmonary hypertension. The necrotizing lesions seem to be commoner in atrial septal defect with severe pulmonary hypertension than in either ventricular septal defect or patent ductus arteriosus. This apparent difference may perhaps be explained by the fact that in atrial septal defect not only may the pulmonary resistance exceed that of the systemic circulation, but the pulmonary pressure may also exceed significantly that in the systemic circulation, since the propelling parts of the circulations are not in communication. In contrast, in ventricular septal defect or patent ductus arteriosus, while the pulmonary vascular resistance may exceed the systemic, the pressures in the 2 circulations cannot be wide apart. The latter phenomenon results from the presence of the communication. As the pulmonary resistance rises above systemic, a right-to-left shunt develops but the 2 pressures will remain at equal levels.

The Effect of the Pulmonary Resistance on Shunts. In contrast to ventricular septal defect, the pulmonary vascular resistance has only an indirect influence on the shunts in atrial septal defect.

To explain this it is first necessary to consider the basis for the shunts in atrial septal defect with normal pulmonary pressure. While in such patients there may be a slightly higher pressure in the left atrium than in the right during parts of the respiratory cycle,[93-95] the 2 atria are, for practical purposes, in free communication through the characteristically large defect.[96] The 2 atria, therefore, operate essentially as a common chamber. The pressure within this functionally common chamber is responsible for filling the 2 ventricles. The right ventricle is thinner than the left. Therefore, the former is more distensible than the latter.[95]

During ventricular diastole when both ventricles are open to the functionally common atrium, a greater volume of blood will flow into the right ventricle than into the left because the former offers a lower resistance to filling. Some of the blood entering the right atrium will be from the anatomic left atrium. This is the blood which constitutes the left-to-right shunt.[97]

Of the blood shunted into the right atrium Swan and associates[98] have shown that there is a greater proportion derived from the right lung than from the left. This is related to the fact that the right pulmonary veins lie closer to the atrial septum and hence to the defect than do the left pulmonary veins. The streams from the right pulmonary veins are thus preferentially shunted through the atrial septal defect.

Even in cases of atrial septal defect with essentially normal pulmonary arterial pressures, there may be a small right-to-left shunt, which is principally derived from the inferior vena cava in contrast to the superior vena cava. This phenomenon is explained by the fact that the inferior caval orifice is directed toward the anterior edge of the atrial septal defect, and the stream of blood is split, some going into the right atrium and some into the left. That which enters the left is, for the most part, directed through the mitral valve into the left ventricle and constitutes the right-to-left shunt. The fact that in this type of atrial septal defect the superior vena cava contributes less to the right-to-left shunt is also explained by anatomic relationships in which the superior caval orifice does not have the close association with the atrial septal defect characteristic of the inferior caval relationships.

Further support for the concept that an anatomic basis underlies the different contribution of the 2 cavae to the right-to-left shunt in the usual variety of atrial septal defect is derived from the fact that when the atrial septal defect lies in an unusual position, such as near the orifice of the superior cava, a preferential right-to-left shunt from the superior vena cava is found.[99]

I have indicated that the basis for the left-to-right shunt in atrial septal defect with normal pulmonary pressures is dependent on the fact that the right ventricle is more distensible than the left. When pulmonary hypertension makes its appearance, the right ventricle hypertrophies in concert with the elevated pulmonary pressure. As the right ventricle becomes thicker, it becomes less distensible, the difference in distensibility between the left and the right ventricles becomes less and the left-to-right shunt diminishes. At the same time, the degree of right-to-left shunt becomes greater.

In an extreme case of atrial septal defect that we have observed, the pulmonary arterial pressures were higher than the systemic pressures and the right ventricle was thicker than the left (fig. 12*b* and *c*). Functional studies did not reveal the presence of any left-to-right shunt, there being only a right-to-left shunt.

Infants and Children

While atrial septal defect as seen in adults is usually not associated with elevated pulmonary resistance, it is well to consider that at the time of birth and during infancy, quite a different situation might have existed. Many facts yet need to be accumulated regarding the hemodynamics in the newborn with atrial septal defect. Certain hypotheses may be developed, however.

Realizing that in the newborn the 2 ventricles are of the same thickness and therefore probably have the same characteristics with respect to distensibility, a shunt through the atrial septal defect might be of very small magnitude, and with an unknown direction. It might be entirely right to left at this early period, as in fetal life. With the normal tendency for the pulmonary vascular resistance to fall after birth, the pulmonary and right ventricular pressures would also tend to fall, leading to the establishment of a left-to-right shunt. Hence while the pulmonary vascular resistance would fall, pulmonary arterial pressure might remain elevated because of the increased pulmonary flow in the presence of pulmonary vessels that have not yet undergone complete postnatal evolution.

While it is reasonable to suspect that in early postnatal life patients with atrial septal defect have an elevated pulmonary arterial pressure, it is realized that in time, at least in the usual instance of this defect, the pulmonary resistance falls to such a degree that the pulmonary pressure is normal in spite of the increased pulmonary flow. What is not known is whether the change from the early stage, when the pulmonary arterial pressure seems to be elevated and the left-to-right shunt small, to the later stage when the pressure is normal and the shunt large represents a sudden or a gradual change. Moreover, the exact dynamics involved in changing from the high-resistance stage of the newborn to the low-resistance stage of the adult are still not known. A further unanswered question remains concerning the occasional child with atrial septal defect and pulmonary hypertension. Does this represent the same phenomenon of intimal occlusive lesions that characterizes the adult who develops pulmonary hypertension, or does this represent the maintenance of the pulmonary hypertension that is hypothesized as being present in the neonatal period?

Obstruction to Pulmonary Venous Flow

Knowledge concerning the pulmonary vascular response to obstruction to pulmonary venous flow was acquired before that concerning the pulmonary vascular responses in the congenital malformations, which I have already discussed. This knowledge was derived initially from the study of acquired mitral stenosis, but it is applicable not only to congenital mitral stenosis, but also to a variety of other congenital conditions that have as a common factor the obstruction to pulmonary venous outflow. In addition to congenital mitral stenosis, which is rare, these include congenital stenosis of the pulmonary veins (principally cor triatriatum), endocardial sclerosis, and chronic failure of the left ventricle from a variety of causes including mitral insufficiency, coarctation of the aorta, and aortic stenosis.

The first approach to an understanding of the interrelationships between the cardiac disease and the response of the pulmonary vessels was obtained by the demonstration that in acquired mitral stenosis the pulmonary arterioles are thickened.

I had the privilege of being an Assistant at the Mallory Institute of Pathology of the Boston City Hospital in training under Dr. Frederic Parker when he and Weiss[100] prepared their now classic and first definitive article on the subject. Subsequent to this demonstration, many other authors have confirmed the observation that in acquired mitral stenosis the pulmonary arteries and arterioles show medial hypertrophy. Henry[101] stressed that segments of arterioles that are normally without a muscular media develop a muscular media. Heath and Whitaker[102] confirmed this. Intimal proliferation may be a secondary phenomenon, although this change may perhaps simply be an aging phenomenon. A number of authors have indicated that controls at comparable ages show similar intimal lesions. Patients with congenital conditions causing obstruction to pulmonary venous flow show qualitatively similar changes, but in general the changes are more severe than in acquired disease.

In congenital cases, not only is there striking medial hypertrophy of arteries and arterioles, but there is unusual prominence of the elastic membranes of the small arteries and of the arterioles.

The functional significance of the hypertrophic changes in the small pulmonary arteries in mitral stenosis was suspected by Borden and associates[103] and supported by further observations of Dexter and associates.[12]

The basic problem involves obstruction to pulmonary venous flow. Unless compensating mechanisms existed, the elevated pressure in the system proximal to the obstructed mitral valve would be similar. This means that the pulmonary capillary pressure would be the same as pulmonary arterial pressure and at a level well above the threshold for development of pulmonary edema. This hypothetical situation, however, does not usually obtain. The fact is that there is a disproportion between the pressures within the pulmonary arteries as opposed to the pulmonary capillaries, the former being considerably higher than the latter. Explanation of such a phenomenon requires the recognition that an obstructive element exists between the pulmonary arteries and the pulmonary capillaries. Such an obstruction could be brought about either by an anatomic or a functional basis for high resistance to flow through the pulmonary arterioles. This correlates well with the anatomic findings in which not only the thickened arterioles could exert a vasoconstrictive effect, but also the thickened vessels can be looked on as being less distensible than thinner vessels, and consequently, as representing a site of increased resistance to flow. The principles given regarding acquired mitral stenosis apply equally to the cases with a congenital basis for obstruction to pulmonary venous flow regardless of the anatomic site of the basic malformation.

The occurrence of pulmonary edema in patients with this functional type of arrangement may perhaps be due to temporary failure of a vasoconstrictive phenomenon at the pulmonary arteriolar level. Were this to occur, the flow through the pulmonary arterioles would increase. Since the pulmonary venous obstructive factor may be looked on as remaining constant and repr senting a high resistance to flow, the increased volume in the pulmonary capillaries would be associated with an increase in pressure at this level. Were this to rise sufficiently high, pulmonary edema would result. With this view in mind, it is possible that some cases of this functional category of congenital malformations may develop pulmonary edema, not from heart failure, but rather from pulmonary arteriolar failure.

I trust that in the foregoing I have conveyed the concept that in many varieties of congenital cardiac disease the responses of the pulmonary vessels are of paramount importance in regulating the circulation.

In some instances the pulmonary vascular responses may be considered an integral part of the cardiac malformation. In other instances they may be complications.

With varying pulmonary vascular response the same anatomic defect is associated with varying functional manifestations.

While certain interrelationships are better recognized today than they were a decade ago, there are doubtless many still to be uncovered.

Particularly wanting are explanations of mechanisms for most of the recognized responses. There is much still to be done.

REFERENCES

1 CONNER, L. A.: A contribution to the symptomatology of thrombophlebitis in typhoid. Arch. Int. Med. **10:** 534, 1912.

[2] —: A pulmonary attack simulating primary lobar pneumonia, caused by pulmonary embolism and infarction from a latent venous thrombosis. Arch. Int. Med. **13:** 349, 1914.

[3] Cournand, A., and Ranges, H. A.: Catheterization of the right auricle in man. Proc. Soc. Exper. Biol. & Med. **46:** 462, 1941.

[4] Blalock, A., and Taussig, H. B.: The surgical treatment of malformations of the heart in which there is pulmonary stenosis or pulmonary atresia. J. A. M. A. **128:** 189, 1945.

[5] Graybiel, A., Strieder, J. W., and Boyer, N. H.: Attempt to obliterate patent ductus arteriosus in patient with subacute bacterial endarteritis. Am. Heart J. **15:** 621, 1938.

[6] Gross, R. E., and Hubbard, J. P.: Surgical ligation of a patent ductus arteriosus: Report of first successful case. J. A. M. A. **112:** 729, 1939.

[7] Abbott, M. E.: Atlas of Congenital Cardiac Disease. New York, The American Heart Association, Inc., 1936, 62 pp.

[8] Moschcowitz, E.: Hypertension of the pulmonary circulation: Its causes, dynamics and relation to other circulatory states. Am. J. M. Sc. **174:** 388, 1927.

[9] Bing, R. J., Vandam, L. D., and Gray, F. D., Jr.: Physiological studies in congenital heart disease. III. Results obtained in five cases of Eisenmenger's complex. Bull. Johns Hopkins Hosp. **80:** 323, 1947.

[10] Handelsman, J. C., Bing, R. J., Campbell, J. A., and Griswold, H. E.: Physiological studies in congenital heart disease. V. The circulation in patients with isolated septal defects. Bull. Johns Hopkins Hosp. **82:** 615, 1948.

[11] Dexter, L., Haynes, F. W., Burwell, C. S., Eppinger, E. C., Sosman, M. C., and Evans, J. M.: Studies of congenital heart disease. III. Venous catheterization as a diagnostic Aid in patent ductus arteriosus, tetralogy of Fallot, ventricular septal defect, and auricular septal defect. J. Clin. Invest. **26:** 561, 1947.

[12] —, Dow, J. W., Haynes, F. W., Whittenberger, J. L., Ferris, B. G., Goodale, W. T., and Hellems, H. K.: Studies of the pulmonary circulation in man at rest. Normal variations and the interrelations between increased pulmonary blood flow, elevated pulmonary arterial pressure, and high pulmonary "capillary" pressures. J. Clin. Invest. **29:** 602, 1950.

[13] Dammann, J. F., Jr., and Muller, W. H., Jr.: The role of the pulmonary vascular bed in congenital heart disease. Pediatrics **12:** 307, 1953.

[14] —, and Ferencz, C.: The significance of the pulmonary vascular bed in congenital heart disease. I. Normal lungs. II. Malformations of the heart in which there is pulmonary stenosis. Am. Heart J. **52:** 7, 1956.

[15] —, and —: The significance of the pulmonary vascular bed in congenital heart disease. III. Defects between the ventricles or great vessels in which both increased pressure and blood flow may act upon the lungs and in which there is a common ejectile force. Am. Heart J. **52:** 210, 1956.

[16] Heath, D., and Whitaker, W.: The pulmonary vessels in patent ductus arteriosus. J. Path. & Bact. **77:** 285, 1955.

[17] Edwards, J. E.: Functional pathology of certain cardiovascular malformations which may be treated surgically. Arch. Surg. **61:** 1103, 1950.

[18] —, James, J. W. and DuShane, J. W.: Congenital malformation of the heart: Origin of transposed great vessels from the right ventricle associated with atresia of the left ventricular outlet, double orifice of the mitral valve, and single coronary artery. Lab. Invest. **1:** 197, 1952.

[19] Selzer, A.: Defects of the cardiac septums. J. A. M. A. **154:** 129, 1954.

[20] Edwards, J. E.: Functional pathology of congenital cardiac disease. Pediat. Clin. North America, February, 1954, pp. 13–49.

[21] Swan, H. J. C., Zapata-Diaz, J., Burchell, H. B., and Wood, E. H.: Pulmonary hypertension in congenital heart disease. Am. J. Med. **16:** 12, 1954.

[22] Blount, S. G., Jr., Mueller, H., and McCord, M. C.: Ventricular septal defect: Clinical and hemodynamic patterns. Am. J. Med. **18:** 871, 1955.

[23] Edwards, J. E., Douglas, J. M., Burchell, H. B., and Christensen, N. A.: Pathology of the intrapulmonary arteries and arterioles in coarctation of the aorta associated with patent ductus arteriosus. Am. Heart J. **38:** 205, 1949.

[24] Barclay, A. E., Franklin, K. J., and Prichard, M. M. L.: The Foetal Circulation and Cardiovascular System, and the Changes That They Undergo at Birth. Springfield, Ill., Charles C Thomas, 1945, 275 pp.

[25] Hamilton, W. F., Woodbury, R. A., and Woods, E. B.: The relation between systemic and pulmonary blood pressures in fetus. Am. J. Physiol. **119:** 206, 1937.

[26] Ardran, G. M., Dawes, G. S., Prichard, M. M. L., Reynolds, S. R. M., and Wyatt, D. G.: The effect of ventilation of the foetal lungs upon the pulmonary circulation. J. Physiol. **118:** 12, 1952.

[27] Reynolds, S. R.: The fetal and neonatal pulmonary vasculature in the guinea pig in relation to hemodynamic changes at birth. Am. J. Anat. **98:** 97, 1956.

[28] Civin, W. H., and Edwards, J. E.: Postnatal structural changes in intrapulmonary arteries and arterioles. Arch. Path. **51:** 192, 1951.

[29] Barclay, A. E., Barcroft, J., Barron, D. H., Franklin, K. J., and Prichard, M. M. L.: Studies of the foetal circulation and of certain

changes that take place after birth. Am. J. Anat. **69:** 383, 1941.

30 CREHAN, E. L.: A Study of the Arterial Oxygen Saturation in Normal Newborn Infants by Means of the Modified Photo-electric Oximeter. Thesis, Graduate School, University of Minnesota, 1950.

31 BURTON, A. C.: Relation of structure to function of the tissues of the wall of blood vessels. Physiol. Rev. **34:** 619, 1954.

32 BRENNER, O.: Pathology of vessels of pulmonary circulation. Arch. Int. Med. **56:** 211, 457, 724, 976, 1189, 1935.

33 MILLER. W. S.: The Lung. Springfield, Ill., Charles C Thomas, 1937, 209 pp.

34 HAMILTON, W. F., WOODBURY, R. A., AND VOGT, E.: Differential pressures in lesser circulation of unanesthetized dog. Am. J. Physiol. **125:** 130, 1939.

35 BLOOMFIELD, R. A., LAUSON, H. D., COURNAND, A., BREED, E. S., AND RICHARDS, D. W., JR.: Recording of right heart pressures in normal subjects and in patients with chronic pulmonary disease and various types of cardio-circulatory disease. J. Clin. Invest. **25:** 639, 1946.

36 HICKAM, J. B., AND CARGILL, W. H.: Effect of exercise on cardiac output and pulmonary arterial pressure in normal persons and in patients with cardiovascular diseases and pulmonary emphysema. J. Clin. Invest. **27:** 10, 1948.

37 —: The pulmonary vascular resistance. Abstracted, J. Clin. Invest. **28:** 788, 1949.

38 COURNAND, A.: Some aspects of the pulmonary circulation in normal man and in chronic cardiopulmonary diseases. Circulation. **2:** 641, 1950.

39 VON EULER, U. S., AND LILJESTRAND, G.: Observations on the pulmonary arterial blood pressure in the cat. Acta physiol. scandinav. **12:** 301, 1946.

40 MOTLEY, H. L., COURNAND, A., WERKO, L., HIMMELSTEIN, A., AND DRESDALE, D.: The influence of short periods of induced acute anoxia upon pulmonary artery pressures in man. Am. J. Physiol. **150:** 315, 1947.

41 RAHN, H., AND BAHNSON, H. T.: Simultaneous determination of bloodflow through each lung. Fed. Proc. **9:** 102, 1950.

42 LEWIS, B. M., AND GORLIN, R.: Effects of hypoxia on pulmonary circulation of the dog. Am. J. Physiol. **170:** 574, 1952.

43 WESTCOTT, R. N., FOWLER, N. O., SCOTT, R. C. HAUENSTEIN, V. D., AND MCGUIRE, J.: Anoxia and human pulmonary vascular resistance. J. Clin. Invest. **30:** 957, 1951.

44 STEAD, E. A., JR., HICKAM, J. B., AND WARREN, J. V.: Mechanism for changing the cardiac output in man. Tr. A. Am. Physicians. **60:** 74, 1947.

45 COURNAND, A.: Recent observations on the dynamics of the pulmonary circulation. Bull. New York Acad. Med. **23:** 27, 1947.

46 NICHOLSON, J. W., III, BURCHELL, H. B., AND WOOD, E. H.: A method for the continuous reading of Evans blue dye curves in arterial blood, and its application to the diagnosis of cardiovascular abnormalities. J. Lab. & Clin. Med. **37:** 353, 1951.

47 BROADBENT, J. C., CLAGETT, O. T., BURCHELL, H. B., AND WOOD, E. H.: Dye-dilution curves in acyanotic congenital heart disease. Abstracted, Am. J. Physiol. **167:** 770, 1951.

48 SWAN, H. J. C., AND WOOD, E. H.: Localization of cardiac defects by dye-dilution curves recorded after injection of T-1824 at multiple sites in the heart and great vessels during cardiac catheterization. Proc. Staff Meet., Mayo Clin. **28:** 95, 1953.

49 ABBOTT, M. E.: Congenital Cardiac Disease. *In* OSLER, W.: Modern Medicine: Its Theory and Practice. *In* Original Contributions by American and Foreign Authors. Vol. IV. Diseases of the Respiratory System—Diseases of the Circulatory System. Ed. 3, Philadelphia, Lea & Febiger, 1927, pp. 612–812.

50 EISENMENGER, V.: Die angeborenen Defekte des Kammerscheiderwand des Herzens. Ztschr. klin. Med. **32:** (Suppl.) 1897.

51 SELZER, A., AND LAQUER, G. L.: The Eisenmenger complex and its relation to the uncomplicated defect of the ventricular septum: Review of thirty-five autopsied cases of Eisenmenger's complex, including two new cases. Arch. Int. Med. **87:** 218, 1951.

52 EISENMENGER, V.: Ursprung der Aorta aus beiden Ventrikeln beim Defect des Septum ventriculorum. Wien. klin. Wchnschr. **11:** 26, 1898.

53 EDWARDS, J. E., DRY, T. J., PARKER, R. L., BURCHELL, H. B., WOOD, E. H., AND BULBULIAN, A. H.: An Atlas of Congenital Anomalies of the Heart and Great Vessels. Springfield, Ill., Charles C Thomas, 1954, 202 pp.

54 HEATH, D., BROWN, J. W., AND WHITAKER, W.: Muscular defects in the ventricular septum. Brit. Heart J. **18:** 1, 1956.

55 BALDWIN, E. DE F., MOORE, L. V., AND NOBLE, R. P.: The demonstration of ventricular septal defect by means of right heart catheterization. Am. Heart J. **32:** 152, 1946.

56 SELZER, A.: Defect of the ventricular septum: Summary of twelve cases and review of the literature. Arch. Int. Med. **84:** 798, 1949.

57 BURCHELL, H. B., AND WOOD, E. H.: Reproducibility of values for arterial oxygen saturations under varying conditions in a patient with an intracardiac venous arterial shunt. Abstracted, Am. J. Physiol. **155:** 429, 1948.

58 HAMILTON, W. F., WINSLOW, J. A., AND HAMILTON, W. F., JR.: Notes on case of congenital

heart disease with cyanotic episodes. J. Clin. Invest. **29:** 20, 1950.

[59] BURCHELL, H. B., TAYLOR, B. E., POLLACK, A. A., DUSHANE, J. W., AND WOOD, E. H.: Ventricular septal defect and pulmonary hypertension without hypoxemia. Proc. Staff Meet., Mayo Clin. **23:** 507, 1948.

[60] ADAMS, F. H.: Pulmonary hypertension in children due to congenital heart disease. J. Pediat. **40:** 42, 1952.

[61] GRIFFIN, G. D. J., AND ESSEX, H. E.: Experimental production of interventricular septal defects: Certain physiologic and pathologic effects. Surg., Gynec. & Obst. **92:** 325, 1951.

[62] DIVERTIE, M. B., AND SWAN, H. J. C.: Unpublished data.

[63] EDWARDS, J. E.: Structural changes of pulmonary vascular bed and their functional significance in congenital cardiac disease: Twenty-sixth Ludvig Hektoen lecture. Proc. Inst. Med. Chicago. **18:** 134, 1950.

[64] ZUR LINDEN, W.: Isolierte Pulmonalsklerose im jüngsten Kindesalter. Arch. path. Anat. **252:** 229, 1924.

[65] SPENCER, H.: Quoted by Brewer, D. B.[71]

[66] KUCSKO, L.: Quoted by Brewer, D. B.[71]

[67] SMITH, G.: Patent ductus arteriosus with pulmonary hypertension and reversed shunt. Brit. Heart J. **16:** 233, 1954.

[68] EVANS, W.: Congenital pulmonary hypertension. Proc. Roy. Soc. Med. **44:** 600, 1951.

[69] WHITAKER, W., HEATH, D., AND BROWN, J. W.: Patent ductus arteriosus with pulmonary hypertension. Brit. Heart J. **17:** 121, 1955.

[70] BROWN, J. W., HEATH, D., AND WHITAKER, W.: Eisenmenger's complex. Brit. Heart J. **17:** 273, 1955.

[71] BREWER, D. B.: Fibrous occlusion and anastomosis of the pulmonary vessels in a case of pulmonary hypertension associated with patent ductus arteriosus. J. Path. & Bact. **70:** 299, 1955.

[72] EDWARDS, J. E.: Pathologic Considerations in Adjustments Between the Systemic and Pulmonary Circulations. *In* Henry Ford Hospital, Detroit International Symposium on Cardiovascular Surgery. Philadelphia, W. B. Saunders Company, 1955, pp. 100–118.

[73] GOLDBERG, H., SILBER, E. N., GORDON, A., AND KATZ, L. N.: The dynamics of Eisenmenger's complex: An integration of the pathologic, physiologic and clinical features. Circulation **4:** 343, 1951.

[74] HEATH, D.: Cor triloculare biatriatum. Circulation. In press.

[75] HULTGREN, H., SELZER, A., PURDY, A., HOLMAN, E., AND GERBODE, F.: The syndrome of patent ductus arteriosus with pulmonary hypertension. Circulation **8:** 15, 1953.

[76] YU, P. N., LOVEJOY, F. W., JR. JOOS. H. A.. NYE, R. E., JR., AND BEATTY, D. E.: Studies of pulmonary hypertension. V. The syndrome of patent ductus arteriosus with marked pulmonary hypertension. Am. Heart J. **48:** 544, 1954.

[77] OLD, J. W., AND RUSSELL, W. O.: Necrotizing pulmonary arteritis occurring with congenital heart disease (Eisenmenger complex): Report of case with necropsy. Am. J. Path. **26:** 789, 1950.

[78] KIPKIE, G. F., AND JOHNSON, D. S.: Possible pathogenic mechanisms responsible for human periarteritis nodosa: as suggested by occurrence of 2 instances of this disease in association with glomerulonephritis. Arch. Path. **51:** 387, 1951.

[79] SYMMERS, W. ST. C.: Necrotizing pulmonary arteriopathy associated with pulmonary hypertension. J. Clin. Path. **5:** 36, 1952.

[80] EDWARDS, J. E., AND CHAMBERLIN, W. B., JR.: Pathology of the pulmonary vascular tree. III. The structure of the intrapulmonary arteries in cor triloculare biatriatum with subaortic stenosis. Circulation **3:** 524, 1951.

[81] COSH, J. A.: Patent ductus arteriosus with pulmonary hypertension. Brit. Heart J. **15:** 423, 1953.

[82] HICKS, J. D.: Acute arterial necrosis in the lungs. J. Path. & Bact. **65:** 333, 1953.

[83] FERGUSON, D. J., AND VARCO, R. L.: The relation of blood pressure and flow to the development and regression of experimentally induced pulmonary arteriosclerosis. Circulation Research **3:** 152, 1955.

[84] HELMHOLZ, H. F., JR., AND EDWARDS, J. E.: Unpublished data.

[85] BURCHELL, H. B., SWAN, H. J. C., AND WOOD, E. H.: Demonstration of differential effects on pulmonary and systemic arterial pressure by variation in oxygen content of inspired air in patients with patent ductus arteriosus and pulmonary hypertension. Circulation **8:** 681, 1953.

[86] DEUCHAR, D. C., AND ZAK, G. A.: Cardiac catheterization in congenital heart disease. I. Four cases of pulmonary stenosis with increased pulmonary blood flow. Guy's Hosp. Rep. **101:** 1, 1952.

[87] SELZER, A., AND CARNES, W. H.: The role of pulmonary stenosis in the production of chronic cyanosis. Am. Heart J. **45:** 382, 1953.

[88] BROADBENT, J. C., WOOD, E. H., AND BURCHELL, H. B.: Left-to-right intracardiac shunts in the presence of pulmonary stenosis. Proc. Staff Meet., Mayo Clin. **28:** 101, 1953.

[89] WOOD, E. H.: Personal communication to the author.

[90] ZIEGLER, R. F.: The importance of patent ductus arteriosus in infants. Am. Heart J. **43:** 553, 1952.

[91] DAMMANN, J. F., JR., AND SELL, C. G. R.: Patent

ductus arteriosus in the absence of a continuous murmur. Circulation **6:** 110, 1952.

[92] —, BERTHRONG, M., AND BING, R. J.: Reverse ductus: A presentation of the syndrome of patency of the ductus arteriosus with pulmonary hypertension and a shunting of blood flow from pulmonary artery to aorta. Bull. Johns Hopkins Hosp. **92:** 128, 1953.

[93] COURNAND, A., MOTLEY, H. L., HIMMELSTEIN, A., and DRESDALE, D.: Recording of blood pressure from the left auricle and the pulmonary veins in human subjects with interauricular septal defect. Am. J. Physiol. **150:** 267, 1947.

[94] HICKAM, J. B.: Atrial septal defect: A study of intracardiac shunts, ventricular outputs, and pulmonary pressure gradient. Am. Heart J. **38:** 801, 1949.

[95] LITTLE, R. C., OPDYKE, D. F., AND HAWLEY, J. G.: Dynamics of experimental atrial septal defects. Am. J. Physiol. **158:** 241, 1949.

[96] DOW, J. W., AND MALONEY, J. V.: Dynamics of experimental atrial septal defect. Abstracted, Am. J. Med. **10:** 235, 1951.

[97] BRANNON, E. S., WEENS, H. S., AND WARREN, J. V.: Atrial septal defect: Study of hemodynamics by the technique of right heart catheterization. Am. J. M. Sc. **210:** 480, 1945.

[98] SWAN, H. J. C., BURCHELL, H. B., AND WOOD, E. H.: Differential diagnosis at cardiac catheterization of anomalous pulmonary venous drainage related to atrial septal defects or abnormal venous connections. Proc. Staff Meet., Mayo Clin. **28:** 452, 1953.

[99] SWAN, H. J. C., KIRKLIN, J. W., BECU, L. M., AND WOOD, E. H.: Anomalous connection of right pulmonary veins to superior vena cava with interatrial communications: A report of hemodynamic findings in eight cases. Unpublished data.

[100] PARKER, F., JR., AND WEISS, S.: Nature and significance of structural changes in lungs in mitral stenosis. Am. J. Path. **12:** 573, 1936.

[101] HENRY, E. W.: The small pulmonary vessels in mitral stenosis. Brit. Heart J. **14:** 406, 1952.

[102] HEATH, D., AND WHITAKER, W.: The pulmonary vessels in mitral stenosis. J. Path & Bact. **70:** 291, 1955.

[103] BORDEN, C. W., EBERT, R. V., WILSON, R. H., AND WELLS, H. S.: Pulmonary hypertension in heart disease. New England J. Med. **242:** 529, 1950.

The Pathology of Hypertensive Pulmonary Vascular Disease

A Description of Six Grades of Structural Changes in the Pulmonary Arteries with Special Reference to Congenital Cardiac Septal Defects

By DONALD HEATH, M.D., AND JESSE E. EDWARDS, M.D.

Progressive histologic changes occur in the pulmonary arteries and arterioles, as a complication of chronically elevated pulmonary arterial blood pressure, in patients with congenital septal defects of the heart. This progression is so stereotyped as to allow a division of the structural effects into 6 grades. The histologic features of each grade are described in detail in this communication. These results afford a basis for comparing the magnitude of these changes to the clinical findings.

PROGRESSIVE histologic changes occur in the pulmonary arteries and arterioles, as a complication of chronically elevated pulmonary arterial blood pressure, in patients with congenital septal defects of the heart. The progression is so stereotyped as to allow a division of the structural effects into 6 grades (table 1), although it is recognized that there is a gradual change from one grade to another. This division is of great practical value, since it enables the pathologist to express a whole group of complex changes in a succinct manner as a grade number. In the present communication, based primarily on the study of 67 cases of congenital septal defects of the heart and 2 cases of idiopathic pulmonary hypertension, a detailed description is given of the histologic changes that characterize each grade. In 55 cases pulmonary hypertension was demonstrated at cardiac catheterization or at cardiotomy; in 9 instances elevated pressure in the pulmonary circulation was inferred from the clinical and pathologic findings. In the remaining 5 cases, the pulmonary artery mean blood pressure was less than 30 mm. of mercury; these were all cases of atrial septal defect studied to illustrate the grade-1 changes in this disease. No cases with pulmonary venous obstruction were studied although at least the earlier changes of hypertensive pulmonary vascular disease and pulmonary arteritis occur in this group of patients. In a companion paper,[1] the relation between each grade and pulmonary artery blood pressure, flow and resistance, and age is demonstrated. In a third study,[2] the relation between each grade and the reversibility of pulmonary hypertension after surgical correction of the cardiac anomaly is considered.

This paper is concerned solely with the changes found in small pulmonary vessels. Structural changes also are found in the intima and media of elastic pulmonary arteries. Atheroma is the characteristic intimal feature related to pulmonary hypertension in these large arteries. The configuration of the elastic tissue of the media of the pulmonary trunk differs in pulmonary hypertension that is acquired from that which is present from birth. These changes in the intima and the media and their relation to pulmonary hypertension are considered in detail elsewhere.[3, 4]

A description is given of the structural changes characteristic of each grade, as found specifically in cases of large ventricular sep-

From the Mayo Clinic and the Mayo Foundation, Rochester, Minn. The Mayo Foundation is a part of the Graduate School of the University of Minnesota.

Dr. Heath was in receipt of a Rockefeller Travelling Fellowship in Medicine while participating in this investigation, which was supported in part by a research grant number H-3531, from the National Heart Institute, U. S. Public Health Service.

tal defect, large patent ductus arteriosus, or any other form of congenital heart disease associated with a free communication between the systemic and pulmonary circulations and pulmonary hypertension from birth. This qualification is necessary because the earliest changes seen in the pulmonary vessels in cases of atrial septal defect (or similar diseases associated with acquired pulmonary hypertension following a long period of high pulmonary blood flow) with increased pulmonary artery blood pressure are not identical with, although in some respects they are similar to, those seen in ventricular septal defect. Furthermore, in acquired idiopathic pulmonary hypertension, the early histologic changes associated with the elevation of blood pressure differ from those associated with ventricular septal defect. The histologic changes defined as grade 1 of hypertensive pulmonary vascular disease in the following section refer to changes seen in patients having congenital heart disease associated with pulmonary hypertension from birth. The corresponding grade of change seen in patients having atrial septal defect and acquired idiopathic pulmonary hypertension is dealt with at the end of the paper. It needs to be stressed, however, that, whereas grade-1 changes are simply an integral part of the various structural and functional alterations in large ventricular septal defect, structural changes of grades 2 and 6 occur as a result of the raised pulmonary artery blood pressure. Grades 2 to 6 are present among all forms of hypertensive pulmonary vascular disease, whatever the etiology, and are found in each of the 2 groups of heart disease referred to herein, as well as in idiopathic pulmonary hypertension.

Before the pathologic aspects of hypertensive pulmonary vascular disease are described, it is necessary to present the histologic features of normal pulmonary blood vessels.

Histologic Features of Normal Pulmonary Blood Vessels

The walls of the pulmonary arterioles consist of a single elastic lamina except proximally at their origin from a muscular artery where serial sections demonstrate their walls to consist of a thin media sandwiched between internal and external elastic laminae.[5] In the majority of patients beyond adolescence studied in this series and in groups of controls studied previously,[6] fine acellular intimal fibrosis was found in arterioles as a normal age change. As already stated, the vast majority of pulmonary arterioles do not have a muscular media beyond their immediate origin from a muscular pulmonary artery, but vessels as small as 80 μ in diameter with a thin but distinct muscular media, bounded by internal and external elastic laminae, can be found after careful search of sections of the normal lung.[7] These tiny vessels, which look like small muscular pulmonary arteries, are found predominantly in the lingula pulmonis.[8] Arterioles arise either as branches, at right angles to the parent stem, which is related to the respective alveolar duct, or as terminations, at an oblique angle, of small muscular pulmonary arteries. Branches of the former type also may arise from quite large muscular arteries near small bronchi and much more proximally in the pulmonary vascular tree than the arterioles that arise as terminations of muscular pulmonary arteries. They have a thin wall with a lumen-to-wall ratio of about 8:1.[5] Brenner[9] defined pulmonary arterioles as arterial vessels in the lung less than 100 μ in diameter, but obviously this is only an approximation. The main criteria employed in the recognition of arterioles apart from size are the structure of their walls and their origin from small muscular arteries.

The muscular pulmonary arteries, usually defined as arterial vessels between 100 and 1,000 μ in diameter,[9] consist of a thin media bounded by internal and external elastic laminae. The media is composed predominantly of smooth muscle with occasional collagenous and elastic fibrils. In small muscular arteries less than 300 μ in diameter the media has a thickness equivalent to 2.8 to 3.1 per cent of the external diameter of the vessel in the upper and lower lobes and 5.5 to 6.8 per cent in the region of the lingula. These figures have been confirmed previously by mensuration of medial thickness in this class

TABLE 1.—*Basis of Grades of Hypertensive Pulmonary Vascular Disease Found in Association with Large Ventricular Septal Defects and Functionally Related Diseases*

		Grade of hypertensive pulmonary vascular disease					
		1	2	3	4	5	6
Type of intimal reaction		←None→					
			←—	——	Cellular	——	—→
				←—	Fibrous and fibroelastic	——	—→
					←—	"Plexiform lesion"	—→
State of media of arteries and arterioles		←—	——	——	Hypertrophied	——	—→
				←—	Some generalized dilatation	——	—→
					←—	Local "dilatation lesions"	—→
						←— P H *	—→
							←N A †→

* Pulmonary hemosiderosis associated with distended, thin-walled, arterial vessels throughout the lung.
† Necrotizing arteritis.

of vessel in series of controls.[8] As in the case of arteries and veins, acellular intimal fibrosis is found as a normal age change beyond adolescence. The adventitia is thin. These vessels are associated with the bronchioles, the respiratory bronchioles, and the alveolar ducts.

The elastic pulmonary arteries, defined as vessels greater than 1,000 μ in diameter,[9] differ from muscular pulmonary arteries in that the elastic arteries show a specific pattern of elastic fibrils that predominate in the media.[4] The media of elastic pulmonary arteries is relatively thicker than that of the muscular pulmonary arteries, so that in normal persons it may account for 10 per cent of the external diameter of the vessel. The thickness of the media of the pulmonary trunk and the configuration of its elastic fibrils in control patients of various ages, in patients with pulmonary hypertension present at birth, and in patients with pulmonary hypertension acquired in adult life are considered in detail elsewhere.[4] Intimal age changes occur less frequently in the pulmonary trunk than in the small pulmonary blood vessels.

The media of the normal venule and small vein up to about 200 μ in diameter consists of a single elastic lamina, and that of the vein, greater than 200 or 300 μ, consists of collagen and smooth muscle fibers with admixed elastic laminae that tend to lie concentrically around the walls of the vein. The clear differentiation of media and inner and outer elastic laminae, so characteristic of arteries, is lacking. Venules move away from the air spaces of their respective units to the interlobular septum to form venous trunks. This location is of great importance in distinguishing them from distended thin-walled veinlike arterial vessels found near small bronchi and bronchioles in the severer forms of hypertensive pulmonary vascular disease. Brenner[9] demonstrated that intimal fibrosis occurs universally in adults in all classes of pulmonary blood vessels, especially veins, as a normal age change.

HISTOLOGIC FEATURES OF GRADES OF HYPERTENSIVE PULMONARY VASCULAR DISEASE (TABLE 1)

Grade 1. The Stage of Retention of Fetal-Type Pulmonary Vessels. The definitive histologic features lie in the pulmonary arterioles and the muscular pulmonary arteries. This grade is the earliest ever found in large ventricular septal defect, wide patent ductus arteriosus, or any other congenital cardiac anomaly that allows the pulmonary vascular bed to be subjected to systemic systolic blood pressures from birth.

In the arterioles that normally have a distinct muscular media with internal and external elastic laminae only in the immediate

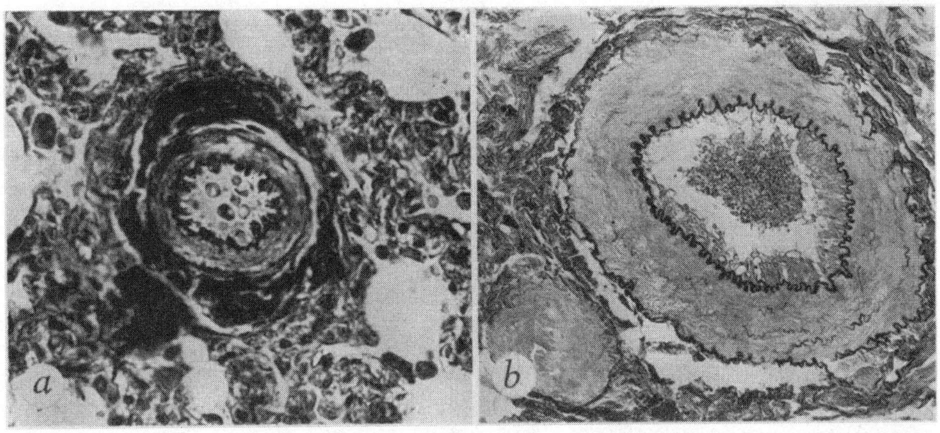

FIG. 1. *a.* Grade 1. Ventricular septal defect type. Transverse section of a pulmonary arteriole with muscular media and internal and external elastic lamina. There is no intimal proliferation. From a boy, aged 1½ years, with ventricular septal defect, corrected transposition, and atrial septal defect. This and all other sections illustrated were stained by Verhoeff's method to demonstrate elastic tissue and counterstained with van Gieson's stain to show muscle and collagen. × 375. *b.* Grade 1. Ventricular septal defect type. Transverse section of a muscular pulmonary artery showing hypertrophy of the media with no intimal reaction. This appearance is characteristic of grade 1, but the dilated, thin-walled branch of the artery containing proliferated endothelium indicates that grade-5 changes were present in this case. This illustrates that the progression of structural changes in pulmonary hypertension is not uniform in individual arteries throughout the lung. From a 34 year old woman having patent ductus arteriosus. × 125.

vicinity of their origins, there is distal extension of muscle. In this way, even arterioles as small as 30 μ look like small muscular pulmonary arteries instead of like veins as they do in the normal lung (fig. 1*a*). The media is relatively thicker than that found in muscular arteries and may be as thick as 25 per cent of the external diameter of the vessel. There is no intimal fibrosis. The adventitia is thick and fibrous. The thickened arterioles also bear a striking resemblance to the intralobular pulmonary arteries of the fetus. It is worthy of comment at this point that comparable classes of vessels differ greatly in size in the fetus and in the adult.

The media of the muscular pulmonary arteries is thickened and may be as thick as 25 per cent of the external diameter (fig. 1*b*). Intimal fibrosis is not present, but the adventitia is thick and fibrous. The medial thickness gradually increases from grade 1 to grade 3, generally speaking, with great variation in the thickness of the individual muscular pulmonary arteries in any one case. As has been suggested previously in a study of the small vessels of the lung in mitral stenosis, this study confirms that there is no clear-cut relation between medial thickness of any one vessel and pulmonary artery blood pressure.[6] The pulmonary veins are normal in ventricular septal defect associated with pulmonary hypertension.

Grade 2. Stage of Medial Hypertrophy with Cellular Intimal Reaction. There is cellular intimal proliferation in the smaller muscular pulmonary arteries, less than about 300 μ in diameter, and the pulmonary arterioles and the lesion may be so marked as to occlude the vessels. There is no intimal reaction elsewhere in the pulmonary arterial tree. Plump endothelial cells that stain brown with van Gieson's stain form only an unduly prominent vascular lining in some arterioles (fig. 2*a*). In other vessels they have proliferated to the extent of forming characteristic eccentric masses with underlying material staining brown with van Gieson's stain (fig. 2*b*). This proliferated intimal material may coalesce

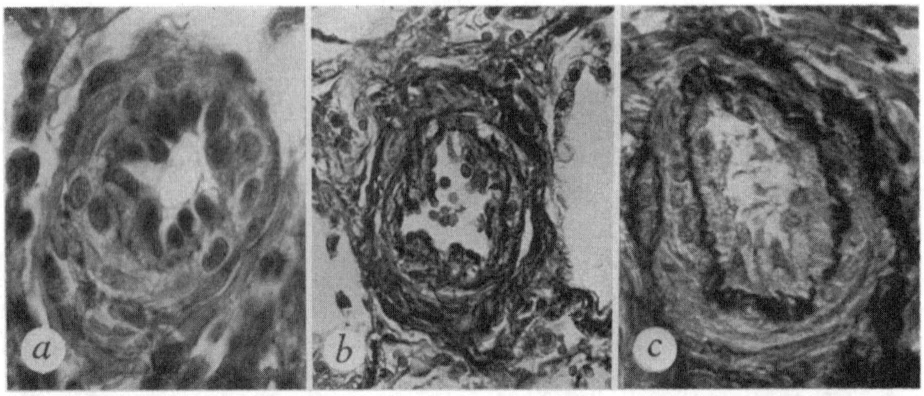

FIG. 2. *a.* Early grade 2. Transverse section of a pulmonary arteriole with plump, endothelial cells that form only an unduly prominent vascular lining. From a 4 year old boy with patent ductus arteriosus. × 700. *b.* Grade 2. Transverse section of a pulmonary arteriole with a muscular media and eccentric endothelial masses with underlying material staining brown with van Gieson's stain. From a 37 year old woman with atrial septal defect. × 375. *c.* Grade 2. Transverse section of a pulmonary arteriole with proliferated endothelium and material staining brown with van Gieson's stain forming a concentric rim around the circumference. From a 4 year old boy with patent ductus arteriosus. × 435.

and lead to vascular occlusion. In some cases the proliferated endothelium and material staining brown with van Gieson's stain may form a concentric rim around the circumference (fig. 2*c*). In time, fibrous tissue, recognizable by its property of staining red with van Gieson's stain, forms beneath the endothelium and this constitutes the earliest stage of grade 3.

Grade 3. Stage of Progressive Fibrous Vascular Occlusion. In this grade there is progressive intimal fibrosis in the smaller (300 μ) muscular pulmonary arteries and pulmonary arterioles with a change in the nature of the intimal proliferation and an extension of it into medium-sized (300 to 500 μ) arteries. The intimal proliferation seen in early lesions of grade 3 represents a change from the predominantly cellular endothelial reaction seen in grade 2 to one that consists of cellular fibrous tissue as judged by its tinctorial properties (fig. 3*a*). Later lesions are characterized by concentric or eccentric masses of less cellular fibrous tissue that stains bright red with van Gieson's stain. Old intimal fibrotic lesions show an admixture of fine or even coarse elastic fibrils and some splitting or elastosis of the internal elastic lamina, while the fibrous tissue may be relatively acellular. Running parallel with these characteristic changes in the histologic structure of the intimal fibrous tissue is its equally characteristic extension.

Most of the intimal lesions are first found in the arterioles and smaller muscular pulmonary arteries and extend back around the mouths of origin of the vessels and involve the parent muscular arteries (fig. 3*b*). In many instances, however, heaped up intimal fibrotic lesions are found early in a muscular pulmonary artery in proximity to the origin of an arteriole. It has already been pointed out that arterioles may rise at a proximal point in the pulmonary vascular tree as right-angled branches of fairly large muscular arteries. They also may arise distally as terminations of the arteries. Intimal fibrosis is found first in both sites. Only in severer cases of pulmonary hypertensive change is widespread intimal fibrosis found in the medium-sized muscular pulmonary arteries.

Serial sections demonstrate the plaques of intimal fibrous tissue in muscular arteries are focal (fig. 3*a*). In some instances these foci of intimal fibrous tissue are continuous with the fibrous tissue in the smallest muscular

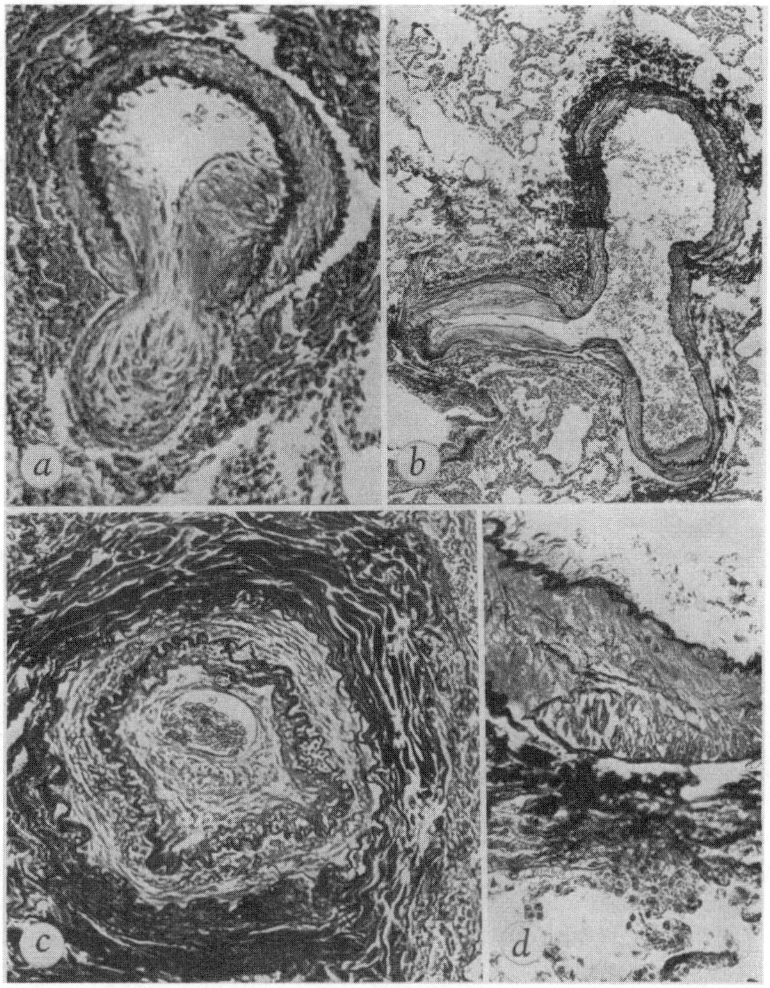

FIG. 3. *a.* Grade 3. Transverse section of a small muscular pulmonary artery with an oblique section of an arteriolar branch. There is medial hypertrophy in the artery. Cellular fibrous tissue forms eccentric masses in the artery and occludes the arteriole. From a 9 year old boy having cor triloculare biatriatum without pulmonary stenosis. × 160. *b.* Grade 3. Transverse section of a medium-sized muscular pulmonary artery and oblique sections of 2 of its branches. The parent artery shows hypertrophy of the media but no intimal reaction. The smaller branch shows some dilatation with thinning of the media and acellular intimal fibrosis. From a 6 year old girl with ventricular septal defect. × 30. *c.* Grade 3. Transverse section of a medium-sized muscular pulmonary artery. There are medial hypertrophy and severe intimal fibrosis so that only a small eccentric endothelium-lined channel remains patent. There is elastosis of the internal elastic lamina. From a girl, aged 6½ years, with ventricular septal defect and patent ductus arteriosus. × 175. *d.* Portion of wall of large muscular pulmonary artery showing fasciculi of longitudinal muscle in close apposition to the external elastic lamina. This case had grade-5 structural changes in the small pulmonary vessels, but the appearances are equally characteristic of any of the grades from 3 to 6. From a 27 year old woman with atrial septal defect. × 200.

arteries and the arterioles but in others there is no connection. Finally, the concentric or eccentric masses of avascular fibrous tissue in the muscular arteries and pulmonary arterioles may completely occlude the vessel, but a small endothelium-lined channel with an irregular course frequently remains patent (fig. 3*c*). Thus the characteristic feature of

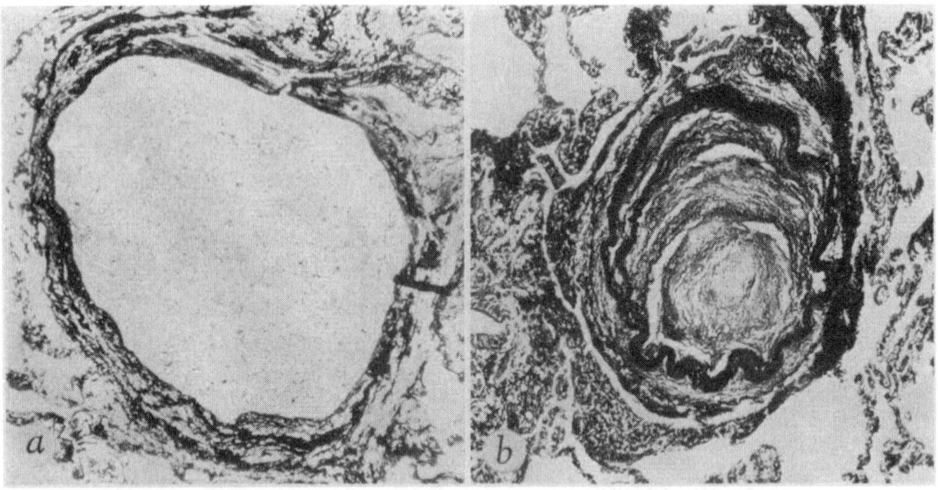

FIG. 4. Generalized dilatation may develop in any of the lesions from severe grade 3 to grade 6. *a*. Grade 3. Transverse section of a dilated muscular pulmonary artery. There is no intimal fibrosis. × 60. *b*. Grade 5. Transverse section of a dilated, muscular pulmonary artery. There is severe intimal fibroelastosis and the internal elastic lamina is grossly thickened. The media is thin and is encroached upon by the intimal fibrosis. From a 24 year old woman with patent ductus arteriosus. × 100.

severe hypertensive pulmonary vascular disease, grade 3, is the widespread occlusion of muscular pulmonary arteries less than about 500 μ in diameter and of arterioles by acellular fibrous tissue admixed with fine elastic fibrils. The large muscular arteries more than about 600 μ in external diameter rarely show intimal fibrosis even when the smallest and medium-sized arteries and arterioles show foci of complete occlusion. Atheroma rather than intimal fibrosis is found in the large muscular and elastic pulmonary arteries in the presence of severe pulmonary hypertension.[3]

In grade 3 the media reaches the limit of its capacity for hypertrophy, so that its thickness may be up to 30 per cent of the external diameter of the vessel. The media of the arteriole is similarly much thickened. In the medium-sized and large muscular arteries the increase in medial thickness is brought about partly by the development of fasciculi of longitudinal muscle which usually lie in close apposition to the internal or external elastic lamina and which are bounded by elastic laminae as shown in figure 3*d*. Occasionally increased numbers of longitudinal muscle fibers, not in distinct fasciculi delineated by elastic fibrils, may be seen in the media itself.

Although the characteristic feature of grade 3 is medial hypertrophy, some thinning of the media is seen also in the severer, late stages of this grade. This dilatation occurs in patent vessels (fig. 4*a*) and those showing focal areas of occlusion (fig. 4*b*). In the latter case, the dilatation of vessels with thinning of the media is found in smaller muscular arteries and arterioles either at or distal to a focus of fibrotic occlusion of a parent muscular artery, and in medium-sized arteries, proximal to the foci of occlusion. In the former site the thinning is probably a type of disuse atrophy subsequent to the lowering of blood pressure distal to the fibrotic occlusion and is analogous to the thinning of pulmonary arteries in pulmonary stenosis. In the latter site the dilatation is an expression of decompensation to the severely elevated pulmonary resistance.

Dilatation Lesions. In addition to the generalized dilatation that occurs in severe examples of grade 3 and in grades 4, 5, and 6, excessive dilatation occurs in some of the smallest muscular pulmonary arteries and the arterioles to form distended sacs. In many of these microaneurysms there is endothelial proliferation and at times superadded throm-

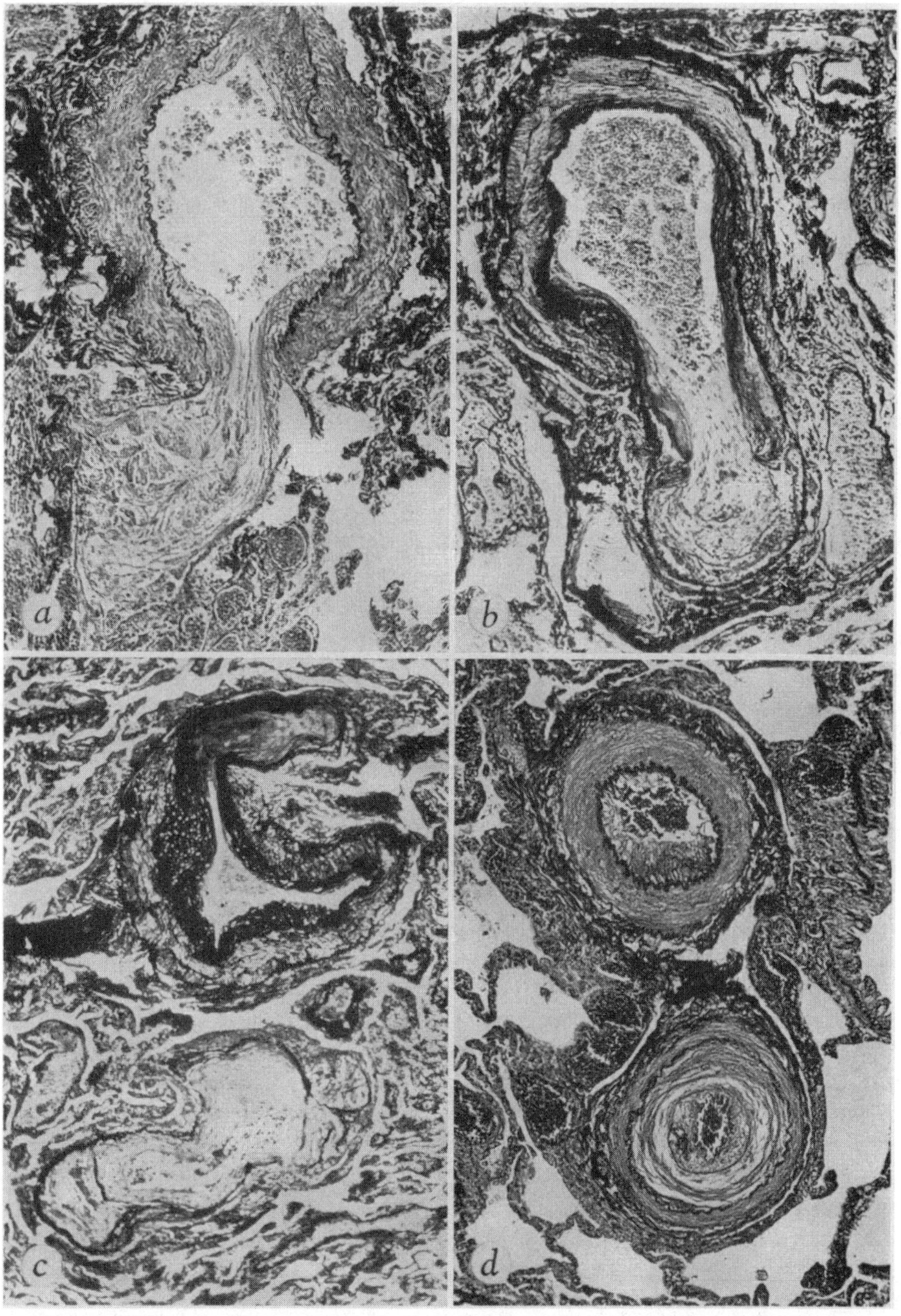

FIG 5. *a.* Grade 5. Section of a muscular pulmonary artery showing hypertrophy of the media and excessive dilatation of an arteriolar branch to form a plexiform lesion. The intimal proliferation in the distended sac is cellular indicating the dilatation lesion to be of recent formation. From a 27 year old woman with atrial septal defect. × 150. *b.* Grade 5. Section of a muscular pulmonary artery showing hypertrophy of the media, with the development of longitudinal muscle, and a plexiform lesion. The cellular proliferation in the dilatation lesion is partially replaced by fibrous tissue indicating that it is older

(Continued on opposite page)

bosis. These complex vascular formations consisting of severely dilated vessels with internal cellular proliferations we term "dilatation lesions," and they are to be distinguished from the generalized dilatation that occurs throughout the pulmonary vasculature in some stages of pulmonary hypertension. These dilatation lesions are seen in 4 main forms: (1) plexiform lesions, (2) veinlike branches of hypertrophied, usually occluded, muscular pulmonary arteries, (3) angiomatoid lesions, and (4) cavernous lesions.

1. The Plexiform Lesion. The pulmonary arterioles and smallest muscular pulmonary arteries are greatly distended to form sacs whose walls are fragile, consisting of a single elastic lamina or an exceedingly thin layer of muscle between 2 ill-defined elastic laminae (fig. 5*a*). Large similarly thin-walled channels leave these dilated sacs and terminate as capillaries that pass to the alveolar walls. In some instances vessels of capillary size leave the sacs and pass directly to the alveolar capillaries. As a result of endothelial proliferation and thrombosis in these dilated vessels, 3 zones, frequently well defined, may be seen in them. Proximally there is fibrous tissue continuous with that in the intima of the patent muscular pulmonary artery. In early lesions this fibrous tissue is cellular; in late lesions it is acellular. There is a central zone of proliferative cellular endothelial tissue which often assumes a characteristic plexiform pattern in the sac so that this lesion might conveniently be termed the "plexiform lesion." It is the hallmark of grade 4. Distally, in the distended sac, there is frequently a thrombus, stimulated probably by the papilliferous endothelial proliferation. As the lesion ages, the fibrosis spreads through it and finally replaces it (fig. 5*b* and *c*).

2. Veinlike Branches of Hypertrophied Muscular Pulmonary Arteries (fig. 6*a* and *b*). Muscular pulmonary arteries, which show medial hypertrophy and gross intimal fibroelastosis, give rise to thin-walled branches resembling veins, and these end as capillaries in the alveolar walls. Such veinlike structures usually emerge from the parent muscular pulmonary artery proximal to the point of obstruction and have been considered to represent a collateral pulmonary blood flow to the alveolar walls.[10] In the present cases, however, some of these dilated branches were found to arise from vessels with patent lumens.

3. The Angiomatoid Lesion (fig. 6*c*). In this instance muscular pulmonary arteries showing intimal fibrosis give rise to thin-walled vessels. The latter show peculiar vascular formations within their lumens. Cross sections of these formations show them to be composed of a series of thin blood vascular structures having walls of simple elastic tissue. These intraluminal vessels leave the arteries containing them to form a surrounding angiomatoid mass. Since the angiomatoid structure surrounds the dilated vessel it lies somewhat removed from the muscular artery that gave rise to the dilated branch. The angiomatoid lesion itself gives rise to many thin-walled vessels which ramify in all directions in the pulmonary substance to supply capillaries to the air spaces. If the intimate connection between parent muscular pulmonary artery, thin-walled branch, and angiomatoid lesion is not established by examination of serial sections, one may mistakenly consider the angiomatoid mass to be an independ-

than the corresponding lesion shown in figure 4*c*. From a 24 year old woman with patent ductus arteriosus. × 75. *c*. Grade 5. Section of a muscular pulmonary artery showing an old plexiform lesion. Gross elastosis of the internal elastic membrane of the artery has developed and the proliferated tissue in the dilated sac has been totally replaced by fibroelastic tissue. From a 20 year old woman with patent ductus arteriosus. × 75. *d*. Transverse section of a parent muscular pulmonary artery that shows hypertrophy of the media and intimal fibrosis, and one of its branches which is dilated and almost totally occluded by fibrous tissue showing a so-called onion-layering configuration. From a 27 year old woman with a common atrioventricular canal with no subvalvular communication. × 75.

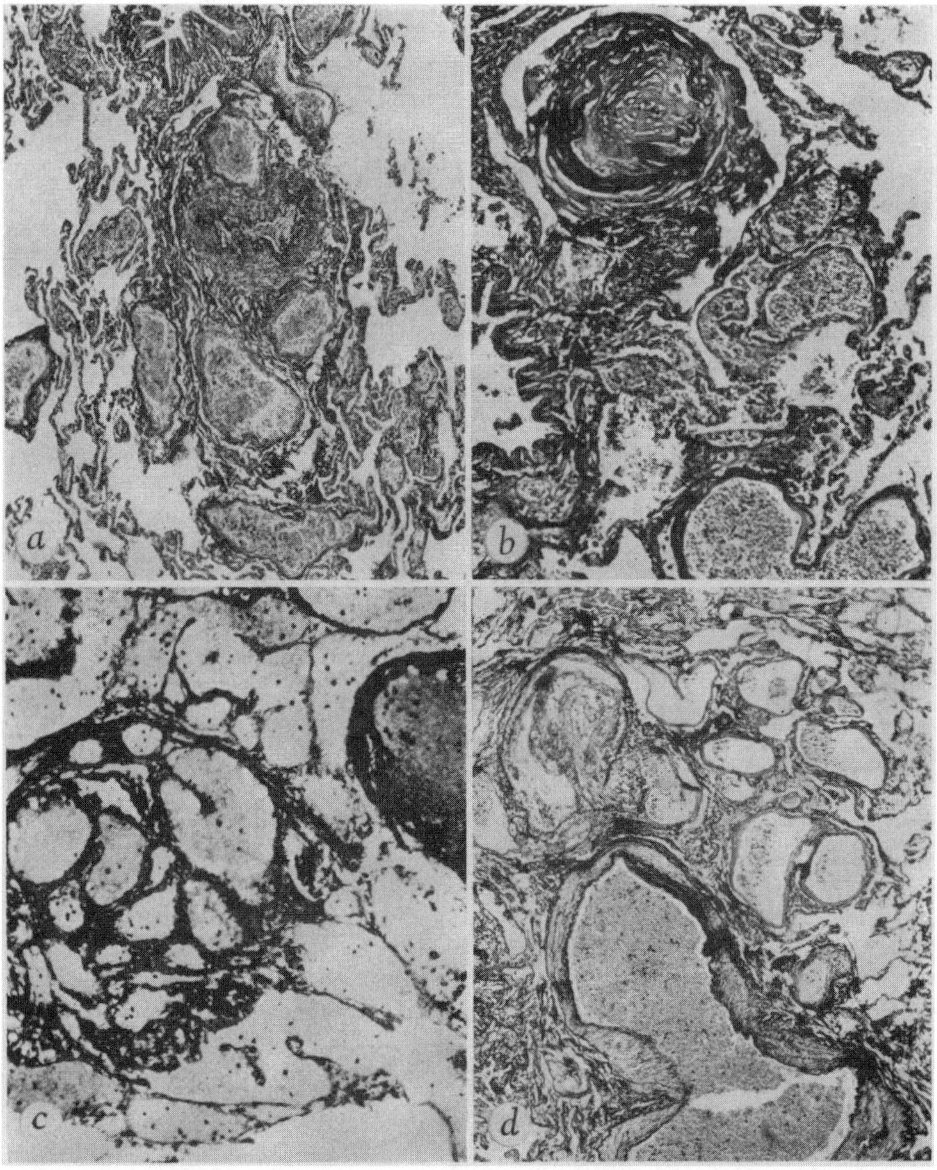

FIG. 6. *a.* Grade 5. Transverse section of a muscular pulmonary artery, showing hypertrophy of the media and obliteration of its lumen by fibrous tissue, and its veinlike, thin-walled branches which cluster characteristically around the parent vessel. From a 24 year old woman with patent ductus arteriosus. × 75. *b.* Grade 5. Transverse section of a muscular pulmonary artery, showing obliteration of its lumen by dense acellular fibrous tissue. There are gross thickening and elastosis of the internal elastic lamina. The media is largely replaced by fibrous tissue. Clustering near the artery are its thin-walled, veinlike branches. From a 24 year old woman with patent ductus arteriosus. × 75. *c.* Grade 5. Transverse section of the angiomatoid form of dilatation lesion. The thin-walled, veinlike branches of a hypertrophied muscular pulmonary artery form an angiomatoid mass in the lungs. From a 32 year old woman with ventricular septal defect. × 100. *d.* Grade 5. Section of lung showing a cavernous dilatation lesion. Cavernous thin-walled branches, one showing endothelial proliferation, are seen clustered around the hypertrophied parent muscular pulmonary artery. From a 24 year old woman with patent ductus arteriosus. × 75.

ent separate entity in the pulmonary substance. The diameter of this structure approaches 1 mm.

4. The Cavernous Lesion (fig. 6*d*). Intermediate between the 2 forms previously described, this form of lesion is composed of cavernous vessels that arise from a thin-walled branch of a muscular pulmonary artery.

All 4 types of dilatation lesions are simply severer and more complex expressions, in the pulmonary arterioles and the smallest pulmonary arteries, of the generalized dilatation that occurs throughout the pulmonary vasculature as a result of the chronically high vascular resistance. Early generalized dilatation is seen in association with the predominantly hypertrophied vessels in a late stage of grade 3, but the appearance of the plexiform lesion is the hallmark of grade 4. In severer examples of grade 4 and in grade 5, the generalized dilatation of pulmonary arteries also proceeds. Grade 5 is characterized by the appearance of many veinlike branches of hypertrophied arteries and the angiomatoid and cavernous lesions, all of which give rise to sinusoid-like vessels throughout the pulmonary substance. The angiomatoid lesion is rare and was not seen in the Mayo Clinic series reported herein. The case included for the sake of completion was one of ventricular septal defect with pulmonary hypertension studied by one of us (D.H.) in association with Dr. D. B. Brewer at the University of Birmingham, England.

Grade 4. Stage of Progressive Generalized Arterial Dilatation with the Formation of Complex Dilatation Lesions (Plexiform Lesions). In grade 4 the emphasis in the histologic picture shifts from predominant signs of hypertrophy to those of dilatation. Both the muscular pulmonary arteries and the arterioles show progression in the dilatation that was seen to originate in the late stages of grade 3. The hallmark of grade 4 is the appearance of the plexiform type of dilatation lesions described in the previous section (fig. 5*a*, *b*, and *c*). In addition, segments of branches of hypertrophied arteries dilate (fig. 5*d*).

A distended sac is formed but the wall consists of a thin but still recognizable arterial structure with a distinct media and internal and external elastic laminae. In such dilated arteries intimal thickening may occur. The intimal tissue is fibrous and the fibers and nuclei tend to be arranged concentrically to give a so-called onion-layering appearance (fig. 5*d*). Beyond the distended segment of the artery, the normal arterial structure is resumed with superadded intimal fibrosis. Many muscular arteries and arterioles in grades 4 to 6 still show marked increase in medial thickness with gross intimal fibroelastosis.

Grade 5. Stage of Chronic Dilatation with Formation of Numerous Dilatation Lesions and Pulmonary Hemosiderosis. This is the stage of dilatation in which the vessels show medial as well as intimal fibrosis and look rigidly dilated. The media of the muscular pulmonary arteries and the arterioles is thinned and fibrosed and in many cases, the intimal fibrous tissue is acellular or even hyaline. In grades 3 and 4, as previously mentioned, arteries with intimal fibrosis show small endothelium-lined channels as the remainder of a lumen all but obliterated by fibrous tissue. In grade 5, however, some of such central channels are widely dilated and surrounded by what appears to be a rigid tube consisting largely of acellular fibrous tissue and a thin, fibrosed media. The arterioles show similar dilatation with fibrosis.

All 4 types of dilatation lesions, that is, the simple veinlike branch of the hypertensive muscular pulmonary artery, the plexiform lesion, the angiomatoid lesion, and the cavernous lesion, are commonly found and give rise to thin-walled, dilated vessels which ramify throughout the lung rendering it highly vascular and filled with sinusoid-like vessels (fig. 7*a*). It would seem that these are fragile and either burst or allow diapedesis of blood, for foci of hemosiderosin-containing macrophages are scattered throughout the lung in grade 5 (fig. 7*b*).

Grade 6. Stage of Necrotizing Arteritis. Few patients with hypertensive pulmonary vascular disease ever show the vascular

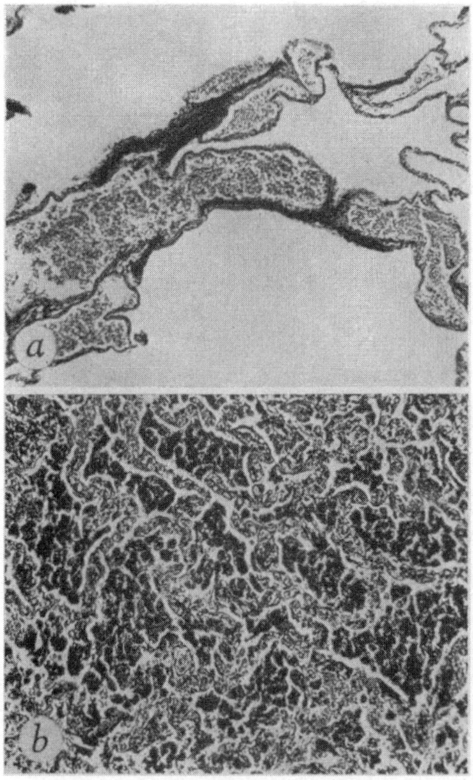

FIG. 7. *a*. Transverse section of a lung showing one of the numerous thin-walled, sinusoid-like vessels which are branches of hypertrophied muscular arteries and which characterize grade 5. From a 21 year old man with ventricular septal defect. ×100. *b*. Grade 5. Transverse section of lung showing the pulmonary hemosiderosis which results from bleeding from thin-walled vessels as shown in figure 7*a*. From a 23 year old man with idiopathic pulmonary hypertension. ×100.

changes in the lung that we include in grade 6. In fact, the only patient of the present series who had this group of histologic features characterized by necrotizing arteritis in its acute and subacute forms was suffering from an unusual form of atrial septal defect associated with pulmonary hypertension from birth. There is justification for including this case at this point to illustrate this grade of hypertensive pulmonary vascular disease, for necrotizing arteritis has been observed in ventricular septal defect with pulmonary hypertension.[11] It is at the same time necessary to point out that necrotizing arteritis is uncommonly reported with any type of cardiac disease; a few cases have been reported in mitral stenosis associated with pulmonary hypertension and in idiopathic pulmonary hypertension.

In necrotizing arteritis some of the muscular pulmonary arteries show acute fibrinoid necrosis. In sections stained with hematoxylin and eosin the muscle has a glassy appearance with loss of nuclei or has smudgy staining. The typical staining reactions for fibrinoid are given. Vessels show complete necrosis of muscle with a surrounding inflammatory reaction consisting predominantly of polymorphonuclear leukocytes with a few eosinophils.

Many arteries exhibit the subacute or healing phase of arteritis with masses of young basophilic cellular fibrous tissue replacing the dead muscle and forming masses in proximity to it in the intima and adventitia. The masses of fibrous tissue in the intima appear to be reactive to the underlying medial necrosis and, being basophilic and cellular, form a striking contrast to the pre-existing intimal fibrous tissue, which is eosinophilic and relatively acellular. Thrombosis is found in some arteries, many of which show gross hypertrophy. The granulation tissue may replace as much as a third of the media (fig. 8*a*) and in exceptional circumstances, the entire vessel may be replaced by granulation tissue, only the elastic laminae retaining partial integrity (fig. 8*b*). In other cases, only a small arc of the media is replaced by fibrous tissue so that, lying between the bulbous expansions in the intima and adventitia, this gives the lesion a dumbbell shape. In the connecting bar of fibrous tissue in the media, the long axes of the fibroblast nuclei are radial.

The adventitial masses of granulation tissue lie around branches of arteriolar size, and endothelium-lined channels of this magnitude enter the fibrotic region but become lost therein. Many small capillaries, lined by plump endothelium and containing erythrocytes, ramify throughout the basophilic fibrous tissue and a few thin-walled vessels leave this tissue to lie between the old acellular collagen fibers of the adventitia (fig. 8*a* to *d*).

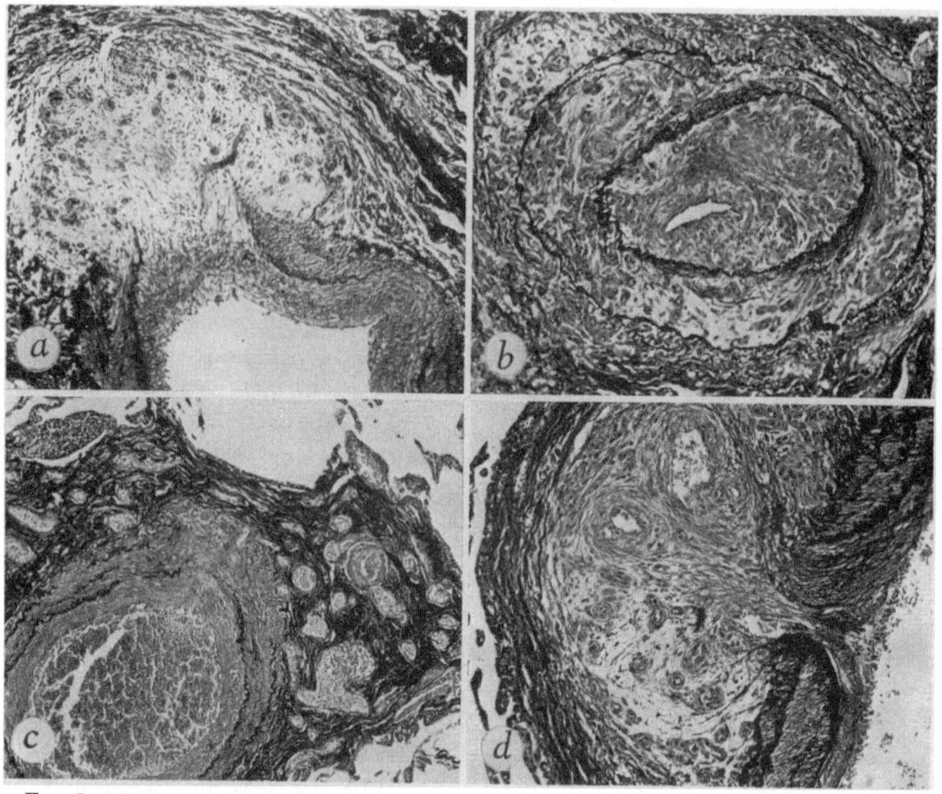

FIG. 8. All photomicrographs are transverse sections of muscular pulmonary arteries from a 27 year old man who had an unusual form of atrial septal defect considered to have been associated with pulmonary hypertension from birth. All show subacute necrotizing arteritis, a change pathognomonic of grade 6. *a.* Section showing medial hypertrophy, acellular intimal fibrosis, and replacement of an arc of the media by granulation tissue with prominent blood capillaries. × 75. *b.* Granulation tissue replaces the media, forms masses in the adventitia, and almost totally occludes the lumen. In this instance the entire media had undergone necrosis × 175. *c.* Prominent, dilated vessels in the adventitia that are derived from granulation tissue. × 125. *d.* The mass of granulation tissue in the adventitia is around the origin of an arteriole, indicating this to be a site of predilection for necrotizing arteritis. The granulation tissue contains large capillary vessels. × 100.

This imparts a characteristic picture of many dilated veinlike structures lying scattered throughout the adventitia of the larger muscular pulmonary arteries (fig. 8*c*).

The site of masses of adventitial fibrous tissue lying around branches of the muscular pulmonary arteries again suggests that the junction of artery and arteriole is a site of predilection for arteritis just as has been found for intimal fibrosis and the so-called dilatation lesions (fig. 8*d*).

Grade 1 in Atrial Septal Defect. In atrial septal defect, and those other forms of congenital heart disease characterized by the presence of high pulmonary blood flow over a prolonged period prior to the onset of pulmonary hypertension, the structural changes in grade 1 differ from those seen in ventricular septal defect. Initially, before the onset of pulmonary hypertension, the pulmonary arterioles are lined by a single elastic lamina as in the normal person.

Both they and the small muscular pulmonary arteries are widely dilated. Even at this stage where the pulmonary arterial blood pressure is normal or only slightly elevated, the pulmonary veins are the site of pronounced, intimal acellular fibrosis. This

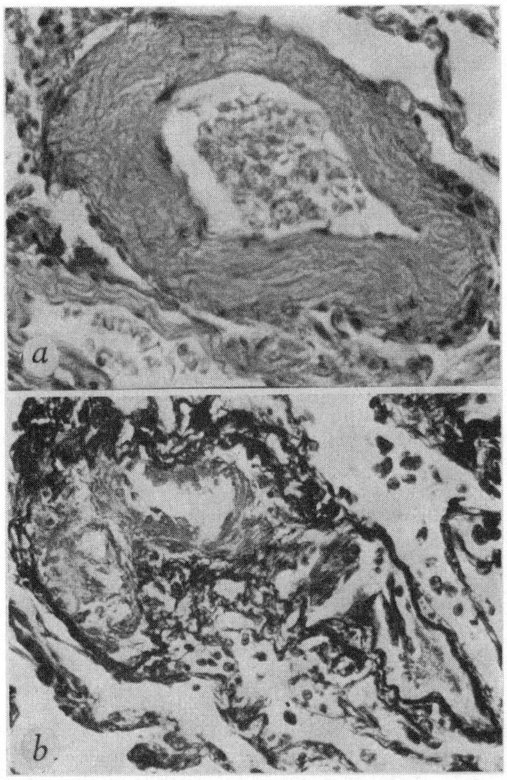

FIG. 9. *a.* Transverse section of a pulmonary vein showing severe acellular intimal fibrosis. From a 50 year old man with atrial septal defect and mitral stenosis. The lesion is characteristic for cases of atrial septal defect. The existing mitral stenosis is considered of incidental significance as regards this lesion. × 365. *b.* Grade 1. Atrial septal defect type. Oblique section of a dilated arteriole showing endothelial proliferation. The arteriole has no muscular media. From a 34 year old man with atrial septal defect and moderate pulmonary hypertension. × 250.

venous intimal change remains characteristic of atrial septal defect with all grades of changes in the pulmonary arteries (fig. 9*a*).

Associated with the onset of pulmonary hypertension is a pronounced cellular endothelial reaction in the arterioles and the smallest muscular pulmonary arteries, so that vascular occlusion by intimal proliferation appears to be the origin of the increased pulmonary vascular resistance (fig. 9*b*). Once pulmonary hypertension is established, a distinct muscular media forms in the arterioles and there is hypertrophy of the media of the muscular pulmonary arteries. These histologic features are the same as those seen in hypertensive pulmonary vascular disease, grade 2, associated with ventricular septal defect, and from this point the progression of structural changes is identical with that already described.

SUMMARY

Progressive histologic changes occur in the media and intima of pulmonary arteries and arterioles in the presence of chronic elevation of pulmonary artery blood pressure complicating congenital septal defects. This progression is so stereotyped as to allow a division of the structural effects of the hypertension into 6 grades. The classification is based on the study of lungs from 67 patients having congenital heart disease, and 2 having idiopathic pulmonary hypertension. Pulmonary arterial hypertension was demonstrated at cardiac catheterization in 55 instances and was inferred from the clinical and pathologic features in 9 others. The classification is as follows:

Grade 1. In large ventricular septal defect and wide patent ductus arteriosus: medial hypertrophy in arteries and arterioles; no intimal changes. In atrial septal defect: cellular, intimal proliferation in the smallest muscular arteries and the arterioles; intimal fibrosis in pulmonary veins.

Grade 2. Medial hypertrophy; cellular intimal proliferation.

Grade 3. Medial hypertrophy; intimal fibrosis; early generalized vascular dilatation in severe instances.

Grade 4. Progressive generalized vascular dilatation and occlusion by intimal fibrosis and fibroelastosis. Appearance of the plexiform lesions, which are one form of the complex dilatation lesions that occur in the pulmonary arterioles and the smaller muscular pulmonary arteries.

Grade 5. Appearance of the other "dilatation lesions," including veinlike branches of hypertrophied muscular arteries, cavernous lesions, and angiomatoid lesions; highly vascular lung due to veinlike arterial branches; pulmonary hemosiderosis.

Grade 6. Necrotizing arteritis.

SUMMARIO IN INTERLINGUA

Progressive alterationes histologic occurre in le tunicas medie e intime del arterias e arteriolas pulmonar in le presentia de elevation chronic del pression de sanguine pulmono-arterial que complica congenite defectos septal. Iste phenomeno es si stereotype que nos pote divider le effectos structural del hypertension in 6 grados successive. Lor definition es basate super le studio del pulmones de 67 patientes con congenite morbo cardiac e de 2 con idiopathic hypertension pulmonar. Hypertension pulmono-arterial esseva demonstrate per catheterisation cardiac in 55 casos e esseva presumite super le base de observationes clinic e pathologic in 9 alteres. Le classification es le sequente:

Grado 1. In casos de grande defectos ventriculo-septal e de marcate patente ducto arteriose: Hypertrophia medial in le arterias e arteriolas; nulle alterationes del intima.– In casos de defecto atrio-septal: Proliferation cellular del intima in le plus micre arterias muscular e in le arteriolas; fibrose intimal in le venas pulmonar.

Grado 2. Hypertrophia medial; proliferation cellular del intima.

Grado 3. Hypertrophia medial; fibrose intimal; precoce generalisate dilatation vascular in casos grave.

Grado 4. Progressive dilatation vascular generalisate e occlusion per fibrose e fibroelastose intimal. Apparition del lesiones plexiforme, le quales representa un del formas del complexe lesiones de dilatation occurrente in le arteriolas pulmonar e in le minor arterias pulmonar muscular.

Grado 5. Apparition del altere "lesiones de dilatation," incluse brancas venoide de hypertrophiate arterias muscular, lesiones cavernose, e lesiones angiomatoide; pulmon altemente vascularisate in consequentia del venoide brancas arterial; hemosiderosis pulmonar.

Grado 6. Arteritis necrotisante.

REFERENCES

1. HEATH, D., HELMHOLZ, H. F., JR., BURCHELL, H. B., DUSHANE, J. W., AND EDWARDS, J. E.: Graded pulmonary vascular changes and hemodynamic findings in cases of atrial and ventricular septal defect and patent ductus arteriosus. Unpublished data.
2. —, —, —, —, KIRKLIN, J. W., AND EDWARDS, J. E.: Relation between structural changes in the small pulmonary arteries and the reversibility of pulmonary hypertension following closure of ventricular and atrial septal defects. Unpublished data.
3. —, WOOD, E. H., DUSHANE, J. W., AND EDWARDS, J. E.: The relation of age and blood pressure to atheroma in the pulmonary arteries and thoracic aorta in congenital heart disease. Unpublished data.
4. —, —, —, AND —: The structure of the pulmonary trunk at different ages and in cases of pulmonary hypertension and pulmonary stenosis. J. Path. & Bact. In press.
5. EDWARDS, J. E.: The Lewis A. Conner memorial lecture. Functional pathology of the pulmonary vascular tree in congenital cardiac disease. Circulation. **15**: 164, 1957.
6. HEATH, D., AND WHITAKER, W.: The pulmonary vessels in mitral stenosis. J. Path. & Bact. **70**: 291, 1955.
7. WADE, G., AND BALL, J.: Unexplained pulmonary hypertension. Quart. J. Med. **26**: 83, 1957.
8. HEATH, D., AND BEST, P. V.: The tunica media of the arteries of the lung in pulmonary hypertension. J. Path. & Bact. **76**: 165, 1958.
9. BRENNER, O.: Pathology of vessels of pulmonary circulation. Arch. Int. Med. **56**: 211; 457; 724; 976; 1189, 1935.
10. BREWER, D. B.: Fibrous occlusion and anastomosis of the pulmonary vessels in a case of pulmonary hypertension associated with patent ductus arteriosus. J. Path. & Bact. **70**: 299, 1955.
11. OLD, J. W., AND RUSSELL, W. O.: Necrotizing pulmonary arteritis occurring with congenital heart disease (Eisenmenger complex). Report of case with necropsy. Am. J. Path. **26**: 789, 1950.

Functional Pathology of the Pulmonary Vascular Tree in Congenital Cardiac Disease

The Pathology of Hypertensive Pulmonary Vascular Disease

Marc Pritzker, M.D.

In 1958 Jesse Edwards and a group of other young luminaries in the then nascent field of pediatric cardiology and cardiac surgery began a series of publications that defined the histological changes in the pulmonary arteries of 67 children with congenital cardiac shunts. From their observations they created taxonomy of histologic lesions that have come to be known as the "Heath Edwards Classification." Subsequent studies using this classification have importantly correlated pathology, hemodynamics and surgical outcomes.

Yet, these seminal studies were not the sometimes-desiccated descriptions of anatomical variants that pathologists not infrequently published, but "living" documents that were in retrospect some of the first outcome studies in modern medicine. These papers had the effect of personalizing medicine by correlating anatomical, hemodynamic and surgical outcome data, thereby allowing for avoidance of interventions where the outcome was predictably poor and encouraging intervention where successful results changed life and fostered the sometimes revolutionary, sometimes incremental insights upon which much of contemporary pediatric cardiology is based.

Never mind that the correlations were imperfect or the receiver operating curves, if constructed, would not be perfect. Surgery at the time carried high risks. The catherization of the pulmonary circulation was in its infancy, subject to wide methodological and technical variation. Angiograms, ultrasound, CT scanning and MRI were hardly dreams of the future. Surgical decisions were made based on rudimentary hemodynamic data, natural history studies of uncorrected lesions as frequently reviewed in retrospect from the pathologist's table, careful physical examination and a good measure of hope. The technology available for intra-cardiac corrections was limited to children of a certain size, and that meant a longer history of exposure to high flows and subsequently high pressures, which in retrospect distorted some of the data.

Never mind that the Heath-Edwards classification created suggested a sequential involvement of and progression through the various arterial layers and stages of disease. This taxonomy focused our attention in an orderly anatomic way at a time when descriptions of pulmonary hypertensive pathology were sporadic and few in number. By creating a consistent anatomic foundation, it allowed those of us in the field to focus on the evolutions in vascular biology and physiology that could be of use in a disease that had no consistent therapies and a dismal prognosis until such focus allowed for determination of vasoactive substances emanating from the vascular wall. Low levels of prostacyclin and nitric oxide, and high levels of endothelin would eventually be augmented or antagonized by new synthetic substances derived from the fruits of systems biology.

By providing an early focus on the distinct anatomies of the intimal and medial layers, the Edwards papers would in effect change a dismal disease of short survival ("2.5 years from diagnosis to death") into an increasingly manageable disease with long-term survival prospects. Never mind that a taxonomy derived from a series of young patients with flow induced pulmonary hypertension imperfectly fit the increasingly diverse universe of disease and pathologies subsequently recognized as having pulmonary arterial hypertension as a core manifestation. Given what we have learned about the redundancies, diversities and convergences of biologic systems, it seems only natural that many roads lead to pulmonary hypertensive pathology, and that different routes do not always demonstrate the exact same scenery.

As I sit writing about the wonderful order and insights to which this platform taxonomy gave rise, I write on every other line of a legal pad to allow for the liberal cutting and pasting all of us of a certain age learned in the basement of Miller Hospital. Off would come his bow tie, up would go his sleeves, the glue bottle would be brought close, and the scissors drawn from the drawer. Not infrequently a comment would come about the only things that he liked better than writing a paper with a student; time with his beloved family and fishing. Then would come the furious editing via the Edwards cut and paste method to which Microsoft, and we whom he trained, owe a great debt.

Much as he crafted our papers, he crafted our careers, providing bold opportunities to meet the existing and soon to be cardiovascular legends of the time. I vividly remember as a fellow encountering Jesse talking with Braunwald, Cooley and Burchell at an AHA meeting. As I passed, Jesse grabbed my sleeve and dragged me into the circle, interrupting the conversation to tell all about a "wonderful" paper I had written. In retrospect it concerned a massive anti-phospholipid antibody mediated thrombosis of the aortic valve in a patient with lupus. I doubt that Braunwald and Cooley cared, but there I was in a comfortable position between Edwards and Burchell, two great teachers and subsequent friends and colleagues, who molded my outlook, thinking and career.

As my teacher, friend, mentor, scholar and exemplar of uncommon kindness and humility in the face of such enormous talent, Jesse modeled all that was good and noble in our profession while providing us with an intellectual underpinnings and personal inspiration upon which much of modern cardiology is predicated.

Clinical Studies

The Developmental Complex of "Parachute Mitral Valve," Supravalvular Ring of Left Atrium, Subaortic Stenosis, and Coarctation of Aorta*

JOHN D. SHONE, M.B., ROBERT D. SELLERS, M.D., RAY C. ANDERSON, M.D., PAUL ADAMS, JR., M.D., C. WALTON LILLEHEI, M.D., F.A.C.C. *and* JESSE E. EDWARDS, M.D.

Minneapolis, Minnesota

IN THE course of studies on the pathology of obstructive anomalies of the left side of the heart, it became apparent that there was a tendency for four obstructive, or potentially obstructive conditions to coexist. These anomalies were a "parachute" deformity of the mitral valve, supravalvular ring of the left atrium, subaortic stenosis and aortic coarctation (Fig. 1).

In the 8 cases reported herein, 2 exhibited all four conditions; in the remaining 6 cases, at least two of these anomalies coexisted. This suggested that the four anomalies formed a developmental complex, the former 2 cases representing the complex in its complete form and the latter 6 cases representing *formes frustes*. In individual cases certain of these anomalies, although present, were not sufficiently developed to cause significant obstruction (Table I).

The primary purpose of this report is to define the individual cardiac anomalies that form this complex, and to indicate what combination was present in each of the 8 cases. Brief reference will be made to the clinical manifestations.

DEFINITION OF THE ANOMALIES OF THE COMPLEX

Parachute Mitral Valve: The deformity called "parachute mitral valve" has the usual two mitral valvular leaflets and commissures but the chordae, instead of diverging to insert into two papillary muscles, converge to insert into one major papillary muscle (Fig. 2 and 3).

The term "parachute" in describing a deformity of an atrioventricular valve was first used, as far as we are aware, in a paper dealing with corrected transposition; one of us (J. E. E.) was co-author.[1] The analogy was suggested by the shape of the deformed valve. The mitral leaflets resemble the canopy of a parachute, the chordae, its shrouds or strings, and the papillary muscle, the harness. The chordae were often short and thick; this, coupled with their convergent papillary insertion, allowed little mobility of the leaflets. The effect was to create a stenotic mitral valve, since the leaflets were held in close apposition. The only effective communication between the left atrium and the left ventricle was through the interchordal spaces. In the aggregate, these spaces did not allow free egress of blood from the left atrium.

The parachute mitral valve, with its chordal and papillary attachments, resembles that localized anomaly termed a "double orifice of the mitral valve." In the latter condition an opening is present within one of the mitral valve leaflets and from the edges of this opening,

* From the Departments of Pediatrics, Surgery and Pathology, University of Minnesota, Minneapolis, Minnesota, and the Department of Pathology, The Charles T. Miller Hospital, St. Paul, Minnesota. This study was supported by Research Grant No. HE-5694 of the National Heart Institute, U. S. Public Health Service.

TABLE I
Summary of Pathologic Findings in 8 Cases Studied

Case	Sex	Age (yrs.)	Supravalvular ring	Sub-aortic stenosis	Parachute mitral	Aortic coarctation	Associated anomalies
1	M	2 3/12	Present & functionally significant	Present & functionally significant	Present & functionally significant	Present & functionally significant	Anomalous m. bundle R.V. L. S.V.C.
2	M	4	Present but not functionally significant	Present & functionally significant	Present & functionally significant	Present & functionally significant	Bicuspid aortic valve
3	F	13 7/12	Present but not functionally significant	Present & functionally significant	Present but not functionally significant	Present but not functionally significant	Aneurysm of memb. sept. c̄ L.V.-R.A. comm. Bicuspid A.V.
4	M	22 6/12	Present & functionally significant	Present & functionally significant	Present & functionally significant	Not present	V.S.D. Bicuspid P.V.
5	F	8/12	Present & functionally significant	Present & functionally significant	Not present	Not present	Short mitral chordae Endocard. scl. L.V. Bicusp. A.V.
6	M	7/12	Present but not functionally significant	Present but not functionally significant	Not present	Not present	Endocard. scl. in L.V.
7	F	3 4/12	Present but not functionally significant	Present but not functionally significant	Not present	Not present	V.S.D. Accessory pouch of Tricuspid valve
8	F	3/12	Present but not functionally significant	Present & functionally significant	Not present	Present & functionally significant	Bicuspid A.V.

Key: (cross-hatched) Present & functionally significant; (hatched) Present but not functionally significant; (blank) Not present.

R.V. = right ventricle; L.S.V.C. = left superior vena cava; L.V.-R.A. Comm. = left ventricular-right atrial communication; A.V. = aortic valve; V.S.D. = ventricular septal defect; P.V. = pulmonic valve; Endocard. scl. = endocardial sclerosis (fibroelastosis); L.V. = left ventricle.

chordae descend to the apex of an underlying papillary muscle.

In one instance (Case 3) two papillary muscles were present, but these were immediately adjacent to each other causing convergence of the chordae at their papillary insertions and yielding the effect of a single papillary muscle (Fig. 4).

Supravalvular Ring of the Left Atrium: This entity is a circumferential ridge of connective tissue that arises at the base of the atrial surfaces of the mitral leaflets and protrudes into the inlet of the mitral valve (Fig. 5.) In the fully developed deformity it acts as a stenosing, perforated diaphragm (Fig. 6A). In some cases it protrudes only slightly and causes no obstruction to the egress of blood from the left atrium (Fig. 6B).

A supravalvular ring was present in each of the 8 cases studied. It was obstructive in 3 and nonobstructive in the remainder.

Subaortic Stenosis: Two types of subaortic stenosis were observed—the muscular and the membranous. The muscular type is characterized by localized protrusion of hypertrophied ventricular septal tissue into the left ventricular outflow tract (Fig. 7B). This type was observed in 5 of the 8 cases studied.

The membranous type is characterized by circumferential endocardial thickening in the left ventricular outflow region (Fig. 7A). In some cases the two types co-existed. In 2 patients (Cases 3 and 4) the zone of endocardial thickening was sufficiently developed to cause obstruction on its own account.

Coarctation of the Aorta: Four of the cases studied had coarctation of the aorta of the clas-

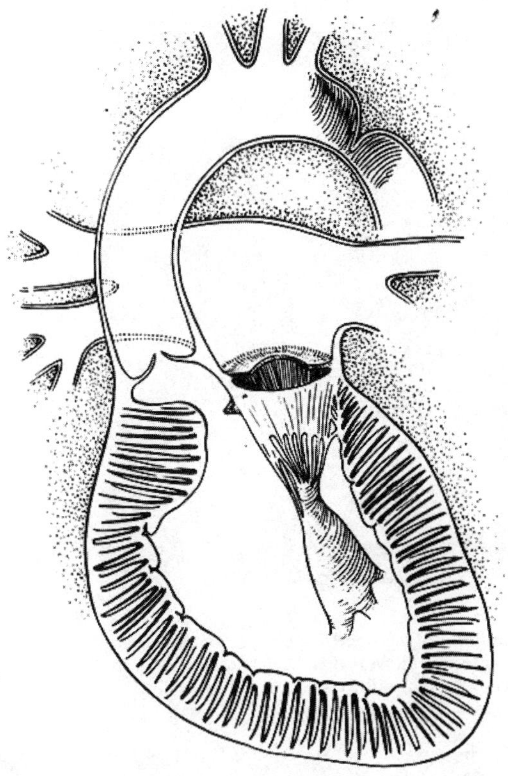

Fig. 1. Diagrammatic representation of the four obstructive anomalies forming the complex: supravalvular ring of left atrium, parachute mitral valve, subaortic stenosis and coarctation of aorta, in that order, according to the direction of flow of blood.

sic type,[2] being located at the junction of the arch and the descending aorta (Fig. 8). In 3 cases the obstruction was significant.

Clinical Manifestations

Review of the clinical records of the 8 cases showed that the multiplicity of obstructive lesions usually was not suspected clinically and that the clinical manifestations in each case were complex and varied. A brief analysis of the clinical features in relation to the pathologic findings in each case will serve to emphasize the problems involved in clinical diagnosis.

Electrocardiograms were available in 7 of the 8 cases. Although no specific pattern diagnostic of the complex could be identified, tracings from 6* of the cases are presented in Figures 9 and 10 because they may prove useful for comparison in future cases.

Case Reports

Case 1. Boy, 2 years, 3 months. *Coarctation of the aorta; obstructive supravalvular ring of left atrium; parachute mitral valve; subaortic stenosis.* (Anomalous muscle bundle of right ventricle was also present.)

Recurrent bouts of congestive cardiac failure had occurred from the age of 5 weeks. "Anginal" attacks accompanied by tachycardia occurred from the age of 9 months. Coarctation of the aorta was resected at the age of 20 months. The child died when he was 2 years and 3 months old at the conclusion of an operation on the mitral valve.

* The electrocardiogram in Case 5 has been published by Rogers and associates.[3] (See footnote, Fig. 10.)

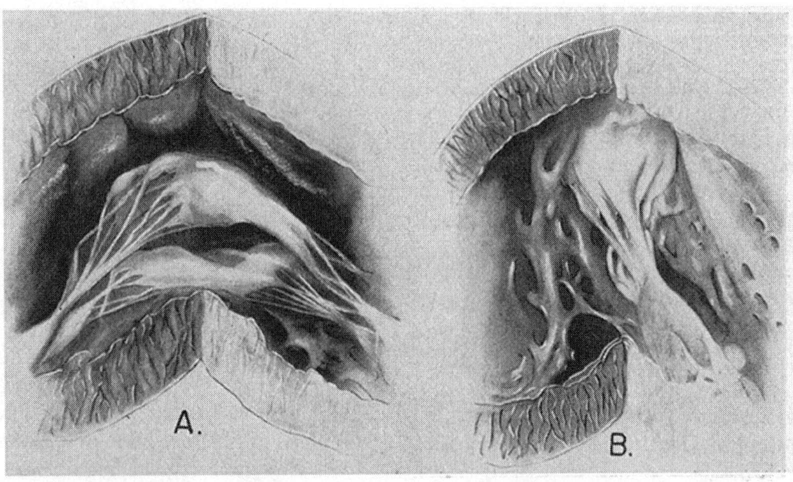

Fig. 2. Artist's representation of mitral valves viewed from below: A, the normal valve. B, the parachute mitral valve. In the normal, the chordae diverge as they insert into two papillary muscles. In the parachute valve, they converge to insert into the single papillary muscle.

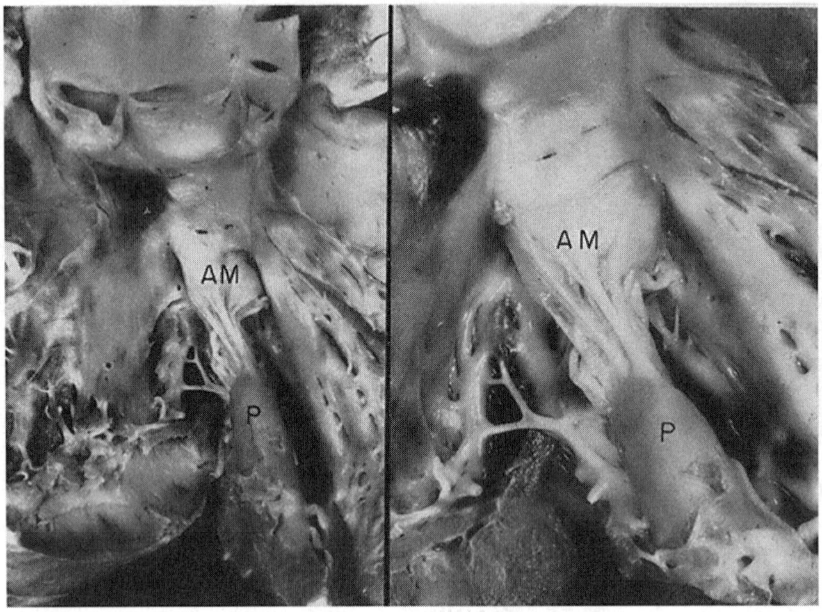

A B

FIG. 3. Case 1. Parachute mitral valve. A, interior of left ventricle and the opened aortic valve. Mitral valve viewed from below. The anterior mitral leaflet (AM) hides most of the posterior leaflet. Chordae of both leaflets insert into the solitary papillary muscle (P). B, close-up view of the mitral valve in the same perspective as shown in A.

The physical findings prior to resection of the coarctation included a grade 3/6 harsh systolic murmur maximal at the third left intercostal space parasternally. There were *radiologic findings* of enlargement of the left atrium, right ventricle and ascending aorta, together with coarctation of aorta. Coarctation of aorta and endocardial sclerosis were the primary diagnoses. Following resection of the coarctation, the appearance of an apical diastolic rumbling murmur and evidence of pulmonary hypertension provided strong evidence of obstruction at the mitral valve. There was also a harsh, ejection-type systolic murmur at the aortic area.

Angiocardiography showed prolonged opacification of the enlarged left atrium. The *electrocardiogram* indicated right axis deviation ($\hat{A}QRS + 150°$) and evidence of biventricular hypertrophy with right ventricular systolic (pressure) overload (Fig. 9A). With a preoperative diagnosis of congenital mitral stenosis, a second operation was done.

At operation it was difficult clearly to relate the structures to those of the normal mitral valve. There was no effective means of overcoming the obvious obstruction, and the patient died at the conclusion of the operation. The parachute mitral valve is seen in Figure 3, the supravalvular ring of left atrium in Figure 6.

Comment: The aortic coarctation initially dominated the clinical picture. It was only

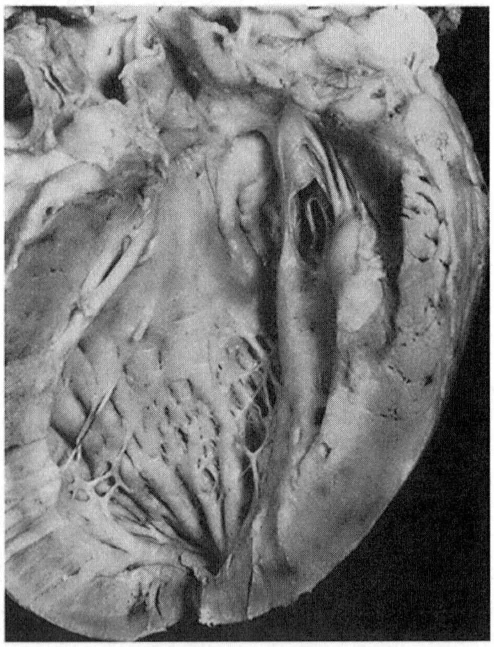

FIG. 4. Case 3. Partial type of parachute mitral valve. Interior of left ventricle. Two papillary muscles are present, but these are immediately adjacent to each other.

A

B

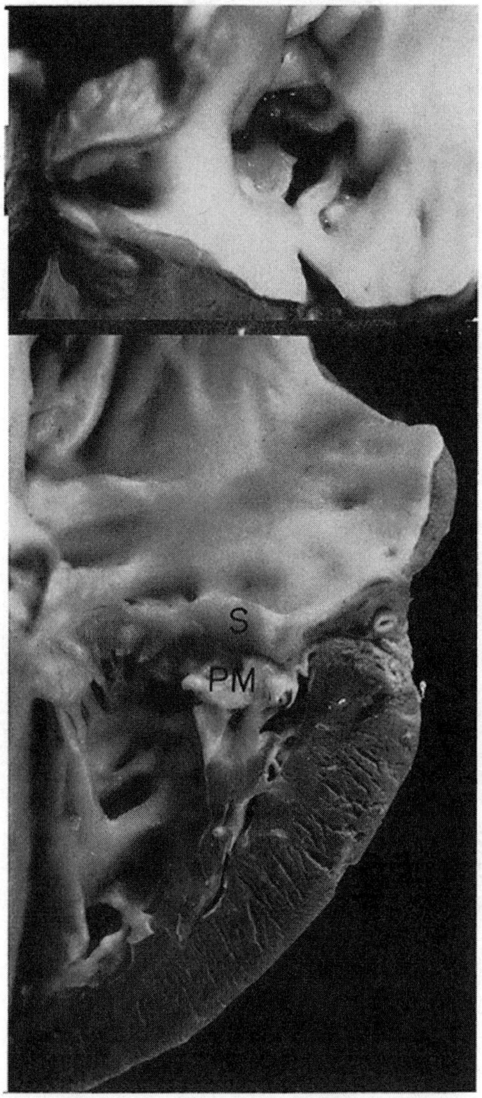

FIG. 5. Case 5. Obstructive supravalvular ring of left atrium. A, the ring is viewed from above. This is stenotic and hides the mitral valve, which lies below. The left atrial endocardium is thick, and the wall is hypertrophied. B, longitudinal section through the posterior leaflet of the mitral valve and adjacent structures. Immediately above the posterior leaflet (PM) is the supravalvular ring (S), which attaches to the base of the mitral valve and protrudes into the cavity of the lowermost portion of the left atrium. (From Rogers and associates[3] with permission of C. V. Mosby Co.)

after resection of the coarctation that obstruction at the mitral valve became clearly apparent. The subaortic stenosis found at necropsy had not been recognized clinically.

CASE 2. Boy, 4 years. *Coarctation of the aorta; parachute mitral valve; subaortic stenosis; nonobstructive supravalvular ring of left atrium.* (A congenitally bicuspid aortic valve was also present.)

During infancy recurrent attacks of congestive cardiac failure and failure to thrive were noted. Sweating and dyspnea occurred during feedings. A coarctation of aorta was resected at the age of 10 months. The child died at 4 years of age, two days after an operation upon the mitral valve.

The physical findings prior to resection of the coarctation included a grade 2/6 systolic murmur at the second left intercostal space and left sternal border. The second sound was single and accentuated at the pulmonic area. The femoral arterial pulsations were diminished. Blood pressures were 100 mm. Hg systolic in the arms, and 70 mm. Hg in the legs. There were *radiologic findings* of moderate cardiomegaly with right ventricular enlargement and of severe left atrial enlargement with normal pulmonary vascular markings. The *electrocardiogram* showed right axis deviation (ÂQRS + 100°) and right ventricular hypertrophy of the systolic (pressure) overload type.

After resection of the coarctation the cardiomegaly and left atrial enlargement persisted, and evidence of obstruction at the mitral valve was indicated by progressive right ventricular enlargement, pulmonary arterial hypertension and the appearance of an apical diastolic rumbling murmur (first detected at age 2 years and 4 months). At age 3 years and 6 months a systolic thrill in the suprasternal notch was noted. The electrocardiogram taken immediately before the second operation is shown in Figure 9B.

With the preoperative diagnosis of congenital mitral stenosis, the patient underwent operation. As in Case 1, it was difficult to identify clearly the components of the mitral valve. However, a commissurotomy was performed, which appeared to relieve the obstruction. The patient died two days after operation.

Comment: In this patient too the aortic coarctation dominated the clinical picture initially. Obstruction at the mitral valve became apparent only after resection of the coarctation. No left ventricular angiocardiographic studies were performed, and the subaortic stenosis found at necropsy was not diagnosed clinically.

CASE 3.* Girl, 13 years and 7 months. *Subaortic stenosis; modified parachute mitral valve; mild aortic coarctation; nonobstructive supravalvular ring of left atrium.* (Also present were a perforated aneurysm of membranous septum with left ventricular-right atrial communication and a mildly stenotic, congenitally bicuspid aortic valve.)

A systolic cardiac murmur was detected when the child was 2 years old, but she was asymptomatic apart from fatigue on exertion. Complete atrio-

* Certain aspects of this case have been reported by Drs. M. J. Levy, R. De Wall and C. W. Lillehei.

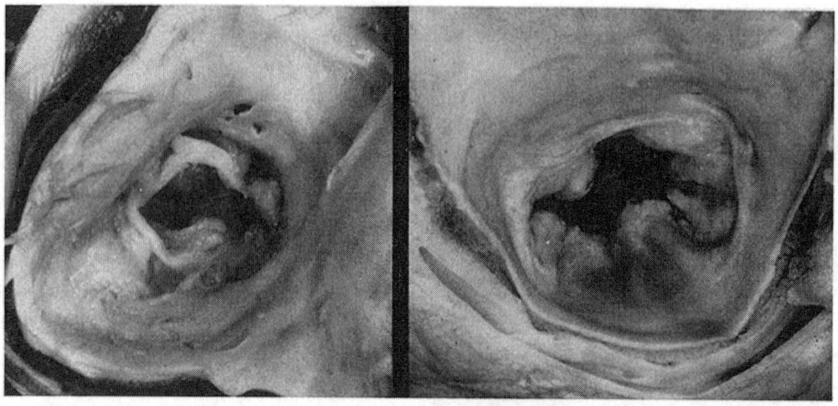

FIG. 6. Supravalvular ring of left atrium in 2 cases, obstructive in one and nonobstructive in the other. A, Case 1. The ring is viewed from the left atrial aspect. It has been partially incised at operation. The mitral valve is obscured beneath it. B, Case 3. The ring between the left atrium and the mitral valve is evident though nonobstructive. A considerable portion of the mitral valve is readily apparent from this perspective.

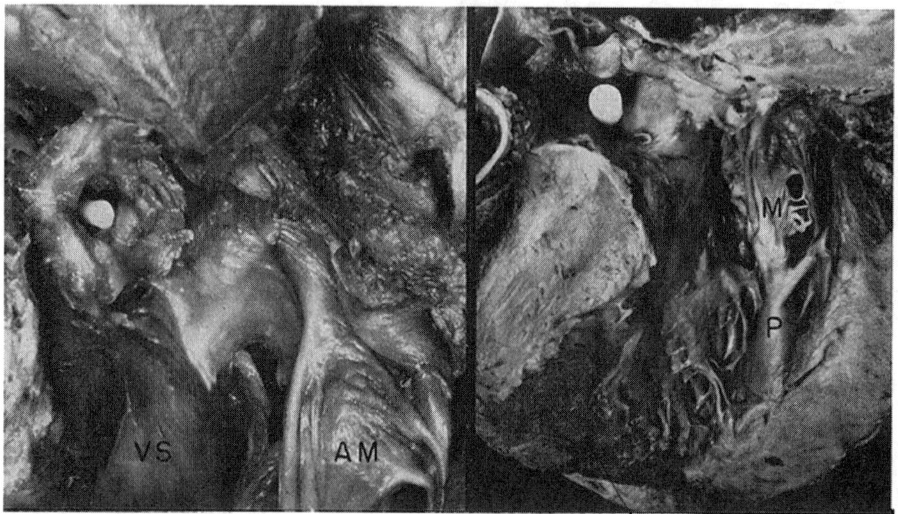

FIG. 7. Case 4. Subaortic stenosis and parachute mitral valve. Ventricular septal defect above the subaortic stenosis is also present. A, the basal aspect of the interior of the left ventricle is exposed. Above a prominent bulge of the ventricular septum (VS) is a fibrous collar which encircles the outflow tract of the left ventricle. The orifice through this area (probe) is severely narrowed. A portion of the anterior leaflet of the mitral valve (AM) is also apparent. B, after the subaortic collar of fibrous tissue illustrated in (A) was excised and the aortic valve opened, the interior of the left ventricle and corresponding valve are exposed. The probe lies in the ventricular septal defect which, in turn, is superior to the zone of subaortic stenosis. The mitral valve (M) shows a typical parachute deformity wherein all the chordae insert into the solitary papillary muscle (P). A stenotic supravalvular ring of the left atrium was also present in this case.

ventricular block occurred following a cardiac operation at the age of 13 years. Death occurred in a Stokes-Adams attack 7 months later.

The physical findings from the age of 4 years included a precordial systolic thrill with a grade 3 to 4/6 harsh, systolic murmur maximal at the third and fourth left intercostal spaces parasternally and at the aortic area. A short, apical diastolic murmur was heard by some observers. The pulmonic component of the second sound was not accentuated. The femoral arterial pulsations were diminished. Blood pressure in the right arm was 120/85 mm. Hg and

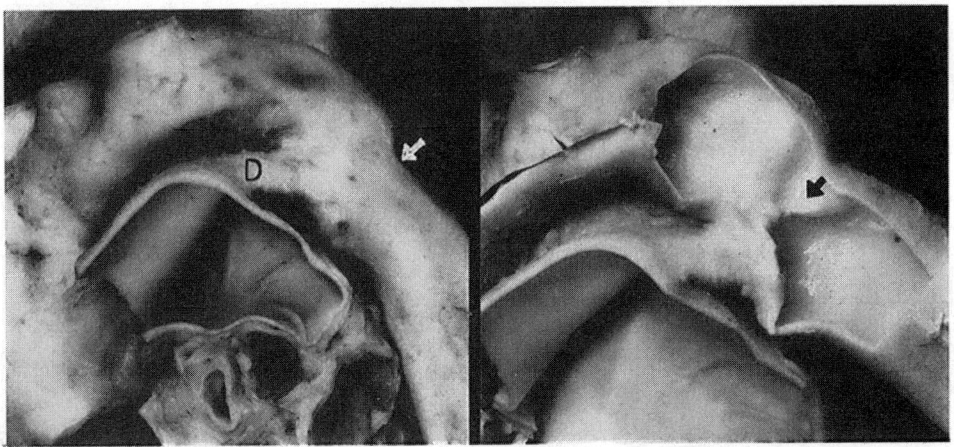

A B

FIG. 8. Case 3. Mild coarctation of aorta. A, external view of the thoracic aorta. Opposite the ligamentum arteriosum (D) is a concave deformity (point of arrow) involving the superior aspect of the aorta. B, interior of the junction of the aortic arch and upper descending aorta. Corresponding to the concavity involving the exterior of the aorta shown in (A) is a curtain-like infolding (point of arrow) which protrudes into the lumen of the aorta. This lesion, characteristic of coarctation of the aorta, caused mild obstruction in this particular instance.

in the right leg, 100/80 mm. Hg. There were *radiologic findings* of marked left atrial enlargement, biventricular enlargement and increased pulmonary vascular markings. The *electrocardiogram* showed a normal QRS axis in the frontal plane and evidence of left ventricular preponderance.

At the age of 6 years the primary diagnoses were ventricular septal defect and mild coarctation of aorta; pulmonary valvular stenosis was considered. At the age of 8 years the patient exhibited a thrill in the suprasternal notch. This was accompanied by a harsh, ejection-type aortic murmur with the paradoxic splitting of the second sound and systolic ejection click of aortic valvular stenosis. The short, apical diastolic murmur was considered that of relative mitral stenosis resulting from the intracardiac left-to-right shunt. At the age of 13 years *selective left ventriculographic studies* revealed a left ventricular-right atrial communication, aortic valvular and subaortic stenosis, and mild aortic coarctation. The electrocardiogram taken prior to operation appears in Figure 9C.

At operation the left ventricular-right atrial communication was closed, and commissurotomy of a stenotic aortic valve and resection of an area of subaortic stenosis were performed. Following operation, the patient exhibited persistent complete atrioventricular dissociation. She died suddenly 7 months following the operation.

Comment: The intracardiac left ventricular-right atrial communication dominated the clinical picture initially. Subsequently definite signs of aortic stenosis developed.

While each of the four anomalies of this complex was represented in this case, one was of major significance. This was the subaortic stenosis which, in conjunction with the left ventricular-right atrial communication, is considered to have been the essential problem to the patient.

In this case, there were two papillary muscles for the mitral valve. Their close apposition contributed to a partial type of parachute deformity (Fig. 4). The nonobstructive ring of left atrium is seen in Figure 6 and the mild aortic coarctation in Figure 8.

CASE 4. Man, 22 years and 6 months. *Parachute mitral valve; obstructive supravalvular ring of left atrium; subaortic stenosis.* (Also present were a ventricular septal defect and a nonstenotic bicuspid pulmonary valve.)

A systolic murmur was noted at the age of 15 months. Dyspnea and fatigue, associated with mild cyanosis of the lips, occurred on exertion. Following an intracardiac operation, the patient died at the age of 22 years and 6 months.

The physical findings at the age of 13 years included left precordial bulging and a systolic thrill accompanied by a grade 4/6, harsh, pansystolic murmur maximal in the third left intercostal space. There was a variable, short, apical diastolic murmur. The second sounds at the aortic and pulmonic areas were equal in intensity. There were *radiologic findings* of left atrial and right ventricular enlargement with increased pulmonary vascular markings. The main pulmonary arterial segment was, however, of normal size. The *electrocardiogram* showed right axis de-

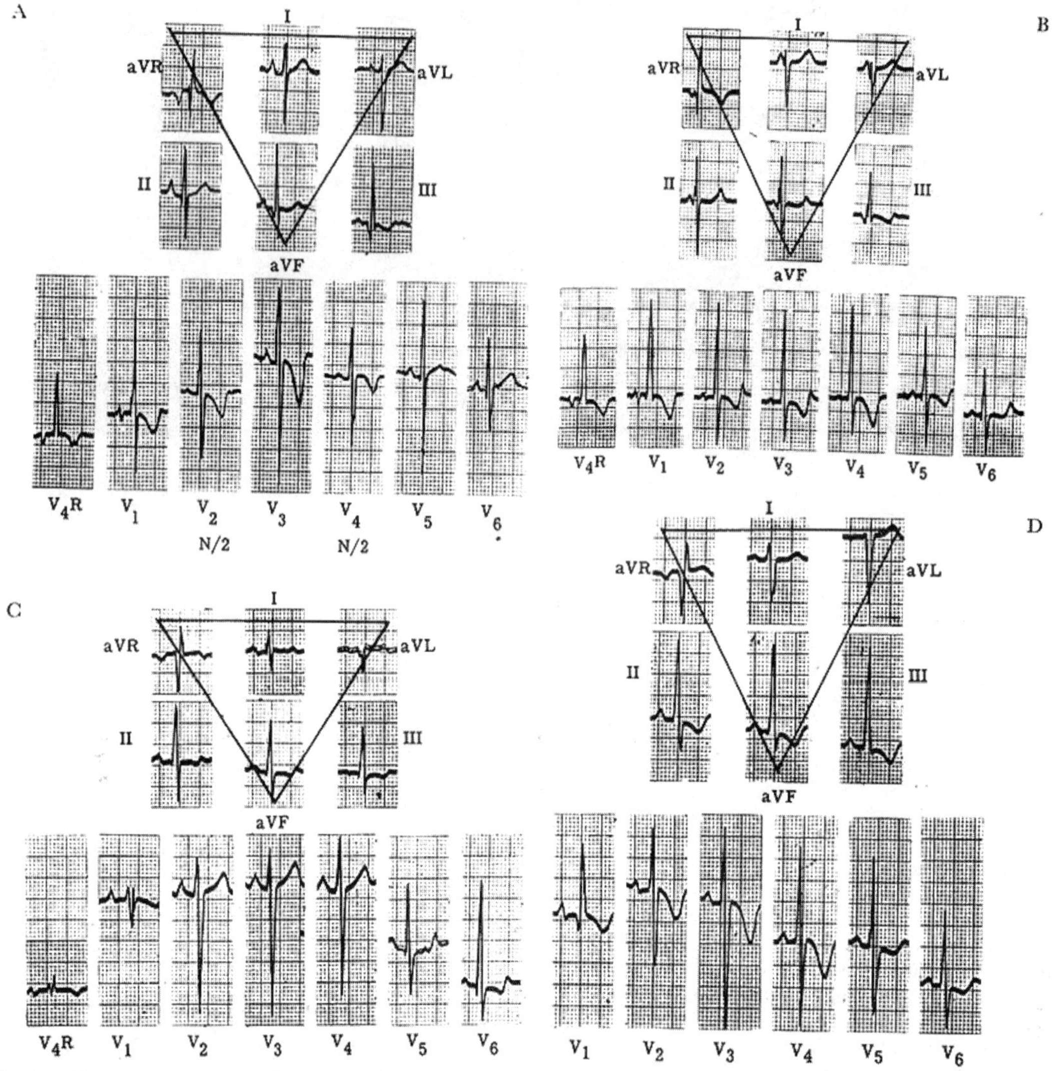

FIG. 9. Electrocardiograms in four cases of the complex. The functionally significant cardiac malformations are indicated. A, Case 1. Supravalvular ring of the left atrium, subaortic stenosis, parachute mitral valve and coarctation of aorta. B, Case 2. Subaortic stenosis, parachute mitral valve and coarctation of aorta. C, Case 3. Subaortic stenosis, left ventricular-right atrial communication. D, Case 4. Parachute mitral valve, supravalvular ring of left atrium, subaortic stenosis and ventricular septal defect.

viation and evidence of right ventricular hypertrophy of the systolic (pressure) overload type.

At this time the diagnoses considered were ventricular septal defect with right-to-left shunt, and a ventricular septal defect with coexisting pulmonic valvular stenosis and patent ductus arteriosus.

Subsequent examination and further studies were refused until the patient was admitted to the hospital at the age of approximately 22 years in a state of congestive cardiac failure associated with atrial flutter. At that time mild cyanosis and digital clubbing were noted. Studies revealed evidence of a large ventricular septal defect with bidirectional shunt (oxygen saturation of systemic arterial blood 84 per cent), pulmonary arterial hypertension and obstruction at the level of the mitral valve. The electrocardiogram taken prior to operation appears in Figure 9D.

At operation the ventricular septal defect was closed. A mitral commissurotomy was done in an attempt to relieve stenosis of the mitral valve. Irreversible ventricular fibrillation occurred, and after intensive efforts at resuscitation the operation was terminated.

Comment: The clinical picture during childhood was dominated by the ventricular septal

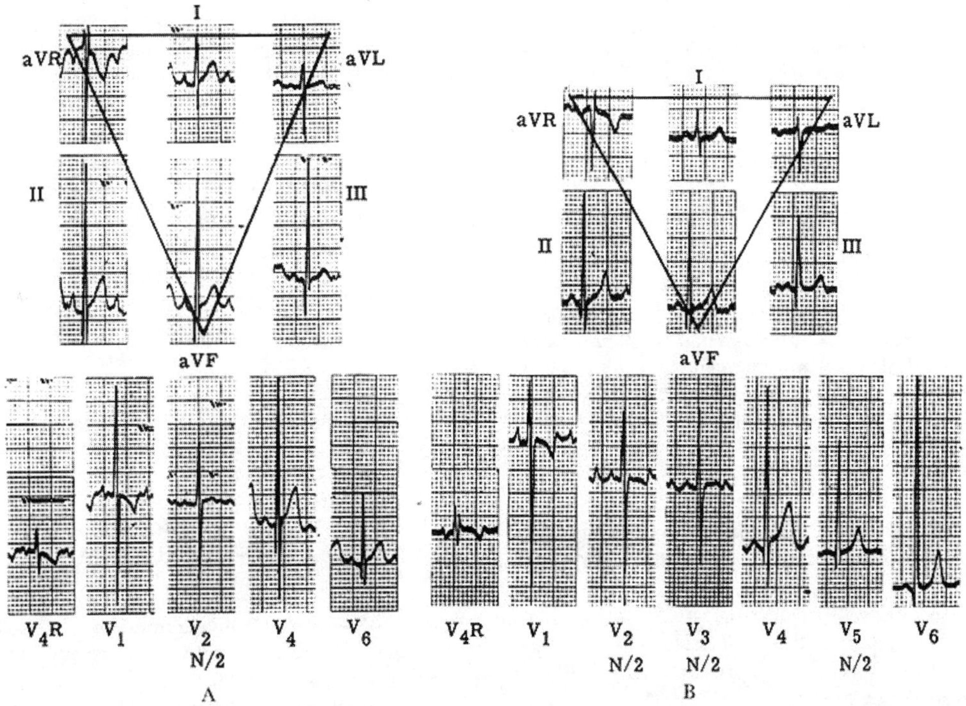

FIG. 10. Electrocardiograms in 2 cases of the complex. Functionally significant cardiac malformations are indicated. A, Case 6. None. B, Case 7. Ventricular septal defect. [Note: The electrocardiogram in Case 5 (supravalvular ring of left atrium and subaortic stenosis) showed a normal QRS frontal plane axis (+100°) with evidence of right ventricular hypertrophy of the systolic (pressure) overload type.[3] No electrocardiogram was obtained in Case 8.]

defect and the associated pulmonary hypertension. When the patient was an adult, studies revealed obstruction at the mitral valve. The severe subaortic stenosis, located proximal to the large ventricular septal defect, was not suspected during life. Had left ventricular studies been done, it is conceivable that this significant anomaly (Fig. 7) might have been identified. The mitral stenosis recognized clinically was the manifestation of a fully developed parachute mitral valve and an obstructive supravalvular ring of the left atrium (Fig. 7). The commissurotomy had not significantly altered the problem of mitral obstruction, so far as could be ascertained from the necropsy. No aortic coarctation was present.

CASE 5.* Female baby, 8 months. *Obstructive supravalvular ring of left atrium; subaortic stenosis.* (Also present were focal endocardial sclerosis of left ventricle with shortening of mitral chordae tendineae and a congenitally bicuspid aortic valve.)

At the age of 6 months the patient was admitted to the hospital with fever. Rales over the upper right hemithorax were noted. A grade 3 systolic murmur was heard over the precordium and transmitted to the back. At the age of 7 months she was readmitted because of cyanosis, dyspnea and fever. No cardiac murmur was identified at that time. The second sound was accentuated at the pulmonic area. There were radiologic findings of severe cardiomegaly, a globular-shaped heart and a rounded, upturned cardiac apex. The electrocardiogram showed right axis deviation and evidence of right ventricular hypertrophy of the systolic (pressure) overload type.[3] Despite treatment the child died at the age of 8 months in a state of congestive cardiac failure.

* Case previously reported by Rogers and associates.[3]

Comment: The most prominent features at necropsy were those of an obstructive supravalvular ring of the left atrium (Fig. 5). The other manifestation of the complex which is the subject of this report was muscular subaortic stenosis. While the mitral chordae were abnormally short and thick, there were two normally located papillary muscles.

The thoracic aorta was not available for study in the specimen at our disposal. It is of interest that a bicuspid aortic valve was present. Although this anomaly has a close developmental association with aortic coarctation, it is recognized that a bicuspid aortic valve may occur in the absence of coarctation.

CASE 6. Male baby, 7 months. *Nonobstructive supravalvular ring of left atrium; mild subaortic stenosis.* (Endocardial sclerosis of left ventricle was also present.)

Hospitalized at the age of 5 months for a persistent periumbilical infection and portal venous obstruction, this patient exhibited a grade 2 to 3/6 systolic murmur at the left sternal border. Roentgenograms showed the cardiac size to be at the upper limits of normal, with increased pulmonary vascular markings. There was mild left atrial enlargement. The electrocardiogram showed a normal axis with equivocal evidence of right atrial enlargement and biventricular hypertrophy (Fig. 10A). The patient developed intractable pneumonia and died at the age of 7 months.

Comment: The two components of the complex, a nonstenotic supravalvular ring of the left atrium and a mild membranous subaortic stenosis, probably were of no functional significance in this patient. Their coexistence suggests that this case represents a mild *forme fruste* of the complex.

CASE 7. Girl, 3 years and 4 months. *Mild subaortic stenosis; nonobstructive supravalvular ring of left atrium.* (Also present were a ventricular septal defect and an accessory pouch of tricuspid valve.)

This patient was first seen at 11 months of age because of a problem in feeding and growth. Following percutaneous left ventricular puncture at the age of 3 years and 4 months, cardiac tamponade developed, and the patient died.

The physical findings at the age of 11 months included minimal precordial bulging, a systolic thrill and grade 4/6 harsh systolic murmur maximal in the fourth left intercostal space at the left sternal border. There was a grade 1 to 2 apical rumbling diastolic murmur. The first sound was accentuated at the mitral area. The pulmonic component of the second sound was accentuated. There were *roentgenographic findings* of marked left atrial enlargement, biventricular enlargement and increased pulmonary vascular markings. The *electrocardiogram* showed a normal QRS axis in the frontal plane and evidence of biventricular hypertrophy with left ventricular preponderance. The primary diagnosis was a ventricular septal defect with pulmonary hypertension. Congenital mitral stenosis was considered also.

Studies at the age of 17 months showed evidence of a large left-to-right shunt at ventricular level with severe pulmonary hypertension. Subsequently the physical signs and the electrocardiogram remained essentially unchanged, although increasing cardiomegaly was evident roentgenographically.

At the age of 3 years and 4 months the patient died of cardiac tamponade which followed percutaneous left ventriculography. The electrocardiogram taken prior to these final studies is shown in Figure 10B.

Comment: Though mitral valvular obstruction was considered clinically, no functionally significant disease at this site was demonstrated.

The rudiments of a supravalvular ring of the left atrium which were found, however, are interesting within the framework of this report. Subaortic stenosis of mild muscular type was the only other manifestation of the complex. This case as was Case 6, is a *forme fruste* of the complex.

CASE 8. Female baby, $3^1/_2$ months. *Coarctation of the aorta; nonobstructive supravalvular ring of left atrium; subaortic stenosis.* (A congenitally bicuspid aortic valve was also present.)

This patient was examined at 1 month of age when no murmur was noted. At $3^1/_2$ months of age the patient was admitted to the hospital in congestive cardiac failure. A precordial systolic murmur was noted. Roentgenographic examination revealed cardiomegaly. Before an electrocardiogram could be obtained, the patient died.

Comment: Although this patient died before adequate clinical evaluation could be made, examination of the necropsy specimen suggested that coarctation was the most clinically significant portion of the complex. It is conceivable that the subaortic stenosis would not have been noted prior to relief of the coarctation. The supravalvular ring was rudimentary.

DISCUSSION

Among the 8 cases reported as belonging to a developmental complex with four obstructive anomalies of the left side of the heart, a supravalvular ring of the left atrium was present in each. It was obstructive in 3 and nonobstructive in 5. Parachute deformity of the mitral valve was observed in 4 cases. In these, the malformation contributed to (2 cases) or was the sole cause (1 case) of mitral stenosis. In the fourth instance, the deformity was of the partial type and caused no obstruction (Case 3).

Subaortic stenosis present in each of the 8 cases caused significant obstruction to left ventricular outflow in 6 cases, but in only one was this condition suspected clinically. Usually the effects of this malformation were masked by the effects of the coexisting anomaly or anomalies. It is of interest that in the 2 cases in which significant coarctation and mitral obstruction coexisted, the latter condition was not readily apparent clinically until the coarctation was resected.

Re-evaluation of previously reported cases of congenital mitral stenosis would probably reveal some examples of parachute deformity of the mitral valve. Swan and associates[4] reported "an unusual form of mitral stenosis" in which the mitral valve was described as "unique." "The chordae tendineae were shortened and fused to form a funnel-shaped, firmly fixed, almost solid sheet of tissue that obstructed the orifice of the valve. This anomalous septum was perforated by fifteen, scattered slit-like openings . . . . The blended chordae were inserted into the apex of the solitary, double-bellied papillary muscle, which arose from the posterior wall of the left ventricle . . . . Viewed from above, the mitral valve resembled the inverted top of a salt shaker." This description, together with Figure 3 of Swan's paper, suggests that this was an example of the parachute mitral valve. This illustration suggests that a supravalvular ring of the left atrium was also present, but this point cannot be established with certainty.

Edwards[5] reported the case of a 4 day old child with mitral stenosis, ventricular septal defect, tubular hypoplasia of the aortic arch and a bicuspid aortic valve. The features of a parachute mitral valve are shown in his Figure VI-91.

In our basic presentation, we emphasized the association of the parachute deformity of the mitral valve with other obstructive anomalies in the arterial side of the heart and vascular system. In the cases herein reported the basic arrangement of the heart and great vessels was normal. In addition to this series, we have observed one example of a parachute deformity of the mitral valve in a 6 month old child with complete transposition of the great vessels and obstruction of the left ventricular outflow tract. In this case the subpulmonary (left ventricular outflow) obstruction was caused by a membranous ring and anomalous attachment of the anterior mitral leaflet to the ventricular septum. Since two of the four anomalies of the developmental complex described herein were present, it is possible that this case with complete transposition belongs to the complex here reported.

Parachute deformity of an atrioventricular valve may be observed in corrected transposition. Among 14 specimens with corrected transposition Schiebler and associates[1] observed this deformity once in the left atrioventricular valve and once in the right. El Sayed and associates[6] illustrated an incomplete form of this anomaly in the right atrioventricular valve of a heart with corrected transposition.

We have had the opportunity of re-examining the specimen in the case reported by Manubens and associates.[7] Significant obstruction at the mitral valve was caused by a supravalvular ring of the left atrium, but none of the other elements of the complex was present. Coexisting malformations were a ventricular septal defect, extreme dextroposition of the aorta and infundibular stenosis of the right ventricle.

An operation on the mitral valve was performed in 3 of our cases, each having significant obstruction caused both by a supravalvular ring of the left atrium and parachute deformity of the mitral valve. Mitral "commisurotomy" did not relieve the obstruction in any of these 3 cases and does not appear to offer a solution to this complicated problem.

Hypothetically, excision of a supravalvular ring should yield a satisfactory relief of obstruction from this cause. The most feasible method of overcoming the obstruction of a parachute deformity of the mitral valve would appear to be excision of the valve with insertion of a prosthesis.

SUMMARY

A developmental complex is described in which four obstructive anomalies of the left side of the heart and aorta coexist. These anomalies are (1) parachute mitral valve; (2) supravalvular ring of left atrium; (3) subaortic stenosis of either the muscular or membranous type; and (4) coarctation of the aorta.

Eight cases form the basis of this report. In 2 cases, each of the four anomalies was present; all of the other 6 cases represent partial forms of the complex, or *formes frustes*, in that only two or three of the anomalies were present.

The clinical picture is compounded of the effects of the several anomalies of the complex and of the frequent association with still other anomalies, including ventricular septal defect.

REFERENCES

1. SCHIEBLER, G. L., EDWARDS, J. E., BURCHELL, H. B., DUSHANE, J. W., ONGLEY, P. A. and WOOD, E. H. Congenital corrected transposition of the great vessels. A study of 33 cases. *Pediatrics (Suppl.)*, 27: 851, 1961.
2. EDWARDS, J. E., CHRISTENSEN, N. A., CLAGETT, O. T. and MCDONALD, J. R. Pathologic considerations in coarctation of the aorta. *Proc. Staff Meet. Mayo Clin.*, 23: 324, 1948.

3. ROGERS, H. M., WALDRON, B. R., MURPHEY, D. F. H. and EDWARDS, J. E. Supravalvular stenosing ring of left atrium in association with endocardial sclerosis (endocardial fibroelastosis) and mitral insufficiency. *Am. Heart J.*, 50: 777, 1955.
4. SWAN, H., TRAPNELL, J. M. and DENST, J. Congenital mitral stenosis and systemic right ventricle with associated pulmonary vascular changes frustrating surgical repair of patent ductus arteriosus and coarctation of the aorta. *Am. Heart J.*, 38: 914, 1949.
5. EDWARDS, J. E. Congenital malformations of the heart. In: GOULD, S. E. Pathology of the Heart, ed. 2, p. 388. Springfield, Ill., 1960. Charles C Thomas.
6. EL SAYED, H. et al. Corrected transposition of the great arterial trunks: surgical treatment of the associated defects. *J. Thoracic & Cardiovas. Surg.*, **44**: 443, 1962.
7. MANUBENS, R., KROVETZ, L. J. and ADAMS, P., JR. Supravalvular stenosing ring of the left atrium. *Am. Heart J.*, 60: 286, 1960.

The Developmental Complex of "Parachute Mitral Valve," Supravalvular Ring of Left Atrium, Subaoritc Stenosis, and Coarctation of Aorta

Kenneth L. Jue, M.D.

At a monthly Cardiac Pathological Correlation Conference conducted by Dr. Jesse Edwards in the 1960s, two cases were reviewed which had been referred from Edmonton, Canada, to the University of Minnesota for operative repair which was unsuccessful. Dr. John Shone, a cardiac fellow originally from Canada, was asked to review the unusual nature of the condition. It was amusingly thought appropriate for a Canadian fellow to review these cases from Edmonton. Dr. Shone observed the presence of two inlet and two outlet obstructions of the left ventricle. Six additional cases were observed from the Jesse Edwards Cardiac Registry at Miller Hospital in St. Paul, Minnesota, for a total of eight cases for study. In each case the inlet obstructions were represented by a supravalvar ring of the left atrium and a parachute mitral valve, while the two outlet obstructions consisted of subaortic stenosis and coarctation of the aorta. In only two instances were all four conditions present while formes frustes was present in the others. This constellation of conditions is now better known as Shone syndrome.

Recent observations have added to our knowledge concerning the entities that comprise this condition. Vaideeswas and associates have recently reported the pathologic findings in 24 cases of supravalvar ring of the mitral valve. They observed the presence of a ridge of connective tissue usually attached to or above the mitral valve annulus and protruding into the inlet of the mitral valve. Eight of the 24 cases (33 percent) were associated with the Shone complex and 16 were not. No difference was observed in the completeness or width of the supra-mitral ridge in those with or without the Shone complex. In seven cases (29 percent), circumferential or complete ridge were observed to be thick and fibrous with a tendency to be obstructive. In the remaining 70 percent of cases an incomplete ring was observed and was either continuous or discontinuous and either annular or suprannaular.

The second inlet obstruction of the left ventricle in the Shone syndrome is the parachute mitral valve. In the normal valve the chordae arise from the mitral valve to insert onto the papillary muscles. In this condition the chordae are foreshortened and thickened, and the interchordal spaces are compromised causing obstruction of blood flow from the left atrium to the left ventricle. In 1974, Rosenquist described a spectrum of mitral valve abnormalities associated with coarctation of the aortic with normally related great vessels and included the parachute mitral valve deformity. In a comprehensive study of 53 specimens he divided them into four categories. In the first three the coarctation of the aorta was associated with hypoplastic but otherwise normal mitral valve. The fourth category was coarctation of the aorta with associated mitral valve anomalies. This last group was further subdivided into cases with: (1) underdevelopment of the space between the papillary muscles which included fusion, separation and accessory muscle bundles, (2) underdevelopment of space between the papillary muscles and ventricular wall, which resulted in one or both muscles becoming indistinct from the left ventricular wall, and (3) attachment of the mitral valve orifice to only one papillary muscle resulting in the parachute mitral valve.

In 1977, Dr. Gittenberger-de Groot and colleagues of the Leiden Group described in 29 cases a condition simulating the parachute mitral valve which they termed the asymmetric mitral valve with two papillary muscles. In this condition usually the anterolateral papillary muscle is elongated with shortened of the chordal attachments to the mitral valve. A spectrum of shortening of the chordae is present so that in the severe cases the mitral valve appears to be directly attached to papillary muscle. This results in an eccentric and oblique orifice which becomes obstructive.

The two left ventricular outflow obstructive conditions include coarctation of the aorta which is paraductal in location with or without an associated patent ductus arteriosus. The other is a subaortic membrane which is usually fibromembrous and less commonly membranous only. Obstruction can be severe if addition to the above valvar stenosis is also present secondary to a bicuspid aortic valve.

Although the constellation of conditions which compromise the Shone syndrome were described more than 40 years ago, we still cannot determine the prognosis or the outcome of treatment. Operative series of this condition are difficult to find in the literature, but the general opinion is that the mortality rate is unsatisfactory with a poor long term prognosis. Bove and the group at the University of Michigan reviewed 30 consecutive patients with this condition between 1966 and 1989. The anatomic diagnoses included: (1) supravalvar ring of the left atrium in 22 patients, (2) mitral valve abnormalities including parachute mitral valve, fused chordae or single papillary muscle in 26 patients, (3) subaortic obstruction in 25 patients and membranous in 1 patient, and (4) coarctation of the aorta in 29 patients. In 19 cases all four conditions were present. Other associated conditions included bicuspid aortic valve in 19 and ventricular septal defect in 20. Operations included coarctation of the aorta repair in 28 patients, mitral valve repair or replacement in 11 patients, ventricular septal defect closure in eight patients, subaortic resection in eight patients, and complex left ventricular reconstruction or bypass in four patients. No operative mortalities were associated with the first operation but the mortality rose to 24 percent after the second operation.

I was a cardiac fellow at the University of Minnesota and worked with Dr. Edwards during my training in the pediatric cardiology and was a graduate of Miller Hospital basement where his registry was located. While a fellow we were taught how to describe cardiac conditions and the use of correct English when writing papers. I subsequently returned to central California and started a clinical pathological conference similar to the one developed by Dr. Edwards but in the Department of Pediatric Cardiology at the University of California in Los Angeles. I was able to utilize many of Dr. Edwards' teachings in this monthly conference, which I conducted for more than 30 years. As a fellow of Dr. Edwards I gained an abundance of scientific knowledge in cardiac pathology to enhance my career, but I also attained great insight into the importance of love of family and colleagues.

Termination of Left Superior Vena Cava in Left Atrium, Atrial Septal Defect, and Absence of Coronary Sinus

A Developmental Complex

By GUNAY RAGHIB, M.D., HERBERT D. RUTTENBERG, M.D., RAY C. ANDERSON, M.D., KURT AMPLATZ, M.D., PAUL ADAMS, JR., M.D., AND JESSE E. EDWARDS, M.D.

EXCLUSIVE of cases of congenital cardiac disease with asplenia[1] we have observed eight cases in which a persistent left superior vena cava terminated in the left atrium. Pathologic study in each of the five cases in which death occurred suggests that when a left superior vena cava joins the left atrium, this vascular anomaly is part of a developmental complex in which absence of the coronary sinus and a defect in the postero-inferior angle of the atrial septum are also a part.

The primary purpose of this communication is to define the individual cardiac anomalies that form this developmental syndrome. Reference is also made to the clinical, physiologic, radiologic, and developmental features.

Anatomic Characteristics

Study of the five cases in which specimens were available form the basis for the anatomic definitions to be given.

Persistent Left Superior Vena Cava Terminating in the Left Atrium

The left jugular venous system and left subclavian vein joined normally to form a large vein, the left superior vena cava. This large vein descended vertically, passing anterior to the aortic arch and to the left pulmonary hilus (fig. 1*a*). The vein terminated in the left atrium, between the left pulmonary veins, posteriorly, and the base of the left atrial appendage, anteriorly. The hemiazygos vein joined the left superior vena cava after arching over the left main bronchus in a mirror-image fashion to the junction of the azygos vein with the superior vena cava on the right side. In four cases, an innominate bridge between the two superior venae cavae was absent. In the fifth case (case 5), wherein the right superior vena cava was absent, the right innominate vein crossed the midline to terminate in the left superior vena cava.

Absent Coronary Sinus

In each of the cases studied, the coronary sinus was absent. The ostium of the left superior vena cava was in the left superior aspect of the left atrium between the base of the atrial appendage and the left superior pulmonary vein. Anteriorly and to the left of this ostium a valve-like structure was seen in three cases and a ridge in a fourth case. The cardiac veins drained individually into the corresponding atria.

Atrial Septal Defect

In three cases there were no malformations of the atrioventricular valves, while in two cases the atrioventricular valves showed clefts characteristic of those in persistent common atrioventricular canal.

In three cases without valvular deformities, the atrial septal defect exhibited certain characteristics, to be described. From the right atrial side (fig. 2*b* and *d*) the atrial septal defect was in the position normally occupied by the right atrial ostium of the coronary

From the Departments of Pediatrics, Radiology, and Pathology, University of Minnesota, Minneapolis, and the Department of Pathology, The Charles T. Miller Hospital, St. Paul, Minnesota.

Supported by Research Grant HE 5694 and Research Training Grant 5 T1 HE 5570 of the National Heart Institute, U. S. Public Health Service.

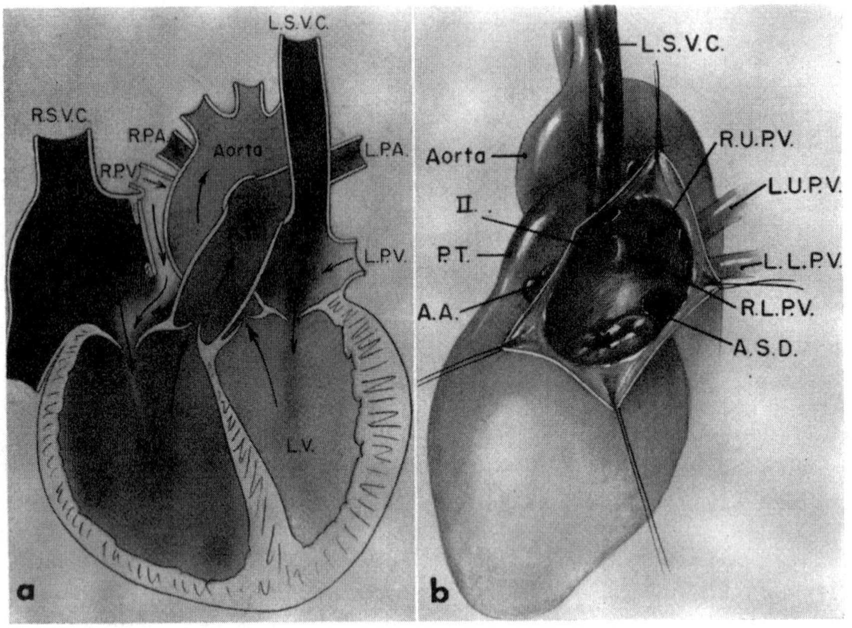

Figure 1

a. *Diagrammatic portrayal of the condition herein reported.* b. *Drawing of interior of the left atrium and the exterior of the left side of the heart and great vessels in the complex described. The atrial septal defect (A.S.D.) lies in the postero-inferior angle of the atrial septum above the posteromedial commissure of the mitral valve and is separated from the valve (M.) by a small amount of septal tissue. The region of the interatrial ostium secundum (II.) is normal. R.U.P.V. and R.L.P.V., right pulmonary veins; L.U.P.V. and L.L.P.V., left pulmonary veins; P.T., pulmonary trunk; L.S.V.C., left superior vena cava.*

sinus. From this view the size and position of the defect might simply suggest an enlarged ostium of a coronary sinus. The defect was located postero-inferiorly to the fossa ovalis, inferior and medial to the ostium of the inferior vena cava, and above the septal leaflet of the tricuspid valve. Some septal tissue lay between the atrial septal defect and the tricuspid valve. The inferior limb of the fossa ovalis separated the fossa ovalis from the atrial septal defect.

When viewed from the left atrial cavity (figs. 1*b*, 2*a* and *c*), the atrial septal defect was above the posteromedial commissure of the mitral valve, and septal tissue separated the defect from the mitral valve. The defect was bounded anteriorly, superiorly, and inferiorly by atrial septal tissue. Posteriorly, it was bounded by the posterior atrial wall.

The defect, as described, possesses three features that distinguish it from the atrial septal defect of persistent common atrioventricular canal. In the latter condition (fig. 3*a*), (1) the atrial septal defect is centered over the central portion of the cleft anterior mitral leaflet, (2) no septal tissue separates the atrial septal defect from the atrioventricular valves, and (3) septal tissue is present between the posterior atrial wall and the defect.

In contrast, the defect of the condition described (1) is centered over the posteromedial commissure of the mitral valve, (2) is separated from the atrioventricular valves by septal tissue, but (3) is not separated from the posterior atrial wall by septal tissue.

In two cases the AV valves showed clefts characteristic of those in persistent common atrioventricular canal. In these, the atrial septal defect was larger and had features different from the three cases in which no valvular malformations were present (fig. 3*b* and *c*). The atrial septal defect appeared to occupy in continuity the positions of both the defect considered specific for the entity being described and the atrial septal defect of classical persistent common atrioventricular canal.

Clinical Observations

The essential clinical findings in the five patients who died and in the three living patients are given in tabular form in table 1.

Initially, when the five patients on whom necropsy was eventually done were studied clinically, no suspicion of connection of a vena cava with the left atrium was entertained. In one patient (case 3), however, cardiac catheterization initially had been attempted through a left antecubital vein. The cardiac catheter was advanced into the

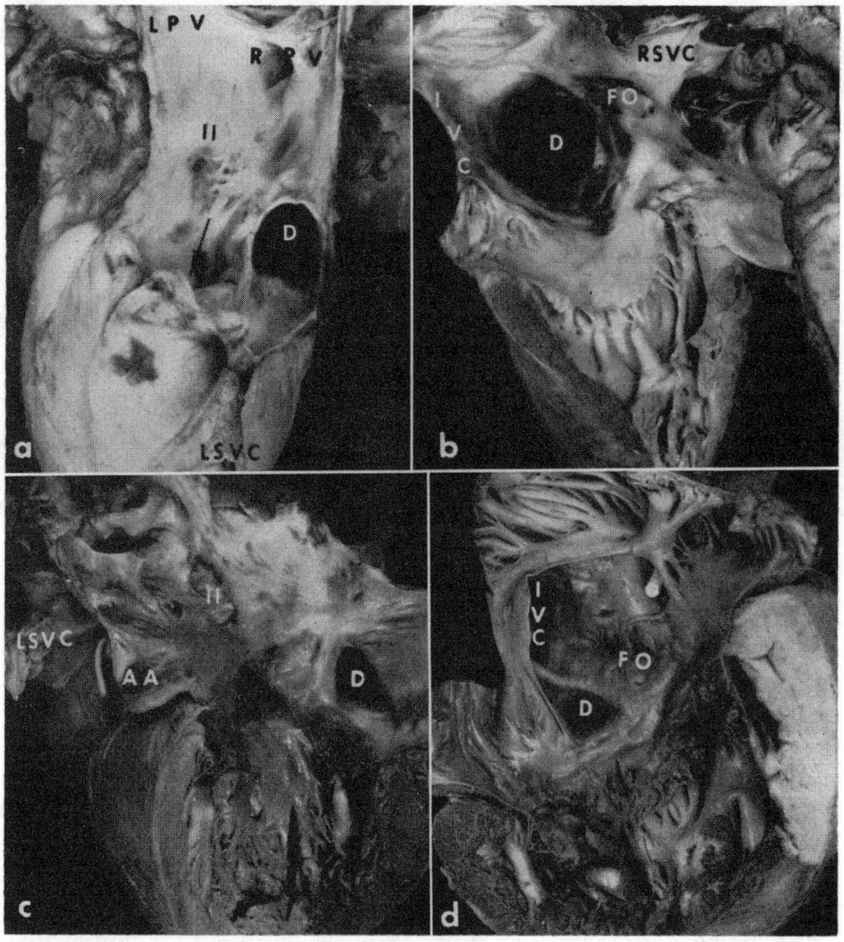

Figure 2

a *and* b. *Case* 3. a. *Left side of the heart exposing the interior of the left atrium. Posterior and superior to the mitral valve* (arrow) *is the atrial septal defect (D) characteristic of the malformation herein described. The left superior vena cava (LSVC) joins the left atrium. The left and right pulmonary veins (LPV; RPV) join the left atrium normally. The interatrial ostium secundum (II) is normal.* b. *Right side of heart. The atrial septal defect (D) lies anterior and inferior to the entrance of the inferior vena cava (IVC) into the right atrium and postero-inferior to the fossa ovalis (FO). RSVC, right superior vena cava joining right atrium.* c *and* d. *Case* 1. c. *Interior of left atrium and left ventricle. The characteristic atrial septal defect (D).* d. *Right atrium and ventricle. The probe lies in the entrance of the superior vena cava. Other abbreviations as in* b.

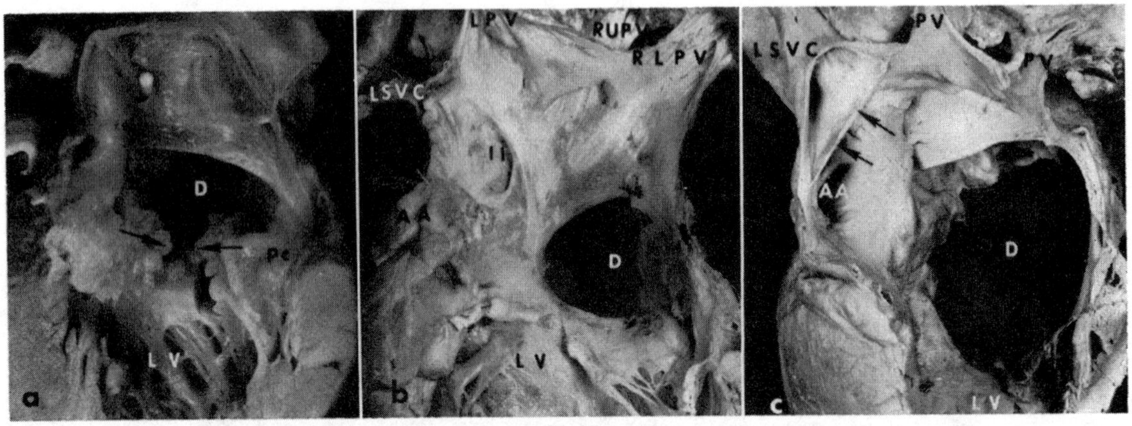

Figure 3

a. Left side of heart in a classic example of persistent common atrioventricular canal. The defect (D) of the atrial septum characteristically lies superior to the cleft (between arrows) in the anterior leaflet of the mitral valve, while above the posteromedial commissure (Pc) of the mitral valve is a small amount of atrial septal tissue. b. Case 4. Left atrium and left ventricle (LV) in a case in which the developmental complex herein described was associated with persistent common atrioventricular canal. In contrast to the atrial septal defect characteristic of isolated persistent common atrioventricular canal shown in a, the defect here extends to the posterior wall of the atrium. The center of the defect lies somewhat posterior to the cleft in the anterior leaflet of the mitral valve. As part of the developmental complex which is the subject of this report, the left superior vena cava (LSVC) joins the left atrium. No coronary sinus was present. c. Case 5. Left atrium and left ventricle (LV). The features in this case are essentially like those of the case illustrated in b. The exception is that the atrial septal defect is larger than in b, but is of the same type in that its posterior boundary is formed by the atrial wall. Along the left margin of the junction of the left superior vena cava (LSVC) and the left atrium is a fold (arrows) resembling a valve-like flap. AA, left atrial ostium of the left atrial appendage.

left superior vena cava, left atrium, and left ventricle. This was subsequently substantiated by angiocardiography. In the remaining patients the clinical findings had been considered as explained by the septal defects present (atrial septal defect in each case; ventricular septal defect in two).

In retrospect, it is interesting to note that, in all but one (case 4) of the five cases, duskiness of the skin was apparent, even though an atrial septal defect was the only intracardiac defect in two of these four patients (cases 2 and 3). In the latter two cases the levels of oxygen saturation were 89 per cent in the left atrium in one (case 2) and 92 per cent in a femoral artery, in the other (case 3).

Similarly, in the three living patients, the initial clinical impression did not include a diagnosis of a systemic venous anomaly, although mild cyanosis was recorded in two cases (cases 6 and 7). Levels of oxygen saturation of the blood, either in a left-sided chamber or in a femoral artery, were 86, 92, and 93 per cent, respectively.

In two (cases 7 and 8) of the three living patients, the clinical diagnosis of termination of the left superior vena cava in the left atrium was made by cardiac catheterization when the heart was explored by a catheter through one of the left brachial veins. In each, suspicion of such a termination was substantiated by angiocardiography. In the third patient (case 6) the initial cardiac catheterization was done through one of the right-sided veins. In this case, however, the diagnosis of left superior vena cava terminating in the left atrium was made after advancing the tip of the catheter through the left atrial cavity, and then into the left superior vena cava. The venous anomaly was substantiated later by angiocardiography performed through a left

Table 1

Clinical and Pathologic Observations

Case no.	Age (yr.)	Diagnoses: Pathologic	Diagnoses: Clinical	Clinical observations	Arterial oxygen saturation (per cent)	Special studies (vein used): Physiologic	Special studies (vein used): Angiocardiogram
1	4/12	ASD Absent coronary sinus LSVC to LA VSD	VSD	Poor weight gain Dusky Grade I-II systolic murmur Died of pul. infection	—	—	—
2	2	ASD Absent coronary sinus LSVC to LA Urogenital anomalies	ASD Urogenital anomalies	Failure to grow Dusky Grade III systolic murmur ASD surgically closed Died of cerebral embolism 8 mos. after operation	LA 89 LV 89	Right saphenous	Rt. saphenous Not diagnostic
3	5	ASD Absent coronary sinus LSVC to LA	ASD LSVC to LA	Small for age Minimal duskiness Grade III systolic murmur Died soon after surgical closure of ASD	FA 92	Left basilic catheter in LSVC to LA	Left basilic Diagnostic
4	8	Persistent CAV canal Absent coronary sinus LSVC to LA Rt. pul. veins to RA	Persistent CAV canal	Poor growth and development Grade III systolic and Grade II diastolic murmurs. Died at conclusion of operation for PC "AV" canal	FA 96	Right saphenous	—
5	9	Persistent CAV canal Absent coronary sinus LSVC to LA Double outlet RV Absent RSVC Rt. pul. veins to RA Levocardia	Persistent CAV canal LSVC to LA Levocardia	Cyanosis Grade III systolic murmur Died at conclusion of operation for PC "AV" canal	FA 79	Left basilic catheter in LSVC to LA	Left basilic Diagnostic

6	9	Living	Single atrium LSVC to LA Mitral insufficiency	Respiratory distress Dusky Grade II systolic and diastolic murmurs Surgical closure of single atrium. Postoperative murmur of mitral insufficiency	Preop. BA 82 Postop. LA 93	Rt. basilic catheter in RA to LA to LSVC	Left basilic Diagnostic
7	10	Living	ASD? LSVC to LA VSD Pul. hypert.	Mild cyanosis Grade III systolic murmur Surgical closure of VSD	Preop. BA 88	Left basilic catheter in LSVC to LA	Left basilic Diagnostic
8	13.5	Living	ASD LSVC to LA	Signs and symptoms of brain abscess Soft systolic murmur Surgical closure of ASD	Preop. LA 93 Postop. BA 93	Left basilic catheter in LSVC to LA	Left basilic Diagnostic

ASD, atrial septal defect; LSVC, left superior vena cava; LA, left atrium; VSD, ventricular septal defect; CAV, common atrioventricular canal; RA, right atrium; FA, femoral artery; BA, brachial artery; LV, left ventricle; —, test not done.

antecubital vein. Each of the latter three cases was operated upon, for closure of an atrial septal defect in two instances, and a ventricular septal defect in the third. In none was the anomalous left superior vena cava surgically interrupted. In one of these latter cases (case 7) uncertainty still exists as to whether an atrial septal defect is present. In this case, the atrial aspect of the heart was not explored at the time of operation.

In the condition under consideration, an intracardiac right-to-left shunt forms part of the functional abnormality. It is of interest that cerebral complications occurred in two of the cases. In one case, involving a 2-year-old girl (case 2), symptoms of cerebral disease began acutely 8 months after the atrial septal defect was closed and 1 day before death. The brain, although not the site of a distinct abscess, showed unilateral acute encephalomalacia with thrombosis of the right internal carotid artery and signs of meningitis.

In the second case (case 8), a brief and self-limited illness suggesting an acute cerebral process had occurred about 1 year before closure of the atrial septal defect. It is of interest that, in this case, the cerebral disease was the initial abnormality leading ultimately to a diagnosis of congenital cardiac disease.

Electrocardiographic Observations

Electrocardiograms were available for study in each of the eight cases.

In two cases (cases 4 and 5), each with associated persistent common atrioventricular canal, the electrocardiographic tracings were classic for this type of cardiac defect.

In four cases (cases 2, 3, 6, and 8) with no intracardiac defects other than the characteristic atrial septal defect, the electrocardiograms were similar to those in the patients with uncomplicated atrial septal defect.

In each of the remaining two patients (cases 1 and 7) with associated ventricular septal defects, the electrocardiograms showed right axis deviation and right ventricular hypertrophy.

Physiologic Observations

Cardiac catheterization was performed in seven of the eight cases. A vein of the right arm was used in three cases, in each of which a transatrial left-to-right shunt was identified. In two of these cases (cases 2 and 4), no unusual course was displayed by the catheter, while in the third case (case 6), the catheter passed from the right atrium through the atrial septal defect into the left atrium and finally into the left superior vena cava.

In each of the four remaining patients (cases 3, 5, 7, and 8), in whom cardiac catheterization was done, the initial catheterization was attempted through a left antecubital vein. In each, the catheter followed a usual course in the thoracic cavity to the level of the left superior mediastinum. At this point, the catheter, instead of crossing to the right side of the superior mediastinum, took an unusual turn and descended in line with the left sternal border to enter the left atrium. From the latter chamber the tip of the catheter was advanced into the left ventricular cavity. In three cases (cases 3, 7, and 8), angiocardiography was performed while the catheter was in the left superior vena cava, and the diagnosis of anomalous termination of this vein in the left atrium was thus confirmed.

Near-simultaneous values for oxygen saturation in both atria were obtained in three subjects (cases 2, 6, and 8). In each of two cases the levels were almost identical. In one case (case 2) the values were 90 per cent in the right atrium and 89 in the left, while in case 6 the values were 85 and 87 per cent, respectively. In the third case the level of oxygen saturation in the right atrium was 89 per cent; in the left atrium, 93 per cent. In each of these cases the left atrial pressure was slightly higher than the right atrial pressure (greatest mean pressure difference being 3 mm. Hg).

In those cases with an intact ventricular septum, the pulmonary arterial pressure was in a normal range. When a ventricular septal defect was also present, the pulmonary pressure was elevated.

The levels of oxygen saturation of blood as measured from a left-sided cardiac chamber or a systemic artery varied from minor degrees of desaturation to values that bordered on the normal (table 1).

Radiologic Observations

Thoracic roentgenograms in each of the eight cases revealed signs consistent with those of a left-to-right shunt, in the form of cardiomegaly and prominent pulmonary vasculature. In those patients with additional cardiac malformations (cases 1, 4, 5, and 7) the signs were more prominent than in the others. In four patients (cases 5, 6, 7, and 8) there was an unusual shadow along the left superior mediastinum corresponding to the left superior vena cava as demonstrated by angiography. The left atrium was not significantly enlarged in any of the cases.

Angiocardiography (fig. 4*a* and *b*) was done through a left antecubital vein in four patients (cases 3, 6, 7, and 8). In each, the unusual shadow noted in plain films became opacified and merged with the left atrial cavity above the level of the left hilum.

At the junction between the left superior vena cava and the left atrium, the cava was quite large. After the opacification of the left atrium, the left ventricle and aorta were opacified normally. In one patient (case 7) the right atrium also opacified, indicating a left-to-right shunt at the atrial level. In the lateral views the dilated left superior vena cava seemed to join the left atrium superiorly.

This appearance is quite different from the more common termination of the left superior vena cava in the coronary sinus, in which the junction with the right atrium is much lower and to the right side of the spine.

Developmental Considerations

The developmental complex described in this report appears to result from faulty development in the sinoatrial region of the heart.

Before attempting an explanation for this

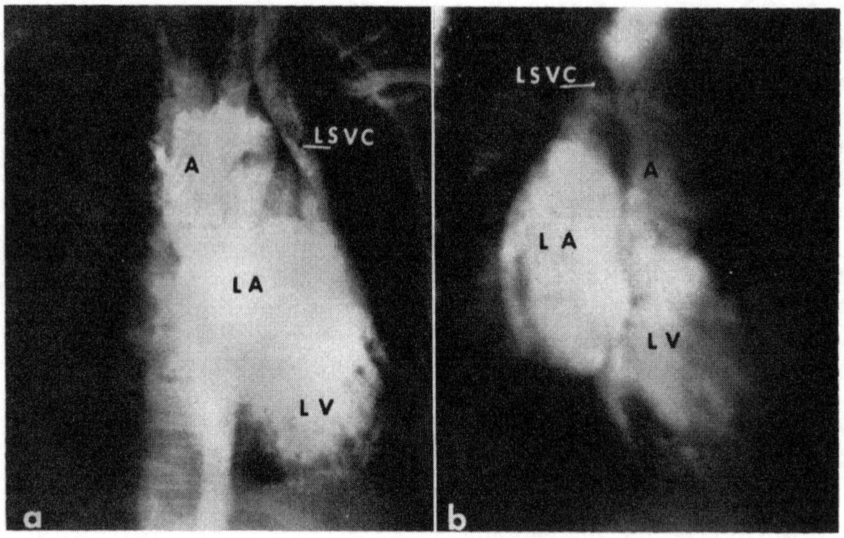

Figure 4

Case 7. Forward angiocardiogram made by injection into a left brachial vein in frontal view, a, *and in lateral view,* b. *In addition to opacification of the left superior vena cava (LSVC) there is dense opacification of the left atrium (LA), the left ventricle (LV), and the aorta (A). In this patient the diagnosis of atrial septal defect could not be conclusively proved, although there is suggestion of faint opacification of the right cardiac chambers and the right pulmonary artery, as might occur if an atrial septal defect were present.*

condition, it is appropriate first to review the features of normal development of the sinoatrial region of the heart and of related structures.

At the 10-11 somite stage, the central cardiovascular system is represented by paired tubes which, in part, ultimately fuse. The fusion begins at the cephalad end and continues toward the caudal end. Thus, a single tubular heart is formed, retaining its paired identity at the caudal end.

The cephalad end of the single tubular heart is the arterial end, which gives rise to the aortic root. Caudal to the aortic root, in turn, are the conus and the ventricle of the tubular heart. More caudal to the ventricle is the venous end, which is composed of paired atria and paired great veins. The paired venous end completes its fusion in the early phase of 11-20 paired-somite stage to form the single atrial cavity and the sinus venosus.

Tandler[2] observed that the sinus venosus never loses its paired condition completely. Thus, he identified three parts of the sinus venosus: (1) the unpaired central part or transverse part (between the orifices of the vitelline veins), and (2) right and (3) left horns which, in turn, receive the respective common cardinal and umbilical veins (fig. 5, I).

Davis'[3] observations were that the cephalic migration and growth of the atrium, which starts when the bulboventricular U loop is formed, becomes significant at the 11-20 paired-somite stage.

As the rapid cephalad growth of the common atrium continues, a sulcus begins to develop (fig. 5, II) at the left side of the junction between the sinus venosus and the common atrium. From within the heart, the site of the sulcus is represented by a fold[4] between the sinus venosus and the left side of the common atrium. With the deepening of the left atriovenous sulcus, this fold progresses from the left side toward the midline of the common atrium. By the completion of 20 paired-somite stage the atriovenous fold separates most of the left side of the common atrium from the sinus venosus. Some communication between the left side of the common atrium and the sinus venosus, however, is still

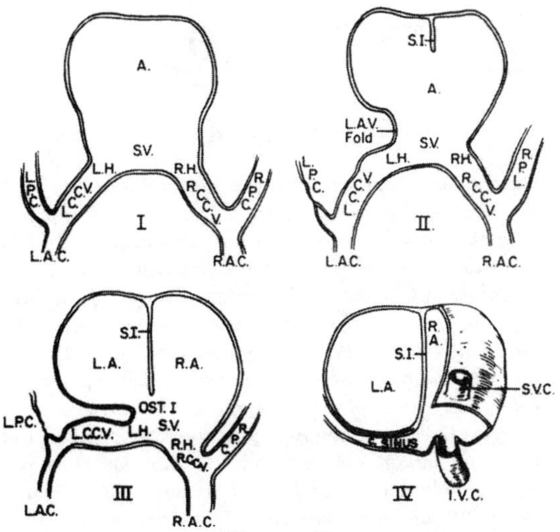

Figure 5

Diagrammatic portrayal of various stages in the development of the sinus venosus and associated structures. I. At an early stage there is a common atrium (A.) which communicates freely with the receiving chamber known as the sinus venosus (S.V.). The latter receives, through its left and right horns, respectively (L.H.; R.H.), the common cardinal vein of the corresponding side (L.C.C.V.; R.C.C.V.). Each common cardinal vein, in turn, receives its corresponding anterior cardinal and posterior cardinal veins (L.A.C.; L.P.C.; R.A.C.; R.P.C.). II. An early indication of partitioning of this portion of the heart into two sides is derived from the appearance of septum primum (S.I.) and the development of a fold (L.A.V. Fold) along the left side of the junction of the common atrium and sinus venosus. III. In the lowermost portion of the atrium, and with further development, the septum primum is approximated by the enlarging left atriovenous fold. At this stage, there is still interatrial communication in the most postero-inferior angle of the common atrium. IV. With further development of the left atriovenous fold, union is made between the fold and the septum primum, thereby obliterating the communication between the sinus venosus and the left atrium. The posterior aspect of the left atriovenous fold contributes to the anterior wall of the newly developed coronary sinus, while the posterior wall of the left horn of the sinus venosus forms the posterior wall of the coronary sinus. Because of the obliteration of the communication between the sinus venosus and the left atrium, the newly formed structure, namely, the coronary sinus, communicates with the right atrium.

present at this stage (fig. 5, II and III).

On the right side, an atriovenous sulcus also develops. This separates the right side of the common atrium from the sinus venosus. In spite of this, the sinus venosus remains connected with the dorsal part of the entire width of the right side of the common atrium.

The left horn of the sinus venosus diminishes in size and, in concert with this, growth of the transverse portion of the sinus venosus becomes retarded. The diminution in size of the left horn results chiefly from the beginning of obliteration of the left umbilical vein. The right horn begins to receive the hepatic veins and thus enlarges.

Along with the changes at the region of the sinus venosus, the common atrium enlarges significantly and it seems that the right half surpasses the left part in volume. By the abutment of the distal portion of the bulbus cordis against the upper and anterior wall of the common atrium, a blunt prominence is formed, which projects into the atrial cavity. Toward the end of the 20-somite to 6-mm. stage, a sickle-shaped protrusion is formed on the aforementioned intraatrial prominence, the protrusion to be known as the interatrial septum primum.

In embryos between 6 and 9 mm., the sinus venosus is completely separated from the left side of the common atrium by progression of the left atriovenous fold toward the right where, in the vicinity of the midline of the common atrium, the fold fuses with the septum primum.

In separating the left side of the common atrium from the sinus venosus, the left atriovenous fold provides part of the posterior wall of the left atrium. It also acts as the anterior wall of the left side of the sinus venosus, thereby creating the coronary sinus. As the anterior wall of the newly formed coronary sinus is the left atriovenous fold, the posterior wall of the coronary sinus is the tissue of the transverse part and left horn of the sinus venosus (fig. 5, IV).

Following development of the coronary sinus by the process described, the left atrium enlarges. This results in compression and stretching of the left horn of the sinus venosus and of the left anterior cardinal vein. This obstruction in the anterior cardinal system stimulates development of collateral channels between the left and right anterior cardinal veins, ultimately leading to establishment of the bridge between the two anterior cardinal veins, known as the left innominate vein. The resulting increased blood flow through the right anterior cardinal vein causes the right horn of the sinus venosus to enlarge and to appear to ascend against the posterior wall of the right atrium. Gradually, the cavities of the right horn of the sinus venosus and the right side of the atrium merge to form a common cavity known as the right atrium.

Accounts on development of the atrial septum do not indicate that the left atriovenous fold plays a role in formation of the final atrial septum. From the nature of the anomalies in the entity being considered, it seems probable that the left atriovenous fold, either by contributing to the atrial septum or by supplying a support to the septum primum at its posterior aspect, participates in closing the postero-inferior angle of the interatrial ostium primum.

More anteriorly, the interatrial ostium primum is closed by fusion of the septum primum with the atrioventricular endocardial cushion, a process that is generally recognized.

From the foregoing, it seems that the fundamental developmental abnormality in the condition reported is failure of completion of the left atriovenous fold (fig. 6). With this deficiency, the left side of the sinus venosus would maintain continuity with the left atrium and would be represented grossly as termination of the left superior vena cava in the left atrium. Failure of the full growth of the left atriovenous fold would deny the septum primum an anchor, posteriorly, and account for the characteristic defect of this condition.

Moreover, as the coronary sinus is derived, in part, from the left atriovenous fold, a deficiency of the fold would result in absence of the anterior wall of the coronary sinus.

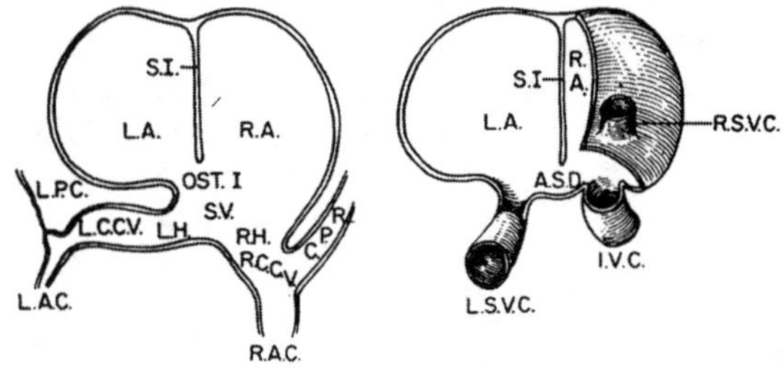

Figure 6

Digrammatic portrayal of the authors' concept as to the basis for the developmental complex here reported, of which the three elements are (1) termination of the left superior vena cava in the left atrium, (2) an atrial septal defect in the postero-inferior angle of the atrial septum, and (3) absence of the coronary sinus. It is envisioned that with incomplete development of the left atriovenous fold, there is failure of union of the fold with the septum primum. Under these circumstances the sinus venosus continues to communicate with the left atrium. As the left superior vena cava has a ready avenue of flow, it remains patent and, in the adult stage, is represented by termination of the left superior vena cava in the left atrium. Failure of union of the left atriovenous fold with the septum primum would explain the presence of an atrial septal defect in the location peculiar for this developmental complex. As the coronary sinus is derived from the normal development of the left atriovenous fold and its junction with the septum primum, failure of the latter process would result in absence of the coronary sinus.

That part of the posterior wall of the definitive left atrium would be derived from that part of the sinus venosus that normally contributes the posterior wall of the coronary sinus. Furthermore, failure of full growth of the left atriovenous fold may be associated with failure of full development of atrioventricular endocardial cushion tissue, the latter accounting for persistence of the common atrioventricular canal. The association of these two developmental anomalies will result in a common atrial septal defect, part of which is in the position of the atrial septal defect in persistent common atrioventricular canal, and part in the position of the atrial septal defect specific for the anomaly being discussed.

Discussion

Among reported instances of termination of the left superior vena cava in the left atrium in which necropsy had been done, atrial septal defect is commonly, though not universally, mentioned.[5–14] When an atrial septal defect is identified, its position is usually not clearly defined. In a case studied clinically by Mankin and associates,[13] an atrial septal defect was considered in association with termination of the left superior vena cava in the left atrium. In that case, the pulmonary veins joined the left superior vena cava.

An atrial septal defect was identified in seven of our eight cases. In the remaining case, an atrial septal defect, although not specifically identified, cannot be excluded.

It is still uncertain whether termination of the left superior vena cava in the left atrium is always associated with an atrial septal defect. Nonetheless, it seems appropriate to consider that a specific developmental complex exists in which the venous anomaly mentioned is associated with a defect in the postero-inferior angle of the atrial septum. This complex appears to be derived from incomplete separation of the sinus venosus from the left atrium.

One of us (J. E. E.) earlier had considered the atrial septal defect of this condition not a true defect of the atrial septum. Rather, it was considered that the anterior wall of the coronary sinus was deficient and therefore allowed an interatrial communication.[15] We are now of the opinion that the interatrial communication in the condition under discussion is to be considered a true atrial septal defect of a specific type and associated with absence of the coronary sinus.

From our material, it is apparent that termination of the left superior vena cava in the left atrium may be associated with persistent common atrioventricular canal (two of eight cases). In such instances, the extensive distribution of the atrial septal defect suggests that the defect represents confluence of the atrial septal defect which is part of persistent common atrioventricular canal and the defect which is specific for the developmental complex here described.

Usually, when the left superior vena cava terminates in the left atrium, the left innominate venous bridge between the two superior venae cavae is absent. This probably reflects absence of obstruction to flow in each superior vena cava. Support for this thesis comes from two cases[11, 12] of termination of the left superior vena cava in the left atrium, in each of which an innominate venous bridge was present. In each of these cases the right superior vena cava was narrow. Obstruction in the latter vessel probably favored the development of collateral flow to the left superior vena cava, the major collateral channel being a developed innominate venous bridge.

Calculations of the venous return to the heart show that under normal conditions about one third of total venous return is through the superior vena cava.[10]

In cases as those herein reported, in which the two superior venae cavae are of about equal size, one may assume that about one sixth of the systemic venous return is to the left atrium. The latter results in desaturation of the left atrial and systemic arterial blood. This may occur to such a degree as to cause cyanosis or duskiness. Such was observed in three of the four patients (cases 2, 3, and 8) in this series in whom there were no additional intracardiac abnormalities.

In our series, the diagnosis of termination of the left superior vena cava in the left atrium was made only when the heart was explored with a catheter through a left antecubital vein; this was substantiated by angiocardiography. In one case, however, during cardiac catheterization, the catheter was easily advanced from the right atrium to the left and into the left superior vena cava. Later studies through a left antecubital vein substantiated the termination of the left superior vena cava in the left atrium. Angiocardiography was the most reliable procedure with which to establish whether a persistent left superior vena cava terminates in the coronary sinus or in the left atrium. In the present series the atrial septal defect has been successfully surgically closed in three instances. One of these patients (case 2) died 8 months after operation, of central nervous system complications; the left superior vena cava had not been interrupted surgically. The other two patients (cases 6 and 8) are living. In each of these cases the arterial oxygen saturation, determined postoperatively, is below normal levels, thus further confirming the drainage of venous blood through the left superior vena cava into the left atrium, even after closure of the atrial septal defect.

In none of the patients in this series in whom surgical closure either of an atrial septal or ventricular septal defect was accomplished had the left superior vena cava been ligated or interrupted.

There are two cases in the literature in which the left superior vena cava was ligated successfully[11, 12] after confirming the presence of the right superior vena cava and an anastomosing vein between the two superior venae cavae.

The occurrence of complications in the central nervous system in two of our patients, which resulted in death of one, suggests that interruption of the left superior vena cava or anastomosis of this vein with the right superior vena cava should be done to avoid complications of a right-to-left shunt.

Summary

Eight cases of termination of the left superior vena cava in the left atrium are reviewed pathologically and clinically.

In three of the five patients who died, pathologic examination revealed three anomalies which, together, are considered to form a developmental complex. The anomalies are (1) termination of the left superior vena cava in the left atrium, (2) absence of the coronary sinus, and (3) an atrial septal defect lying in the postero-inferior angle of the atrial septum. In the two remaining fatal cases, the aforementioned anomalies were associated with persistent common atrioventricular canal. In this situation, the atrial septal defect of the latter malformation was confluent with the atrial septal defect of the anomalous complex described.

The coexistence of three anomalies—the left superior vena cava terminating in the left atrium, absent coronary sinus, and atrial septal defect—is considered to result from a single developmental abnormality. This takes the form of failure of complete formation of the left atriovenous fold, that fold which normally develops along the left side of the junction of the sinus venosus and the atrial portion of the heart.

Clinically, features of increased pulmonary blood flow, coupled with duskiness of the skin, were the significant abnormalities.

When cardiac catheterization was attempted through a right-sided vein, the data revealed a left-to-right shunt at atrial level, while levels of arterial oxygen desaturation were present.

Except in cases with coexistent ventricular septal defect, pulmonary hypertension was absent.

In each of the four patients in whom cardiac catheterization was performed through a left antecubital vein, the catheter was advanced into the left superior vena cava, left atrium, and left ventricle. This was substantiated by angiocardiography in three of the four patients. In our experience, angiocardiography was the most reliable procedure to substantiate the termination of the left superior vena cava in the left atrium.

The present study suggests that, in the absence of pulmonary hypertension, a left-to-right transatrial shunt associated with systemic arterial oxygen desaturation may indicate the presence of a persistent left superior vena cava terminating in the left atrium. Moreover, an atrial septal defect identified surgically as lying in the postero-inferior angle of the atrial septum should suggest that an additional anomaly may be present in the form of termination of the left superior vena cava in the left atrium.

References

1. RUTTENBERG, H. D., NEUFELD, H. N., AND EDWARDS, J. E.: Syndrome of congenital cardiac disease with asplenia. Distinction from other forms of congenital cyanotic cardiac disease. Am. J. Cardiol. 13: 387, 1964.
2. TANDLER, J.: The development of the human heart. *In* Kiebel and Mall: Human Embryol-

ogy. Philadelphia, J. B. Lippincott, 1912, vol. 2, p. 534.

3. DAVIS, C. L.: Development of the human heart from its first appearance to the stage found in embryos of twenty paired somites. Carnegie Institution. Contributions to Embryology **19:** 247, 1937.
4. VAN MIEROP, L. H. S., AND WIGLESWORTH, F. W.: Isomerism of the cardiac atria in the asplenia syndrome. Lab. Invest. **11:** 1303, 1962.
5. FRASER, R. S., DOORKEN, J., ROSSALL, R. E., AND EIDEM, R.: Left superior vena cava. A review of associated congenital heart lesions, catheterization data and roentgenologic findings. Am. J. Med. **31:** 711, 1961.
6. CAMPBELL, M., AND DEUCHER, D. C.: The left-sided superior vena cava. Brit. Heart J. **16:** 423, 1954.
7. WINTER, F. S.: Persistent left superior vena cava. Survey of world literature and report of thirty additional cases. Angiology **5:** 90, 1954.
8. POTTER, E. L.: Diffuse angiectasis of cerebral meninges of the newborn infant. Report of three cases. Arch. Path. **46:** 87, 1948.
9. MCCOTTER, R. E.: Three cases of the persistence of the left superior vena cava. Anat. Rec. **10:** 371, 1916.
10. TUCHMAN, H., BROWN, J. F., HUSTON, J. H., WEINSTEIN, A. B., ROWE, G. G., AND CRUMPTON, C. W.: Superior vena cava draining into left atrium. Another cause for left ventricular hypertrophy with cyanotic congenital heart disease. Am. J. Med. **21:** 481, 1956.
11. HURWITT, E. S., ESCHER, J. W., DORIS, M., AND CITRIN, L. I.: Surgical correction of cyanosis due to entrance of left superior vena cava into left auricle. Surgery **38:** 903, 1955.
12. DAVIS, W. H., JORDAAN, F. R., AND SNYMAN, H. W.: Persistent left superior vena cava draining into the left atrium, as an isolated anomaly. Am. Heart J. **57:** 616, 1959.
13. MANKIN, H. T., AND BURCHELL, H. B.: Clinical considerations in partial anomalous pulmonary venous connection: Report of 2 unusual cases. Proc. Staff Meet., Mayo Clin. **28:** 463, 1953.
14. DIAZ, A. R., AND ANIDO, H.: Tetralogy of Fallot: Surgical treatment. Dis. Chest. **15:** 684, 1949.
15. EDWARDS, J. E.: Malformations of the atrial septal complex. *In* Gould, S. E., editor.: Pathology of the Heart. Ed. 2. Springfield, Illinois, Charles C Thomas, Publisher, 1960, p. 275.

Termination of Left Superior Vena Cava in Left Atrium, Atrial Septal Defect, and Absence of Coronary Sinus. A Developmental Complex.

Robert H. Anderson BSc, MD, FRCPath

I did not have the privilege of working directly, and studying, with Jesse. I was, of course, influenced to huge extent by his writings, not least by the monumental chapter he produced for Gould's edited volume entitled "Pathology of the Heart." This fundamental resource is cited as the 15th reference in this account of the complex involving connection of the left superior caval vein to the roof of the left atrium, and an interatrial communication at the anticipated site of the orifice of the coronary sinus. It was, however, my privilege to obtain vicarious access to his teachings through my lifelong collaborations with Anton Becker. And, together with Anton, it was my pleasure to be entertained by Jesse on several occasions, both professionally and socially. These all-too-brief associations were sufficient to confirm to me that not only was Jesse the consummate observer and scientist, but also a true gentleman.

The account given by Raghib, and several others of Jesse's own lifelong collaborators, gives a superb overview of the entity we would now describe as a coronary sinus interatrial communication. The paper illustrates the huge care taken by Jesse to ensure that all available clinical findings were correlated with the pathological observations. The account of the pathological findings themselves, and the excellent illustrations, still serves as an example of the very best of morphologic studies. The number of cases assembled with the described combination of lesions is remarkable. We were able to collect and describe several examples ourselves, but did not find any in which the coronary sinus defect was confluent with an atrioventricular septal defect, as was the situation in two of the autopsied cases described in this study. It is noteworthy that the authors excluded all cases with asplenia, or isomerism of the right atrial appendages as we would describe them nowadays, recognizing that the coronary sinus is always absent in this latter setting.

The areas in which we might now improve on this account are confined to whether or not the hole at the site of the expected orifice of the coronary sinus is a true atrial septal defect, and the story provided to explain the morphogenesis of the lesion. With regard to the septal nature of the defect, it is noteworthy that Jesse explains that, previously, he had believed the hole to represent the orifice of the coronary sinus, citing his chapter in Gould's textbook as the source of this opinion. For myself, I much prefer this earlier account, most notably because the so-called Raghib complex can be seen in incomplete forms with fenestration of the wall of the coronary sinus, a lesion also described in great detail by Jess in association with the late lamented Alan Rose. With regard to the embryology, we have learned much in the last decade that calls into question the description given for formation of the left sinuatrial fold. It is certainly the case that the left sinus horn becomes incorporated into the developing left atrioventricular junction, but the eventual sealing and closure of the primary interatrial communication is now known to involve growth into the heart of the vestibular spine, or dorsal mesenchymal protrusion. Evidence is also accruing rapidly that it is failure of growth of the spine, rather than abnormal formation of the endocardial cushions, which is the essential feature of retention of the common atrioventricular junction, this being the essence of the so-called atrioventricular canal malformation. These differences, however, are mere bagatelles when set against the overall strength of this superb account of the Raghib complex.

Surgical Clinics of North America, August 1949

PERSISTENT TRUNCUS ARTERIOSUS: A CLASSIFICATION ACCORDING TO ANATOMIC TYPES

ROBERT W. COLLETT AND JESSE E. EDWARDS

There has always been considerable confusion concerning the pathologic criteria for the diagnosis of persistent truncus arteriosus. In order to clarify the pathologic diagnosis of persistent truncus arteriosus and to arrive at an applicable classification of this congenital anomaly, an analysis was made of reports of 116 cases of a congenitally defective heart characterized by a single functioning arterial trunk. Ninety-three of these cases were considered to be examples of either persistent truncus arteriosus or partial persistent truncus arteriosus. Of the other 23 cases, 12 were not true examples of this entity even though they had formerly been considered as such by other authors. The remaining 11 cases could not be classified because of inadequate information.

The chief sources of information used were the classic reviews of this type of congenital heart disease made by Taruffi in 1875, Vierordt in 1898, Herxheimer in 1910, Abbott in 1927, Humphreys in 1932 and Lev and Saphir in 1942. However, numerous other reports of cases not included in these reviews were discovered and included in our analysis. Since 1942, at least 11 cases have been reported as examples of the malformation under consideration. However, only 6 of these have been included in the present series as true examples of persistent truncus arteriosus.

From the analysis of the 93 cases of persistent truncus arteriosus, an anatomic classification has been developed on the basis of the embryology of the human heart and great arterial vessels.

Pathologically, a persistent truncus arteriosus consists of a single arterial trunk arising from the ventricular part of the heart. Complete or partial failure of the septum, which normally divides the embryonic truncus arteriosus into the aortic and pulmonary trunk, to form, results in such an anomaly. The single trunk receives blood from both ventricles and supplies the coronary, pulmonary and systemic circulations.

This anomaly may assume numerous variations, and from this fact stems most of the controversy concerning the pathologic diagnosis of persistent truncus arteriosus. In order to clarify the confusion concerning this entity, one must understand the embryologic basis for its development.

EMBRYOLOGIC CONSIDERATIONS

The Truncus Arteriosus and Conus Arteriosus.—Kramer in 1942 published an excellent description of the partitioning of the truncus arteriosus and conus arteriosus and of the formation of the ventricular septum in the embryonic human heart. The truncus arteriosus is the single arterial vessel which passes cephalad as the main outlet from the heart. The conus arteriosus is the conically shaped part of the heart which joins the ventricle with the truncus arteriosus. The line of division between the conus and truncus lies at the level of the formation of the pulmonary and aortic valves. This continuous channel made up of the truncus arteriosus and the conus arteriosus may be called the trun-

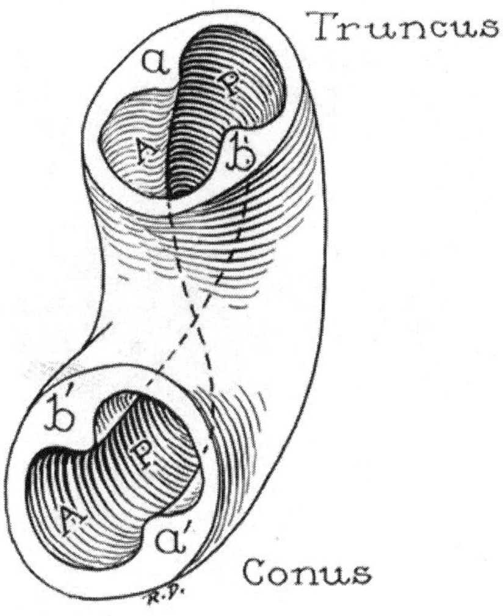

Fig. 460.—The truncoconal channel showing the two truncoconal ridges (*a*, *a'* and *b*, *b'*). *a*, Truncus ridge in dextrodorsal position; *b*, truncus ridge in sinistroventral position; *a'*, conal ridge in sinistroventral position; *b'*, conal ridge in dextrodorsal position; *A*, aortic channel; and *P*, pulmonary channel.

coconal channel. In the lining of this channel, two opposed and spiraled rows of swellings, the truncoconal ridges, develop (fig. 460). As each ridge is followed caudally, it spirals in a clockwise manner. At the lower level of the conus arteriosus the relations of the opposing ridges are exactly reversed.

As a result of normal growth, these ridges meet in the central axis of the truncoconal channel and fuse to form a spiral septum that divides the channel into two vessels, the pulmonary trunk and the ascending aorta. The septum which results from the fusion of these spiraled ridges is itself spiraled so that the two vessels which result from this division are also spiraled. Thus, the spiraled nature of the truncoconal ridges is responsible for the spiraling of the pulmonary trunk and aorta about each other and for the communication of the aorta with the left ventricle and the pulmonary trunk with the right ventricle.[30]

Below the level of the semilunar valves the conus ridges unite to separate that part of the right ventricle known as the conus pulmonalis from the more modified corresponding portion of the left ventricle that serves as the outlet into the aorta. Complete or partial absence of the truncoconal ridges results in failure of division of the truncoconal channel into the pulmonary trunk and ascending aorta, thus resulting in the congenital anomaly classified as persistent truncus arteriosus.

The Semilunar Valve Cusps.—At the junction of the truncus arteriosus and conus arteriosus, swellings develop on the parietal wall of the truncoconal channel and on the truncoconal septum (fig. 461). From

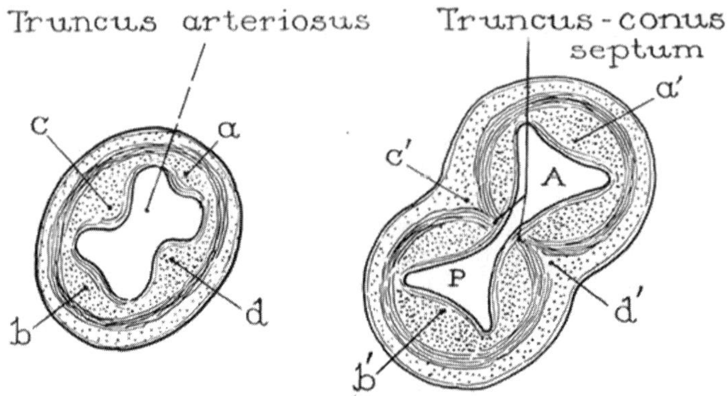

Fig. 461.—Development of the semilunar valve cusps from the parietal wall of the truncoconal channel and on the truncoconal septum. *a*, Intercalated valve swelling which becomes the dorsal cusp of the aortic valve, *a′*; *b*, intercalated valve swelling which becomes the ventral cusp of the pulmonary valve, *b′*; and *c* and *d*, the truncoconal ridge swellings which unite to form the truncoconal septum, *c′* and *d′*, and serve to form the two ventral aortic semilunar valve leaflets and the two dorsal pulmonary valve leaflets (modified from Kramer).

these the usual number of semilunar cusps are formed. However, if the truncoconal ridges fail to form and no other tissue develops into valvular tissue, the only valve leaflets that develop are derived from the parietal wall of the truncoconal channel. Only two semilunar cusps then result. The case of persistent truncus arteriosus reported by Carr, Goodale and Rockwell, in which there were only two semilunar cusps, illustrates such a maldevelopment.

If the truncoconal ridges develop incompletely without the completion of the truncoconal septum, the number of cusps may vary from four to six. In 9 cases of the series reviewed there were four semilunar cusps. In the case reported by Rizzi there were six semilunar cusps.

On the other hand, when there is an eccentric alignment of the truncoconal ridges, three or four valve cusps may result. The size of these may vary with the degree of eccentricity of the ridges. In the majority of the cases included in the series, there were three cusps, and in 6 of these cases there was partial division of one of the three cusps.

It readily can be seen that the number of valve leaflets present in persistent truncus arteriosus may vary between two and six. In contrast to the statement that four cusps are necessary for the diagnosis of persistent truncus arteriosus,[57,106] the number of valve cusps present cannot be employed as a significant criterion for the diagnosis of persistent truncus arteriosus.

Pars Membranacea Septi.—The formation of the uppermost portion of the ventricular septum, the membranous portion, is brought about in the region of the conus arteriosus of the ventricles. This is accomplished by the merging of the lower portions of the conus ridges with the right tubercles of the endocardial cushions of the atrioventricular canal and the crest of the muscular ventricular septum. This does not take place, however, through direct fusion of these elements, for, as pointed out by Frazer, Odgers, and Kramer, the embryonic interventricular foramen never completely closes. Rather, the original interventricular foramen above the primary muscular septum is partially remolded into the subaortic conus and the final steps in the partitioning of the ventricle and conus take place where this foramen opens into the right ventricle. The right tubercle of the ventral atrioventricular cushion plays a most important role in this final closure of the interventricular foramen.

As the conus septum, which has developed by the fusing of the conus ridges, grows caudad, it extends toward the right border of the ventricular septum. However, the dextrodorsal conus ridge diverges toward the orifice of the right atrioventricular canal while the sinistroventral conus ridge becomes continuous with the right border of the ventricular septum. The dextrodorsal conus ridge merges with the right tubercle of the atrioventricular canal cushion, thus straddling the right atrioventricular orifice. The fusion of the basal portion of this conus ridge with the right tubercle of the ventral cushion of the atrioventricular canal closes the communication between the right ventricle and the subaortic conus of the left ventricle. With further fusion of (1) the right and left conus ridges, (2) the endocardial cushion tissue at the crest of the ventricular septum and (3) the right tubercle of the ventral atrioventricular canal cushion, the opening between the subaortic conus and the right ventricle is occluded.[90] This is the final step in the separation of the aortic and pulmonary channels. At least three reports[20, 62, 74] in the literature concern hearts in which congenital defects occurred in this final closure. They should be considered as examples of partial persistent conus arteriosus.

In accordance with this concept, it is found that ventricular septal defects of varying magnitude may be associated with persistent truncus arteriosus. The defect may represent complete absence of the entire ventricular septum as in cases of cor biloculare or cor triloculare biatriatum. This occurred in 19 of the cases of persistent truncus arteriosus in the series reviewed. A complete ventricular septum may be present, with the defect only in the upper part of the conus or truncus septum. Four such cases have been reported in which a complete pars membranacea septi was present (Preisz, cases 15 and 16, Kettler, and Graham and Montgomery). There were also cases of a single localized defect in the truncus septum that gave communication between the aorta and pulmonary trunk.

The Pulmonary Arteries.—An understanding of the manner of origin of the pulmonary circulation from the truncus arteriosus involves a consideration of the development of the sixth aortic arches. In vertebrate embryos, six pairs of aortic arches are formed; these connect the ventral aorta with the dorsal aortae. In human embryos the entire series of aortic arches are never present simultaneously. The two most cephalad arches disappear as main chanels before the more caudad arches are well established. The fifth arch, if indeed it appears, does so transitorily as a vestigial vessel appended to one of the neighboring arches. Only the ventral and dorsal aortic roots and the third, fourth and sixth arches play an important role in the formation of the permanent vessels. The sixth arches give rise to the right and left pulmonary arteries.

Bremer in 1902 and Llorca in 1933 demonstrated that when the sixth aortic arches are first formed they branch off laterally from the ascending primitive trunk (fig. 462, *a*) to meet the descending dorsal aortic roots. From the caudal aspect of each of the sixth arches buds develop which are the anlagen of the pulmonary arteries. That part of the left sixth arch between the developing left pulmonary artery and its connection with the left dorsal aortic root remains as the ductus arteriosus. Normally, the corresponding portion on the right side disappears.

Llorca, in his study of a series of eight human embryos that varied from 5 to 13 mm. in length, was able to show that the right sixth arch shifts dorsally toward the left sixth arch (fig. 462, *b*). By the time these two arches have become closely aligned, the truncus septum has partially formed, thus separating the aortic and pulmonary circulations as shown in figure 462, *c*. Both Bremer and Llorca emphasized that the right sixth arch shifts so completely to the left, apparently owing to differential growth, that it may appear to spring from the left arch. With the completion of the truncus septum, the circulation appears as it does in figure 462, *d* with a single pulmonary trunk and persistent ductus arteriosus on the left.

It is upon the recognition of these stages in the development of the pulmonary circulation that the anatomic classification of the cases of persistent truncus arteriosus reviewed by us is based. It was found that the cases could be typed according to the origin of the pulmonary arteries, each type representing different stages in the evolution of the sixth aortic arches as shown in figure 462, *a*, *b*, *c* and *d*.

CRITERIA FOR THE PATHOLOGIC DIAGNOSIS OF PERSISTENT TRUNCUS ARTERIOSUS

Vierordt in 1898 was one of the first to classify cases of persistent truncus arteriosus. He classified 28 cases into three groups according to the following gross anatomic characteristics: (1) partial persistence of the embryonic truncus arteriosus as a single trunk from which the aorta and pulmonary trunks arose, (2) a single arterial trunk with the characteristics of the aorta and (3) a single arterial trunk with the characteristics of the pulmonary artery. This same classification was accepted by Herxheimer in 1910 and Mönckeberg in 1924. The latter author suggested that cases be classified as to "partial" or "complete" persistence of the common arterial trunk on the basis of the degree of septal formation.

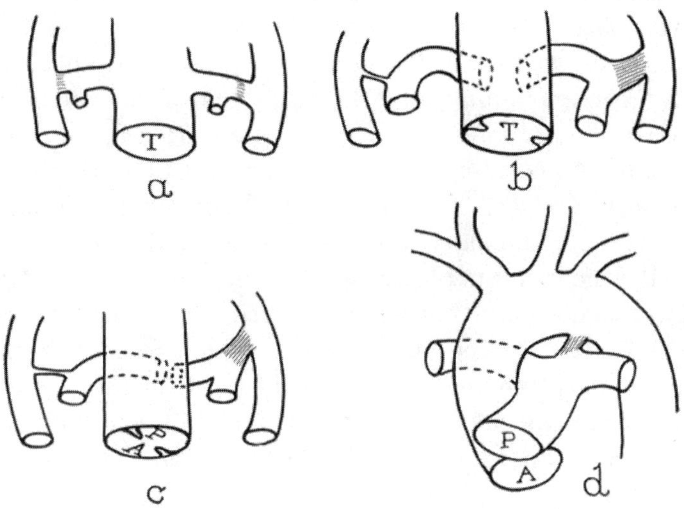

Fig. 462.—*a* to *d*, Development of the sixth aortic arches to form the pulmonary arteries and pulmonary trunk from the primitive truncus arteriosus. *Shaded part*, the ductus arteriosus, distal portion of the sixth aortic arch; *T*, truncus arteriosus; *A*, aorta, and *P*, pulmonary trunk. See text.

Humphreys in 1932 classified the reported cases according to the number of semilunar cusps. She set down eight criteria for the identification of persistent truncus arteriosus. Her first two criteria are acceptable to us and are included in the list of criteria to follow; her last six criteria do not seem valid. She included as criteria the presence of four semilunar valve leaflets, an abnormal topography of the cardiac musculature, an atrial septal defect and abnormal atrioventricular valves.

The number and position of the semilunar valve cusps of the truncus are not significant because, as shown in the discussion on their development, they may vary from only two cusps to as many as six. In 8 cases that met our criteria, there was no atrial septal defect. In the majority of cases the mitral and tricuspid valves were normal.

Lev and Saphir in 1942 stated that the only criterion necessary for diagnosis of persistent truncus was the presence of one large trunk emanating from the heart and giving off the coronary arteries, the pulmonary arteries and the systemic arteries. They referred to their definite cases as "partial," "almost complete" and "complete" types of persistent truncus, in accordance with Mönckeberg's suggestion.

After reviewing numerous descriptions of hearts with a single arterial trunk in which there were no remnants of an atretic second vessel and after investigating the embryologic development of the truncus and conus arteriosus, we have come to the conclusion that only two absolute criteria are necessary for the pathologic diagnosis of persistent truncus arteriosus: (1) there must be only one main arterial trunk leaving the base of the heart and there must be no remnant of an atretic pulmonary artery or aorta and (2) this single arterial trunk must supply branches to the coronary, pulmonary and systemic circulations.

Frequent concomitants of persistent truncus cases but not criteria for pathologic diagnosis are (1) an interventricular septal defect, varying from a small defect of the membranous portion to complete absence of the ventricular septum and (2) an overriding of the interventricular septal defect by the truncus arteriosus, which at times arises more from the right ventricle than from the left. With extreme dextroposition, the truncus may arise solely from the right ventricle.

ANATOMIC CLASSIFICATION OF THE REPORTED CASES OF PERSISTENT TRUNCUS ARTERIOSUS

The most applicable classification of the different types of persistent truncus arteriosus which meet the necessary criteria for a pathologic diagnosis is based on the embryologic stages in the development of the pulmonary arteries from the sixth aortic arches. There are four major types of cases of persistent truncus arteriosus (fig. 463):

Type 1. A single pulmonary trunk and ascending aorta arise from the truncus arteriosus.

Type 2. The right and left pulmonary arteries arise close together from the dorsal wall of the truncus arteriosus.

Type 3. One or both pulmonary arteries arise independently from either side of the truncus arteriosus.

Type 4. There are no pulmonary arteries and there is apparent congenital absence of the sixth aortic arches. The arterial circulation to the lungs is by way of bronchial arteries.

1252 ROBERT W. COLLETT, JESSE E. EDWARDS

These four major types represent the various stages of arrested development (fig. 462). Type 4 signifies the earliest stage, since no representation of the sixth aortic arches is present. Type 3 represents the next earliest stage in which the sixth aortic arches branch laterally from the truncus (fig. 462, *a*). Type 2 represents a later stage in which the right pulmonary artery has shifted dorsally and to the left to become more closely allied with the left sixth arch (fig. 462, *b* and *c*). Type 1 indicates a much later stage in which the two pulmonary arteries branch from a common pulmonary trunk that in turn takes its origin from the truncus arteriosus. The various types are subdivided on the basis of the direction

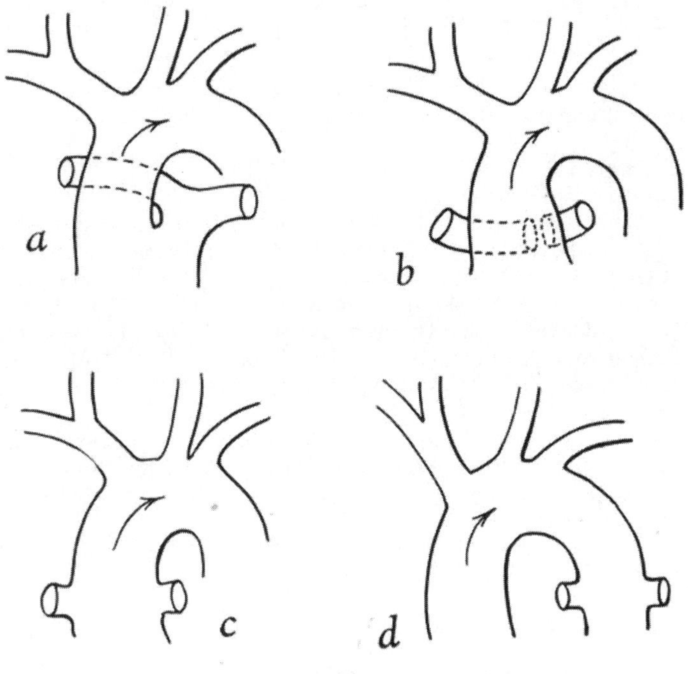

Fig. 463.—The four major anatomic types of persistent truncus arteriosus. *a*, Type 1; *b*, type 2; *c*, type 3; and *d*, type 4. Arrow indicates the direction of flow of blood from the heart.

and condition of the aortic arch and the presence or absence of the ductus arteriosus. These types and subtypes are illustrated in figures 464 to 469, which were drawn by Mr. Russell Drake.

Type 1.—Type 1 is represented by 38 cases which are subdivided according to seven different anatomic variations (fig. 464). In each case a short pulmonary trunk and ascending aorta arise from the truncus arteriosus. The first subdivision includes 21 cases, in which the aortic arch turns to the left, the ductus arteriosus is absent and the pulmonary trunk springs from the left side of the truncus (fig. 464, *a*). This subtype represents the largest single group of cases of the series. The second subtype differs from the first in that the pulmonary trunk arises from the

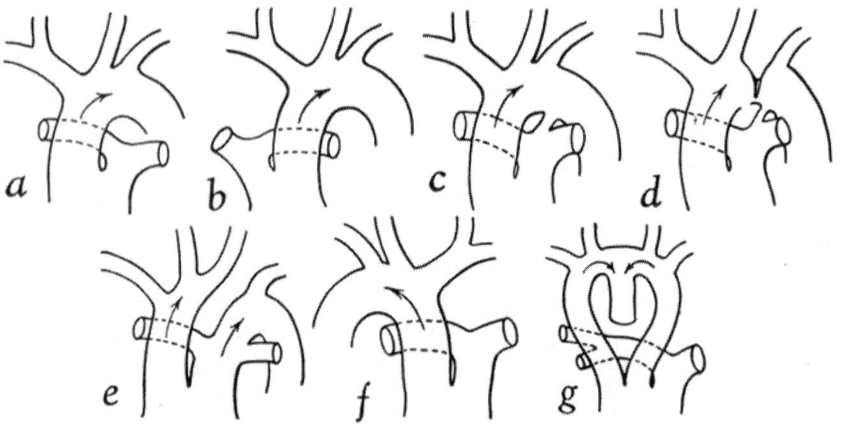

Fig. 464.—Type 1 persistent truncus arteriosus.

Type 1. Single pulmonary trunk and ascending aorta arise from truncus arteriosus (38 cases)

- A. Left aortic arch
  - 1. Ductus arteriosus absent
    - a. Pulmonary trunk from left side (subtype 1, 21 cases) (fig. 464, *a*). Case reports: Wilson (1798)*; Mansfeld (1843)†‡; Hyernaux (1851)§; Deutsch (1851)*†; Green (1868)†; Pott, case 9 (1879)†; Clarke (1885)†; Klipstein, case 1 (1890)‡; Klipstein, case 2 (1890)†; Cade (1897)†; Santa Cruz (1925); Beaver (1933); Davison (1935); Cardelle and co-workers (1935)†; Pierret and Lelebure (1937) †; Rizzi, case 3 (1938) *; Mannheimer and Nordenfelt (1938)*; Kettler (1939); Doerr (1943); Marshall (1943); Taussig (1947)
    - b. Pulmonary trunk from right side (subtype 2, 5 cases) (fig. 464, *b*). Case reports: Preisz, case 15 (1890); Valdes Diaz and Perez de Los Reyes (1936); Szypulski (1937)†; Walls (1941)*†; Michelson (1943)
  - 2. Ductus arteriosus present
    - a. Coarctation of aortic arch not present (subtype 3, 3 cases) (fig. 464, *c*). Case reports: Feller, case 4 (1931); Humphreys (1932); Van Brown (1942)
    - b. Coarctation of aortic arch present (subtype 4, 1 case) (fig. 464, *d*). Case report: Feller, case 2 (1931)
    - c. Complete atresia of part of aortic arch (subtype 5, 1 case) (fig. 464, *e*). Case report: Preisz, case 16 (1890)
- B. Right aortic arch (subtype 6, 6 cases) (fig. 464, *f*). Case reports: Rokitansky (1852); Epstein (1886)*; Krausse (1905)*; Feller, case 1 (1931); Roos (1935); Bredt (1935)
- C. Double aortic arch (subtype 7, 1 case) (fig. 464, *g*). Case report: Kerwin (1936)

---

* Single ventricle.
† Direction of arch assumed to be normal.
‡ Stenosis of pulmonary trunk.
§ Origin of pulmonary trunk high.

right side of the truncus (fig. 464, *b*). There are 5 cases of this subtype. The third subtype, represented by 3 cases, differs from the first only in that the ductus arteriosus is present and patent (fig. 464, *c*).

There is only 1 case each of the fourth and fifth subtypes, but they are closely related. In the former case, reported by Feller, there is an associated coarctation of the aorta between the origin of the left common carotid and the left subclavian arteries (fig. 464, *d*). In the latter case, reported by Priesz, there is complete interruption of the aorta at approximately the same site as the coarctation in the former case (fig. 464, *e*). In each the ductus arteriosus is functioning. Recently, Sewart reported a case of congenital interruption of the aortic arch in which the

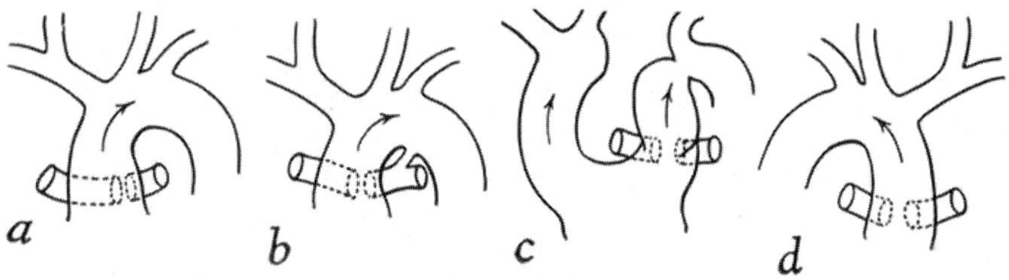

Fig. 465—Type 2 persistent truncus arteriosus.

Type 2. The right and left pulmonary arteries arise close together from the dorsal wall of the truncus arteriosus (23 cases)

- A. Left aortic arch
  - 1. Ductus arteriosus absent
    - a. (Subtype 1, 18 cases) (fig. 465, *a*). Case reports: Forster (1846)*; Vernon (1856)†; Bradley (1873)†; Pott, case 1 (1879)†‡; Grant (1883)*; Wenner, case 5 (1909); Wenner, case 6 (1909)*†; Ingalls (1915); Klemke (1925); Pezzi and Agostoni (1928); Siegmund, case 2 (1928); Dagnini, case 2 (1931); Dagnini, case 1, (1931)†; Hunter and Mackey (1935); Carr and co-workers (1935); Giustra and Tosti, case 1, (1939)†; Giustra and Tosti, case 2, (1939)†; Lev and Saphir (1942)
  - 2. Ductus arteriosus present
    - a. Coarctation and atresia of aortic arch not present (subtype 2, 2 cases) (fig. 465, *b*). Case reports: Motta (1932); Harris and Thomson (1937)
    - b. Complete interruption of aortic arch (subtype 3, 1 case) (fig. 465, *c*). Case report: Tiedemann (1831)
- B. Right aortic arch (subtype 4, 2 cases) (fig. 465, *d*). Case reports: Buchanan (1864); Abbott (1931)

---

* Direction of arch assumed to be normal.
† Single ventricle.
‡ Stenosis of truncus arteriosus.

ascending aorta and pulmonary trunk were perfectly formed. In her case the interruption was distal to the left subclavian artery. It is of passing interest that there are 6 similar cases reported in the literature.

The sixth subtype is represented by 6 cases (fig. 464, *f*). In these the pulmonary trunk arises from the left side of the truncus but the aortic arch is on the right side. They are almost mirror images of the cases of the second subtype.

In the last case of type 1, representing the seventh subtype, there is a double aortic arch (fig. 464*g*). The single pulmonary trunk springs from the left side of the truncus.

Type 2.—Twenty-three cases represent type 2 (fig. 465). They are subdivided into four anatomic subtypes according to the same pattern as type 1. In all of these cases both the right and left pulmonary arteries arise directly from the truncus, their orifices being very close to each other. The 18 cases of the first subtype are comparable to those of the first subtype of type 1 in that the aortic arch is on the left and there is no ductus arteriosus (fig. 465, *a*). Only 2 cases are of the second subtype

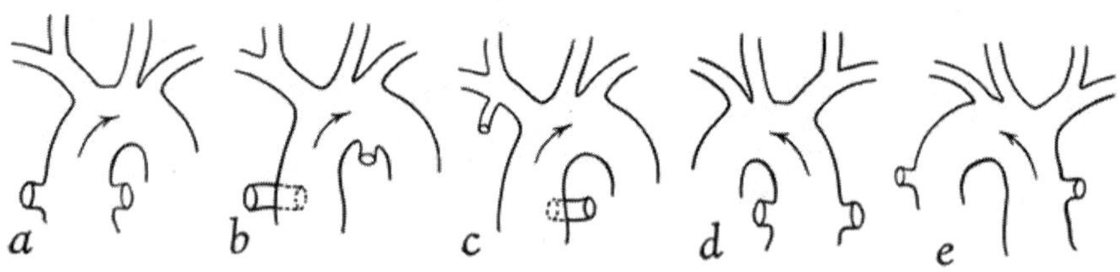

Fig. 466.—Type 3 persistent truncus arteriosus.

Type 3. The right and left pulmonary arteries arise independently from the right and left lateral walls of the truncus arteriosus (9 cases)
- A. Left aortic arch
  - 1. Ductus arteriosus not present
    - a. Both sixth arches present (subtype 1, 4 cases) (fig. 466, *a*). Case reports: Heath and Power (1865); Feller, case 3 (1931); Tow (1931)*†; Goltman and Stern (1939)
  - 2. Ductus arteriosus present
    - a. Only one sixth arch present, supplying one lung; other lung supplied by way of ductus arteriosus or bronchial arteries (subtype 2, 3 cases) (fig. 466, *b* and *c*). Case reports: Pott, case 10 (1879) (fig. 466, *b*); Dickson and Fraser (1914)‡; Shapiro (1930) (fig. 466, *c*)
- B. Right aortic arch
  - a. Both sixth arches present (subtype 3, 1 case) (fig. 466, *d*). Case report: Mallory (1948)
  - b. One sixth arch present, bronchial supply to other lung (subtype 4, 1 case) (fig. 466, *e*). Case report: Wirth (1912)§

* Direction of arch assumed to be normal.

† Single ventricle.

‡ Right pulmonary artery arose from left side of truncus. Left lung supplied by bronchial artery from descending aorta.

§ Origin of pulmonary artery high.

(fig. 465, *b*). In these the ductus arteriosus is present and patent and the aortic arch is normal. The case reported by Tiedemann representing the third subtype of type 2 (fig. 465, *c*) is similar, with respect to the structure of the aortic arch to the Priesz case 16. There is complete interruption of the aortic arch. In the 2 remaining cases of type 2, the aortic arch curves to the right (fig. 465, *d*).

Type 3.—Nine cases are of type 3 (fig. 466). They are divided into four anatomic subtypes. The pulmonary arteries arise independently from the right and left lateral walls of the truncus. The first subtype is represented by 4 cases in which the aortic arch is on the left (fig. 466, *a*). In cases of the second (fig. 466, *b* and *c*) and fourth (fig. 466, *e*) subtypes, only one pulmonary artery is present and it supplies only one lung; the other lung is supplied by enlarged bronchial arteries or a persistent ductus arteriosus. These two subtypes differ from each other in the direction of the aortic arch. The 1 case of the third subtype was reported recently by Mallory and associates (fig. 466, *d*). They described it as a case in which the fifth aortic arches were persistent. More logically, it seems that this case is comparable to those in the first subtype of type 3 ex-

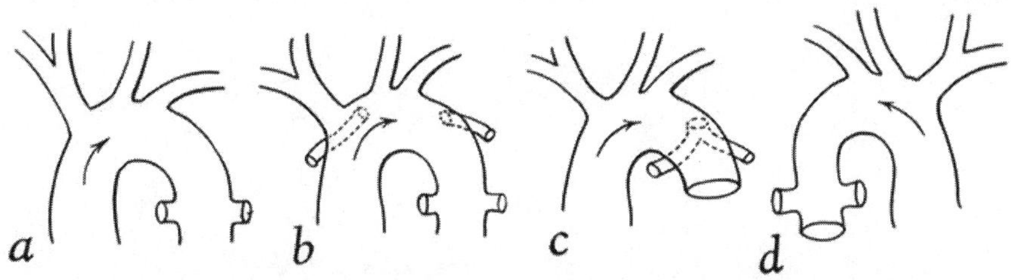

Fig. 467.—Type 4 persistent truncus arteriosus.

Type 4. No pulmonary arteries. Absence of sixth arch derivatives. Arterial circulation to lungs by way of bronchial arteries (10 cases)

- A. Left aortic arch
  - 1. Bronchial supply to lungs
    - a. From descending aorta (subtype 1, 7 cases) (fig. 467, *a*). Case reports: Calori (1843)*; Charrin and Le Noir (1891)*; Hülse (1918); Zimmerman (1927); Finley (1930); Miller and Lyon (1931); Greenspon and Leaman (1939)
    - b. From descending aorta and arch of aorta (subtype 2, 1 case) (fig. 467, *b*). Case report: Gallois (1896)
    - c. From arch of aorta (subtype 3, 1 case) (fig. 467, *c*). Case report: Graham and Montgomery (1938)
- B. Right aortic arch
  - 1. Bronchial supply to lungs
    - a. From descending aorta (subtype 4, 1 case) (fig. 467, *d*). Case report: Siegmund, case 1 (1928)

* Direction of arch assumed to be normal.

cept for the right-sided aortic arch. It resembles a mirror image of the first subtype of type 3.

Type 4.—The cases of type 4 are those in which neither right nor left pulmonary arteries nor a pulmonary trunk is present (fig. 467). The ungs are supplied solely by bronchial arteries arising from either the arch of the aorta or the descending aorta. There are 10 cases of this type which are subdivided into four subtypes. The first subtype is represented by 7 cases, in all of which there is a left aortic arch and in which the bronchial arteries arise from the descending aorta (fig. 467, *a*). Each of the remaining three subtypes is represented by 1 case. The case of Gallois (second subtype, fig. 467, *b*) and Graham and associates (third subtype, fig. 467, *c*) differ from each other only in the location and number of bronchial arteries. In each there is a left aortic arch. In the first case reported by Siegmund, comprising the fourth subtype, there is a right aortic arch, and the bronchial supply to the lungs is from the descending aorta (fig. 467, *d*).

The 80 cases that represent the first four major types in this classification are unequivocally examples of persistent truncus arteriosus. Eleven additional cases of probable persistent truncus arteriosus could not be classified because insufficient information was given. The exact mode of arterial supply to the lungs was not stated specifically. Therefore, these

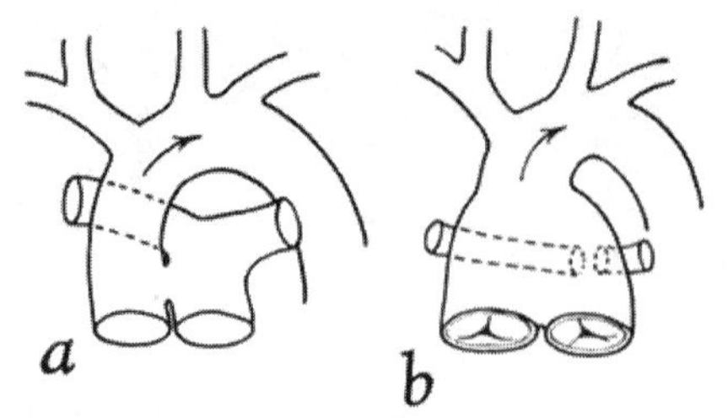

Fig. 468.—Type 5 persistent truncus arteriosus.

Type 5. Partial persistent truncus arteriosus. Localized defect in truncus-conus septum. Communication between aorta and pulmonary trunk (congenital) (13 cases)

A. Small defect. Left aortic arch. Right and left pulmonary arteries from pulmonary trunk (subtype 1, 11 cases) (fig. 468, *a*). Case reports: Elliotson (1830)*; Wilks (1860)*; Fraentzel (1868)*; Rauchfuss (1878)*; Baginsky (1879)*; Caesar (1880)†; Gerhardt (1881)*; Rickards (1881)†; Girard (1895)†; Fisher (1901)†; Moorhead and Smith (1923)‡

B. Large defect. Left aortic arch. Right and left pulmonary arteries from sinistrodorsal aspect of persistent truncus (subtype 2, 2 cases) (fig. 468, *b*). Case reports: Hektoen (1899)§; Bain (1943)‡

---

* Ductus arteriosus closed.
† Condition of ductus arteriosus not known.
‡ Ductus arteriosus absent.
§ Ductus arteriosus fully developed.

11 cases are listed under "Unclassified group" after data pertaining to figure 469.

There is an interesting group of cases which may seem at first not to meet the required criteria for the diagnosis of persistent truncus arteriosus. These are cases in which the pulmonary and aortic channels are separated at the level of the semilunar valves, but in which there are various localized defects in the septal system either above, at or below this level giving communication between the two circulations.

The localized defects are due either to absence of development of the truncoconal septum at the level of the defect or to localized fenestration of the septum after it has formed. There may be a large defect between the pulmonary trunk and aorta even though their respective semilunar valves are well formed and the ventricular septum is intact.

Since persistent truncus arteriosus, by definition, is manifested by incomplete division of the truncoconal channel by the truncoconal septum, these cases represent partial persistence of the truncus. Therefore, such cases are described in the classification as type 5.

Type 5.—This type is characterized by partial persistent truncus arteriosus, localized defect in the truncoconal septum and a communication between the aorta and the pulmonary trunk (congenital) (fig. 468).

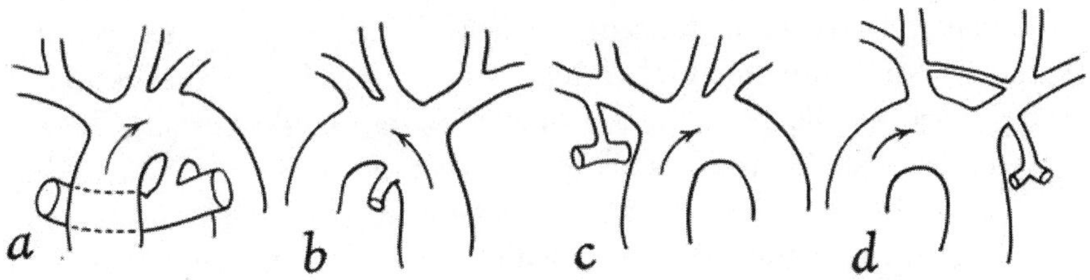

Fig. 469.—So-called persistent truncus arteriosus.

Anomalies considered not to be persistent truncus arteriosus which have been considered as such by other authors (12 cases)

- A. Single arterial trunk
  1. Left aortic arch. Pulmonary supply by way of ductus arteriosus (8 cases) (fig. 469 *a*). Case reports: Ramsbotham (1848)*†; Peacock and Reed (1880); Wright and Drake (1903); Knape (1912); Bókay (1914); Popjak (1942); Hunter (1944); Webb (1946)
  2. Right aortic arch. Pulmonary supply by way of right ductus arteriosus (?) (1 case) (fig. 469, *b*). Case report: Harris (1926)
- B. Single arterial trunk
  1. Left aortic arch
     - a. Pulmonary supply by way of remnant of ductus arteriosus through innominate artery (right) (2 cases) (fig. 469, *c*). Case reports: Herxheimer (1910)*; Mehta and Hewlett (1945)
     - b. By way of left innominant artery (1 case) (fig. 469, *d*). Case report: Wood and Williams (1928)

Unclassified group (11 cases)

(Insufficient information—neither direction of aortic arch nor means of circulation to lungs known)

Case reports: Crisp (1846); Hervieux (1861); Nunneley (1871); Richardière and Huber (1912); Abbott, case 2 (1927); Luis de Cubas (1931); Dancourt and Bastien (1935); Leech, case 61 (1935); Leech, case 63 (1935); Cordier and coworkers (1938); Solis-Cohen and co-workers (1944).

---

* Direction of arch assumed to be normal.

† Single ventricle.

Thirteen cases of this type are reported in the literature. They can be subdivided according to the relative size of the truncoconal septal defect. Small localized defects in the truncus septum were found in 11 cases comprising the first subtype (fig. 468, *a*). The defects varied in location from a site just above the anterior aortic sinus to a site at the beginning of the arch of the aorta. Those communications in or near the arch of the aorta should not be confused with the so-called window type of persistent ductus arteriosus such as in the case reported by Lutembacher. It is emphasized that it may be difficult to rule out acquired communications in some of these cases.

In a case reported by Rickards the defect lay behind the anterior semilunar cusp of a bicuspid aortic valve. Below this communication between the pulmonary trunk and the aorta, there was a defect in the membranous portion of the ventricular septum.

In 2 cases, one reported by Charteris and another by Jacobi and Heinrich, there was a communication between the aorta and the conus of the right ventricle representing a defect in the final step in the separation of the aortic and pulmonary channels as described in the discussion of the embryology of the pars membranacea. These could be classed as cases representing partial persistence of the conus arteriosus due to lack of completion of the conus septum in localized areas.

Livingston reported a case in which there was a defect between the aorta and right ventricle at the level of the tricuspid valve; this defect represented the lack of fusion of the basal portion of the dextrodorsal conus ridge with the right tubercle of the ventral cushion of the atrioventricular canal.

Localized weakness in the completed truncoconal septum may result in an aneurysm of that particular portion of the septum. Ten cases of such aneurysms[1, 8, 43, 51, 69, 71, 107, 112, 114, 124] have been reported. It is questionable if these can all be considered to be congenital defects because only 1 of the patients died at an age of less than 26 years. This was the case reported by White in a boy aged 15 years.

In the remaining 2 cases of type 5 there was a large defect in the truncus septum (fig. 468, *b*). The right and left pulmonary arteries arose from the posterior left aspect of the partial persisting truncus. Except for the presence of the intact aortic and pulmonary semilunar valves, these cases resemble those of type 2.

In 6 of the cases of type 5, the ductus arteriosus had formed but was closed at the time of necropsy. The ductus arteriosus was absent in 2 cases, 1 of which was reported by Moorhead and Smith in 1923 and the other by Bain and Parkinson in 1943. In Hektoen's case, the ductus arteriosus was persistent and patent.

CASES CONSIDERED NOT TO BE PERSISTENT TRUNCUS ARTERIOSUS WHICH HAVE FORMERLY BEEN CONSIDERED AS SUCH

The remaining 12 cases of the 116 in this series are considered not to be cases of persistent truncus arteriosus (fig. 469). The essential features of these cases include the presence of a single arterial trunk that follows the course of the aorta and a pulmonary arterial supply that is acquired by means of a persistent ductus arteriosus. There are 8 cases in which the source of blood to the lungs is by a normally located ductus, that is, the right and left pulmonary arteries appear to branch from the ductus arteriosus (fig. 469, *a*). Such cases have been included as typical examples in former series of cases of persistent truncus arteriosus. However, since the right and left pulmonary arteries are derived as branches of the proximal portions of the right and left sixth aortic arches, the presence of both of them presupposes that the proximal portion of the right and left sixth aortic arches were present at one time. Since the right and left pulmonary arteries showed no connection with the truncus or a derivative of it, those parts of the sixth arches must have been present at one time but must have subsequently disappeared. Under these circumstances it is impossible to state whether they had arisen from a truncus arteriosus or from a pulmonary trunk which had developed from partitioning of the truncus. There are numerous cases in the literature which resemble these 8 cases in that the pulmonary supply was obtained through a ductus arteriosus, but in which an atretic pulmonary trunk is present and connected with the functioning ductus. Inasmuch as it is impossible to determine in these 8 cases whether or not the truncus had in fact been partitioned at one time, it is impossible to include them unequivocally as examples of persistent truncus arteriosus.

In the case of a right aortic arch reported by Harris in 1926 there was complete absence of the left lung. The arterial supply to the right lung appeared to be by way of a right-sided ductus arteriosus (fig. 469, *b*). Thus interpreted, a right-sided pulmonary trunk might have developed at one time but subsequently disappeared. The stillborn infant which Harris described was markedly deformed. It was a case of phocomelus with congenital cystic elephantiasis.

In the last 3 cases a single arterial trunk arose from the base of the heart but the pulmonary arterial supply was by means of an anomalous ductus arteriosus that branched from the innominate artery. The anomaly described in the cases reported by Herxheimer, and Mehta and Hewlett is illustrated in figure 469, *c*. The anomaly described by Wood and Williams is illustrated in figure 469, *d*.

ANOMALIES ASSOCIATED WITH PERSISTENT TRUNCUS ARTERIOSUS

Associated with persistent truncus arteriosus in the 93 cases of the five types given in the classification were numerous other cardiac and vascular anomalies (table 1). The origin of the truncus arteriosus in the first four types and the variation in the number of semilunar valve cusps are shown in table 2. The direction of the aortic arch and the variation in number and position of the coronary arteries are shown in table 3.

Various noncardiac congenital anomalies that were coexistent with persistent truncus are listed in table 4.

The age of the patients at the time of death in the cases reviewed are

TABLE 1

CARDIAC AND VASCULAR ANOMALIES ASSOCIATED WITH PERSISTENT TRUNCUS ARTERIOSUS (93 CASES)

Anomaly	Cases
Atrial septal defect	8
Common atrioventricular valve	19
Single ventricle	19
Bilocular heart	14
Trilocular heart	5
Stenosis of truncus	1
Stenosis of pulmonary trunk	2
Ectopic coronary arteries	6
One present	7
Three present	1
One from pulmonary artery	1
Right aortic arch	11
Double aortic arch	1
Absent ductus arteriosus	71
Functioning ductus arteriosus	12
Coarctation of aortic arch	1
Complete interruption of aortic arch	2
Two superior venae cavae	2
Abnormal number of pulmonary veins	20
Two pulmonary veins	9
One pulmonary vein	7
Three pulmonary veins	4
Abnormal brachiocephalic vessels	11
Four brachiocephalic vessels	6

TABLE 2

ORIGIN OF THE TRUNCUS ARTERIOSUS AND THE NUMBER OF SEMILUNAR VALVES ACCORDING TO THE VARIOUS TYPES

	Type				Total
	1	2	3	4	
Origin of truncus					
Both ventricles (overriding septal defect)	17	11	3	7	38
Right ventricle	7	3	4	2	16
Left ventricle	2	0	0	0	2
Single ventricle	8	9	2	0	19
Unknown	4	0	0	1	5
Number of semilunar cusps					
Two	0	1	0	0	1
Three	14	15	7	7	43
Three plus*	1	4	1	0	6
Four	9	0	0	0	9
Six	1	0	0	0	1
Not given	13	3	1	3	20

* Evidence of partial division of one of the three cusps.

shown in table 5. It is interesting to note that of the four major types, only in the cases of type 2, in which the right and left pulmonary

TABLE 3

The Direction of the Aortic Arch and the Variation in Number and Position of the Coronary Arteries According to the Types of Persistent Truncus Arteriosus

	Type					Total
	1	2	3	4	5	
Direction of aortic arch						
To the left	20	18	6	7	13	64
To the right	6	2	2	1	0	11
Double arch	1	0	0	0	0	1
Not known	11	3	1	2	0	17
Totals	38	23	9	10	13	93
Number of coronary arteries						
Number given	19	17	7	7	4	54
Three	1	0	0	0	0	1
Two	16	14	6	6	4	46
One	2	3	1	1	0	7
Number not given	19	6	2	3	9	39
Ectopic coronary arteries	2	3	1	0	0	6

TABLE 4

Noncardiac Congenital Anomalies and Inflammatory Conditions Associated with Persistent Truncus Arteriosus

Anomaly or Inflammatory Condition	Cases
Situs inversus	3
Sympus apus	1
Aplasia of spleen	2
Aplasia of anus	1
Aplasia of kidneys and ureters	1
Aplasia of testes	1
Horseshoe kidney	2
Polycystic kidney	1
Spina bifida	2
Cleft palate	1
Omphalocele and ectopia cordis	1
Absent diaphragm	1
Polydactylism	1
Microphthalmus	1
Bone defects (arm, digits)	3
Subacute bacterial endocarditis	1
"Fetal endocarditis"	4
Fibrous endocarditis	1
Cerebral abscess	3

arteries arose close together from the dorsal wall of the truncus, and in cases of type 4, in which no pulmonary arteries were present, did any persons reach maturity. In the cases of type 2, 3 persons died between the ages of 16 and 36 years. Five with type 4 lesions died between the ages of 18 and 36 years. It is also interesting that few deaths occurred between the ages of 5 and 16 years; only 3 patients with lesions of the first four major types died in this period, at ages 5,[48] $5\frac{1}{2}$[60] and 13[81] years respectively. Twenty-six of the 85 patients for whom the age of death was given died during the first week of life (30.6 per cent). Thirty persons died in the age period of 8 days to 6 months inclusive and 8 from the ages of 7 to 14 months inclusive. Nearly a third of the patients lived to be more than 6 months of age. About 10 per cent of the patients lived to the age of 20 years or more.

The inflammatory conditions stated as being commonly associated with congenital heart disease were conspicuous by their paucity. In only 1 of the 80 cases of the four major types was the patient reported to have had subacute bacterial endocarditis. In 4 cases there were warty vegetations on the atrioventricular valves. These were considered by the respective authors to be evidence of fetal endocarditis. Fibrous endocarditis was described in 1 case (Santa Cruz). Three patients reported on by Greenspon and Leaman, Hülse and Caesar, respectively, died of cerebral abscesses as a complication of the congenital heart disease.

TABLE 5

AGE OF PATIENTS WITH PERSISTENT TRUNCUS ARTERIOSUS AT THE TIME OF DEATH

AGE AT DEATH	TOTAL	CASES BY TYPE				
		1	2	3	4	5
Stillborn–7 days	26	11	10	3	1	1
8 days–6 mo	30	17	7	2	3	1
7–14 mo.	8	3	1	3	0	1
15 mo.–9 yr.	6	2	0	0	1	3
10–19 yr.	5	1	2	0	2	0
20 yr. or more	10	0	2	0	3	5
Age not given	8	4	1	1	0	2
Totals	93	38	23	9	10	13
Range of ages		(1 hr.–13 yr.)	(Stillborn–36 yr.)	(1 hr.–14 mo.)	(1 hr.–33 yr.)	(Newborn–48 yr.)

SUMMARY

A review is made of the embryology of the human heart, with emphasis on the development of the septal system which divides the ventricles, the conus arteriosus and the truncus arteriosus to form two separate circulations. This review is based fundamentally upon work done by Kramer and Patten. It is pointed out that by defective growth of the truncoconal ridges which normally unite to form the truncoconal septum, the original truncoconal channel remains as a persistent truncus arteriosus.

On the basis of this review, the two absolute criteria set up for the pathologic diagnosis of persistent truncus arteriosus are (1) that there must be only one main arterial trunk leaving the base of the heart and there must be no remnant of an atretic pulmonary trunk or aorta and (2) that this single arterial trunk must supply branches to the coronary, pulmonary and systemic circulations. The contribution of the sixth aortic arches in the formation of the pulmonary arteries is pointed out. On the basis of the embryologic development of the pulmonary arteries from the sixth aortic arches, an anatomic classification of the cases of persistent truncus arteriosus into four major types and one minor type is made, grouping the cases by types according to various stages of arrested development in this embryologic process.

In this classification, type 4 (10 cases) signifies the earliest stage, since no representation of the sixth aortic arches is present. Type 3 (9 cases) represents the next earliest stage, in which the sixth aortic arches branch laterally from the truncus. Type 2 (23 cases) represents a later stage in which the right pulmonary artery has shifted dorsally and to the left to become more closely allied with the left sixth arch. Type 1 (38 cases) indicates a much later stage in which the two pulmonary arteries branch from a common pulmonary trunk that in turn takes its origin from the truncus arteriosus. These various types are subdivided on the basis of the direction and condition of the aortic arch and the presence or absence of the ductus arteriosus.

REFERENCES

1. Abbott, Maude E.: Clinical and Developmental Study of a Case of Ruptured Aneurysm of the Right Anterior Aortic Sinus of Valsalva Leading to Communication Between the Aorta and Base of the Right Ventricle, Diagnosed During Life. Opening in Anterior Interventricular Septum (Probably Bulbar Septal Defect). Malignant Endocarditis. In: Contributions to Medical and Biological Research, Dedicated to Sir William Osler. New York, Paul B. Hoeber, Inc., 1919, vol. 2, pp. 899–914.
2. Abbott, Maude E.: Congenital Heart Disease. Complete Defect of the Aortic Septum: Persistent Truncus Arteriosus. In Nelson Loose-leaf Medicine. New York, Thomas Nelson & Sons, 1931, vol. 4, pp. 280–284.
3. Abbott, Maude E.: Quoted by Bauer, D. de F., and Astbury, Effie C.: Congenital Cardiac Disease. Bibliography of the 1,000 Cases Analyzed in Maude Abbott's Atlas. Am. Heart J. *27*:688–732 (May) 1944.
4. Abbott, Maude E.: Quoted by Osler, William and McCrae, Thomas: Modern Medicine; Its Theory and Practice. Philadelphia, Lea & Febiger, 1927, vol. 4, pp. 707–710.
5. Baginsky, B.: Verhandlungen ärztlicher Gesellschaften. Berl. klin. Wchnschr. *16*:439–440 (July 21) 1879.
6. Bain, C. W. C. and Parkinson, John: Common Aorto-pulmonary Trunk: A Rare Congenital Defect. Brit. Heart J. *5*:97–100, 1943.
7. Beaver, D. C.: Persistent Truncus Arteriosus and Congenital Absence of One Kidney With Other Developmental Defects. Arch. Path. *15*:51–54 (Jan.) 1933.

8. Beck, T. S.: Case of Aneurism of the Ascending Aorta, Bursting Into the Right Ventricle: With a Communication Between the Two Ventricles. Med. Chir. Tr. London. *25*:15–20, 1842.
9. Bókay, Zoltán: Case of Truncus Arteriosus Communis Persistens. Orvosi hétil. *58*:39–41, 1914.
10. Bradley, S. M.: Tricoelian Human Heart. Brit. M. J. *1*:33–34 (Jan. 11) 1873.
11. Bredt, Heinrich: Formdeutung und Entstehung des missgebildeten menschlichen Herzens. Kennzeichnung und Eintilung des sog. Truncus arteriosus communis persistens. Virchows Arch. f. path. Anat. *296*:130–138 (Nov. 25) 1935.
12. Bremer, J. L.: On the Origin of the Pulmonary Arteries in Mammals. Am. J. Anat. *1*:137–144 (Feb. 28) 1902.
13. Buchanan: Malformation of Heart. Undivided Truncus Arteriosus. Heart Otherwise Double. Tr. Path. Soc. London. *15*:89–91, 1864.
14. Cade, M.: Malformation du coeur; maladie bleue. Lyon méd. *85*:413 (July 18) 1897.
15. Caesar, Julius: Case of Malformation of Heart and Abscess of Brain; Unusual Contents. Lancet. *2*:768 (Nov. 13) 1880.
16. Calori, Juigi: Quoted by Taruffi, Cesare.[111]
17. Cardelle, Gustavo, Artola, Ellis, Perez de Los Reyes, R.: Dos casos de cardiopatias congenitas. Arch. de med. inf. *4*:286–296, 1935.
18. Carr, F. B., Goodale, R. H. and Rockwell, A. E. P.: Persistent Truncus Arteriosus in a Man Aged Thirty-six Years. Arch. Path. *19*:833–837 (June) 1935.
19. Charrin and Le Noir: Des phénomenès physiologiques et cliniques, dans un cas de maladie bleue. Arch. de physiol. norm. et path. *3*:206–212, 1891.
20. Charteris: Quoted by Hektoen, Ludvig.[53]
21. Clarke, Ernest: Malformation of Heart. Tr. Path. Soc. London. *36*:178, 1885.
22. Cordier, Devos, Gellé and Marcelle: A propos d'un coeur a deux cavités, absence complète de cloisonnement du tube cardiaque. Ann. d'anat. path. *15*:1034–1040 (Dec. 1) 1938.
23. Crisp: Malformation of the Heart Consisting in an Imperfect Separation of the Two Ventricles, With Absence of the Pulmonary Artery. Tr. Path. Soc. London. *1*:50–51, 1846–1848.
24. Dagnini, Giovanni: Due casi di tronco arterioso commune persistente. Clin. paediat. *13*:601–614, 1931.
25. Dancourt and Bastien, P.: Sur un cas de persistance du bulbe artériel. Echo méd. du Nord. *3*:445–447 (Mar. 24) 1935.
26. Davison, George: A Case of Congenital Heart Disease With Single Arterial Trunk. J. Anat. *69*:423–426 (July) 1935.
27. Deutsch: Ueber Cyanosis. Günsb. Ztschr. II. 2, 1851. (Abstr.) Schmidt's Jahrb. *71*:54–56, 1851.
28. Dickson, W. E. C. and Fraser, John: A Congenital Abnormality of the Heart and Blood-vessels. J. Anat. & Physiol. London. *48*:210–214 (Jan.) 1914.
29. Doerr, Wilhelm: Über Missbildungen des menschlichen Herzens mit besonderer Berücksichtigung von Bulbus und Truncus. Virchows Arch. f. path. Anat. *310*:304–368 (May 4) 1943.
30. Edwards, J. E., Bulbulian, A. H. and Rogers, H. M.: Pathologic and Embryologic Considerations in Tetralogy of Fallot. Proc. Staff Meet., Mayo Clin. *22*:166–172 (Apr. 30) 1947.
31. Elliotson: Case of Malformation of the Pulmonary Artery and Aorta. Lancet. *1*:247–248 (Nov. 13) 1830.
32. Epstein, A.: Beitrag zu den Bildungsfehlern des Herzens. Ztsch. f. Heilk. *7*:293, 1886. (Abstr.) Schmidt's Jahrb. *212*:20–21, 1886.
33. Feller, A.: Zur Kenntnis der angeborenen Herzkrankheiten. I. Truncus arteriosus communis persistens und seine formale Entstehung. Virchows Arch. f. path. Anat. *279*:869–910 (Jan. 10) 1931.

34. Finley, K. H.: A Congenital Anomaly of the Heart (Truncus Arteriosus Communis With Subacute Endocarditis). Am. J. Path. *6*:317–323 (May) 1930.
35. Fisher, Theodore: Quoted by Bauer, D. de F., and Astbury, Effie C.: Congenital Cardiac Disease. Bibliography of the 1,000 Cases Analyzed in Maude Abbott's Atlas. Am. Heart J. *27*:688–732 (May) 1944.
36. Forster, J. C.: A Heart Consisting of Only Two Cavities. Tr. Path. Soc. London. *1*:48–49, 1846–1848.
37. Fraentzel, O.: Ein Fall von abnormer Communication der Aorta mit der Arteria pulmonalis. Virchows Arch. f. path. Anat. *43*:420–426 (May 27) 1868.
38. Frazer, J. E.: The Formation of the Pars Membranacea Septi. J. Anat. *51*:19–29 (Oct.) 1916.
39. Gallois, M. E.: Forme rare de malformation cardiaque congenitale. Lyon méd. *83*:469–476 (Dec. 6) 1896.
40. Gerhardt, C.: Quoted by Hektoen, Ludvig.[53]
41. Girard, E.: Quoted by Hektoen, Ludvig.[53]
42. Giustra, F. X. and Tosti, V. G.: True Cor Biloculare in Identical Twins. Am. Heart J. *17*:249–250 (Feb.) 1939.
43. Goehring, Carl: Congenital Aneurysm of the Aortic Sinus of Valsalva. J. M. Research. *42*:49–59 (July–Sept.) 1920.
44. Goltman, D. W. and Stern, N. S.: Congenital Heart Disease. Report of a Case of Dextroposition, Persistence of an Early Stage of Embryonic Development of the Heart, Persistent Truncus Arteriosus, Abnormal Systemic and Pulmonary Veins, and Subdiaphragmatic Situs Inversus. Am. Heart J. *18*:176–187 (Aug.) 1939.
45. Graham, Stanley and Montgomery, G. L.: Congenital Malformation of Heart: Persistent Truncus Arteriosus. J. Tech. Methods. *18*:97–100 (Oct.) 1938.
46. Grant, H. H.: An Anomaly of the Human Heart. Am. J. M. Sc. *86*:149–151 (July) 1883.
47. Green, T. H.: Malformation of Heart; Absence of Pulmonary Artery; Aorta Springing from Right Ventricle; Incomplete Septum Ventriculorum; Patent Foramen Ovale. Tr. Path. Soc. London. *19*:188, 1868.
48. Greenspon, Samuel and Leaman, W. G., Jr.: Complete Pulmonary Atresia. Report of a Case With Hypertrophy of the Bronchial Arteries Simulating the Tetralogy of Fallot. Internat. Clin. *4*:208–212, 1939.
49. Harris, H. A.: Phocomelus With Congenital Cystic Elephantiasis. Am. J. Obst. & Gynec. *11*:767–778 (June) 1926.
50. Harris, H. A. and Thomson, G. C.: Persistent Truncus Arteriosus Communis With Microphthalmos, Orbital Cyst and Polydactyly. Arch. Dis. Childhood. *12*:59–66, 1937.
51. Hart, Karl: Über das Aneurysma des rechten Sinus Valsalvae der Aorta und seine Beziehungen zum oberen Ventrikelseptum. Virchows Arch. f. path. Anat. *182*:167–178 (Nov. 4) 1905.
52. Heath, Christopher and Power, H.: Case of Opening in Septum Ventriculorum. Pulmonary Artery and Aorta Given Off From the Heart as One Trunk. Tr. Path. Soc. London. *16*:62–63, 1865.
53. Hektoen, Ludvig: Rare Cardiac Anomalies. Congenital Aortico-pulmonary Communication; Communication Between the Aorta and the Left Ventricle Under a Semilunar Valve. Tr. Chicago Path. Soc. *4*:97–113, 1899–1901.
54: Hervieux: Communication des cavités du coeur entre elles; absence de l'artère pulmonair.—Dyspnée et accès de suffocation pendant la vie; mort a la suite d'un de ces accès. Bull. Soc. méd. d. hôp. de Paris. *5*:19–27 (Apr. 10) 1861.
55. Herxheimer, Gotthold: Missbildungen des Herzens und der grossun Gefässe, (b) Truncus arteriosus communis persistens. In Schwalbe, Ernst: Die Morphologie der Missbildungen des Menschen und der Tiere, Schwalbe, Jena. Gustav Fischer, 1910, vol. 3, pt. 2, chap. 4, pp. 427–431.

56. Hülse, Walter: Beitrag zur Kenntnis der totalen Persistenz des Truncus arteriosus communis. Virchows Arch. f. path. Anat. *225:*16–23 (May 29) 1918.
57. Humphreys, Eleanor M.: Truncus Arteriosus Communis Persistens. Arch. Path. *14:*671–700 (Nov.) 1932.
58. Hunter, O. B., Jr.: Truncus Arteriosus Communis Persistens. Arch. Path. *37:*328–330 (May) 1944.
59. Hunter, W. C. and Mackey, H. E.: Sympus Apus, With Associated Truncus Arteriosus Communis. Am. J. Obst. & Gynec. *29:*726–730 (May) 1935.
60. Hyernaux: Cyanose, Communication der beiden Herzventrikel mit der Aorta. Jr. de Bruxelles, Sept., 1851. (Abstr.) Schmidt's Jahrb. *75:*306, 1852.
61. Ingalls, N. W.: Truncus Arteriosus Communis Persistens. Anat. Rec. *10:*9–14 (Nov.) 1915.
62. Jacobi, Mendel and Heinrich, Abraham: Congenital Aorticoventricular Fistula With Engrafted Acute Suppurative Endocarditis. Am. J. M. Sc. *186:* 364–372 (Sept.) 1933.
63. Kerwin, A. J.: Persistent (Partial) Truncus Arteriosus Associated With Double Aortic Arch. J. Tech. Methods. *15:*142–147 (Mar.) 1936.
64. Kettler, L.H.: Zur Frage der Persistenz des Truncus arteriosus communis. Virchows Arch. f. path. Anat. *304:*513–525 (Oct. 18) 1939.
65. Klemke, W.: Ein klassischer Fall von totaler Persistenz des Truncus arteriosus communis. Zentralbl. f. allg. Path. u. path. Anat. *36:*307–312 (July 15) 1925.
66. Klipstein, Ludwig: Zwei Fälle von congenitaler Herzmissbildung. Arch. f. Kinderh. *11:*361–379, 1890.
67. Knape, Walter: Eine seltene Herzmissbildung bei Situs inversus abdominis. Virchows Arch. f. path. Anat. *209:*473–476 (Sept. 7) 1912.
68. Kramer, T. C.: The Partitioning of the Truncus and Conus and the Formation of the Membranous Portion of the Interventricular Septum in the Human Heart. Am. J. Anat. *71:*343–370 (Nov.) 1942.
69. Kraus, F.: Ueber wahres Aneurysma des Sinus Valsalvae Aortae dexter. Berl. klin. Wchnschr. *39:* 1161–1164 (Dec. 15) 1902.
70. Krausse, O.: Ein Beitrag zur Lehre von den kongenitalen Herzfehlern und ihrer Koinzidenz mit andern Missbildungen. Jahrb. f. Kinderh. *62:*35–49, 1905.
71. von Krzywicki, C.: Das Septum membranaceum ventriculorum cordis, sein Verhältniss zum Sinus Valsalvae dexter Aortae und die aneurysmatischen Veränderungen beider. Beitr. z. path. Anat. u. z. allg. Path. *6:*463–484, 1889.
72. Leech, C. B.: Congenital Heart Disease. Clinical Analysis of Seventy-five Cases From the Johns Hopkins Hospital. J. Pediat. *7:*802–839 (Dec.) 1935.
73. Lev, Maurice and Saphir, Otto: Truncus Arteriosus Communis Persistens. J. Pediat. *20:*74–88 (Jan.) 1942.
74. Livingston, Beverly: Congenital Communication Between the Right Side of the Heart and the Beginning of the Aorta. M. Rec. *24:*249 (Sept. 1) 1883.
75. Llorca, F. O.: Quelques remarques a propos du développement des arterès pulmonaires chez l'embryon humain. Ann. d'anat. path. *10:*935–936 (July) 1933.
76. Luis de Cubas, José: Un caso de corazon bilocular. Vida Nueva. *28:*221–226 (Aug. 15) 1931.
77. Lutembacher, R.: Communication entre l'aorte et l'artère pulmonaire. Presse méd. *2:*577–578 (Oct. 27) 1945.
78. Massachusetts General Hospital: Case 34161. New England J. Med. *238:*567–570 (Apr. 15) 1948.
79. Mannheimer, Edgar and Nordenfelt, P. J.: Four Cases of Congenital Cardiac Disease. Case I. Cor Bilocular With Persistent Truncus Arteriosus. Acta paediat. *23:*200–204, 1938–1939.

80. Mansfeld: Ein Fall von Blausucht. Hamburg Zeitsch. f. d. ges. Med. *23*:2, 1843. (Abstr.) Schmidt's Jahrb. *41*:278, 1844.
81. Marshall, Robert: Persistent Truncus Arteriosus. Brit. Heart J. *5*:194–196, 1943.
82. Mehta, J. B. and Hewlett, R. F. L.: Cor Triloculare Biauriculare. Brit. Heart J. *7*:41–44 (Jan.) 1945.
83. Michelson, R. P.: Report of a Case of Cor Biloculare With Persistent Truncus Arteriosus. Am. Heart J. *25*:112–115 (Jan.) 1943.
84. Miller, M. K. and Lyon, M. W., Jr.: Persistent Truncus Arteriosus: Cardiac Hypertrophy, Dysphagia, Death on Eleventh Day. Am. Heart J. *7*:106–109 (Oct.) 1931.
85. Mönckeberg, J. G.: Die Missbildungen des Herzens. In Henke, F. and Lubarsch, O.: Handbuch der speziellen pathologischen Anatomie und Histologie. Berlin, Julius Springer, 1924, vol. 2, p. 38.
86. Moorhead, T. G. and Smith, E. C.: Congenital Cardiac Anomaly—Abnormal Opening Between Aorta and Pulmonary Artery. Irish J. M. Sc. *1*:545–549 (Feb.) 1923.
87. Motta, Cunha: Troncos arteriosos communum permanente com endocardite chronica fetal. Ann. Fac. de med. de São Paulo. *7*:125–132, 1932.
88. Nunneley, F. B.: Observations on Palpitation of the Heart and Its Treatment. Lancet. *1*:228–265 (Feb. 25) 1871.
89. Odgers, P. N. B.: The Development of the Pars Membranacea Septi in the Human Heart. J. Anat. *72*:247–259 (Jan.) 1938.
90. Patten, B. M.: Human Embryology. Philadelphia, The Blakiston Company, 1946, p. 679.
91. Peacock, T. B. and Reed, W. C.: Malformation of the Heart; Absence of the Pulmonary Artery. (Card Specimen) Tr. Path. Soc. London. *31*:91–92, 1880.
92. Pezzi, C. and Agostoni, G.: Considérations cliniques anatomiques et radiogiques a propos d'un cas de maladie congénitale du coeur contralée a l'autopsie persistance du tronc artériel commun. Arch. d. mal. du coeur. *21*:19–29, 1928.
93. Pierret, Rene and Lelebure, G.: Apnée avec cyanose chez un vourrisson porteur d'un tronc commun aortico-pulmonaire absolument latent. Echo méd. du Nord. *8*:371–375 (Sept. 19) 1937.
94. Popjak, George: Two Cases of Congenital Cardiac Disease: (I) Cor Biloculare with Solitary Aortic Trunk, (II) Atresia of the Aorta with Hypoplasia of the Left Ventricle. J. Path. & Bact. *54*:67–73 (Jan.) 1942.
95. Pott, Richard: Ein Beitrag zu den Bildungsfehlern und foetalen Erkrankungen des Herzens. Jahrb. f. Kinderh. *13*:11–34, 1879.
96. Preisz, Hugo: Beiträge zur Lehre von den angeborenen Herzanomalien. Beitr. z. path. Anat. u. z. allg. Path. *7*:245–298, 1890.
97. Ramsbotham: The Heart of an Infant Consisting of Only One Auricle and Ventricle. Tr. Path. Soc. London. *1*:48, 1846–1848.
98. Rauchfuss: Quoted by Hektoen, Ludvig.[53]
99. Richardière and Huber: Inocclusion de la cloison interventriculaire avec absence d'artère pulmonaire. Bull. Soc. de pédiat. de Paris. *14*: 29–31 (Jan. 15) 1912.
100. Rickards, Edwin: Six Cardiac and Vascular Cases: With Remarks and Engravings. Brit. M. J. *2*:71–72 (July 16) 1881.
101. Rizzi, I.: Contributo allo studio di- varie malformazioni cardiache. (Stenosi dell 'aorta-tronco arterioso commune—trasposizione dei grossi vasi) Gior. di clin. med. *19*:863–882 (Sept. 20) 1938.
102. Rokitansky: Quoted by Kieth, Arthur: Malformations of the Heart. Lancet. *2*:433–435 (Aug. 14) 1909.
103. Roos, Allan: Persistent Truncus Arteriosus Communis. Report of a Case With Four Semilunar Cusps and Aortic Arch on the Right Side. Am. J. Dis. Child. *50*:966–978 (Oct.) 1935.

104. Santa Cruz, J. Z.: A Case of Common Ventricular Opening for the Aorta and Pulmonary Artery. J. Philippine Islands M. A. *5:*295–300 (Oct.) 1925.
105. Sewart, Margaret: Congenital Interruption of the Aortic Arch. Arch. Dis. Childhood. *23:*63–64 (Mar.) 1948.
106. Shapiro, P. F.: Detorsion Defects in Congenital Cardiac Anomalies. Report of Three Cases, With an Analysis of the Mechanism of Their Formation. Arch. Path. *9:*54–68 (Jan.) 1930.
107. Shepherd, S. G., Park, F. R. and Kitchell, J. R.: A Case of Aorto-pulmonic Communication Incident to a Congenital Aortic Septal Defect: Discussion of Embryologic Changes Involved. Am. Heart J. *27:*733–738 (May) 1944.
108. Siegmund, H.: Totale Persistenz des Truncus arteriosus communis (bei einer 33 jährigen Frau und einem neugeborenen Mädchen). Ztschr. f. Kreislaufforsch. *20:*65–73 (Feb.) 1928.
109. Solis-Cohen, Myer, Zaslow, Jerry and Rolnick, M. H.: A Rare Case of Congenital Heart Disease, With Interventricular Septal Defect, Atretic Pulmonary Artery, Dextroposition of the Aorta, Bicuspid Right Atrioventricular Valve and Superimposed Subacute Vegetative Endocarditis. Am. Heart J. *28:*115–123 (July) 1944.
110. Szypulski, J. T.: A Study of Congenital Heart Disease at the Philadelphia General Hospital. J. Tech. Methods. *17:*119–126 (Sept. 15) 1937.
111. Taruffi, Cesare: Sulle malattie congenite e sulle anomalie del cuore. Mem. Soc. med.-chir. di. Bologna. *8:*215–218, 1875.
112. Tate, W. W. H.: Case of Malformation of the Heart. Tr. Path. Soc. London. *43:*36, 1892.
113. Taussig, Helen B.: Clinical and Pathological Findings in Cases of Truncus Arteriosus in Infancy. Am. J. Med. *2:*26–34 (Jan.) 1947.
114. Thurnam, John: On Aneurisms, and Especially Spontaneous Varicose Aneurisms of the Ascending Aorta and Sinuses of Valsalva, With Cases. Med. Chir. Tr. London. *23:*323–384, 1840.
115. Tiedemann, Friedrich: Abweichende Anordnung der Pulsaderstämme des Herzens. Ztschr. f. Physiol. *4:*287, 1831.
116. Tow, Abraham: Cor Biloculáre With Truncus Arteriosus and Endocarditis. Am. J. Dis. Child. *42:*1413–1416 (Dec.) 1931.
117. Valdes Diaz, R. and Perez de Los Reyes, R.: Cardiopatia congenita con cianosis, corazon trilocular biventriculado tronco arterial unico persistencia del seno venoso. Arch. de med. inf. *5:*51–68, 1936.
118. Van Brown, David: Cardiovascular Anomalies; Truncus Arteriosus Communis Persistens. J. Tech. Methods. *22:*101–109 (July) 1942.
119. Vernon, H. H.: Angeborne Herzfehler. Med.-Chir. Transact. *39:*1856. (Abstr.) Schmidt's Jahrb. *96:*298–299, 1857.
120. Vierordt, Hermann: Die angeborenen Herzkrankheiten: Unvollständige Theilung und einseitige Umbildung des primären Truncus. Persistenz des Truncus arteriosus. Specielle Pathologie u. Therapie. *15:*132–138, 1898.
121. Walls, E. W.: Biatrial Trilocular Heart; With Atresia of the Mitral Valve. Lancet. *2:*668 (Nov. 29) 1941.
122. Webb, A. C.: Truncus Arteriosus Communis Persistens. Arch. Path. *42:*427–432 (Oct.) 1946.
123. Wenner, Otto: Beiträge zur Lehre der Herzmissbildunge. Virchows Arch. f. path. Anat. *196:*127–168 (Apr. 1) 1909.
124. White, W. H.: A Case of Patent Ventricular Septum, Together With an Aneurism of the Base of the Aorta Opening Into the Right Ventricle. Tr. Path. Soc. London. *43:*34–36, 1892.
125. Wilks: Communication Between Pulmonary Artery and Aorta. Tr. Path. Soc. London. *11:*57–58, 1860.
126. Wilson, J.: On a Very Unusual Formation of the Human Heart. Phil. Tr. Roy. Soc. London. *18:*332–337, 1798.

127. Wirth, Amandus: Quoted by Mönckeberg, J. G.[85]
128. Wood, R. H. and Williams, G. A.: Primitive Human Hearts. Cor. "Biloculare" and Triloculare; Report of Cases. Am. J. M. Sc. *175*:242–255 (Feb.) 1928.
129. Wright, J. H. and Drake, A. K.: A Case of Extreme Malformation of the Heart. Tr. A. Am. Physicians. *18*:272–274, 1903.
130. Zimmerman, H. M.: A Congenital Anomaly of the Heart: Truncus Arteriosus Communis. Am. J. Path. *3*:617–621 (Nov.) 1927.

Persistent Truncus: A Classification According to Anatomic Types

Mary Ella Pierpont, M.D., Ph.D.

The Collett and Edwards classification of the anatomy of persistent truncus arteriosus (TA) has been and still is the most widely quoted in the literature and used by clinicians. This landmark anatomic scheme, developed in 1949, placed most of the emphasis of the differential anatomies of TA on the specific configuration and location of the pulmonary arteries. In each of Types 1, 2, and 3, careful descriptions were also provided regarding the aortic arch (right or left), presence or absence of the ductus arteriosus, vascular anomalies such as aortic coarctation or interruption, ventricular origin of the truncus, number and integrity of the truncal valve cusps, and coronary artery variations. These anatomic descriptions provided a critical base for the evolution of surgical procedures to repair TA, with the first successful surgical repair by McGoon and coworkers in 1967.

As Dr. Edwards (or Chief as I preferred to call him) and I examined a cardiac specimen with TA in the first few days of my pediatric cardiology fellowship, we discussed the observation that some hearts with TA had the origin of the truncus predominately from the right ventricle. Stimulated by that finding, Dr. Edwards later evaluated 54 specimens with TA and found 30 percent with a right aortic arch and 42.5 percent with the origin of the truncus predominately from the right ventricle. The primary location of the truncus from the right ventricle was described as possibly predisposing to subaortic obstruction at the time of VSD closure with complete correction. Overall, there was a group of hearts with TA where the anatomy was simple, and a group associated with other vascular anomalies such as interruption of the aortic arch, coronary artery abnormality, right aortic arch, double aortic arch, or other cardiac abnormalities. There appeared to be a higher mortality in those with associated vascular anomalies.

In the mid 1980s, Dr. Edwards and I examined the hearts of two siblings with TA. We began to wonder what the familial recurrence risks of TA would be, and what factors might predispose to the development of congenital heart disease in families of children with TA. At that time, most recurrence risks for the various types of congenital heart disease were considered to be 1 to 4 percent and no value was known for TA due to its rarity. We were able to locate 49 index cases of TA spanning a 30 year time period and found the recurrence risk of heart disease in siblings to be 6.6 percent. When the TA had complex anatomy in the index case (such as associated with vascular anomalies), the recurrence risk in siblings was 13.6 percent. These studies foreshadowed the breakthroughs in understanding the genetics of TA which would occur almost a decade later.

The advent of the molecular genetic technique fluorescence-in-situ-hybridization (FISH) in the 1990's unlocked some of the mystery of the genetic aspects of TA. Using the FISH technique, a submicroscopic deletion of a portion of the long arm of chromosome 22 (del22q11.2) was found in children with TA and other conotruncal cardiac malformations. Children with DiGeorge syndrome or Velocardiofacial syndrome, two well known genetic syndromes, had deletions of 22q11.2 together with a high incidence of conotruncal cardiac malformations, including TA. Goldmuntz and coworkers in 1998 later found that 30 to 40 percent of children with TA had a 22q11.2 deletion. Furthermore they also showed that those with associated anomalies of the aortic arch or other vessels had an increased incidence of the 22q11.2 deletion (45 to 50 percent for all conotruncal cardiac anomalies). In retrospect, the 22q11.2 deletion was likely a major factor in our findings of relatives of children with TA also affected by cardiac anomalies.

The designation of TA as a conotruncal cardiac malformation arose from chick embryo studies where the ablation of neural crest cells was found to cause TA and other cardiac anomalies (ML Kirby). Thus the embryonic neural crest cells are greatly affected by the absence of genetic input from the 22q11.2 chromosome region. Ongoing genetic studies are focusing on other genes which affect the neural crest cells such as TBX1. Additional genes currently being evaluated in relevant animal models include Alk5, Sox4, Fgf8 and the gene for retinaldehyde dehydrogenase 2. These studies likely will add to our understanding of the heterogeneous causes of TA, perhaps including the specific anatomical types described by Dr. Edwards.

As predicted by Dr. Edwards, the surgical repair of TA has been and remains very challenging due to the variety of associated abnormalities. The VSD must be repaired and continuity established between the right ventricle and the pulmonary circulation. As delineated by Collett and Edwards, abnormalities of the truncal valve, ventricular location of the origin of the truncus, and association of other vascular anomalies like interruption of the aortic arch, are factors contributing to increased mortality of children with TA. An early surgical approach included pulmonary artery banding shortly after birth followed by later surgical correction, but this proved to have high mortality. Some surgeons have favored an approach to surgical repair at the age of 3-6 months when a VSD has often been repaired. Currently, the preferred surgery for TA is neonatal corrective repair within the first 2 weeks of life, if possible. Subsequent conduit or homograft replacement is a certainty with this approach. In many centers, the overall survival of children with TA has improved to 75 to 85 percent long term with an early mortality of 5 to 10 percent and late mortality of 10 to 15 percent.

There is reason to be optimistic about the future of specialized care for children with TA. Development of new techniques improving early fetal echocardiography and new research on fetal surgical approaches based on understanding of the multiple anatomical types of TA is ongoing. Surgeons are utilizing more sophisticated techniques with conduits and homografts, and potential gene therapies are on the horizon.

Thank you, Chief, for your encouragement of what has turned out to be a career-long interest in the genetics of congenital cardiac malformations.

Persistent Truncus: A Classification According to Anatomic Types

Anton E. Becker, M.D.

TRUNCUS ARTERIOSUS OR ELSE?

The classical paper by Collett and Edwards is an amazing piece of work to read again, certainly since it is based solely on a review of cases reported in the literature. It is hard to imagine anyone nowadays even starting such an enterprise. It is important also to keep in mind that this work was accomplished at a time that surgical intervention was not available. So, what are the merits of this work today?

First of all we have to consider the fact that their review is based on the premise that defective development of the truncoconal ridges creates persistence of the truncus arteriosus. Taking embryology as point of departure, albeit very understandable, at the same time creates an Achilles heel. Why is that? Because the aficionados in cardiac embryology quarrel about almost everything. What is the conus? And what is its septum? And where does a truncus start and end? New classifications were born based on insights of one group, but not necessarily shared by others. The naming game was on, but does it really improve matters if we call the thing a common arterial trunk rather than a persistent truncus arteriosus? And, does it really matter? After all, it all boils down to the definition used. Collett and Edwards were very clear about that. They defined two absolute criteria for the pathologic diagnosis of persistent truncus arteriosus: (1) there must be one main arterial trunk leaving the base of the heart and (2) this single arterial trunk must supply branches to the coronary, pulmonary and systemic circulations. On the basis of the 93 cases collected from the literature they then propose a subdivision in four major categories, taking the anatomy of the origin of the pulmonary arteries as point of departure. The rationale for doing that was based on the premise of various stages of developmental arrest of the sixth aortic arches resulting in different anatomic types. It is interesting to look back at that, because basically what they recognized were different anatomic configurations, which they afterwards "explained" by referring to different stages in developmental arrest.

Is the Collett and Edwards classification of persistent truncus arteriosus still of practical value, now that we have entered an era where surgical intervention is an option? I would say that the answer could be yes and no.

YES, because it is simple, and everybody can understand it and remember it. The mode of origin of the pulmonary arteries from the single arterial trunk, moreover, is of major surgical significance. Whether it is a type 1, with a common pulmonary trunk, or a type 2, 3 with both pulmonary arteries originating directly from the single trunk, does make a difference for the surgeon. It is interesting, on a personal note, that when my wife and I had the privilege to study with Jesse in 1969-70, he expressed serious doubt whether type 3 really existed. He had never seen it himself, and the literature review in 1949 had revealed only nine cases to be interpreted as such. And, I have to say, in my own experience since then I have never seen a type 3 either. Be that as it may, the fact that type 3 may not exist after all should not detract from the usefulness of a distinction between types 1 and 2.

NO, because the type 4, where there are no pulmonary arteries nor a pulmonary trunk, has a very different surgical outlook and these cases basically fit within the spectrum of pulmonary atresia with VSD. Another drawback comes from the fact that in all its simplicity the classification is insufficient because of its incompleteness. Collett and Edwards were well aware of that, since they further subcategorized their four types according to additional features, such as right aortic arch, aortic coarctation or interruption, etc. At the same time they had the wisdom not to put forward a classification like type 1a,b,c,d,e,f,g and type 2a,b,c,d,e, realizing that it would be the kiss of death. I had wished that others in the arena of classification of congenital heart malformations had thought about that as well! The message is, of course, that only a full evaluation of any congenital heart malformation can provide the necessary details for successful intervention. And this should not necessarily reflect in a classification.

So even today, starting a full evaluation of a patient with persistent truncus arteriosus by categorizing it as either type 1 or 2 is a useful first step.

Origin of Both Great Vessels from the Right Ventricle

I. Without Pulmonary Stenosis

By HENRY N. NEUFELD, M.D., JAMES W. DUSHANE, M.D., EARL H. WOOD, M.D., JOHN W. KIRKLIN, M.D., AND JESSE E. EDWARDS, M.D.

AMONG the congenital malformations in which an abnormal relationship exists between the aorta and pulmonary trunk is that in which both of these vessels arise from the right ventricle. The only outlet for the left ventricle is a ventricular septal defect. Right ventricular infundibular stenosis may or may not be associated. These cases apparently are extremely rare,[1-3] and only a few have been reported in the last 25 years.[4-7] A few cases were documented in the last century.[1, 3]

Many terms have been used for this malformation, including "partial transposition,"[2] "double-outlet right ventricle,"[7] and "origin of both great vessels from the right ventricle."[8]

Witham,[7] in 1957, summarized six cases reported in detail in the literature and added four cases. He divided these cases into two groups and called them the "Fallot type" and the "Eisenmenger type," depending on the presence or absence of pulmonary stenosis.

One of the patients in his study was seen at the Mayo Clinic.[9] This case was not included in the present analysis because additional multiple intracardiac malformations were present, and it appeared to us that different embryologic as well as hemodynamic problems were involved.

In a study of the pathologic and clinical material from the Mayo Clinic, we found 14 cases in which both great vessels originated from the right ventricle. Three main categories of this malformation occurred as follows: (1) without pulmonary stenosis (eight cases); (2) with pulmonary stenosis (five cases) and (3) with other intracardiac malformations (one case).

The purpose of this investigation is to correlate the anatomic findings (pathologicoanatomic or surgical) with the clinical and hemodynamic data and to discuss the possibilities of clinical diagnosis.

The three groups, although probably related embryologically, present different anatomic, clinical, hemodynamic, and surgical problems; therefore, we will discuss them in two separate communications.

The present paper is concerned with the eight cases of this malformation without pulmonary stenosis. The diagnosis in five instances was proved at necropsy, whereas it was established during operation in the other three. In two cases, patent ductus arteriosus, mitral insufficiency, and some degree of coarctation of the aorta were present. Pulmonary hypertension was present in all eight cases.

Pathologicoanatomic Features

The anatomic features in the five cases studied at necropsy fell into two subgroups that could be distinguished from each other by the relationship of the aortic and mitral valves. In the first subgroup (three cases), these two valves lacked the element of continuity found in normal hearts; the second subgroup (two cases) was marked by continuity between aortic and mitral valvular tissue.

In the first subgroup, the ascending aorta and the pulmonary artery appeared from the exterior to have a normal relationship, the ascending aorta lying to the right of the pulmonary trunk. The interior of the heart, however, revealed a profound abnormality of the aorta. Instead of extending inferiorly from the base of the heart to a position

From the Mayo Clinic and the Mayo Foundation, Rochester, Minnesota.

Supported in part by research grants no. H4014 and no. H3532 from the National Heart Institute, U. S. Public Health Service.

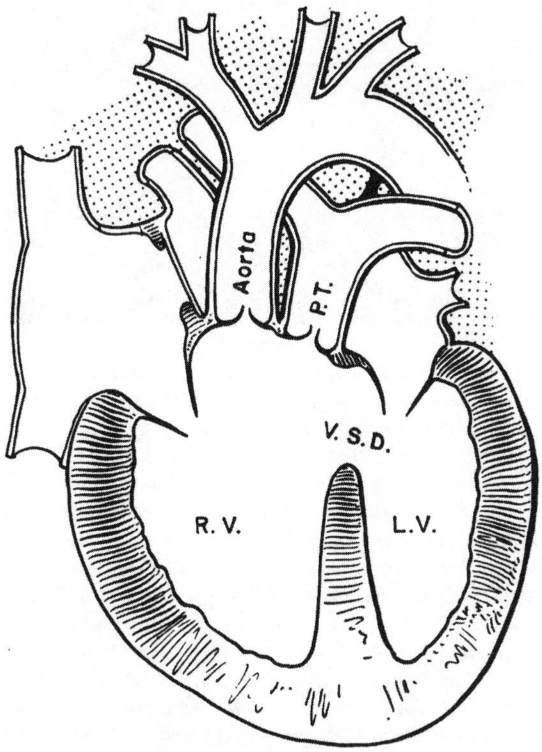

Figure 1
Diagrammatic representation of origin of both great vessels from right ventricle without pulmonary stenosis and with ventricular septal defect.

dorsal and caudal to the pulmonary valve, the aortic orifice communicated only with the right ventricle and lay to the right of and in the same coronal body plane as the pulmonary valve (figs. 1 and 2).

The interior of the right ventricle showed a prominent horizontal crista supraventricularis, with the aortic orifice lying between two branches of this structure. A ventricular septal defect was present in the basal part of the septum, caudal to the crista supraventricularis. Dorsally, this defect was bounded by the junction of the anterior mitral leaflet and the septal tricuspid leaflet. The caudad, ventral, and cephalad edges of the defect were composed of muscle; the muscle forming the cephalad boundary was the crista supraventricularis. By means of right ventricular landmarks, the position of the ventricular septal defect could be identified as lying dorsally and caudal to the crista supraventricularis and being caudal to the tricuspid valve.

The anatomic relationships of the mitral valve were abnormal because of the aforementioned lack of continuity between the aortic and mitral valves. Although the basal attachments of the posterior mitral leaflet were normal, those of the anterior leaflet were abnormal. The main basal attachment of the anterior mitral leaflet was to the septal tricuspid leaflet, with which, as already noted, it was continuous behind the septal defect. Anteriorly, the base of the anterior mitral leaflet attached to the muscle forming the superior boundary of the ventricular septal defect (fig. 3).

Two of the three hearts in this first subgroup corresponded to the above description. A second type in this first subgroup of cases was represented by one case (fig. 4). In this instance, the ventricular septal defect was cephalad to the crista supraventricularis and beneath the pulmonary valve. The aorta arose entirely from the right ventricle, being to the right of and slightly dorsal to the pulmonary valve. The aortic and pulmonary valves were in the same cross-sectional body plane. The ventricular septal defect was separated from the tricuspid valve by the crista supraventricularis, which lay in a horizontal position. The septal defect was surrounded on all sides by muscle. Dorsally, this muscle made up the left extremity of the crista supraventricularis.

The posterior mitral leaflet had normal attachments. The anterior mitral leaflet was attached to the posterior edge of the ventricular septal defect, being separated from the aortic valve and the tricuspid valve by the aforementioned muscle, which formed the posterior wall of the ventricular septal defect.

From the viewpoint of anatomic classification, it is of significance in these cases that, if an incision is made through the left ventricular wall into the aorta, one initially gains the impression that the aorta is in direct continuity with the left ventricle. However, this is an illusion since, in order to reach the aorta from the left ventricle, one must pass through the ventricular septal defect (fig. 5).

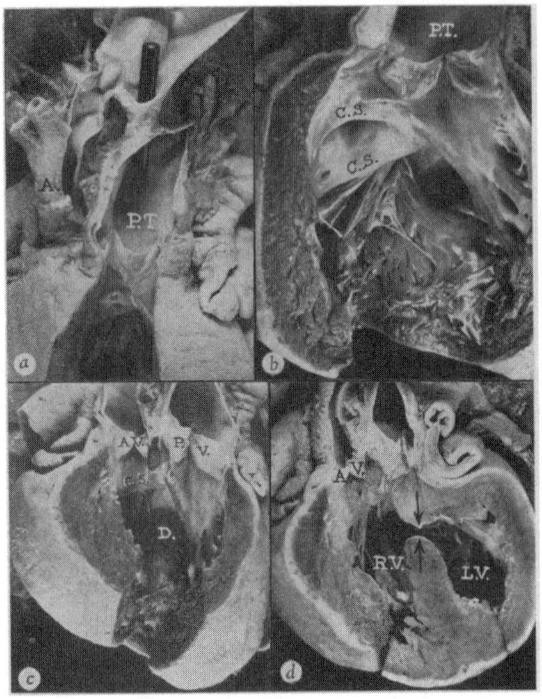

Figure 2

Case 3. First subgroup of origin of both great vessels from right ventricle without pulmonary stenosis and with ventricular septal defect. a. *Outflow portion of right ventricle and great vessels. The ascending aorta (A.) lies beside the pulmonary trunk (P.T.). Exteriorly, the relationship between the two great vessels did not appear abnormal. A probe lies in a patent ductus arteriosus.* b. *Interior of right ventricle and origin of pulmonary trunk (P.T.). Between the two limbs of the crista supraventricularis (C.S.) is a channel leading to the origin of the aorta. The ventricular septal defect lies below the lower limb of the crista.* c. *Interior of right ventricle in similar perspective to that in* b. *A sagittal section has been made through the valves and great vessels. The ventral limb of the crista supraventricularis has been removed, leaving the dorsal limb (C.S.). The aortic valve (A.V.) lies to the right of and in the same body plane as the pulmonary valve (P.V.). The ventricular septal defect (D.) lies dorsal to both the aortic and pulmonary valves and below the crista supraventricularis.* d. *Section made in right ventricle in* c *carried across ventricular septum and through lateral wall of left ventricle, exposing left ventricular cavity (L.V.). The ventricular septal defect lies between the arrows. It is the only outlet for the left ventricle and it leads directly into the right ventricle (R.V.).*

As already noted, the second subgroup of these five cases studied at necropsy comprises

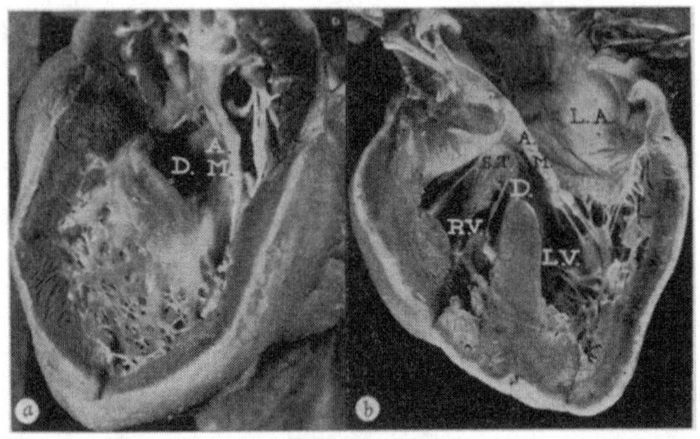

Figure 3

Case 3. Relationships of ventricular septal defect and mitral valve. a. *Interior of left ventricle. The only outlet for the left ventricle is the ventricular septal defect (D.). The anterior leaflet of the mitral valve (A.M.) forms part of the dorsal wall of the ventricular septal defect.* b. *Section through heart parallel to that shown in figure* 2d *but on a more dorsal plane that lies dorsal to the semilunar valves. The anterior leaflet of the mitral valve has continuity with the septal leaflet of the tricuspid valve (S.T.) behind the ventricular septal defect. The anterior leaflet of the mitral valve attaches anteriorly with the muscular edge of the ventricular septal defect and does not have continuity with the aortic valve. This is in striking contrast to the normal situation. L.A. = left atrium.*

the two cases in which the aortic and mitral valves were continuous. This normal relationship existed not by virtue of a normal position of the aortic valve but as the result of an unusually long anterior mitral leaflet. The latter ascended through the ventricular septal defect to join the aortic valve. The latter lay entirely over the right ventricle and to the right of the ventricular septal defect.

From the exterior, the relationships of the aorta and pulmonary trunk appeared to be normal (fig. 6). The interior of the right ventricle revealed a large ventricular septal defect dorsal to the horizontal crista supraventricularis. In the usual instance in which a ventricular septal defect lies dorsal to the crista, the defect also is caudal to the septal leaflet of the tricuspid valve. In these two cases, the relationship of the defect to the tricuspid valve was unusual. It was not related closely to the septal leaflet of the tricuspid valve but instead lay cephalad and medial to the commissure between the anterior

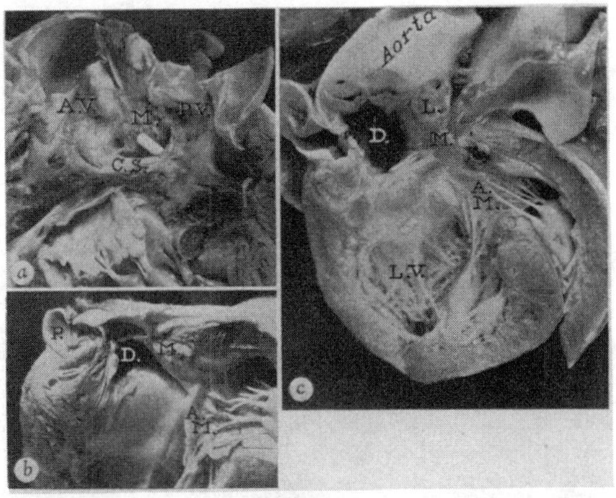

Figure 4

Case 5. a. *Right ventricular aspect viewed laterally. The ventricular septal defect (probe) lies above the crista supraventricularis and dorsocaudal to the pulmonary valve. The ventricular septal defect is surrounded on all sides by muscle; that forming the dorsal wall is designated by "M." The origin of the aortic valve lies dorsal to and to the right of the pulmonary valve but at the same cross-sectional body plane. The aorta originates entirely from the right ventricle and does not straddle the defect.* b. *Base of left ventricle viewed laterally. The ventricular septal defect (D.) lies behind the pulmonary valve (P.). The aortic valve lies beyond the ventricular septal defect and is separated from the anterior leaflet of the mitral valve (A.M.) by the muscle (M.), which forms the dorsal wall of the ventricular septal defect.* c. *Left ventricle, ventricular septal defect, and aorta. This perspective is the result of an incision made through the anterior wall of the left ventricle and carried into the aorta. The impression of continuity between the aorta and the left ventricle is an illusion. No continuity exists between aortic and mitral valves. The ventricular septal defect is surrounded on all sides by muscle, and the aortic origin lies on the right ventricular side of the ventricular septal defect. Interposed between the aortic valve and the anterior mitral leaflet (A.M.) is the mass of muscle (M.) that forms the dorsal wall of the ventricular septal defect. L. = left aortic cusp.*

and septal tricuspid leaflets. The defect in one case extended upward toward the right to lie cephalad to the major portion of the anterior tricuspid leaflet (fig. 6*a*).

Forming the lower dorsal boundary of the ventricular septal defect was the anterior leaflet of the mitral valve where it was continuous with the septal tricuspid leaflet.

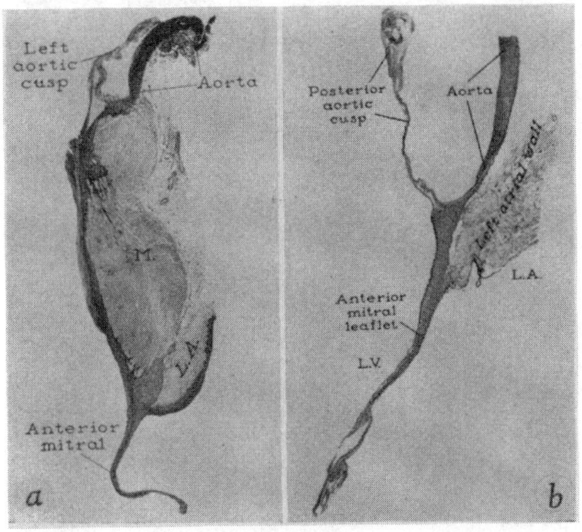

Figure 5

Case 5. a. *From case illustrated in figure 4. This low-power photomicrograph of a section made through the left aortic cusp and anterior mitral leaflets shows the mass of muscle (M.) interposed between the two valves. This muscle represents the dorsal wall of the ventricular septal defect and is abnormal in position. L.A. = left atrial wall.* b. *Section through aortic and mitral valves of normal heart in essentially the same plane for comparison with* a. *The normal heart shows continuity between aortic and mitral valves, in contrast to the abnormal heart.*

Cephalodorsally, the anterior mitral leaflet extended upward to form the cephalodorsal boundary of the ventricular septal defect, and then it joined the root of the aorta and the aortic valve.

When the left ventricular incision was extended into the aorta during dissection of these hearts, the incision cut through the elongated anterior mitral valve and aorta. Muscular tissue did not intervene between these two valvular structures (fig. 7), as was present in the second type of the first subgroup of hearts.

It might be asked justifiably how the hearts of the second subgroup differ from those with the common variety of ventricular septal defect. The following differences may be pointed out: In the hearts of this subgroup, the aorta does not connect directly with the left ventricle or straddle the ventricular septal defect; rather, it lies to the right of the defect. The aortic valve connects with the

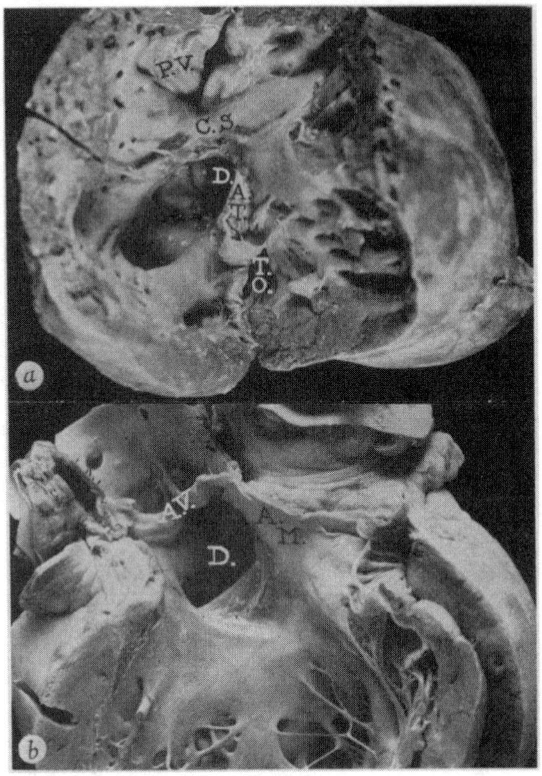

Figure 6

Case 1. Second subgroup of origin of both great vessels from right ventricle without pulmonary stenosis. a. *Interior of right ventricle. The ventricular septal defect (D.) is separated from the pulmonary valve (P.V.) by the horizontal crista supraventricularis (C.S.). The defect, although lying posteroinferior to the crista, has an abnormal relationship to the tricuspid valve, lying ventral to the anterior tricuspid leaflet (A.T.). The aortic valve lies immediately above the defect and communicates entirely with the right ventricle, although it has continuity with the anterior leaflet of the mitral valve.* b. *Left ventricle and aortic valve (A.V.). The dorsal wall of the ventricular septal defect (D.) is formed by the anterior leaflet of the mitral valve (A.M.) as it becomes continuous with the septal leaflet of the tricuspid valve below and with the aortic valve above. Continuity is present between aortic valvular tissue and tissue of the anterior leaflet of the mitral valve, but it does not result from a normal position of the aorta but rather because of an abnormally long anterior mitral leaflet, which ascends through the ventricular septal defect to become continuous with the aortic valve. An additional abnormality is that the portion of the heart in which the aortic and mitral valves are continuous has an epicardial relationship; in normal hearts, on the contrary, the zone of continuity between the mitral and aortic valves is entirely intracardiac.*

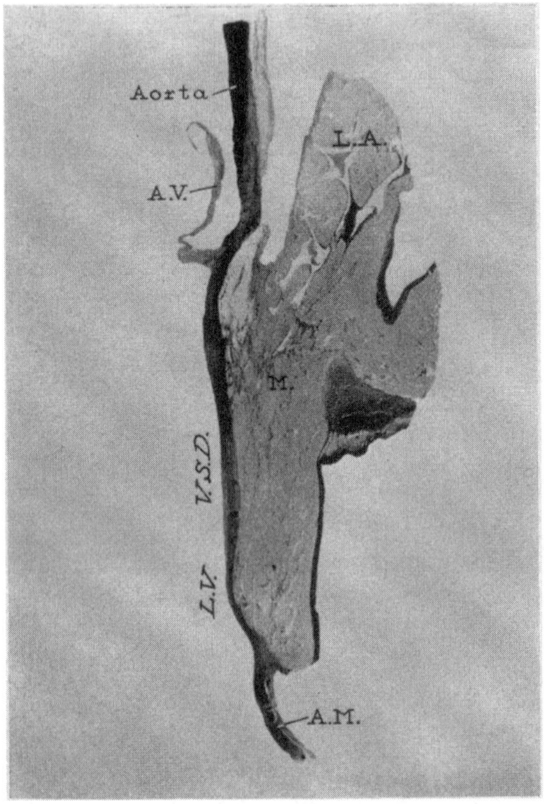

Figure 7

*Case 6. Low-power photomicrograph showing continuity between aortic valve and anterior leaflet of mitral valve. The relationship between the two valves is profoundly different from that in the first sub-group (fig. 5). Although the relationship in this case bears some similarity to the normal, the zone of continuity between the two valves has a close epicardial relationship. Under normal conditions, this zone is entirely in an intracardiac position. The recess between the aortic wall and the left atrial wall is the pericardial cavity. Contrast this with the normal in figure 5*b.

mitral valve not because of a normal position but because an elongated anterior mitral leaflet extends upward and to the right to join the aortic valve. The aortic valve is not caudal to the pulmonary valve but lies at the same level. The ventricular septal defect does not extend caudally dorsal to the septal tricuspid leaflet but rather extends cephalad ventral to the anterior tricuspid leaflet.

Clinical Findings

The clinical findings (table 1) were similar to those in cases of ventricular septal defect with associated pulmonary hypertension.

Table 1

Clinical Data in Eight Cases of Origin of Both Great Vessels from Right Ventricle

			History				Physical findings*					
Case	Age, yrs.	Sex	Cyanosis	Shortness of breath	Congestive failure	Respiratory infections	Systolic thrill, location	Systolic murmur, grade and location†	Other murmurs: type, grade and location	Second pulmonic sound	Blood pressure, mm. of Hg	Femoral pulses
1	14	F	–	+	–	+	LICS (2-4)	III (3)	–	+++ Split	98/68	+
2	4	F	–	+	+	+	Left sternal border	III (3-4)	Mid diastolic	+++ Split	92/60	+
3	15	F	–	+	–	+	LICS (2-3)	II (2-4)	SM, I, apex; DM, I, apex	++	110/60	+
4	6	M	When crying	+	–	+	Supra-sternal notch	III (3-4)	SM, I, apex	+++	94/60	±
5	2	M	–	–	–	–	LICS (3-4)	IV (3-4)	DM, apex	+++ Split	90/50	+
6	9	M	–	+	–	–	+	III (2-4)	DM, I, LICS (2-4)	+++	88/60	+
7	3	F	–	+	+	+	–	II (4)	–	+	94/50	+
8	2	M	Since age 3 mo. when crying	+	+	++	Lower sternum	III (4)	DM, I, apex	+ Split	95/45	+

*LICS, left intercostal space; DM, diastolic murmur; SM, systolic murmur.

†Roman numerals indicate grade of murmur; arabic numbers in parentheses indicate those left intercostal spaces where the murmur was heard.

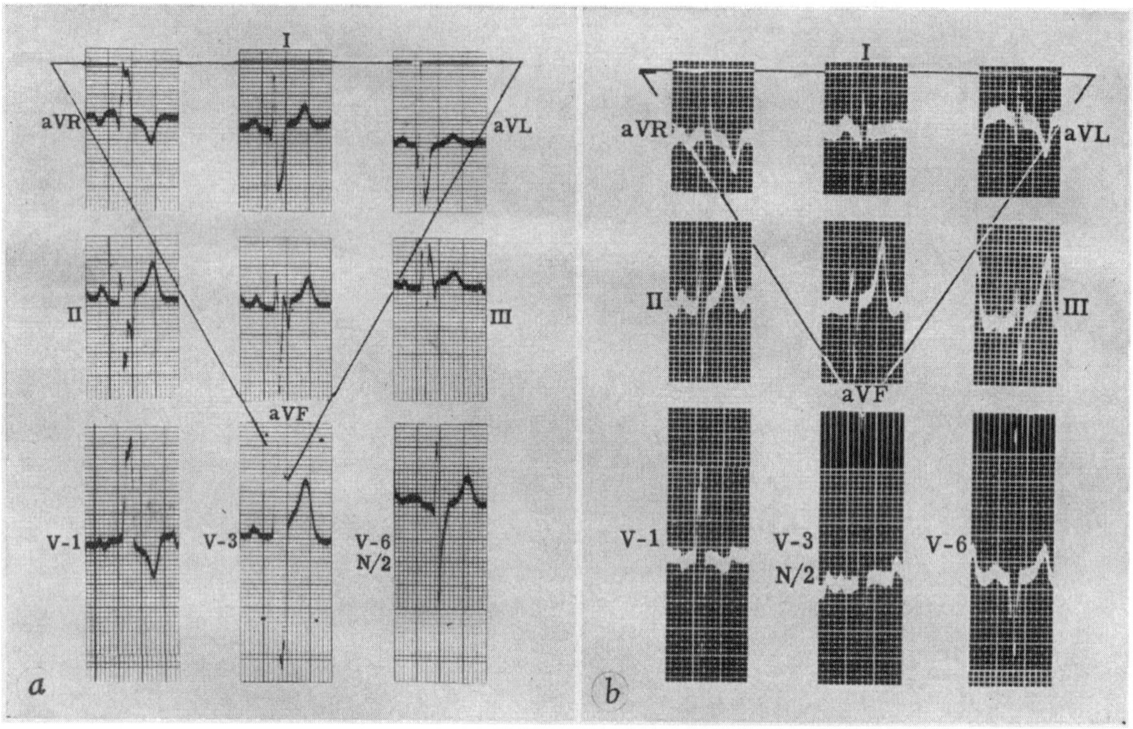

Figure 8

Electrocardiograms in two cases. a. *Case 1.* b. *Case 7. See table 2 for details.*

There were four boys and four girls, with ages ranging from 2 to 15 years.

Slight cyanosis had been noted after effort in two patients. All but one had experienced dyspnea after effort. In three patients, congestive heart failure had been present in the past or was noted at the time of observation. Six patients had a history of recurrent respiratory infection.

Examination at the clinic did not show cyanosis or clubbing in any of the patients. A systolic thrill was present in all but one patient. A systolic murmur was present in all eight cases, varying from grade II to grade IV (on the basis of grades I to VI established by the New York Heart Association).

A grade I apical diastolic murmur was heard in three patients, and two had a Graham Steell murmur. An apical systolic murmur suggesting mitral insufficiency was noted in two patients (cases 3 and 4); this lesion subsequently was found at necropsy. The second pulmonic sound was accentuated in all eight patients. Femoral arterial pulsations were palpable in all instances, being somewhat diminished in one patient (case 4) because of an associated coarctation of the aorta. The blood pressure was in the normal range in all patients.

Electrocardiographic Findings

All eight patients had normal sinus rhythm (fig. 8). The P-R interval was greatly prolonged in case 3 and slightly prolonged in all the other cases, as based on the assumed P-R interval for age and heart rate (Ziegler).[10]

The P waves were high and notched in leads I, II, and aV_F, suggesting left atrial enlargement, in the two patients (cases 3 and 4) in whom mitral insufficiency was found at necropsy.

The most striking electrocardiographic features in these eight cases were the manifest mean electric axes and the vectors of the QRS complexes in the frontal plane as projected from the scalar electrocardiograms (table 2). The manifest mean electric axes of the QRS complexes in seven of the patients

Table 2

Electrocardiographic Findings in Eight Cases of Origin of Both Great Vessels from Right Ventricle

Case	Age, yrs.	Rate, beats per min.	QRS axis, degrees	QRS vector loop, frontal plane*	P waves, mm.	P-R interval, sec.	QRS complex, sec.	QRS in lead V_1, mm.	R in aV_R, mm.	R:S ratio in aV_R	QRS in lead V_6, mm.
1	14	90	−160	CCL	High, notched; 3 mm. in I; 4 mm. in II	0.20	0.14	r R′ R′ = 22	10	>1	Q = 2 R = 13 S = 22
2	4	120	− 70	CCL	High; 3 mm. in II	0.16	0.08	R = 25	9.5	>1	Q = 2 R = 30 S = 4.5
3	15	83	−120	CCL	Notched in I, II and aV_F	0.24	0.12	r R′ R′ = 23	12	>1	Q = 2 R = 22 S = 9
4	6	112	−170	CCL; figure-of-eight	High and notched in I, II and aV_F	0.17	0.14	R = 25	8	>1	Q = 10 R = 28 S = 19
5	2	142	− 30	CCL	Notched in I and aV_F	0.16	0.07	RS R = 32 S = 14	2.5	<1	Q = 6 R = 20
6	9	100	−130	CCL	2 mm. in II	0.16	0.10	RS R = 25 S = 14	16	>1	Q = 4 R = 28 S = 18
7	3	120	− 90	CCL	Normal	0.16	0.08	RS R = 13 S = 17 Slurred R	12	>1	Q = 5 R = 27 S = 13
8	2	136	+120	CL	3 mm. in II	0.14	0.08	RS R = 33 S = 10	9	=1	Q = 12 R = 33 S = 6

*CCL, counterclockwise; CL, clockwise.

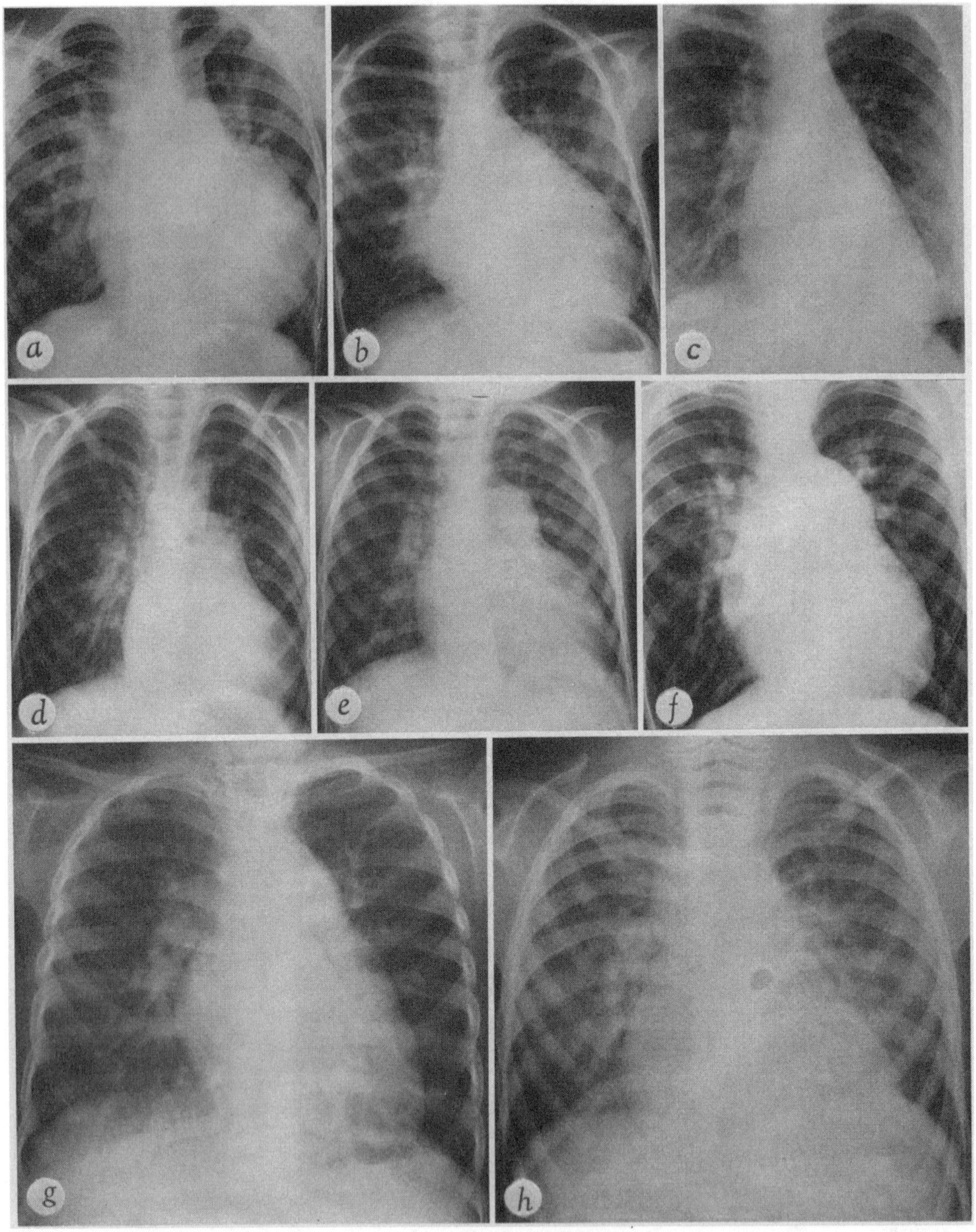

Figure 9

a-h. *Posteroanterior thoracic roentgenograms in cases 1 through 8, respectively. See text for details.*

Table 3

Hemodynamic Data in Eight Cases of Origin of Both Great Vessels from Right Ventricle

Case*	Pressure, mm. Hg†						Blood oxygen saturation, per cent‡						O₂ capacity, vol. per cent
	RA	RV	PA	Radial artery	Aorta	LA	IVC	MRA	SVC	RV	PA	Radial artery	
1 A	14/8	103/16	100/44	—	—	—	—	63	—	94	90	96.7 FA	17.4
1 B	15/9	82/8	—	—	89/47	21/12							
2 (B)	8/5	85/6	—	—	LV 88/7	16/8							
3 (A)	9/3	110/15	110/68 135/75	119/54	102/60 via (ductus) 130/75	—	70	71	70	80	89	91	18.0
4 (A)	20/14	124/10	129/60	131/79	121/96	—	38	38	46	43	45	66	19.6
	—	80/70	—	—	LV 98/10	—							
5 (A)	4	70/5	60/15	—	70/40	—	—	50	50	80	80	89 Aorta	—
6 A	7	92/0	85/41	—	—	—	—	65	68	82	83	88	14.9
6 B	9/6	75/6	74/23	73/47	—								
7 A	10/0	80/0	—	—	—	10/0							
7 B	7	77/4	—	83/51 FA	—	19/9							
8 (B)	9/5	86/6	73/19	91/43	LV 119/8	—							

*A, catheterization performed elsewhere; B, data obtained during operation.
†RA, right atrium; RV, right ventricle; PA, pulmonary artery; LA, left atrium; LV, left ventricle; FA, femoral artery.
‡IVC, inferior vena cava; MRA, mid right atrium; SVC, superior vena cava.

lay between −30 and −170 degrees; the frontal QRS vector described a counterclockwise loop in seven of these patients, and its major portion was superiorly oriented. Only one patient (case 8) had a different vector and axis. All patients showed a certain degree of right ventricular hypertrophy. The R waves in lead V_1 were high in all instances. The R:S ratio in lead aV_R was 1 or more in seven patients (fig. 8).

A QRS or QR pattern was present in lead V_6 in all cases, with the Q waves ranging from 2 to 12 mm. (0.2 to 1.2 mv.), the R waves from 13 to 33 mm. (1.3 to 3.3 mv.), and the S waves from 4.5 to 22 mm. (0.45 to 2.2 mv.).

Roentgenologic Appearance

Roentgenologic examination revealed enlargement of the cardiac shadow and increased pulmonary vasculature as evidence of pulmonary arterial hypertension in all patients (fig. 9). In two instances (cases 1 and 8), the supracardiac shadow was widened.

Hemodynamics

The cardiac catheterization data are shown in table 3. In two of the patients (cases 3 and 4), complete data were obtained in our laboratory; case 3 will be discussed in greater detail. Most important is the fact that the pulmonary arterial pressure was equal to the systemic arterial pressure in all of the patients.

The peripheral systemic arterial oxygen saturation varied from slightly below normal (88 per cent) to normal (96.7 per cent) in four of the five patients in whom it was obtained, while the fifth patient (case 4) showed severe arterial hypoxemia. This patient had congestive heart failure and was studied while he was under anesthesia. Values for the oxygen saturation of pulmonary arterial blood were obtained in the same five patients; in two (cases 3 and 6), the values in the pulmonary artery and the aorta were closely similar.

Sufficient data were obtained in four patients to exclude the presence of a large left-to-right shunt at the atrial level.

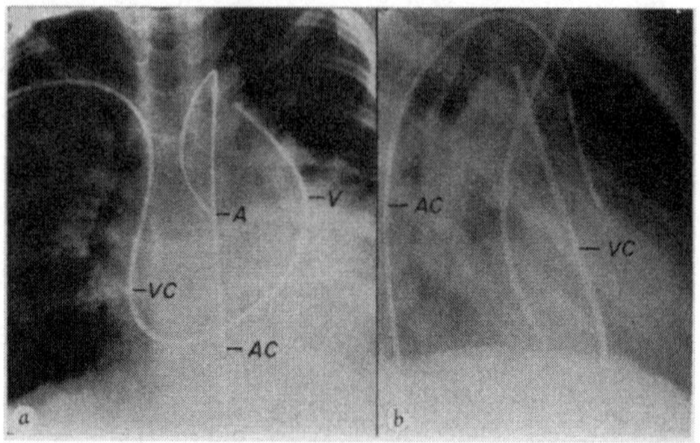

Figure 10

Case 4. a. *Position of catheter in posteroanterior view. VC = venous catheter; AC = aortic catheter; A = aortic valve; V = pulmonary valve. Note that both valves are at approximately the same level.* b. *Lateral view. Note that the distal part of the aortic catheter is positioned anterior to the venous catheter.*

Data in Case 3

The data obtained during cardiac catheterization in case 3 established the presence of an interventricular communication and an aorticopulmonic communication, the latter being interpreted as a patent ductus arteriosus. The catheter traversed the ductus on numerous occasions and was advanced into the abdominal aorta.

The oxygen saturation of right radial arterial blood (91 per cent) was 2 per cent greater than that of blood withdrawn simultaneously from the femoral artery. The oxygen saturation of femoral and pulmonary arterial blood apparently was identical. Dye-dilution curves recorded simultaneously at the right radial and femoral arteries after injection into the superior vena cava were similar, each showing a right-to-left shunt that was approximately 35 per cent at the radial artery and slightly greater at the femoral artery.

The pulmonary blood flow of 15.0 liters per minute was considerably greater than the systemic blood flow of 5.8 liters. The estimated pulmonary resistance of 380 dynes sec. $cm.^{-5}$ was significantly less than the total systemic resistance of 1035 dynes sec. $cm.^{-5}$.

The data were interpreted to indicate a large left-to-right shunt at the ventricular level. The identity of the oxygen saturation levels in the pulmonary and femoral arteries is compatible with the interpretation that partial or complete interruption of the aortic arch was present, with all, or a large portion, of the descending thoracic aorta originating from the ductus arteriosus. Partial interruption of the aortic arch was found at operation. The systolic pressure in the aortic arch was significantly higher than that in the descending aorta (table 4).

Table 4

Effect of Temporary Closure of Patent Ductus Arteriosus on Central Arterial Pressures (Case 3)

	Pressure, mm. Hg		
	Aortic arch	Descending aorta	Pulmonary artery
Ductus open	137/57	124/58	128/66*
Ductus closed	143/74	111/75	149/58*

*Pressures in pulmonary artery not recorded simultaneously with those in aorta.

Temporary closure of the ductus during operation resulted in a decrease in systolic pressure in the descending aorta and an increase in systolic pressure in the pulmonary artery, indicating the presence of a significant flow of blood via the ductus into the descending aorta (table 4).

This patient had practically uniform mixing of systemic venous and pulmonary venous blood in the outflow tract of the right ventricle and in the pulmonary artery, since the oxygen saturation of blood in the pulmonary, right radial, and femoral arteries was closely similar.

Discussion

The clinical picture in these patients was that of a large ventricular septal defect with pulmonary hypertension. Electrocardiography showed features that could be of some diagnostic help. To our knowledge, the electrocardiographic changes in this anomaly have not been previously described in detail. Witham[7] included an electrocardiographic tracing in one case of his "Eisenmenger group," but it is difficult from the reproductions to judge the exact portion of the electric axis and the vectorial QRS loop in the frontal plane; the axis was described as left and the P-R interval as being prolonged.

As already noted, all of our patients had prolonged P-R intervals, and the manifest mean electric QRS axis ranged between −30 and −170 degrees in all but one instance. The QRS loop as projected on the frontal plane rotated in a counterclockwise direction in six patients, and its major portion was superiorly oriented. The universal presence of right ventricular hypertrophy was indicated by the magnitude of the R waves in leads aV_R and V_1 and of the S waves in V_6. In cases 1, 3, and 4, a typical pattern of right bundle-branch block was observed.

The combination of the QRS electric axis lying above the superior point and a counterclockwise rotation of the QRS vector in the presence of signs of right ventricular hypertrophy has been described as an important electrocardiographic sign in persistent common atrioventricular canal by Toscano-Barboza and associates.[11] Toscano-Barboza and DuShane[12] found such electrocardiographic findings in nine of 59 anatomically proved cases of ventricular septal defect. According to Keith and co-workers,[13] and Char and associates,[14] the combination of left axis deviation in the standard leads and right ventricular hypertrophy in the precordial leads in cases with ventricular septal defect is rare.

Toscano-Barboza and associates,[11] in their explanation of the electrocardiographic changes in common atrioventricular canal, suggested that the defect at the top of the ventricular septum causes a fundamental alteration in the excitation pathway into the ventricles.

Neufeld and co-workers[15] found similar electrocardiographic alterations in excitation with ventricular septal defects of the persistent common atrioventricular canal type. Histologic studies showed that the conduction tissue lay dorsal to and skirted the ventricular septal defect. Similar changes were found by Lev[16] in cases of common atrioventricular canal.

Since the defect in cases in which both great vessels originate from the right ventricle is positioned dorsally, the same changes in the position of the conduction system might be expected. At present, these changes in conduction are thought to be on the same embryologic basis as the defect and are a possible cause of the electrocardiographic alterations.

In the presence of clinical signs of ventricular septal defect with pulmonary hypertension and the electrocardiographic changes already described, the possibility of both great vessels originating from the right ventricle should be considered, as well as the possibility of a ventricular septal defect of the persistent common atrioventricular canal type.

Hemodynamics

Measurements of pressure obtained during catheterization or operation or both disclosed closely similar systolic pressures in the right and left ventricles. In case 3, the oxygen saturation in the pulmonary artery was almost equal to that in the radial artery, which may be attributed to nearly complete mixing of systemic venous and left ventricular blood in the right ventricle. The pulmonary blood flow depends on the relative levels of pulmonary and systemic vascular resistance. With a lower pulmonary resistance, the pulmonary flow will be greater than the systemic flow, as in case 3.

In the presence of both an extremely high pulmonary flow and good mixing in the right ventricle, the oxygen saturation of pulmonary arterial blood can be equal to that in the systemic arterial system, and the systemic arterial blood oxygen saturation can approach normal values. If, during cardiac catheterization, a left-to-right shunt at the ventricular level is found and the oxygen saturation in the pulmonary artery is equal to that in one of the systemic arteries, the diagnosis of a single ventricle[17, 18] or the origin of both great vessels from the right ventricle is suggested. Determination of the anatomic positions of the semilunar valves and the great vessels may help to differentiate these two conditions.

In a single ventricle without pulmonary stenosis,[17] the relative positions of the aorta and pulmonary artery frequently are reversed. The ascending aorta lies ventral and parallel to the pulmonary artery, with the aortic valve occupying a position that is ventral and cephalad to and to the left of the pulmonary valve.

When both great vessels take origin from the right ventricle, the ascending aorta lies to the right of the pulmonary artery and the two semilunar valves lie in approximately the same coronal and cross-sectional body planes.

The relationship of the great vessels to each other may be demonstrated by positioning two catheters simultaneously in the aorta and pulmonary artery, which demonstrates that the aorta is to the right of the pulmonary artery, with both lying parallel in posteroanterior as well as lateral views. This procedure also shows that the cephalocaudal levels of the aortic and pulmonic valves are similar (fig. 10*a*). In the lateral view, the catheters appear to be approximately in the same coronal body plane (fig. 10*b*).

Some cases of origin of both great vessels from the right ventricle (as well as some cases of single ventricle)[17] show poor mixing of venous and arterial blood in the ventricle. In these instances, a streaming effect apparently exists,[14] the left ventricular blood being shunted preferentially through the ventricular septal defect directly into the aorta and the right ventricular blood being directed into the pulmonary artery. When this occurs, the oxygen saturation of the pulmonary arterial blood is significantly less than that of the systemic arterial blood. Such patients present a difficult diagnostic problem at cardiac catheterization, because the data on blood oxygen saturation obtained from the cardiac chambers and great vessels resemble those in patients who have the usual type of ventricular septal defect with a large left-to-right shunt.

A clue to the correct diagnosis of common origin of the great vessels from the right ventricle can be obtained at cardiac catheterization in such patients by recognizing the unusual positions of the aorta and pulmonary arteries in relationship to each other, as well as the anatomic relationships of the semilunar valves. Demonstration of these unusual anatomic relationships can be particularly clear cut if the two-catheter technic (fig. 10) or biplanar selective angiocardiography is used.

Summary and Conclusions

Clinical, hemodynamic, and pathologicoanatomic findings were studied in eight cases in which both great vessels took origin from the right ventricle in the absence of pulmonary stenosis. In each case, a ventricular septal defect constituted the only outlet for the left ventricle. The aortic and pulmonary valves were in approximately the same cross-sectional and coronal body planes, which contrasts to the situation in the usual ventricular septal defect, in which the aortic valve lies in a normal position, being caudal to the pulmonary valve.

The clinical features simulated those of a large ventricular septal defect associated with pulmonary hypertension. The importance of distinguishing these two anomalies is emphasized, since the surgical methods for repair are different.

The following findings aid in the differential diagnosis: (1) electrocardiography shows a manifest mean electric axis above the zero line, with the frontal-plane vectorial loop of the QRS directed in a counterclockwise direction and its main portion lying above the zero line; (2) cardiac catheterization or angiocardiography or both demonstrate that the aortic valve lies at the same cross-sectional body level as the pulmonary valve in the anteroposterior view and at the same coronal plane in the lateral view; (3) in some cases, the oxygen saturation of blood in the pulmonary artery approaches or equals that in the aorta, indicating that relatively complete mixing of pulmonary venous and systemic venous blood has occurred in the outflow tract of the right ventricle.

References

1. ROKITANSKY, K.: Die Defecte der Scheidewände des Herzens: Pathologisch-anatomische Abhandlung. Wein, Wilhelm Braümuller, 1875, 156 pp.
2. SPITZER, A.: The Architecture of Normal and Malformed Hearts: A Phylogenetic Theory of Their Development. Springfield, Illinois, Charles C Thomas, 1951, 145 pp.
3. PEACOCK, T. B.: Quoted by Witham, A. C.[7]
4. ABBOTT, M. E. S.: Atlas of Congenital Heart Disease. New York, The American Heart Association, 1936, 62 pp.
5. INGHAM, D. W., AND WILLIUS, F. A.: Congenital transposition of great arterial trunks. Am. Heart J. 15: 482, 1938.
6. SAPHIR, O., AND LEV, M.: The tetralogy of Eisenmenger. Am. Heart J. 21: 31, 1941.
7. WITHAM, A. C.: Double outlet right ventricle: A partial transposition complex. Am. Heart J. 53: 928, 1957.
8. EDWARDS, J. E.: Congenital Malformations of the Heart and Great Vessels. *In* Gould, S. E.: Pathology of the Heart. Ed. 2, Springfield, Illinois, Charles C Thomas, 1960, pp. 260-496.
9. EDWARDS, J. E., JAMES, J. W., AND DUSHANE, J. W.: Congenital malformation of the heart: Origin of transposed great vessels from the right ventricle associated with atresia of the left ventricular outlet, double orifice of the mitral valve, and single coronary artery. Lad. Invest. 1: 197, 1952.
10. ZIEGLER, R. F.: Electrocardiographic Studies in Normal Infants and Children. Springfield, Illinois, Charles C Thomas, 1951, 207 pp.
11. TOSCANO-BARBOZA, E., BRANDENBURG, R. O., AND BURCHELL, H. B.: Electrocardiographic studies of cases with intracardiac malformations of the atrioventricular canal. Proc. Staff. Meet., Mayo Clin. 31: 513, 1956.
12. TOSCANO-BARBOZA, E., AND DUSHANE, J. W.: Ventricular septal defect: Correlation of electrocardiographic and hemodynamic findings in 60 proved cases. Am. J. Cardiol. 3: 721, 1959.
13. KEITH, J. D., ROWE, R. D., AND VLAD, P.: Heart Disease in Infancy and Childhood. New York, Macmillan Company, 1958, 877 pp.
14. CHAR, F., ADAMS, P., JR., AND ANDERSON, R. C.: Electrocardiographic findings in one hundred verified cases of ventricular septal defect. A.M.A. J. Dis. Child. 97: 48, 1959.
15. NEUFELD, H. N., TITUS, J. L., DUSHANE, J. W., BURCHELL, H. B., AND EDWARDS, J. E.: Unpublished data.
16. LEV, M.: The architecture of the conduction system in congenital heart disease. I. Common atrioventricular orifice. A.M.A. Arch. Path. 65: 174, 1958.
17. BROW, R. E., SWAN, H. J. C., AND WOOD, E. H.: Unpublished data.
18. VAN BUCHEM, F. S. P., NIEVEEN, J., AND MARRING, W.: Cor triloculare biatriatum. Cardiologia 24: 135, 1954.

Origin of Both Great Vessels from the Right Ventricle

II. With Pulmonary Stenosis

By HENRY N. NEUFELD, M.D., JAMES W. DUSHANE, M.D., AND JESSE E. EDWARDS, M.D.

THE FIRST PAPER[1] of this series dealt with the origin of both great vessels from the right ventricle in the absence of pulmonary stenosis. It was indicated that the clinical picture in that condition might be confused with that of a large ventricular septal defect. Electrocardiographically, such an anomaly might be confused with either a persistent common atrioventricular canal[2] or the "AV commune" type of ventricular septal defect.[3]

The condition forming the basis for the present communication anatomically has in common with the foregoing anomaly the origin of both great vessels from the right ventricle, but pulmonary stenosis is also present. The hemodynamic, clinical, and electrocardiographic data resemble those in the tetralogy of Fallot.

This part of the study includes five cases in which both great vessels originated from the right ventricle associated with ventricular septal defect and pulmonic stenosis, and a sixth case, in which both great vessels took origin from the right ventricle and in which a common atrioventricular canal and pulmonic stenosis were associated.

The purpose of this paper is to summarize the clinical, hemodynamic, and anatomic findings in these cases. The differentiation of this anomaly from the tetralogy of Fallot with cyanosis is important because of the more complicated surgical approach in the former.

This anomaly has been described before in articles devoted to pathology, but only in recent years have a few cases been reported clinically.[1, 4-9]

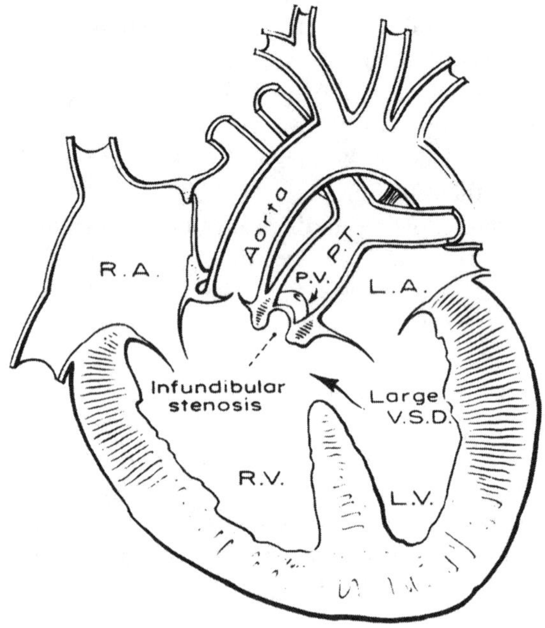

Figure 1

Diagrammatic representation of origin of both great vessels from right ventricle, with pulmonary stenosis and ventricular septal defect.

Witham,[10] in 1957, summarized reports of three cases from the literature and added two of his own, calling them "double outlet right ventricle, Fallot type."

Pathologico-anatomic Features

As in the cases in which both great vessels took origin from the right ventricle without pulmonary stenosis, the external view of the relationship of the great vessels in cases with pulmonary stenosis is very similar to the normal appearance, but important differences exist at lower levels within the heart (figs. 1-4).

The origin of the aorta lies to the right of the origin of the pulmonary artery, both

From the Mayo Clinic and the Mayo Foundation, Rochester, Minnesota. The Mayo Foundation is a part of the Graduate School of the University of Minnesota.

Supported in part by research grant no. H4014 of the National Heart Institute, U. S. Public Health Service.

Table 1

Clinical Data in Five Cases of Origin of Both Great Vessels from Right Ventricle, with Pulmonary Stenosis

Case	Age, yrs.	Sex	History: Cyanosis, age at onset	History: Shortness of breath	History: Palpitation	Physical findings: Cyanosis	Clubbing	Systolic thrill	Systolic murmur, grade and location*	Other murmurs	Second pulmonic sound	Blood pressure, mm. of Hg	Femoral pulses	Hemoglobin Gm./100 ml.
1	7/12	M	2 mos.	−	−	+	−	−	+	−			+	
2†	3	F	6 mos.	−	−	++	++	−	I (3)	−	Single, not diminished	115/75	+	19
3‡	13	M	2½ mos.	+	+	+	−	+	IV (4-5)	−	Single, not diminished	110/75	+	15.9
4†	8	M	8 mos.	+	+	+	+	+	III (3-4)	Machinery murmur; syst. ejection click	Accentuated	100/80	+	15.8
5	3½	M	Birth	+	+	+++	++	+	IV (3-4)	−	Diminished	100/75	+	18.2

*Roman numerals indicate grade of murmur; Arabic numbers in parentheses indicate those left intercostal spaces where the murmur was heard.
†Previous Blalock's procedure; a Potts operation also was done in case 4.
‡Previous Brock's procedure.

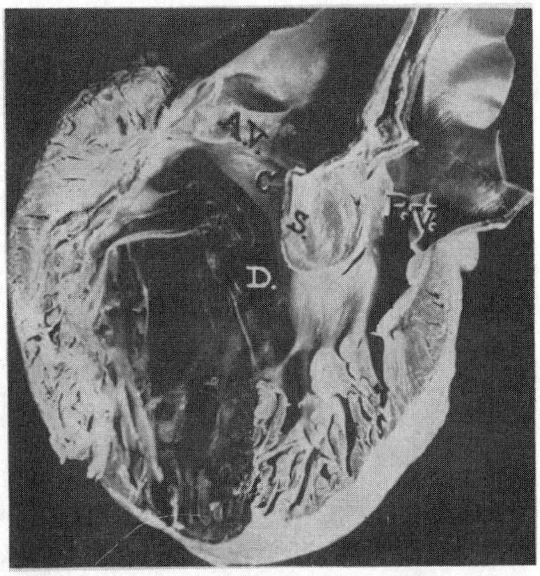

Figure 2

Origin of both great vessels from right ventricle, with infundibular stenosis, seen from right ventricular aspect. The ventricular septal defect (D.) lies caudal to the horizontal limb of the crista supraventricularis (C.S.). The vertical limb of the crista supraventricularis creates an infundibular chamber that is moderately stenotic and above which rises the pulmonary artery. P.V. = pulmonary valve. The aortic origin (A.V.) lies to the right of the pulmonary origin and at about the same body cross-sectional and coronal plane. The aortic valve lies above the horizontal limb of the crista supraventricularis, which separates the valves from the ventricular septal defect.

vessels being at about the same cross-sectional body plane. Internal views of the heart show that the aorta does not communicate with the left ventricle but arises completely from the right ventricle. The only outlet for the left ventricle is a ventricular septal defect.

The aortic valve lies above the horizontal limb of the crista supraventricularis, which separates the valve from the ventricular septal defect and from the atrioventricular valvular tissue. The aortic valve lies in the same coronal body plane as does the pulmonary valve.

Infundibular stenosis is created by a vertical limb of the crista supraventricularis.

One specimen (case 5) showed different features (fig. 5). The aorta originated from the right ventricle, lying to the right of the

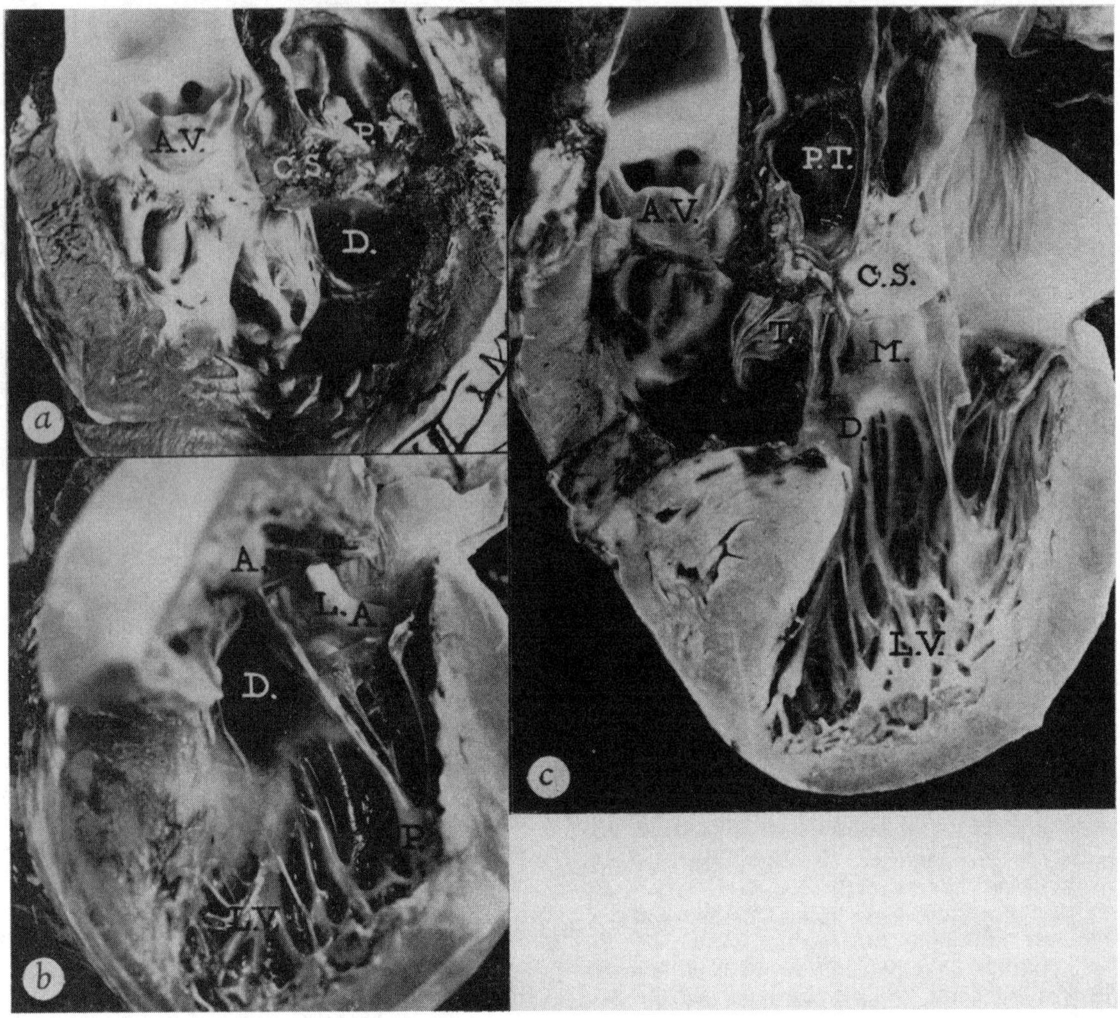

Figure 3

Origin of both great vessels from right ventricle, with infundibular stenosis. The specimen in this case resembles the one shown in figure 1. a. *Right ventricular aspect. A section has been made through the infundibular zone. The ventricular septal defect lies caudal to the crista supraventricularis (C. S.). A portion of the stenotic infundibular channel is present and lies below the pulmonary valve (P.V.). The aortic valve (A.V.) lies at the same cross-sectional body plane and to the right of the pulmonary valve, being separated from the atrioventricular valvular tissue by the horizontal limb of the crista ventricularis.* b. *Left atrium (L.A.) and left ventricle (L.V.). The anterior leaflet of the mitral valve has been stretched to prepare this illustration; it shows a normal caudal connection with the anterolateral papillary muscle (A.) and the posteromedial papillary muscle (P.). The ventricular septal defect (D.) lies ventral to the anterior leaflet of the mitral valve.* c. *Sagittal section through both ventricles and anterior leaflet of mitral valve. The posterior boundary of the ventricular septal defect (D.) is formed by the tissue of the septal leaflet of the tricuspid valve (T.) and the anterior leaflet of the mitral valve (M.), which joins the crista supraventricularis (C.S.). No continuity exists between the aortic valve and the atrioventricular valvular tissue. L.V. = left ventricle; P.T. = pulmonary trunk.*

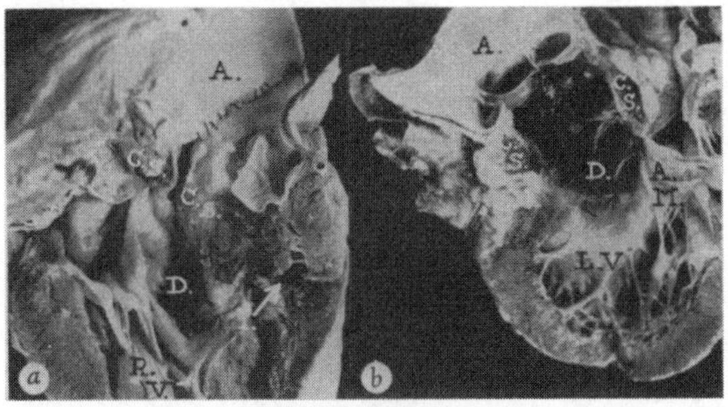

Figure 4

Origin of both great vessels from right ventricle, with infundibular stenosis. The ventricular septal defect is caudal to the crista supraventricularis. These illustrations show the relations of the aortic valve to the ventricular septal defect and the anterior leaflet of the mitral valve. They emphasize that, in the usual dissection, the fact that the aorta does not communicate with the left ventricle may be obscured by an illusion, which makes it appear to originate from the left ventricle when in fact it does not. a. *Right ventricular aspect. The aorta (A.) arises from the right ventricle. The aortic valve is separated from the ventricular septal defect (D.) by a horizontal limb of the crista supraventricularis (C.S.). A vertical limb of the crista supraventricularis creates an infundibular chamber(I.), which is stenotic. In this specimen, the incision has been carried from the left ventricle to the aorta, the crista supraventricularis being divided. The postmortem incision in the aorta has been sutured.* b. *Left ventricle and aortic valve. The specimen has been opened in the line of section shown in* a. *This figure shows apparent continuity between the aorta and the left ventricle, but this is an illusion because between the aorta, the left ventricle and the anterior leaflet of the mitral valve (A.M.) is a mass of muscle (C.S.), the crista supraventricularis, which lies above the ventricular septal defect (D.) and below the aortic valve. In normal hearts, a section through the left ventricle into the aorta in this perspective shows continuity between the aortic valve and the anterior leaflet of the mitral valve. In this heart, the crista supraventricularis separates these two valvular structures.*

origin of the pulmonary trunk. The posterior wall of the ventricular septal defect was formed by the septal leaflet of the tricuspid valve and the anterior mitral leaflet. Continuity was present between the mitral valvular tissue and the aortic valve, but the latter was positioned farther to the right than it is in the classic anatomic tetralogy of Fallot.

Table 2

Cardiac Catheterization Data in Case 2

Site	Pressure, mm. Hg	Oxygen saturation, per cent
Inferior vena cava	—	53
Superior vena cava	8/5	57
Right atrium	8/5	54-56
Right ventricular outflow	115/7	55
Main pulmonary artery	15/7	56
Right femoral artery	125/71	61

Clinical Findings

The clinical data in the first five cases are summarized in table 1. There were four boys and one girl; the youngest patient was 7 months of age and the oldest was 13 years. The first patient in this study was seen at the Mayo Clinic in 1936 (case 1 in table 1). All the patients had been cyanotic since the first months of life. Clubbing of the fingers was present in three instances. Three patients had a systolic thrill. The second sound at the pulmonary area was accentuated in one patient (case 4), on whom both a Blalock and a Potts operation had been done in the past. Squatting was not observed in any of the patients. None of the patients had experienced congestive cardiac failure or undue respiratory infections.

Electrocardiographic tracings were obtained in four of these five cases, and they were compatible with right ventricular hypertrophy of the type seen in the tetralogy of Fallot (fig. 6).

Roentgenograms were obtained in the same four cases (fig. 7). They revealed moderate enlargement of the heart and diminished pulmonary vasculature.

Hemodynamics*

Catheterization of the right side of the heart was performed in one instance (case 2). The data are shown in table 2. Severe desaturation of the peripheral arterial blood

*The authors gratefully acknowledge the assistance of Dr. E. H. Wood, who made available the hemodynamic data. Support for the latter was derived from grant no. H3532 of the National Heart Institute.

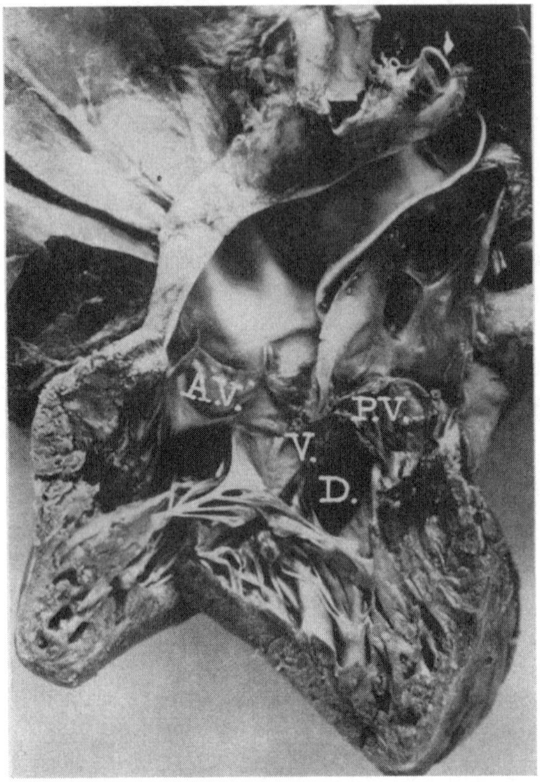

Figure 5

Case 5. A variant of the tetralogy of Fallot that in certain respects presents problems and anatomic relations more similar to those in origin of both great vessels from the right ventricle than to those in the classic tetralogy. The specimen shows the aortic origin (A.V.) from the right ventricle and to the right of the origin of the pulmonary trunk (P.T.). The left aspect of the aorta is at about the same plane as the ventricular septal defect (D.). The dorsal wall of the ventricular septal defect is formed by the septal leaflet of the tricuspid valve and the anterior mitral leaflet (V.). This specimen shows continuity between the mitral valvular tissue and the aortic valve, but the position of the aortic valve is considerably farther to the right than it is in the classic tetralogy of Fallot.

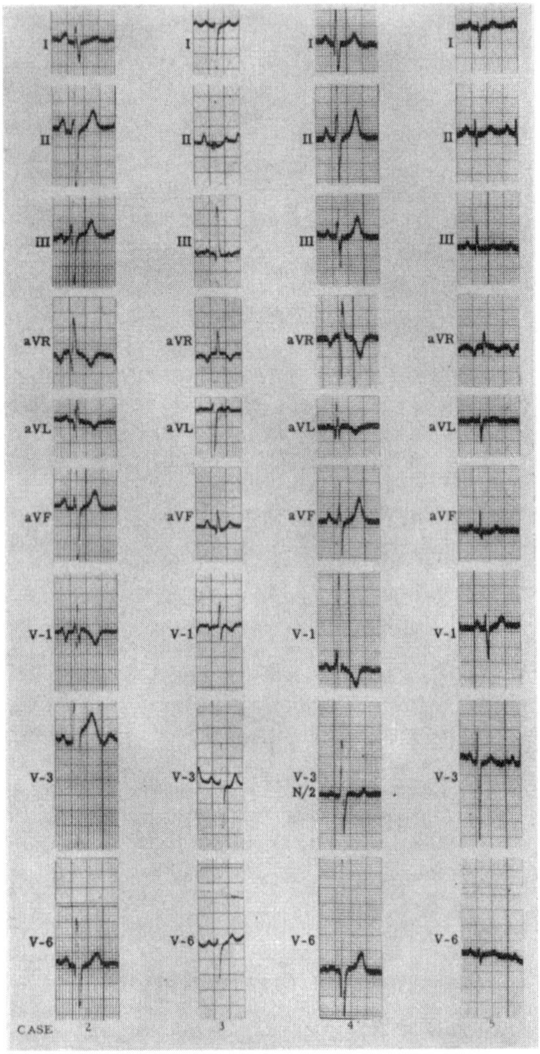

Figure 6

Electrocardiograms in cases 2 through 5.

was present. The oxygen saturation of right ventricular blood taken at the same time was 6 percentage points less than that of systemic arterial blood. The saturation of mixed venous blood ranged between 53 and 57 per cent. Pressures in the great veins and right atrium were normal. The right ventricular pressure was 115/7, expressed as millimeters of mercury. The catheter was manipulated to enter the pulmonary artery and was passed into the right lung field to the wedge position. The pressure in the right pulmonary artery was 10-15/0-5, and the wedge pressure was 2-4 mm. No significant difference was noted between the oxygen saturation in the main pulmonary artery and that in the outflow portion of the right ventricle. When the catheter was withdrawn across the pulmonary valve, the region of obstruction appeared to be sharply localized to a region at or near the pulmonary valve, since a high systolic ventricular pressure was recorded immediately upstream to the pulmonary valve. Further changes in pressure were not

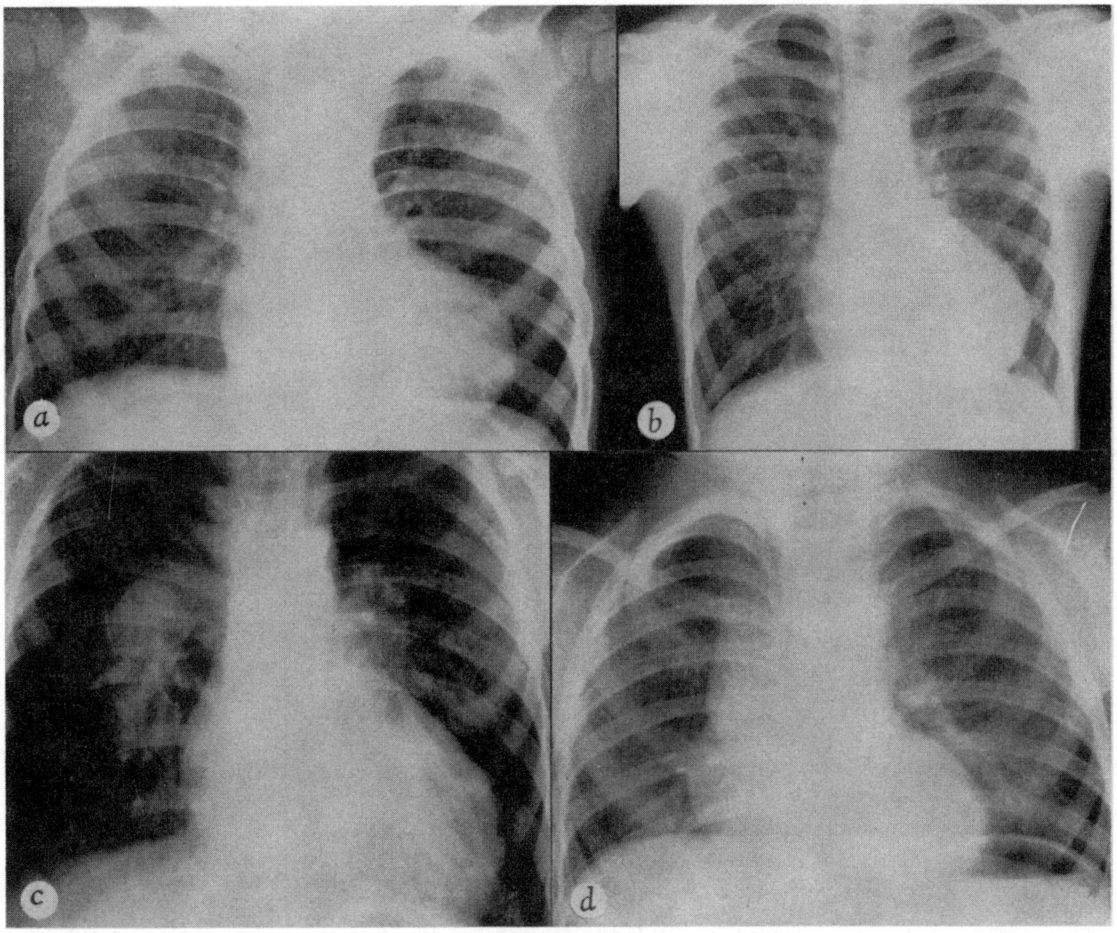

Figure 7

a-d. *Thoracic roentgenograms in cases 2 through 5.*

Table 3

Cardiac Catheterization Data in Case 6

Site	Pressure, mm. Hg	Oxygen saturation, per cent
Superior vena cava	—	53
Right atrium	8/3	57
Left atrium	11/7	79-85
Right ventricle	116/4	65-67
Femoral artery	121/63	72
Pulmonary vein	10/5	99

observed when the catheter was withdrawn from this position to the lower part of the right ventricle.

The catheter was then advanced, and it entered the aorta. The aortic arch was located on the left.

Indicator-dilution curves were recorded at the right radial artery after injections of cardio-green dye into the main pulmonary artery, the lower part of the right ventricle, the aorta and the superior vena cava. The contours of the curves obtained after injection into the superior vena cava, right ventricle, and aorta were similar or almost identical. The similarity of the contours of curves recorded after injections into the superior vena cava and right ventricle excluded the possibility of preferential injection into the aorta from the right ventricle. The close similarity of the curves indicated an extremely large right-to-left shunt and practically an absence of flow from the right ventricle directly to the pulmonary artery.[10]

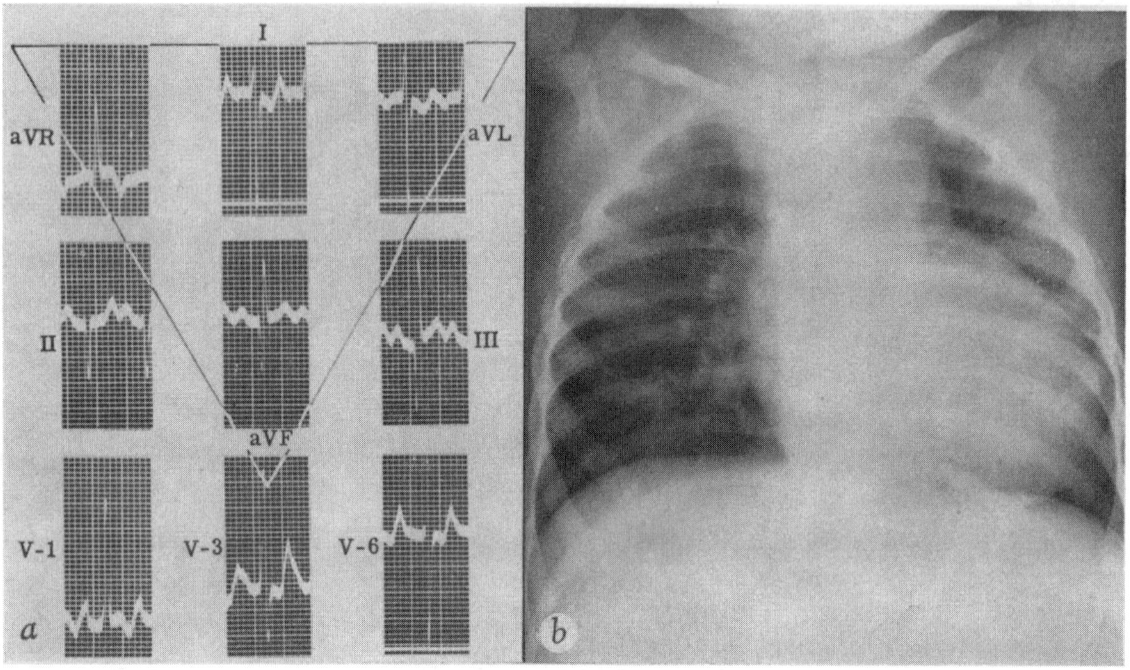

Figure 8

Case 6. a. *Electrocardiogram of a 3-year-old girl who had persistent common atrioventricular canal.* b. *Thoracic roentgenogram in same case.*

The hemodynamic state in this anomaly is similar to that present in severe tetralogy of Fallot with cyanosis. The pressures in both ventricles are equal, and a pressure gradient exists between the right ventricle and the pulmonary artery. Peripheral oxygen desaturation is present in all cases.

In some instances, relatively complete mixing of systemic venous and left ventricular blood in the right ventricle might be expected to occur; when this is present, closely similar values for oxygen saturation in the systemic and pulmonary arteries would be found. On the other hand, some of the patients will show poor mixing in the right ventricle. In such instances, a streaming effect apparently exists, the left ventricular blood being shunted preferentially through the ventricular septal defect directly into the aorta, and the right ventricular blood being directed into the pulmonary artery. In these cases, the oxygen saturation of the pulmonary arterial blood will be significantly less than that of the systemic arterial blood. This situation prevailed in case 2 (table 2).

Diagnostic Clues

A clue to the correct diagnosis of the origin of both great vessels from the right ventricle with pulmonary stenosis can be obtained during cardiac catheterization or angiocardiography or both. Utilizing a two-catheter technic (venous and aortic) and bearing in mind the anatomic relationship of the semilunar valves, one might prove that both semilunar valves are in the same cross-sectional and coronal body planes. The same applies to biplanar selective angiocardiography. Another clue that can be obtained in angiocardiography is the relationship of the ventricular septal defect to the crista supraventricularis. In the tetralogy of Fallot, the crista supraventricularis is ventral to the ventricular septal defect; in origin of both great vessels from the right ventricle with pulmonary stenosis, the crista supraventricularis is cephalad to the ventricular septal defect.

Report of Unusual Case

The afore-mentioned sixth case showed additional interesting pathologic features.

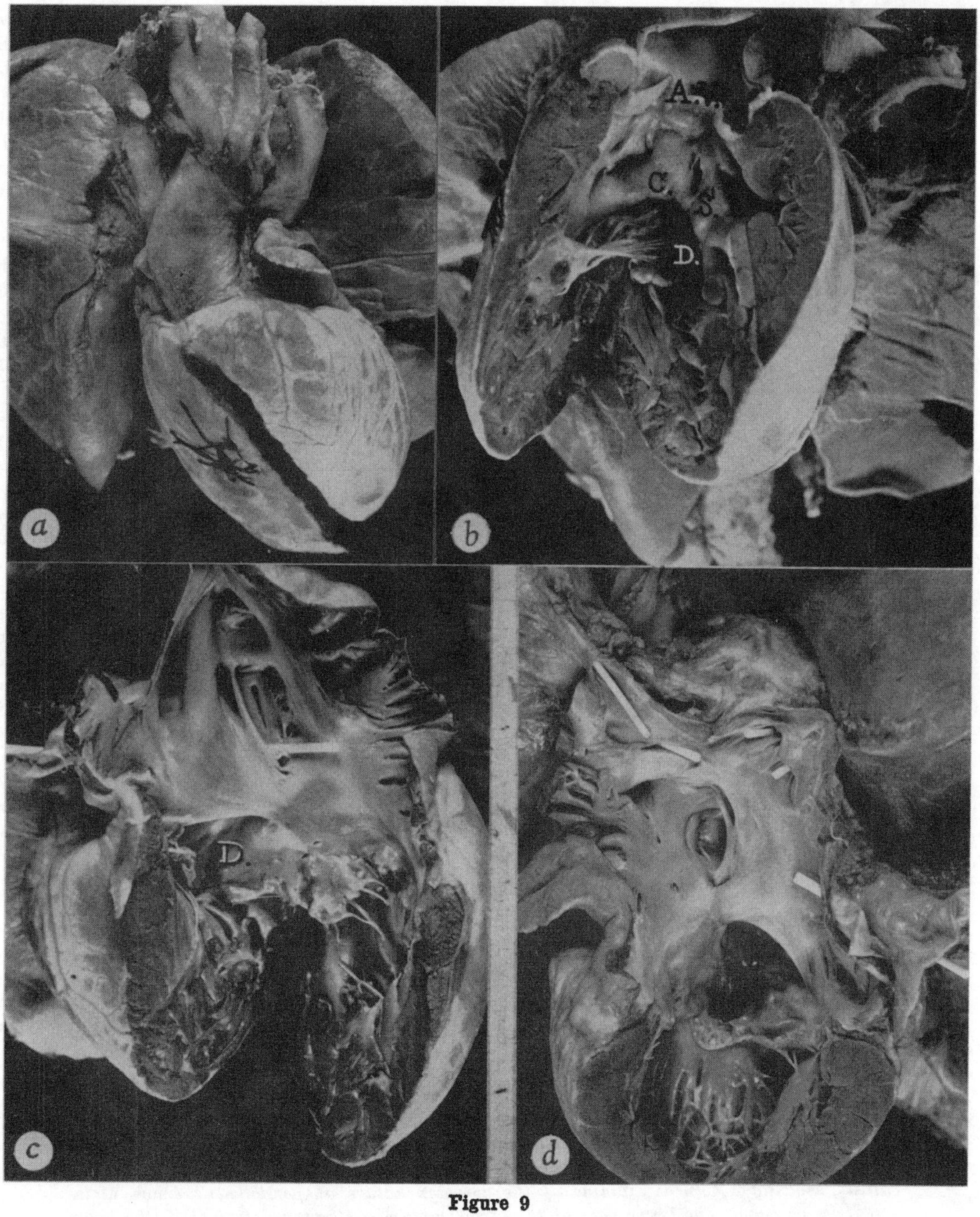

Figure 9

Case 6. Origin of both great vessels from right ventricle, with persistent common atrioventricular canal. In this unusual heart, the relative positions of the aorta and the pulmonary trunk are contrary to those in the usual examples of origin of both great vessels from the right ventricle. In the latter condition, the aortic origin lies to the right of the pulmonary trunk; in this specimen, the aortic origin lies ventral to the pulmonary trunk. a. External view of heart and great vessels, showing prominent ventral position of aorta. b. Interior of right ventricle. The aorta (A.V.) arises from the right ventricle above the crista supraventricularis (C.S.), which creates an infundi-

Case 6. A 3-year-old girl was brought to the clinic in June 1958, for evaluation of a cardiac lesion and the possibilities of surgical intervention. The child had been cyanotic since birth, and her physical and mental development was impaired.

Cyanosis and clubbing were present. The heart was quiet, and a harsh systolic murmur (grade 2) was best heard at the second and third left intercostal spaces. The second cardiac sound in the pulmonic area was single and diminished. The femoral pulsations were normal.

The electrocardiogram showed a normal sinus rhythm. The mean manifest QRS electric axis was —170 degrees, with a figure-of-eight loop in the frontal plane, the initial portion of the loop being counterclockwise. Signs of right ventricular hypertrophy were present in the thoracic leads (fig. 8*a*).

Roentgenologic examination revealed cardiac enlargement and decreased pulmonary vasculature (fig. 8*b*).

Cardiac catheterization was performed (table 3). The pulmonary artery was not entered. The left atrium was entered in a retrograde fashion from the ventricle, suggesting either an anatomically common ventricle or a persistent common atrioventricular canal type of defect. The pulmonary venous saturation was greater than the left atrial saturation, indicating a right-to-left shunt at the atrial level. The most likely diagnosis considered from the catheterization data was a common ventricle or a persistent common atrioventricular canal associated with pulmonic stenosis.

An infundibular resection was performed at operation. The patient died on the same day.

Pathologic Findings. Necropsy revealed that the great vessels were transposed; both vessels originated from the right ventricle, but the pulmonary trunk lay dorsal to and to the right of the ascending aorta (fig. 9). The ascending aorta was considerably wider than normal, while the pulmonary trunk was thin-walled and narrow, measuring only about 8 mm. in diameter.

Significant venous anomalies were present. Bilateral superior venae cavae were present; the bridge between the two that is present under normal conditions also existed in this case. The right superior vena cava entered the right atrium in the normal position, while the left superior vena cava entered the left atrium at a position comparable to that at which the right one entered the right atrium. Two inferior venae cavae were present that perforated the diaphragm on either side of the esophagus. The right one measured about 1.5 cm. in diameter, while the left measured 1 cm. The right inferior vena cava entered the right atrium in a normal position, while the left inferior vena cava entered the left atrium in the posteroinferior aspect, inferior to the left inferior pulmonary vein. The pulmonary veins entered the left atrium normally.

The interior of the heart showed an atrial septal defect measuring about 1 by 0.5 cm. involving the fossa ovalis. No lower limbus of the fossa ovalis could be identified. The lowermost portion of the atrial septum contained a large defect characteristic of that associated with a persistent common atrioventricular canal. A common atrioventricular valve served both sides of the heart. The lowermost part of the defect in this region was formed by the crest of the underlying ventricular septum. Thus, the defect presented a picture of the complete variety of persistent common atrioventricular canal. Beneath the posterior leaflet were many interchordal spaces that allowed interventricular communication. A small number of interchordal spaces were found beneath the anterior leaflet of the common atrioventricular valve. The coronary sinus was absent. Two ventricles were present, each being about the same size, although the right ventricular muscle appeared somewhat thicker than the left. The left ventricle did not have any vessel of egress. This chamber communicated with the right side by way of the subvalvular communications in relation to the persistent common atrioventricular canal that already has been described; in addition, a defect about 8 mm. in diameter was present in the muscular part of the most superior anterior portion of the ventricular septum.

bular chamber that leads to the origin of the transposed pulmonary artery. The ventricular septal defect (D.) lies caudal to the crista supraventricularis. c. *Right side of the heart, showing a typical example of the complex nature of persistent common atrioventricular canal. The lower part of the atrial septum contains a defect (D.), the lower border of which is formed by atrioventricular valvular tissue. The latter is represented by a valve common to both sides of the heart, representing the complete variety of persistent common atrioventricular canal. In this case, the inferior vena cava entered the left atrium. The probe shows an additional atrioseptal defect at the fossa ovalis.* d. *Left side of heart, showing the typical deformities of persistent common atrioventricular canal. The upper probes are in normally situated pulmonary venous connections with the left atrium. A probe in the right lower part of the photograph shows the entrance of the inferior vena cava into the left atrium.*

The aorta arose entirely from the right ventricle. Posterior to the origin of the aorta was a narrow muscle-walled tract measuring only about 3 mm. in diameter that led to the pulmonary artery beyond. Evidence of recent surgical intervention in relationship to the subpulmonary stenosis was present. The aortic arch was on the left side. The ductus arteriosus was closed. The bronchial arteries appeared to be enlarged.

The pathologic diagnoses included origin of both great vessels from the right ventricle, with pulmonary stenosis; persistent atrioventricular canal (complete variety); anomalous connection of a persistent left superior vena cava with the left atrium; bilateral inferior venae cavae, the left one communicating with the left atrium; absence of the coronary sinus.

Comment. Despite the pathologico-anatomic findings of significant pulmonary stenosis, the initial vectors in the electrocardiogram in the frontal plane were directed to the left, as they are in persistent common atrioventricular canal, which was present in this patient.

Summary and Conclusions

Clinical, hemodynamic, and pathologico-anatomic findings were studied in six cases in which both great vessels took origin from the right ventricle in the presence of pulmonary stenosis. This condition is indistinguishable from the tetralogy of Fallot, with cyanosis on the basis of clinical, electrocardiographic, and radiologic findings. The hemodynamics are also similar in both conditions.

The more complicated surgical approach in the condition under consideration emphasizes the importance of its differentiation from the usual case of tetralogy of Fallot with cyanosis.

Only angiocardiography and cardiac catheterization might be of diagnostic help, if one bears in mind the anatomic characteristics of this condition. The fact that both the aortic and pulmonary valves are at the same horizontal body level in this anomaly must be considered at angiocardiography. Also, the fact that the crista supraventricularis is cranial and more dorsal to the ventricular septal defect may be of some diagnostic help at angiocardiography. Careful analysis of the exact position of the semilunar valves during combined catheterization of the right side of the heart and the aorta is of some diagnostic importance.

References

1. NEUFELD, H. N., DUSHANE, J. W., WOOD, E. H., KIRKLIN, J. W., AND EDWARDS, J. E.: Origin of both great vessels from the right ventricle. I. Without pulmonary stenosis. Circulation 23: 399, 1961.
2. TOSCANO-BARBOSA, E., BRANDENBURG, R. O., AND BURCHELL, H. B.: Electrocardiographic studies of cases with intracardiac malformations of the atrioventricular canal. Proc. Staff. Meet., Mayo Clin. 31: 513, 1956.
3. NEUFELD, H. N., TITUS, J. L., DUSHANE, J. W., BURCHELL, H. B., AND EDWARDS, J. E.: Isolated ventricular septal defect of the persistent common atrioventricular canal type. Unpublished data.
4. SPITZER, A.: The Architecture of Normal and Malformed Hearts: A Phylogenetic Theory of Their Development. Springfield, Illinois, Charles C Thomas, 1951, 145 pp.
5. PEACOCK, T. B.: Malformations of the Human Heart. Ed. 2, London, J. Churchill & Sons, 1866, 204 pp.
6. ABBOTT, M. E. S.: Atlas of Congenital Cardiac Disease. New York, American Heart Association, 1936, 62 pp.
7. EDWARDS, J. E.: Congenital Malformations of the Heart and Great Vessels. *In* Gould, S. E.: Pathology of the Heart. Ed. 2, Springfield, Illinois, Charles C Thomas, 1960, pp. 260-496.
8. LEV, M.: Autopsy Diagnosis of Congenitally Malformed Hearts. Springfield, Illinois, Charles C Thomas, 1953, 194 pp.
9. BRAUN, K., DE VRIES, A., FEINGOLD, D. S., EHRENFELD, N. E., FELDMAN, J., AND SCHORR, S.: Complete dextroposition of the aorta, pulmonary stenosis, interventricular septal defect, and patent foramen ovale. Am. Heart J. 43: 773, 1952.
10. WITHAM, A. C.: Double outlet right ventricle: A partial transposition complex. Am. Heart J. 53: 928, 1957.

Origin of Both Great Vessels From the Right Ventricle.

I. Without pulmonary stenosis

II. Origin of Both Great Vessels from the Right Ventricle.

II. With Pulmonary Stenosis

Richard Van Praagh, M.D.

Why were the publications in 1961 by Edwards and his colleagues on what would become known as double-outlet right ventricle (DORV) such bomb shells? Having survived my 80th birthday this year, I am old enough to remember and to understand their impact. There were two papers, DORV without pulmonary stenosis (PS)[1], and DORV with PS[2], written by an all-star cast:

Henry Neufeld, the lead author, subsequently to win renown as Israel's leading cardiologist;

Jim DuShane, head of Pediatric Cardiology at the Mayo Clinic in Rochester, Minnesota;

Earl Wood, resident genius of the Medical Sciences Building at Mayo, developer of the G-suit (gravity-suit) to prevent blacking out from cerebral ischemia during high-speed aerial maneuvers, and intimately involved in the American space program; I met our first astronauts — rhesus monkeys that were trained and instrumented by Earl Wood and his colleagues; the cover story, that none of the house staff (I was a fellow in Dr. Jeremy Swan's Cath Lab) saw through, was that these monkeys were taking part in a neuropsychiatric stress test — a ruse that contained much truth;

John Kirklin, regarded by many as the best congenital heart surgeon of his era; and

Jesse Edwards, the senior author, widely considered to be the best cardiovascular pathologist of his time, with a special talent for clinico-pathologic correlation.

These papers[1, 2] were bomb shells because they represented a radical but necessary departure from the earlier understanding, terminology, and classification of congenital heart disease. In 1927, Maude Abbott[3] had defined transposition of the great arteries (TGA) as "an alteration in the position of the two great vessels relative to the ventricles of the heart or to each other at their origin."

Thus, *any* abnormality in the relations between the great arteries themselves or between the great arteries and the ventricles was regarded as some form of TGA. The problem was that there were so many different kinds!

Accurate diagnosis and successful surgery required greater precision, as Edwards and his colleagues knew. And there was already a move in that direction:

In 1952, Braun et al[4] reported a patient in whom "the right ventricle serves as a '*double-outlet' ventricle*."

In 1957, A. Calhoun Witham[5] introduced the designation *double–outlet right ventricle*, an anomaly that had previously been called *partial transposition* of the great arteries because only one great artery (the aorta) was transposed, i.e., placed across (*trans ponere*, Latin) the ventricular septum, and hence arose above the morphologically inappropriate ventricle.

In 1960, Alois Beuren[6] pointed out that the

Taussig-Bing malformation[7], a form of DORV described in 1949, could be distinguished from typical TGA by the location of the main pulmonary artery: posterior in typical TGA, but side-by-side in the Taussig-Bing type of DORV.

In 1961, Dwight McGoon[8] — a prince of a man and a brilliant surgeon at the Mayo Clinic — described repair of DORV surgically. With characteristic generosity and honesty, Dwight McGoon wrote that the techniques he described had first been utilized at the Mayo Clinic by his senior surgical colleague John W. Kirklin.

So by 1961, Edwards and his colleagues knew that it was high time that the pathologic anatomy and the clinical diagnosis of DORV be described and clarified, which is precisely what they did.[1, 2] In describing the largest series of cases of DORV reported up to that time, Neufeld et al[1, 2] used the somewhat longer diagnostic term *origin of both great vessels from the right ventricle.*

These two studies were of considerable importance because **Edwards and his colleagues took DORV out of the category of TGA**. From then on, DORV was diagnosed and treated as such. What Edwards and his colleagues did for DORV[1, 2] then made it possible for *double-outlet left ventricle (DOLV)*[9, 10], and *anatomically corrected malposition of the great arteries (ACM)*[11, 12] also to be diagnosed and treated specifically. Moreover, *TGA1*[3] became a specific, discrete anomaly – not a whole category of many different malformations — that could be diagnosed and treated specifically.

Thus Edwards and his colleagues[1, 2] in 1961 led the advance that resulted in the modern specific diagnosis of the various different anatomic types of abnormally related great arteries: TGA, DORV, DOLV, and ACM, etc. Since the classical pioneering studies of Neufeld and colleagues,[1, 2] much has been learned concerning the various anatomic types of DORV.[14]

What of the future? Although a reluctant prophet, I would suggest the following:

(1) Normally related great arteries are characterized by completely asymmetrical (opposite) right-left development of the subarterial conal free walls.[15, 16]

(2) Abnormally related great arteries of all anatomic types are characterized by anomalies of complete right-left asymmetry in the development of the subarterial conal free walls.[15, 16]

(3) "Mother nature" normally does an embryonic aortic switch procedure by 35 to 44 days of age in utero.[15, 16]

(4) There is only one way to do the developmental aortic switch right: complete resorption of the right-sided subaortic conal free wall (permitting aortic-mitral fibrous continuity), and left-sided subpulmonary conal free wall growth and expansion (elevating the pulmonary valve superiorly, away from the interventricular foramen [IVF], permitting the aortic valve to pass mostly through the IVF to override the left ventricle).[15, 16]

(5) There are many ways of doing the embryonic aortic switch wrong, resulting in abnormally related great arteries. In typical DORV, for example, both subarterial conal free walls grow and expand, preventing semilunar – mitral fibrous continuity, with both great arteries remaining above the right ventricle.[15, 16]

(6) Abnormally related great arteries appear to have a molecular genetic etiology. Mutations in the highly conserved Nodal gene cascade[17] appear to be very important in the causation of anomalies of right-left asymmetry in man. Clarification of the genetic etiology of conal (not conotruncal) malformations such as DORV is one of the most important challenges facing our field in the 21st century.

References

1.) Neufeld HN, DuShane JW, Wood EH, Kirklin JW, Edwards JE: Origin of both great vessels from the right ventricle: I. Without pulmonary stenosis. Circulation 1961; 23: 399.

2.) Neufeld HN, DuShane JW, Edwards JE: Origin of both great vessels from the right ventricle: II. With pulmonary stenosis. Circulation 1961; 23: 603.

3.) Abbott ME: Transposition or reversed torsion of the arterial trunks. *In*, Modern Medicine, Osler & McCrae (eds), Philadelphia, Lea and Febiger Co 1927; 4: 716.

4.) Braun K, de Vries A, Feingold DS, Ehrenfeld NE, Feldman J, Schorr S: Complete dextroposition of the aorta, pulmonary stenosis, interventricular septal defect, and patent foramen ovale. Am Heart J 1952; 43: 773.

5.) Witham AC: Double outlet right ventricle, a partial transposition complex. Am Heart J 1957; 53: 928.

6.) Beuren A: Differential diagnosis of the Taussig-Bing heart from complete transposition of the great vessels with a posteriorly overriding pulmonary artery. Circulation 1960; 21: 1071.

7.) Taussig HB, Bing RJ: Complete transposition of the aorta and a levoposition of the pulmonary artery. Am Heart J 1949; 37: 551.

8.) McGoon DC: Origin of both great vessels from the right ventricle. Surg Clin N America 1961; 41: 1113.

9.) Sakakibara S, Takao A, Arai T, Hashimoto A, Nogi M: Both great vessels arising from the left ventricle (double outlet left ventricle) (origin of both great vessels from the left ventricle). Bull Heart Inst Japan, 1967, p 66.

10.) Paul MH, Sinha SN, Muster AJ, Cole RB, Van Praagh R: Double outlet left ventricle. Report of an autopsy case with an intact ventricular septum and consideration of its developmental implications. Circulation 1970; 41: 129.

11.) Harris JS, Farber S: Transposition of the great cardiac vessels, with special reference to the phylogenetic theory of Spitzer. Arch Path 1939; 28: 427.

12.) Van Praagh R, Durnin RE, Jockin H, Wagner HR, Korns M, Garabedian H, Ando M, Calder AL: Anatomically corrected malposition of the great arteries {S, D, L}. Circulation 1975; 51: 20.

Coronary Arterial Patterns in Transposition Complexes

Anatomic and Angiocardiographic Studies*

LARRY P. ELLIOTT, M.D., KURT AMPLATZ, M.D. *and* JESSE E. EDWARDS, M.D.

Minneapolis and St. Paul, Minnesota

ANATOMIC studies indicate that for each of the major transposition complexes there is a tendency for association of a particular pattern of coronary arterial origin and branching. On this basis, the pattern of the coronary arteries may yield helpful points when a transposition complex is analyzed angiocardiographically.

The purposes of this report are twofold: (1) to bring together published and unpublished anatomic observations from our institutions on the coronary arterial patterns in 115 specimens, each exhibiting one of the four common transposition complexes, including (a) origin of both great vessels from the right ventricle, (b) complete transposition, (c) corrected transposition, and (d) common ventricle with transposition; and (2) to correlate the coronary arterial patterns with the type of transposition as seen in angiocardiograms in 17 available cases.

The study was divided into anatomic and angiocardiographic aspects. For the anatomic part of the study 115 pathologic specimens of heart, each having one of the transposition complexes concerned, were examined for the type of transposition and the patterns of origin and distribution of the coronary arteries.

The 115 specimens were obtained from 14 cases of origin of both great vessels from the right ventricle, 60 cases of complete transposition,† 15 cases of corrected transposition and 26 cases of common cardiac ventricle with transposition.

† The anatomic details of coronary arterial patterns in these cases were described earlier.[1]

For the angiocardiographic part of this study, each of the four transposition complexes considered was represented among the 17 cases available. In 4 of these (3 of origin of both great vessels from the right ventricle; 1 of complete transposition) necropsy specimens were also available. The 13 remaining patients were living at the time of this study. In each, the type of transposition was identified by selective angiocardiography, and in 7 of these there was further confirmation by surgical observation.

AORTIC VALVE AND CORONARY ARTERIES IN THE NORMAL SUBJECT

Each of the transposition complexes studied will be defined when considered. First, it seems appropriate to summarize, as a basis for reference, the essential features of origin and distribution of the coronary arteries in the normal subject.

Of the three aortic cusps, one is oriented posteriorly (termed the posterior or noncoronary cusp) and two are oriented anteriorly. One of the latter two is oriented toward the right and called the right aortic cusp; the other is oriented toward the left and called the left aortic cusp. Between each cusp and the corresponding part of the aortic wall is a specialized part of the aortic lumen termed a sinus of Valsalva or an aortic sinus. The sinuses are named to correspond with the cusps to which they are related.

The plane of the aortic valve is oblique, the right side being lower than the left and the posterior aspect slightly lower than the anterior (Fig. 1). In the frontal projection of the

* From the Departments of Radiology and Pathology, University of Minnesota, Minneapolis, Minn., and the Department of Pathology, The Charles T. Miller Hospital, St. Paul, Minn.

This study was supported by Research Grant HE-5694 and Training Grant 5 T1 HE-5570 of the National Heart Institute, National Institutes of Health, U. S. Public Health Service.

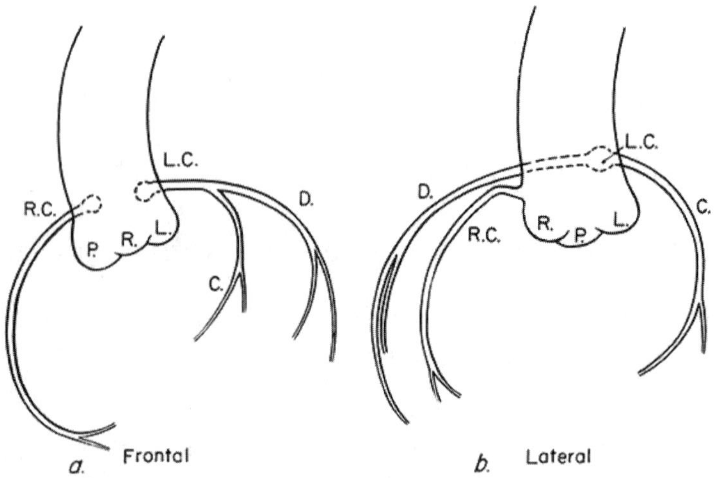

FIG. 1. *Diagrammatic representation of the essential features of origin and distribution of the coronary arteries in the normal.* a and b, frontal and lateral views, respectively. R.C. = right coronary artery; L.C. = left coronary artery; D. = anterior descending coronary artery; C. = left circumflex coronary artery; P. = posterior aortic sinus; R. = right aortic sinus; and L. = left aortic sinus.

aortogram, the posterior and left aortic cusps are seen on their respective sides of the valve (Fig. 1). In some instances the right aortic cusp is seen *en face* between the posterior and left cusps. In the lateral projection, the right cusp is anterior, the left cusp is posterior and the posterior cusp lies midway between the right and left cusps. In this position the lower margin of the posterior cusp lies below the inferior margin of the other two cusps.

The right coronary artery arises above the right aortic sinus and enters the right atrioventricular sulcus where it runs laterally and then turns to reach the posterior surface of the heart (Fig. 1). The left coronary artery arises above the left aortic sinus and runs laterally and ventrally between the root of the pulmonary trunk and the left atrium (Fig. 1). After a short course it gives rise to its anterior descending and left circumflex branches. The anterior descending branch courses inferiorly in the anterior interventricular sulcus to the cardiac apex. The left circumflex branch courses in the left atrioventricular sulcus until it reaches the posterior surface of the heart.

Origin of Both Great Vessels from the Right Ventricle

Origin of both great vessels from the right ventricle, as the name implies, is characterized by both the aorta and pulmonary trunk arising from the right ventricle. The only outlet for the left ventricle is a ventricular septal defect. The condition has also been called *partial transposition* or *double outlet right ventricle.* Studies by Neufeld and associates[2] suggested the value of recognizing two subdivisions, depending on the position of the ventricular septal defect. These two subdivisions are as follows: *Type I.* The ventricular septal defect is below the crista supraventricularis (Fig. 2*a*). *Type II.* The ventricular septal defect is above the crista supraventricularis (Fig. 2*b*). This latter type is synonomous with the *Taussig-Bing complex.*

Certain anatomic similarities in all cases of origin of both great vessels from the right ventricle, regardless of subdivision, are as follows: (1) The pulmonary trunk and aorta show a near-normal relation externally; (2) the aorta arises entirely from the right ventricle lying to the right of the pulmonary trunk; (3) the semilunar valves lie in the same horizontal body plane; (4) the pulmonary trunk is in normal position, and (5) there is discontinuity of mitral and aortic valvular tissue.

Anatomic relation of aorta to pulmonary trunk

In 13 of the 14 cases of this condition available for anatomic study, one type of relation between the two great vessels was present. In these 13, from external examination, the aorta and pulmonary trunk occupied near-normal positions, and the pulmonary trunk, a normal position. The aorta, however, was situated slightly more anteriorly than normal and, at the base of the

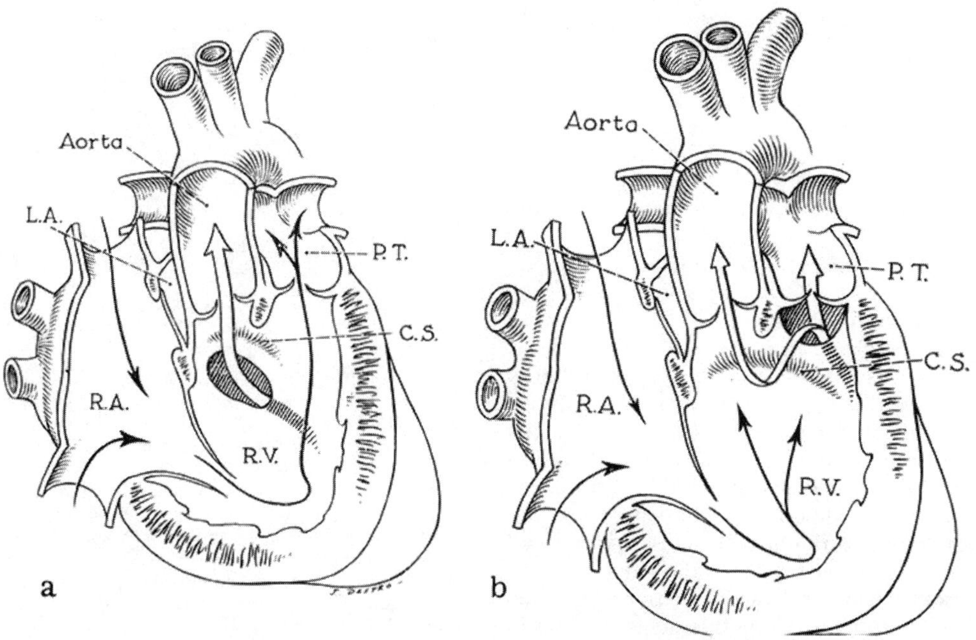

FIG. 2. *Diagrammatic representation of origin of both great vessels from the right ventricle.* (Reproduced with permission from Neufeld et al.[2]) *a, Type I.* The ventricular septal defect is below the crista supraventricularis (C.S.). *b, Type II* (Taussig-Bing complex). The specific anatomic feature is that the ventricular septal defect is above the crista supraventricularis.

heart, the aorta failed to curve posteriorly behind the pulmonary trunk. In the fourteenth case, the relation of the great vessels was atypical and resembled that of complete transposition. The ascending aorta lay anteriorly and to the right of the pulmonary trunk.

ANATOMY OF THE CORONARY ARTERIES

In 13 of the 14 cases, regardless of the position of the ventricular septal defect or the position of the two great vessels, the origin and the course of the two main coronary arteries were essentially identical to that in the normal heart. In

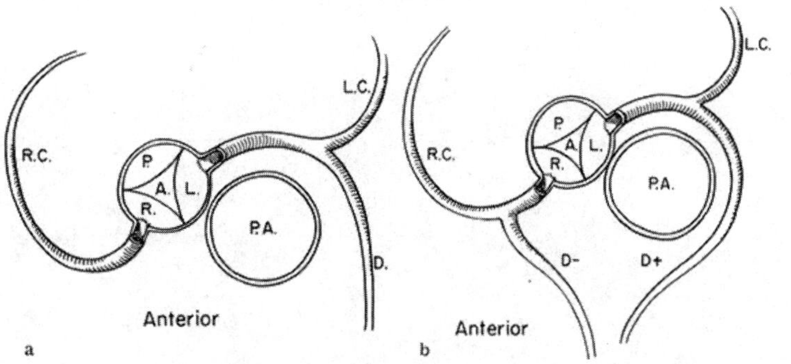

FIG. 3. *Patterns of origin and course of the coronary arteries in origin of both great vessels from the right ventricle. a, pattern occurring predominantly in both Types I and II.* The right coronary artery (R.C.) arises above the right aortic sinus (R.), and the left coronary artery arises above the left aortic sinus (L.). The posterior aortic sinus (P.) is the *noncoronary* sinus. This pattern is essentially identical to that of the normal heart. *b, one case; Type I.* In this pattern two anterior descending coronary arteries were present. The major one (D+) arose from the left coronary artery while the minor one (D−) arose from the right coronary artery.

the fourteenth case, the right coronary artery arose from the left coronary artery.

In each of the 14 cases, as in the normal, the posterior aortic sinus was the noncoronary one. In 13 cases, the left coronary artery arose above the left aortic sinus and the right coronary artery arose above the right aortic sinus (Fig. 3*a*). In 1 case, two anterior descending coronary arteries were present (Fig. 3*b*). One anterior descending coronary artery arose from the right coronary artery and the other arose from the left coronary artery.

In the fourteenth case, a large left coronary artery arose above the left aortic sinus, and shortly after its origin, it gave origin to an anomalously arising right coronary artery (Fig. 4). The left coronary artery then continued for a short distance before branching into the left circumflex and anterior descending coronary arteries. From above the right aortic sinus arose a small branch which coursed down the anterior interventricular sulcus as a minor anterior descending artery. Further details of this unusual case will be discussed with the angiocardiographic findings.

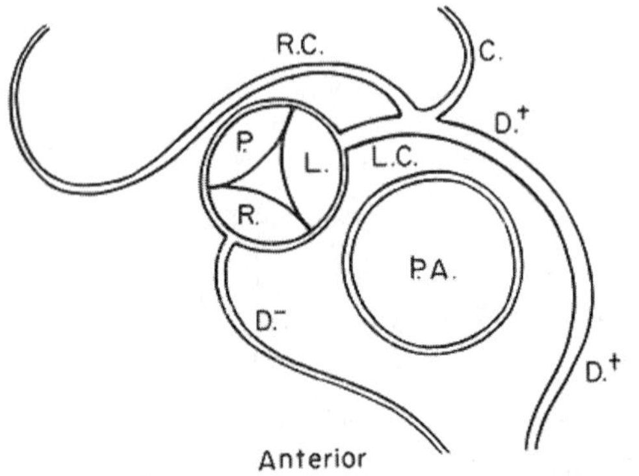

FIG. 4. *Atypical coronary arterial pattern in case of origin of both great vessels from the right ventricle.* The left coronary artery (L.C.) arises above the left aortic sinus. The right coronary artery (R.C.) is the first branch which courses posterior to the aorta and enters the right atrioventricular sulcus. The left coronary then gives rise to the left circumflex (C.) and the major anterior descending coronary arteries (D^+). Above the right aortic sinus (R.) arises a small minor anterior descending coronary artery (D-F), which enters the anterior interventricular sulcus along side of the major anterior descending coronary artery (D^+).

ANGIOCARDIOGRAPHIC OBSERVATIONS

Six cases were studied angiocardiographically: The coronary arteries were visualized in 5 by retrograde aortography and in 1 by selective right ventriculography. The first 5 cases are of the Type I variety and the latter of the Type II (Taussig-Bing) variety.

In the 5 cases studied by selective aortography and in a sixth case studied by right ventriculography, the aortic cusps lay in normal relation to each other. In 5 of these, the right coronary artery arose just above the right aortic sinus, its origin being clearly visible in the lateral projection (Fig. 5). (The sixth case, studied by aortography, is represented by the one with the anomalously arising right coronary artery and

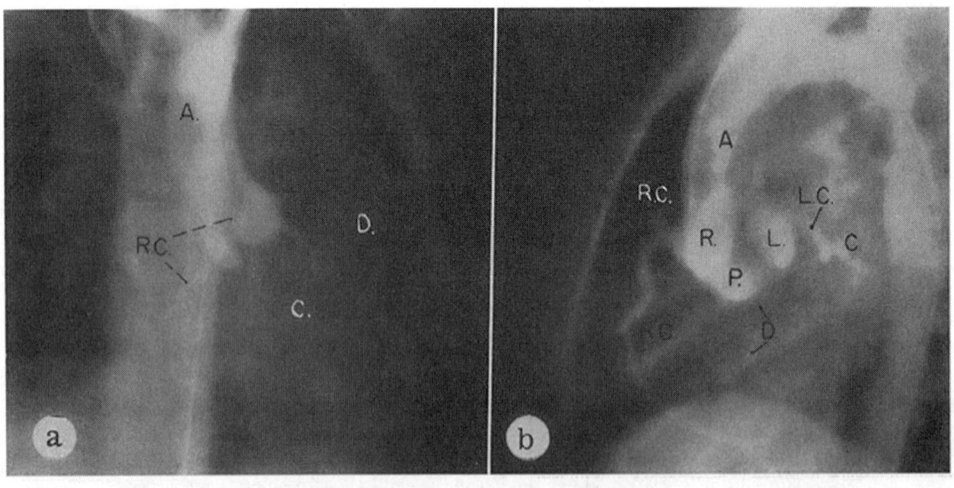

FIG. 5. *Selective thoracic aortogram in case of origin of both great vessels from the right ventricle* (*Type II*) confirmed by necropsy. *a, anterior view* showing the right coronary (R.C.) *en face* arising above the right aortic cusp. The left coronary (L.C.) arises normally and divides into the anterior descending (D.) and left circumflex (C.) branches. *b, lateral view* showing the right coronary arising normally above the right aortic cusp (R.). Its origin is seen in profile. L. = left cusp; P. = posterior cusp; and A. = ascending aorta.

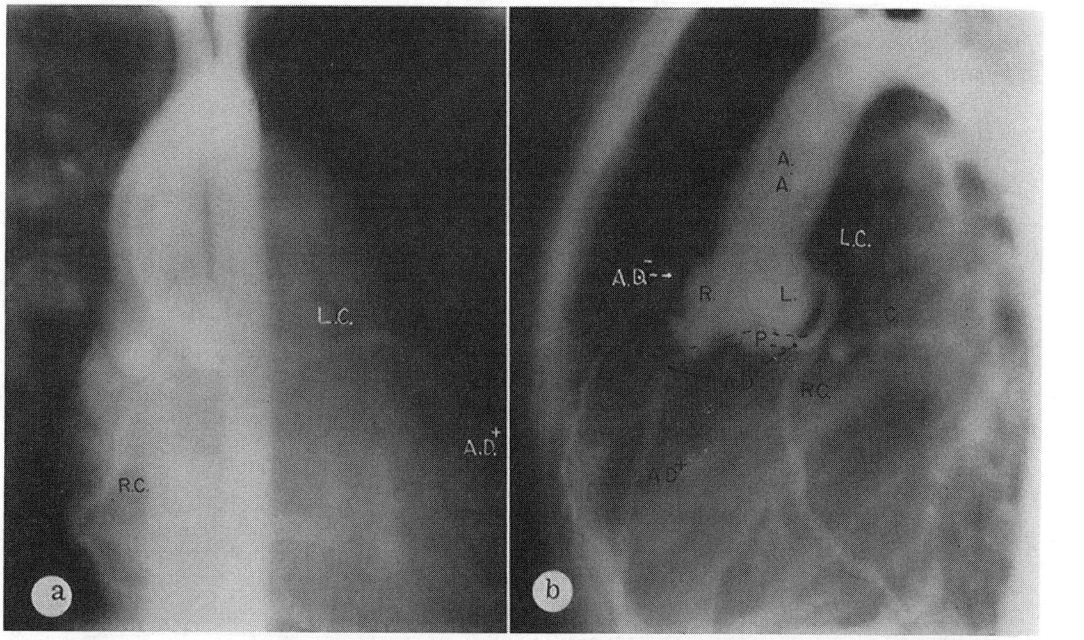

FIG. 6. *Atypical form of Type I origin of both great vessels from the right ventricle. Selective thoracic aortogram* of coronary arterial pattern studied pathologically and shown in Figure 4. Abbreviations same as in Figure 4. *a, frontal view and b, lateral view.* The left coronary artery (L.C.) arises normally above the left aortic sinus (L.). A large right coronary (R.C.) is the first branch of the left coronary artery. The right coronary artery continues posteriorly behind the aorta to course in the right atrioventricular sulcus. The left circumflex (C.) and major anterior descending (D+) coronary arteries are a continuation of the left coronary artery. A small minor anterior descending coronary artery (D−) arises above the right aortic sinus (R.).

will be discussed separately.) The right coronary artery assumed a normal concave shape in an upward and outward direction. The vessel was seen best in the lateral view (Fig. 5*b*). The right coronary artery continued in the atrioventricular sulcus to the posterior aspect of the heart. In 1 case the conus branch was prominent and well visualized in the lateral view.

In the normal heart the right coronary artery, when viewed in the lateral projection, lies between the two branches of the left coronary artery, the anterior descending branch lying anteriorly and the circumflex branch, posteriorly. In these 5 cases, an alteration from the normal was observed. In each case the right coronary artery was enlarged and lay anterior to the anterior descending branch (Fig. 5), an anatomic situation indicating hypertrophy of the right ventricle. In 1 case (previously described in the section dealing with pathologic description), two anterior descending coronary arteries were present. The larger anterior descending artery arose from the right coronary artery and was well visualized in the lateral view. The other anterior descending branch arose normally from the left coronary artery but was barely visible in the aortogram.

The left coronary artery in each case arose in a position identical to that in the normal heart and gave origin to its two main branches. In the lateral view, the site of origin was seen on end and formed a dense circular shadow situated above the left aortic cusp toward the left posterior aspect of the aortic root. In each case, the anterior descending coronary artery, when viewed in the lateral projection, lay posterior to the right coronary artery (Fig. 5*b*). As mentioned, this is different from the normal.

In the sixth case, in which aortography had been done, the left coronary artery arose above the left aortic sinus (Fig. 6). This artery was unusually wide and, in contrast to normal, its origin was seen in profile rather than on end (Fig. 6). Its initial portion coursed in a posterior direction and gave origin to a large right coronary artery which coursed inferiorly and posteriorly to the aorta to reach the right atrioventricular sulcus. Following origin of the right coronary artery, the left coronary artery gave rise to a wide anterior descending and normal-sized left circumflex artery. The anterior descending branch coursed anteriorly and laterally along the interventricular sulcus (Fig. 6*b*). From above the posterior aspect of the right aortic sinus, a small coronary artery arose. As a result, the site of origin was not seen in profile. This artery coursed along the anterior surface of the heart whereupon it joined the major anterior descending coronary artery at the apex of the heart.

Complete Transposition

In complete transposition of the great vessels there are two ventricles (although a defect may be present in the ventricular septum). The aorta, from which the coronary arteries arise, takes origin from the right ventricle, while the pulmonary trunk takes origin exclusively from the left ventricle (Fig. 7). Both atrioventricular valves are patent. The connections of the systemic, pulmonary and coronary veins are normal.

ANATOMIC RELATION OF AORTA AND PULMONARY TRUNK

The previously reported[1] anatomic details of the 60 cases of this condition identified three possible patterns of relation between the ascending aorta and pulmonary trunk as follows:

Type I (Oblique Relation; 39 Cases): In this type the aorta was situated obliquely with respect to the pulmonary trunk, and it was more anterior than the latter vessel. The left side of the ascending aorta lay anterior to the right side of the pulmonary trunk (Fig. 8*a*).

Type II (Side-to-Side Relation; 19 Cases): In this type the ascending aorta was situated to the right of the pulmonary trunk (Fig. 8*b*).

Type III (Anteroposterior Relation; 2 Cases): In this type the pulmonary trunk lay directly posteriorly to the aorta.

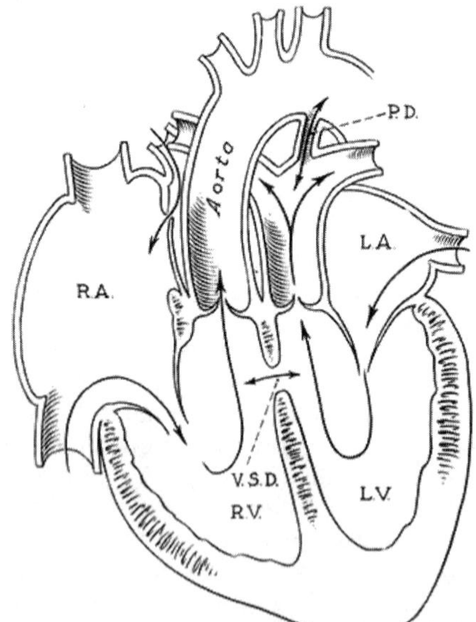

FIG. 7. *Diagrammatic representation of complete transposition of the great vessels.* The aorta arises exclusively from the right ventricle (R.V.) and the pulmonary trunk from the left ventricle (L.V.). Communications between the systemic and pulmonary circulations may exist as a patent ductus arteriosus (P.D.), patent foramen ovale and ventricular septal defect (V.S.D.). Both atrioventricular valves are patent. R.A. = right atrium and L.A. = left atrium.

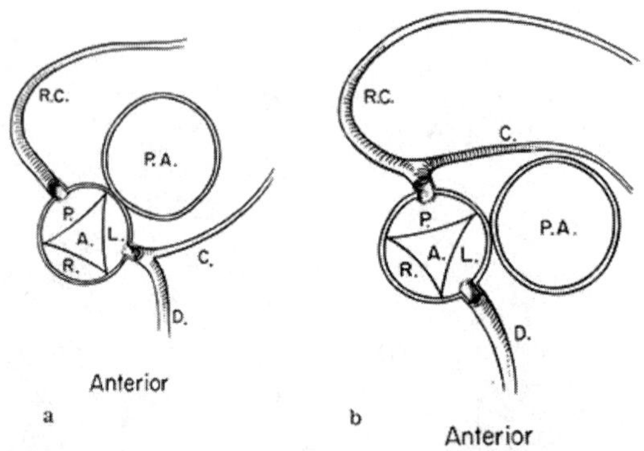

FIG. 8. *The two common patterns of origin and course of the coronary arteries in complete transposition of the great vessels.* (Reproduced with permission from Elliott et al.[1]) *a, pattern occurring predominantly in cases in which the relationship of the aorta and pulmonary artery is oblique.* In this pattern, the anterior descending coronary artery (D.) and the left circumflex coronary artery (C.) arise from the left coronary artery which, in turn, arises above the left aortic sinus (L.). The right coronary artery (R.C.) arises above the posterior (P.) sinus. No coronary artery arises above the right aortic sinus (R.). A. = aorta; P.A. = pulmonary trunk. *b, prevalent coronary arterial pattern in cases in which the relation of the aorta and pulmonary artery is side-to-side.* A vessel that arises above the posterior aortic sinus (P.) divides into the circumflex coronary artery (C.) and the right coronary artery (R.C.). The anterior descending coronary artery arises independently above the left aortic sinus (L.).

ANATOMY OF THE CORONARY ARTERIES

In all but 1 of the 60 cases reviewed the right aortic sinus was the noncoronary one. In 59 of the 60 cases the right coronary artery arose above the *posterior* aortic sinus. In each case the left coronary artery arose above the left aortic sinus. Among the 60 cases two major coronary arterial patterns were observed.

The first and most common arterial pattern was seen in 40 of the 60 cases and tended to be associated with an oblique relation of the great

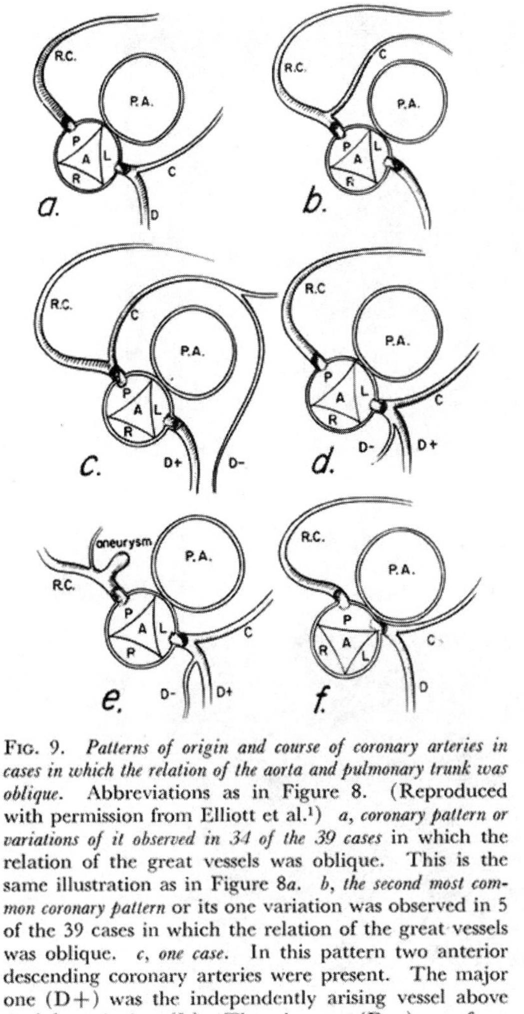

FIG. 9. *Patterns of origin and course of coronary arteries in cases in which the relation of the aorta and pulmonary trunk was oblique.* Abbreviations as in Figure 8. (Reproduced with permission from Elliott et al.[1]) *a, coronary pattern or variations of it observed in 34 of the 39 cases* in which the relation of the great vessels was oblique. This is the same illustration as in Figure 8*a*. *b, the second most common coronary pattern* or its one variation was observed in 5 of the 39 cases in which the relation of the great vessels was oblique. *c, one case.* In this pattern two anterior descending coronary arteries were present. The major one (D+) was the independently arising vessel above the left aortic sinus (L). The minor one (D−) arose from the left circumflex coronary artery (C). *d, 2 cases.* A variation of the prevailing coronary pattern observed in 1 case. Shortly after its origin from the left coronary artery the anterior vessel bifurcated (D+, D−). *e, 1 case.* Two anterior descending coronary arteries are present and there is an aneurysmal dilatation of the right coronary artery. *f, 1 case.* Both coronary arteries arose above the same (posterior) aortic sinus.

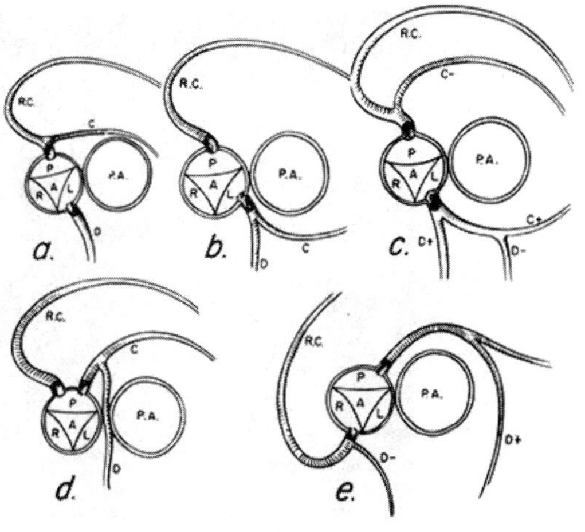

FIG. 10. *Coronary arterial patterns in 19 cases in which the relation of the great vessels was side-to-side.* Abbreviations same as in Figure 8. (Reproduced with permission from Elliott et al.[1]) *a, this coronary arterial pattern or modifications of it were observed in 13 of 19 cases.* The circumflex branch arises from the right coronary artery. *b, 4 cases.* Coronary arterial pattern similar to the prevailing pattern in cases in which the relation of the great vessels was oblique. *c, 2 cases.* A coronary arterial pattern considered a variation of that shown in *a*. Two circumflex arteries (C+ and C−) are present. One (C−) arises from the right coronary artery (R.C.) and the other (C+) arises from the left coronary artery. In addition, two anterior descending coronary arteries (D+ and D−) are present. *d, 1 case.* Both coronary arteries arise above the posterior aortic sinus (P). The anterior descending coronary artery (D) passes between the aorta and the pulmonary trunk to reach the anterior interventricular sulcus. *e, 1 case.* The right coronary artery (R.C.) arises above the right anterior aortic sinus (R). The left coronary artery arises above the right anterior aortic sinus (R). The left coronary artery arises above the posterior aortic sinus (P) and gives rise to the circumflex coronary artery and the anterior descending branch (D+). A minor descending coronary artery (D−) arises from the right coronary artery.

vessels. The left coronary artery gave rise to the anterior descending branch and the left circumflex branch (Fig. 8*a*). In contrast to the normal the stem of the left coronary artery passed anterior to the pulmonary trunk rather than posterior to it. Moreover, the right coronary artery arose above the posterior aortic sinus rather than the right and then entered the right atrioventricular sulcus, whereupon it followed a normal course.

The second and less common coronary arterial pattern was observed in 20 of the 60 cases and tended to be associated with a side-to-side relation of the great vessels. The anterior descending coronary artery arose above the left aortic sinus while the left circumflex coronary artery arose as a branch of the right coronary artery (Fig. 8*b*). The latter vessel, in turn, arose above the posterior aortic sinus.

Certain variations from the prevailing coronary arterial pattern were observed in 5 of the 39 cases with Type I (oblique) relation of the great vessels and in 4 of the 19 cases with Type II (side-to-side) relation of the great vessels. These variations are illustrated in Figures 9 and 10.

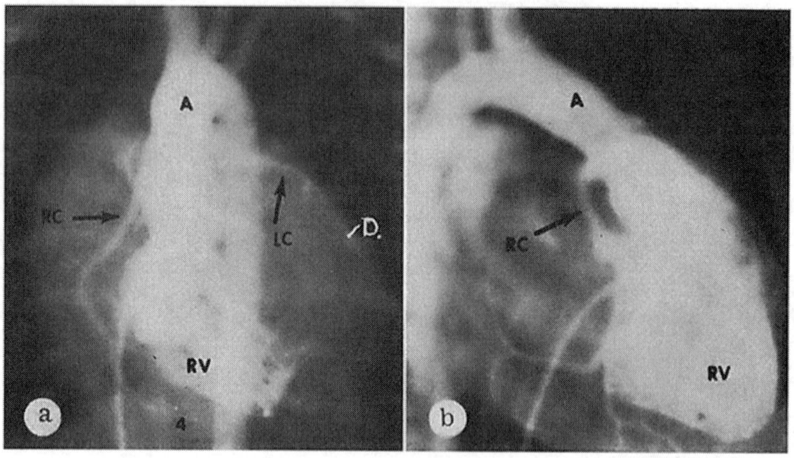

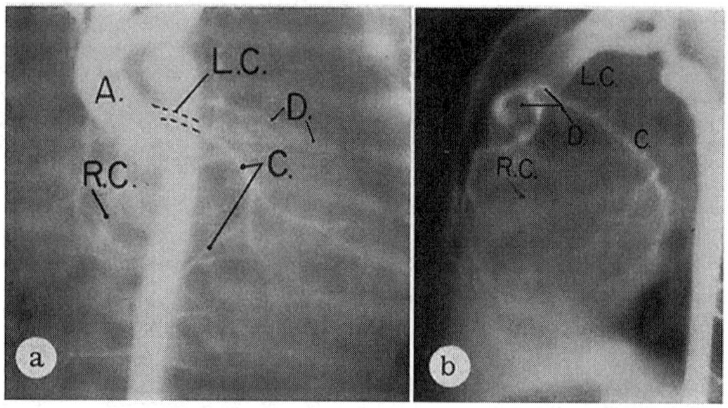

ANGIOCARDIOGRAPHIC OBSERVATIONS

The coronary arteries were visualized in 4 cases of complete transposition, 1 by aortography and 3 by selective right ventriculography. In 3 of these cases the relation between the two great vessels was of the "oblique" variety and of the anteroposterior variety in the fourth case.

In contrast to the normal situation, the right coronary artery arose in a rightward and posterior position above the posterior aortic sinus (Fig. 11 and 12). As seen in the lateral view following its rightward-posterior site of origin, the right coronary artery coursed either directly inferiorly to reach the atrioventricular sulcus (2 cases; Fig. 11*a*), or deviated in a slightly anterior direction before entering the atrioventricular sulcus (1 case, Fig. 12*b*).

In the one case in which selective aortography

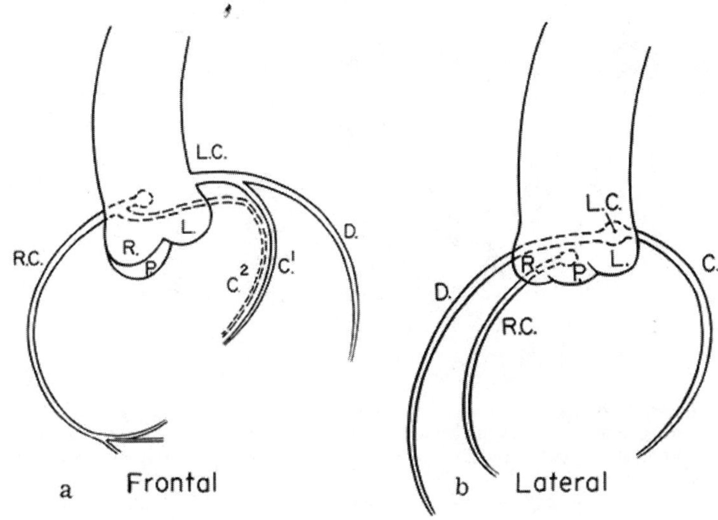

FIG. 13. *Diagrammatic representation of the typical coronary arterial pattern viewed angiocardiographically in complete transposition of the great vessels. a and b, frontal and lateral views, respectively.* The anticipated site of origin and course pursued by the left circumflex coronary artery ($C.^2$) as it arises from the right coronary artery (R.C.) is represented by broken lines in the frontal view. Abbreviations as in Figure 1.

was performed, the left coronary artery was seen to arise from the left lateral side of the aorta above the left aortic sinus (Fig. 12). It gave rise to a small, barely perceptible anterior descending branch and to the left circumflex branch (Fig. 12). In none of the 4 cases was the left circumflex branch seen to arise from the right coronary artery, a feature that was seen in several pathologic specimens. Figure 13 shows a schematic diagram of the origin and course of the coronary arteries in a typical case of complete transposition as might be seen in frontal and lateral angiocardiographic projections.

CORRECTED TRANSPOSITION

Corrected transposition is an established entity in which two ventricles and two atrioventricular valves are present, and except for associated anomalies (i.e., ventricular septal defect), the heart could function normally (Fig. 14*a*). In this condition the left-sided ventricle (i.e., the arterial ventricle) resembles a normal right ventricle and the right-sided ventricle, i.e., the venous ventricle, resembles a normal left ventricle (Fig. 14*a*). The aorta is situated at the left basal aspect of the heart and arises from the infundibulum of the left-sided arterial ventricle. The pulmonary trunk arises posteriorly and to the right of the transposed ascending aorta.

ANATOMIC RELATION BETWEEN AORTA AND PULMONARY TRUNK

Among the 15 specimens of heart with corrected transposition two types of relation between the aorta and pulmonary trunk were noted. In each, the ascending aorta arose from the left anterior basal aspect of the heart. In the first and more common type of relation (9 of 15 cases), the aorta was situated obliquely with respect to the pulmonary trunk. The aorta was anterior and to the left of the pulmonary trunk. The second relation (6 cases) showed the aortic origin directly anterior to the pulmonary trunk.

Of the three aortic cusps, one was oriented directly anteriorly (and will be termed the "anterior" aortic cusp, Fig. 14*b*) and two were oriented posteriorly. One of the latter two was oriented predominantly toward the right and called the right aortic cusp. The other was oriented toward the left and called the left aortic cusp. When the aortic cusps are viewed in the sagittal plane, the posteriorly lying right and left aortic sinuses are superimposed on one another. In the normal heart, the posteriorly lying aortic cusps do not overlie one another. In the normal subject, the posterior cusp, when viewed in the sagittal plane, lies midway between the "right" and "left" aortic cusps (Fig.

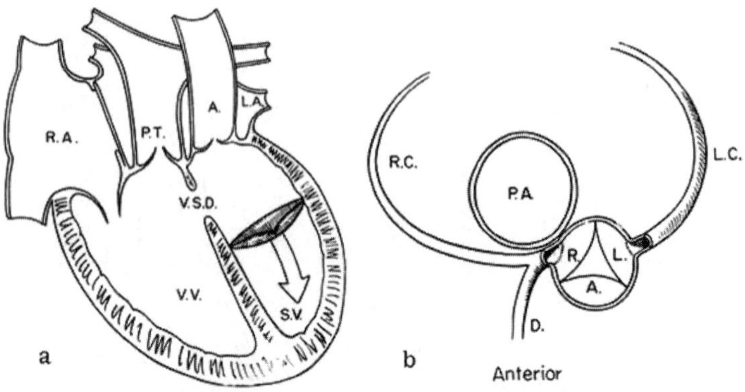

FIG. 14. *Corrected transposition. a, diagrammatic representation of the heart.* Two ventricles and two atrioventricular valves are present. The right-sided (venous) ventricle (V.V.) anatomically resembles a left ventricle and the left-sided (systemic) ventricle (S.V.) resembles a right ventricle. The aorta (A.) is situated at the left basal aspect of the heart and arises from the infundibulum of the left-sided (arterial) ventricle. The pulmonary trunk (P.T.) arises posteriorly and to the right from the right-sided (venous) ventricle. The right-sided atrioventricular valve is bicuspid and the left-sided atrioventricular valve is tricuspid. *b, patterns of origin and course of the coronary arteries.* The right coronary artery (R.C.) arises above the right aortic sinus (R.), gives rise to the anterior descending (D.) branch and then continues in the right atrioventricular sulcus. The left coronary artery (L.C.) arises independently above the left aortic sinus (L.). The anterior aortic sinus (A.) is the noncoronary one.

1*b*). It is important to realize, however, that the relations regarding the aortic cusps are never precise and may be altered in any patient owing to rotation of the heart.

In 14 of the 15 cases of corrected transposition the anterior aortic cusp was the noncoronary one (Fig. 14*b*), whereas in the fifteenth case, the right aortic cusp was noncoronary.

In each of the 15 cases, the right coronary artery arose in a right lateral-posterior position above the *right* aortic sinus and branched into the anterior descending branch (which coursed in the anterior interventricular sulcus) and a second vessel which proceeded into the right atrioventricular sulcus to the posterior aspect of the heart (Fig. 14*b*). In no instance did the right coronary artery show a normal origin as in cases of origin of both great vessels from the right ventricle.

The left coronary artery in each case arose above the left aortic sinus and proceeded into the left atrioventricular sulcus as the left circumflex artery, giving off a marginal branch and the posterior descending coronary artery (Fig. 14 *b*).

ANGIOCARDIOGRAPHIC OBSERVATIONS

The coronary arteries were studied by selective aortography in 3 cases. The plane of the aortic valve was less oblique than that of the normal aortic valve. In contrast to the normal, the plane of the aortic valve, as seen in the lateral view, showed the anterior aspect of the valve to be situated higher than the posterior aspect (Fig. 15). The anterior cusp was situated directly in front of the right and left aortic cusps (Figs. 15*c* and 16*a*). In the lateral projection, the right and left aortic cusps were superimposed over one another.

In each case the origin of the right coronary artery was abnormal. This artery arose above the right aortic sinus in a right-lateral position whereby its origin was seen in profile in the frontal view and *en face* as a dense circular shadow in the lateral view (Fig. 15, *a* and *b*). The normal concave shape of the right coronary artery shortly after its origin was absent.

A short distance from its origin the right coronary artery divided into two main branches. One was the *anterior descending branch*, which continued across the base of the heart in a left-inferior direction to descend in the anterior interventricular sulcus. In the lateral view the anterior descending artery was the most anterior branch (Fig. 15*c*). The second branch ran along the right atrioventricular sulcus.

The origin of the left coronary artery could be seen in profile in the lateral view (Fig. 15*b*). It arose as a single branch and spread laterally

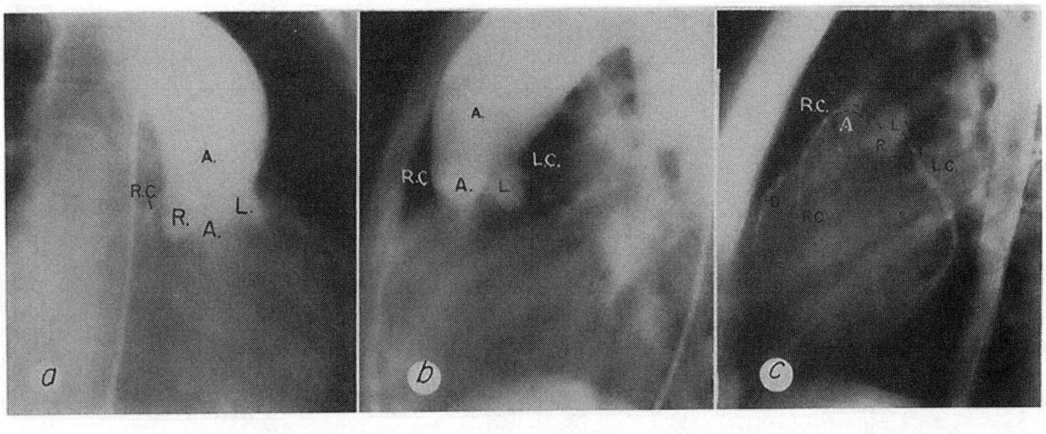

FIG. 15. *Selective aortogram in 2 cases of corrected transposition. a, frontal view, and b, lateral view in case with pulmonary stenosis. a,* the right coronary artery (R.C.) arises above the right aortic sinus and is seen in profile. *b,* the left coronary artery (L.C.) is shown arising in profile above the left aortic sinus. *c, lateral view in an additional case* shows the right coronary artery (R.C.) arising above the right aortic sinus (R.). It branches into the anterior descending branch (D) and then continues in the right atrioventricular sulcus to the posterior surface of the heart. The left coronary artery (L.) arises above the left aortic sinus and proceeds as the left circumflex (L.C.) artery.

first, then posteriorly and inferiorly to course along the left atrioventricular sulcus, whereupon it gave off the posterior descending coronary artery. Diagrammatic representation of the coronary arteries in corrected transposition, as seen in angiocardiograms, is shown in Figure 16.

COMMON CARDIAC VENTRICLE WITH TRANSPOSITION

In this condition there is one ventricular chamber into which both (when there are two) atrioventricular valves empty (Fig. 17). Lying anteriorly at the basal portion of the ventricle a subdivision of the common ventricle, the infundibular chamber, communicates with the main part of the ventricle. The pulmonary trunk arises from the common ventricular chamber, while the aorta arises in a transposed position from the infundibulum. The atrioventricular valves (when there are two) do not communicate with the infundibular chamber. The infundibulum located at the base of the heart lies in one of two positions. When the infundibulum is located at the right superior aspect of the base of the heart it is considered to be "non-inverted" (Fig. 17*a*). When the infundibulum is located at the left aspect of the base of the heart it is considered "inverted" (Fig. 17*b*). Thus, there are two major groups comprising the condition common cardiac ventricle.

In some cases of common ventricle there are two near-normal atrioventricular valves, while in others, there is significant malformation of these valves; the latter includes common atrioventricular valve and atresia of either the mitral or tricuspid valves. Specific anatomic details of the 26 cases of common ventricle studied herein were reported previously.[3]

ANATOMIC RELATIONSHIP OF AORTA AND PULMONARY TRUNK

Among the 26 cases of common ventricle used in this study the infundibulum was inverted in 13 and non-inverted in a like number. The relation between the aorta and the pulmonary trunk and the anatomy of the coronary arteries will be considered according to these two subdivisions.

Noninversion of Infundibulum: In the 13 cases of common ventricle with non-inversion, the transposed aorta arose from the infundibulum at the right-anterior aspect of the cardiac base. The sweep of the ascending aorta was convex toward the right (Fig. 17*a*).

The external relationship of the ascending aorta to the pulmonary trunk showed two main anatomic patterns. Of the 13 cases, eight showed a great vessel relationship similar to that of the Type I (oblique) pattern of the great vessels of complete transposition (Fig. 17*a*). In the remaining 5 cases the great vessel relation was similar to that of the Type III (anteroposterior) pattern of complete transposition.

Inversion of the Infundibulum: In these 13 cases the external relation of the ascending aorta to the pulmonary trunk was identical to that described for corrected transposition (Fig. 17*b*).

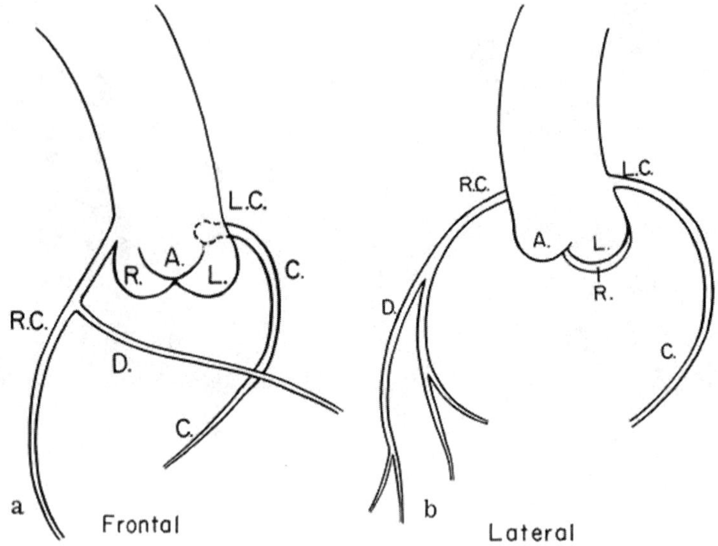

FIG. 16. *Diagrammatic representation of the typical coronary arterial pattern in corrected transposition* as seen in aortograms. *a*, frontal view. *b*, lateral view. Abbreviations as in Figure 14.

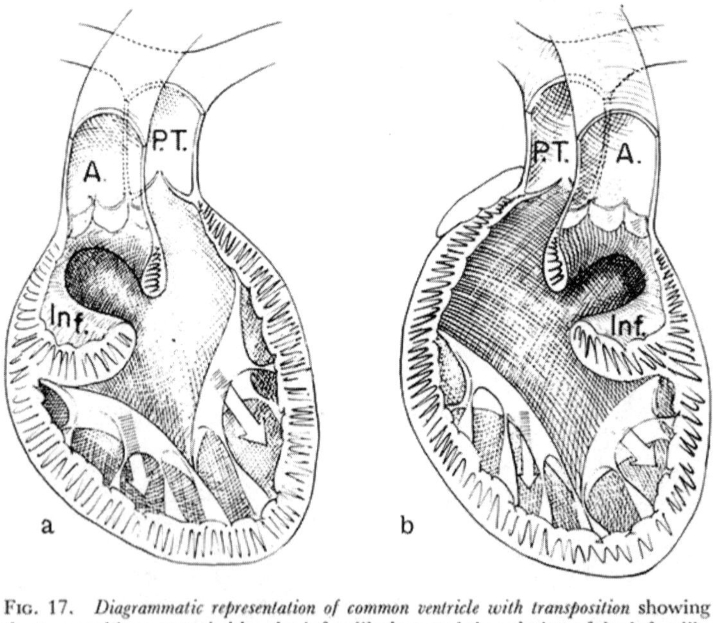

FIG. 17. *Diagrammatic representation of common ventricle with transposition* showing the two positions occupied by the infundibulum and the relation of the infundibulum to the common ventricle itself. (Reproduced with permission from Elliott et al.[3]). *a, the infundibulum* (inf.) *is located at the right side of the base of the heart* in the so-called "non-inverted" position. The transposed aorta arises from the infundibulum, and the pulmonary trunk (P.T.), which is posterior and to the left of the aorta (A.) arises from the main portion of the common ventricle. Both atrioventricular valves (when there are two) empty into the common ventricle. *b, the infundibular chamber* (inf.) *is located at the left side of the base of the heart* and is considered to occupy an "inverted" position. The transposed aorta arises from the infundibulum.

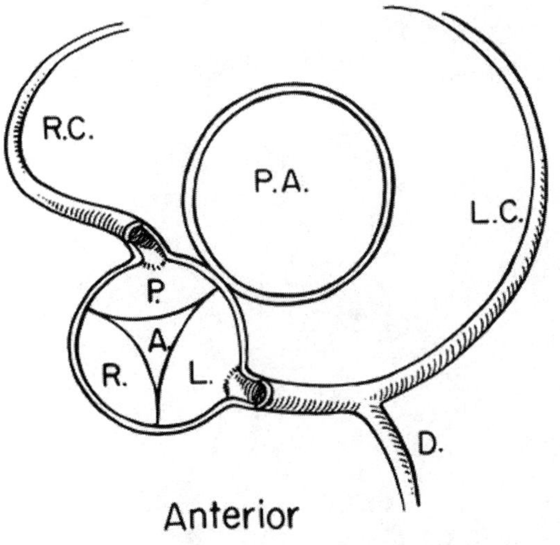

FIG. 18. *The patterns of origin and course of the coronary arteries in common ventricle with "noninversion" of the infundibulum.* The coronary pattern in this condition was essentially identical to that in complete transposition of the great vessels in which there is an oblique relation between the great vessels as shown in Figure 8*a*.

ANATOMY OF THE CORONARY ARTERIES

Noninversion of the Infundibulum: In these 13 cases the aortic sinuses were similar in position to that in complete transposition and the anatomic terms applying to the aortic sinuses will be the same.

In each case, the right aortic sinus was the noncoronary one. In these 13 cases the left coronary artery arose in a left anterior position above the left aortic sinus and gave rise to the anterior descending and the left circumflex branches (Fig. 18). As in complete transposition and in contrast to the normal pattern, the stem of the left coronary artery and the left circumflex coronary artery passed anterior to the pulmonary trunk rather than posterior to it. The right coronary artery in each case arose in a right posterior position and coursed in the right atrioventricular sulcus (Fig. 18).

Inversion of the Infundibulum: In these 13 cases, the position of the aortic sinuses was identical to that in corrected transposition (Fig. 19*a*). As a result, the same terminology which applies to the position of the aortic cusps in the latter condition will apply in this condition.

In each of the 13 cases the anterior aortic sinus was the noncoronary one. The coronary arterial pattern in nine was identical to that seen in common ventricle with noninversion of the infundibulum (Fig. 19*a*). In the remaining 4 the coronary arterial pattern differed from the foregoing with respect to the origin of the anterior descending coronary artery. In each this branch arose from the vessel that arose above the right aortic sinus (Fig. 19*b*) in a manner identical to that seen in corrected transposition. The artery arising above the left aortic sinus proceeded in the left atrioventricular sulcus simply as the left circumflex coronary artery (Fig. 19*b*).

ANGIOCARDIOGRAPHIC OBSERVATIONS

The coronary arteries were studied by selective aortography in 4 cases of common ventricle, one with noninversion of the infundibulum and in three cases with inversion of the infundibulum.

In the patient with noninversion of the infundibulum

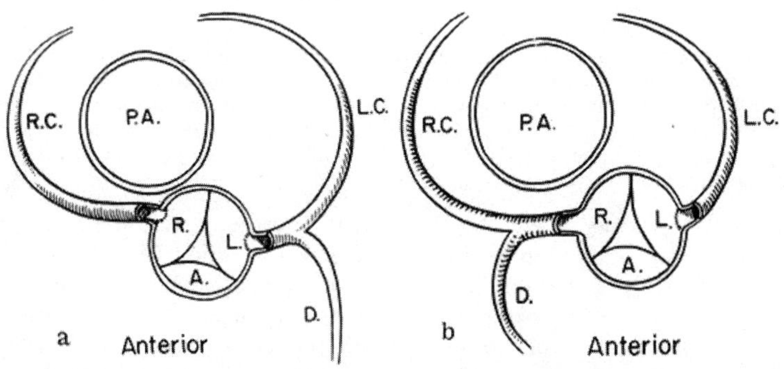

FIG. 19. *The two patterns of origin and course of the coronary arteries in common ventricle with "inversion" of the infundibulum. a, coronary arterial pattern in 9 of 13 cases.* The most important finding is that the anterior descending coronary artery (D.) arises from the left coronary artery. This anatomic feature, when present, distinguishes this condition from corrected transposition. *b, this coronary arterial pattern* was observed in 4 of 13 cases studied pathologically and is identical to that in corrected transposition.

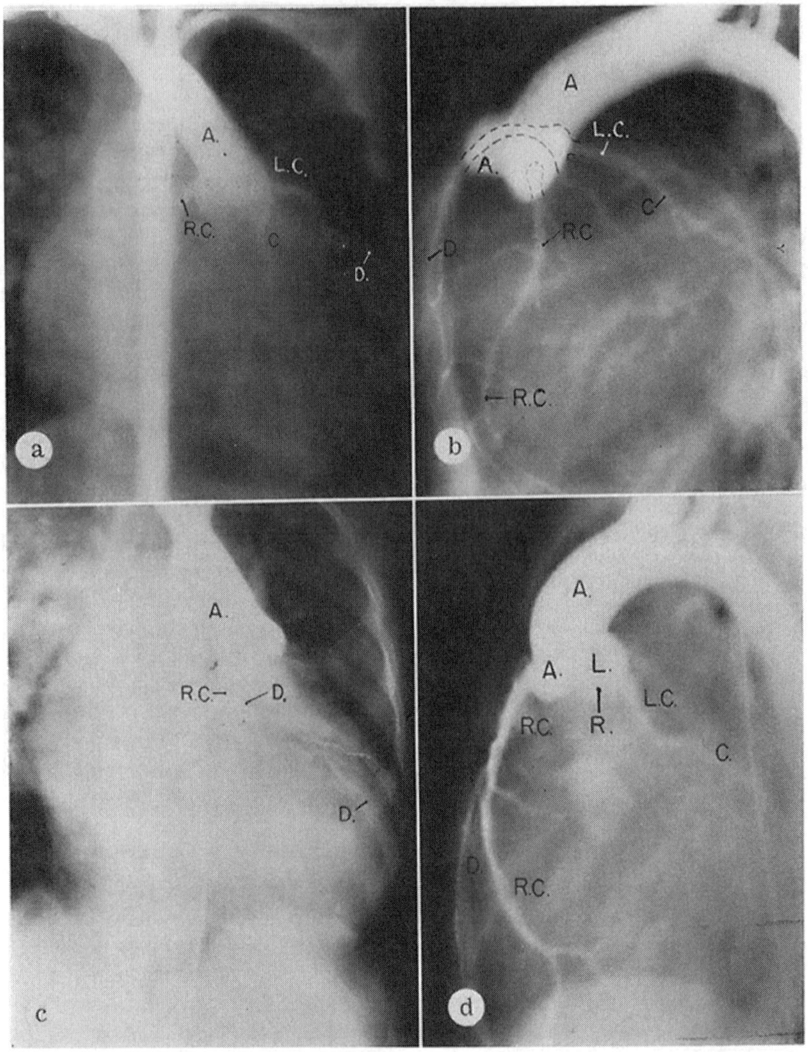

FIG. 20. *Selective aortogram in 2 cases of common ventricle with "inversion" of the infundibulum.* (Abbreviations as in Figure 14.) *a and b, frontal and lateral views, respectively,* showing typical pattern in common ventricle. The anterior descending coronary artery (D.) arises from the left coronary artery (L.C.). The right coronary artery (R.C.) arises above the right aortic sinus and courses along the right atrioventricular sulcus. *c and d, frontal and lateral views, respectively,* from a second case showing the atypical pattern for common ventricle. The anterior descending (D.) coronary artery arises as a branch of the right coronary artery (R.C.). The left coronary artery (L.C.) arises above the left aortic cusp (L.) and courses in the left atrioventricular sulcus as the left circumflex artery.

the left coronary artery arising above the left aortic sinus in a left anterior position gave rise to the anterior descending and left circumflex arteries. The second coronary artery arose above the posterior aortic sinus in a right posterior position and coursed as the right coronary artery. The right aortic sinus was the noncoronary one.

Three cases with inversion of the infundibulum were examined angiocardiographically. The position of the aortic sinuses and the tilt of the aortic valvular plane were identical to those of corrected transposition (Fig. 20 and 21).

The right aortic sinus gave rise to the right coronary artery in a right lateral position. The right laterally situated aortic cusp (right cusp) was superimposed over the left aortic cusp when viewed in the lateral projection (Fig. 20*b*). The left coronary artery arose above the left aortic sinus and gave rise to the anterior descending and left circumflex coronary arteries.

In the third case with infundibular inversion,

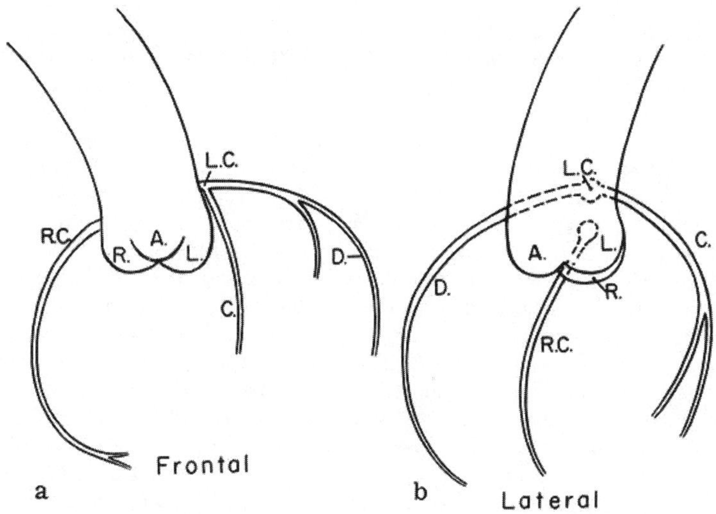

FIG. 21. *Diagrammatic representation* of the prevalent pattern of origin and course of the coronary arteries in common ventricle with "inversion" of the infundibulum as seen in aortograms. *a, frontal and b, lateral views, respectively.*

the coronary arterial pattern was identical to that in corrected transposition (Fig. 20, *c* and *d*). As mentioned in the section dealing with pathologic findings, this was an *uncommon* pattern.

COMMENT

The roentgenologist dealing with congenital cardiac disease is frequently confronted with cases in which there is some abnormal relation between the two great vessels (transposition). In the majority of cases correlation of the clinical, physiologic and angiocardiographic findings yields the correct diagnosis. In some instances, however, conditions characterized by some form of transposition are not readily accessible to precise anatomic diagnosis even after conventional studies have been performed. For example, in complete transposition the two great vessels may lie in a side-to-side (Type II) relation and differentiation from origin of both great vessels from the right ventricle of the Taussig-Bing variety may be difficult. Moreover, in the course of study of a given case with transposition determination of the presence of two functioning ventricles may be difficult. As a result, complete transposition or corrected transposition may be difficult to differentiate from common cardiac ventricle with transposition. The present study was concerned with determining whether or not precise angiocardiographic knowledge of the coronary arterial pattern in a given case of "transposition" could serve to differentiate one transposition complex from another.

The essential and important differential diagnostic features that may be gained from this study as to the relation of coronary arterial patterns to specific transposition complexes follows.

Origin and Course of the Right Coronary Artery: One of the essential pieces of information in differentiating origin of both great vessels from the right ventricle from all other transposition complexes depends upon a knowledge of the origin of the right coronary artery. In 13 of 14 cases of this condition studied pathologically or angiocardiographically, the right coronary artery arose in a normal position. This vessel originated just above the right aortic sinus, its site of origin being clearly visible in profile in the lateral view in aortograms (Fig. 5). Among the vast majority of other cases of transposition studied pathologically (99 of 101) and in each case studied angiocardiographically, the right coronary artery arose in an abnormal right-lateral or right-posterior position, depending on the type of transposition. As a result of this abnormal origin, the anteriorly situated aortic sinus became the noncoronary sinus and the site of origin of the right coronary artery in these latter conditions was not seen in profile in the lateral view. Therefore, when the roentgenologist is dealing with a case in which he suspects some form of transposition, angiocardiographic evidence that the right coronary artery arises in a normal position should rule out complete transposition, corrected transposition and common ventricle. Origin of both great vessels from the right ventricle should be favored.

Origin and Course of the Anterior Descending Coronary Artery: Knowledge of the site of origin of the anterior descending coronary artery is extremely valuable in differentiating between corrected transposition and common cardiac ventricle with inversion of the infundibulum since the external relation of the great vessels in these two conditions are identical.

In all cases of corrected transposition studied by us, both pathologically and angiocardiographically, the anterior descending coronary artery arose as a branch of the right coronary artery. On the other hand, in the majority of cases of common ventricle with inversion of the infundibulum, the anterior descending coronary artery arose from the left coronary artery. Therefore, when the roentgenologist is confronted with a case in which the arrangement of the great vessels is that seen in corrected transposition or common ventricle, the finding of the anterior descending coronary artery arising from the left coronary artery rules out corrected transposition and tends to favor common ventricle with inverted infundibulum. Moreover, it is important to realize that the anterior descending artery arises from the left coronary artery in the other forms of transposition also studied, including common ventricle with noninverted infundibulum.

Origin of Left Circumflex Coronary Artery: An important anatomic observation involving the left circumflex coronary artery in complete transposition was observed.

In specimens of 60 cases of complete transposition there were two basic patterns of origin and course of the coronary arteries. The pattern of coronary arterial origin, in which the left circumflex and anterior descending coronary arteries had a common stem, occurred most often when the two great vessels exhibited an oblique relation. A more important observation regarding differential diagnosis was the prevailing coronary arterial pattern when the two great vessels were side-to-side. In this situation the tendency was for the anterior descending to arise above the left aortic sinus as the sole vessel and the left circumflex to arise as a branch of the right coronary artery and to pass behind the pulmonary trunk. In no other transposition complex studied did this pattern occur. Thus, if the roentgenologist can demonstrate a single anterior descending coronary artery arising above the left aortic sinus and the left circumflex artery as a branch of the right coronary artery the diagnosis of complete transposition may be strongly suspected. The angiocardiographic demonstration, however, of the left circumflex arising from the right coronary artery in an infant with complete transposition may be difficult.

Origin of the Left Coronary Artery: In each of the 115 cases comprising the anatomic part of this study and in each case studied angiocardiographically, the left coronary artery arose above the left aortic sinus.

In 13 of 14 cases of origin of both great vessels from the right ventricle the origin and main trunk of the left coronary artery when viewed angiocardiographically in the lateral view showed this artery on end as a dense circular shadow originating from the upper portion of the left aortic sinus. As mentioned above, this is a normal pattern.

In contrast to the normal pattern just described in origin of both great vessels from the right ventricle, the left coronary artery in several cases of corrected transposition and common ventricle showed a somewhat different origin. Lateral views of aortograms in both these conditions not infrequently showed the origin and main trunk of the left coronary artery in profile as it arose just above the left aortic cusp. Whether this same relation exists angiocardiographically in complete transposition could not be determined from this study.

SUMMARY

The coronary arterial patterns were studied at necropsy in each of 115 cases with one of four transposition complexes as follows: (1) origin of both great vessels from the right ventricle (14 cases); (2) complete transposition of the great vessels (60 cases); (3) corrected transposition of the great vessels (15 cases); and (4) common ventricle with transposition of the great vessels (26 cases). These findings were correlated in 17 additional cases studied angiocardiographically. The important anatomic and angiocardiographic features were as follows:

The right coronary artery arose in a normal position in 13 of the 14 cases of origin of both great vessels from the right ventricle studied anatomically and angiocardiographically. Among the other three entities studied the right coronary artery arose in an abnormal right posterior or right lateral position.

The anterior descending coronary artery arose from the right coronary artery in each case of corrected transposition. In the majority of cases of common ventricle and in all cases of complete transposition and origin of both great vessels from the right ventricle, the anterior descending coronary artery arose as a branch of the left coronary artery.

The left circumflex coronary artery arose from the right coronary artery in one third of the cases of complete transposition. In no other form of transposition was this pattern observed.

The left coronary artery arose above the left aortic cusp in each condition studied. In common ventricle and corrected transposition, however, the left coronary artery arose in a more posterior position than in the other conditions.

It is concluded that the coronary arterial pattern in the transposition complexes is frequently specific for certain conditions. Angiocardiography may be a valuable aid in differentiating one form of transposition from another.

REFERENCES

1. ELLIOTT, L. P., NEUFELD, H. N., ANDERSON, R. C., ADAMS, P., JR. and EDWARDS, J. E. Complete transposition of the great vessels. I. An anatomic study of sixty cases. *Circulation*, 27: 1105, 1963.
2. NEUFELD, H. N. et al. Origin of both great vessels from the right ventricle without pulmonary stenosis. *Brit. Heart J.*, 24: 393, 1962.
3. ELLIOTT, L. P., ANDERSON, R. C. and EDWARDS, J. E. The common cardiac ventricle with transposition of the great vessels. *Brit. Heart J.*, 26: 289, 1964.

Coronary Arterial Patterns in Transposition Complexes. Anatomic and Angiocardiographic Studies.

Julien I. E. Hoffman, M.D.

When this article was written, it was often difficult by angiography of the ventricles and great arteries to differentiate between several transposition complexes: double outlet right ventricle, complete (d-) transposition of the great arteries, corrected (l-) transposition of the great arteries, and single ventricle with transposition. Jesse Edwards, working with two eminent radiologists, applied the study of cardiac pathology to provide details of coronary anatomy to help the diagnostic process.

Double outlet (N=14)

The concept of double outlet right ventricle has been extended since the article was written, and now encompasses a greater diversity of positions of the great arteries, ventricular septal defects and outlet septums than recognized at that time. Rather than normal relations of the aorta and main pulmonary artery that Elliott and co-workers described, side-by-side great arteries predominate, and both d-transposition and l-transposition of the aorta have been described. They were correct in stating that the coronary arteries usually originated normally from their appropriate sinuses, but did not have a large enough series to detect less common variations.

Complete transposition (N=60)

The authors were ahead of their time in defining transposition by the discordant ventriculo-arterial connections rather than by the anatomic positions of the great arteries. It took years before the dispute was settled in their favor. They correctly described the coronary arteries as arising from the facing sinuses (the two aortic sinuses adjacent to the main pulmonary artery), with the left coronary artery arising from the anterior aortic sinus and the right coronary artery from the posterior sinus. They observed that in about one-third of patients the left circumflex coronary artery arose from the right coronary artery, and in these the roots of the two great arteries were side-by-side rather than obliquely related. They described many variations among the peripheral branches. Those interested in arterial switch surgery have added some details, but the main findings remain unchanged.

Corrected transposition (N=15)

They described the non-coronary sinus as being usually anterior, with the right and left coronary arteries arising from the right and left posterior sinuses. In keeping with ventricular inversion, the coronary arteries were distributed to their appropriate ventricles. Consequently the right coronary artery supplied the left ventricle and the anterior descending coronary artery, whereas the left coronary artery gave rise to the posterior descending artery.

Single ventricle with transposition (N=26)

In 13 of these the infundibulum from which the aorta arose was not inverted, and in 13 it was inverted. In the former, the coronary pattern resembled that of a typical complete transposition, with the left coronary artery arising from the left anterior sinus and dividing into left circumflex and anterior descending branches. In the latter, the sinuses resembled those seen in corrected transposition. In 9 of 13 hearts the coronary arteries were like those in the non-inverted group, and the other four were like those in corrected transposition.

Although advances in imaging techniques have made differentiation between these complexes easier, for many years it was the contributions of the pathologist that facilitated diagnosis during life.

Congenital Cardiac Disease Associated with Polysplenia

A Developmental Complex of Bilateral "Left-Sidedness"

By JAMES H. MOLLER, M.D., AHMAD NAKIB, M.D., RAY C. ANDERSON, M.D., PH.D., AND JESSE E. EDWARDS, M.D.

SUMMARY

The well-recognized association of congenital cardiac disease with asplenia has been termed "bilateral right-sidedness" or dextro-isomerism, since the spleen is absent, the liver is symmetrical, and each lung has three lobes and an epiarterial bronchus. In a study of pathological material from 12 patients with congenital cardiac disease associated with multiple spleens (as contrasted to accessory spleen), we found a definite tendency for the symmetrical development of organs but with a tendency for bilateral left-sidedness or levo-isomerism.

The abnormalities assumed one of three forms as follows: (1) absence of a normal right-sided structure, (2) bilateral organs, each with the structure of a left-sided organ, or (3) excessive tissue of a left-sided organ. Thus, in polysplenia we observed a tendency for (1) absence of the hepatic segment of the inferior vena cava and absence of the gallbladder, (2) two lobes in each lung with hyparterial bronchi, and (3) multiple spleens. Other noncardiac abnormalities were partial or complete abdominal heterotaxia and partial malrotation of the bowel. The cardiac malformations included dextrocardia, bilateral superior venae cavae, anomalous pulmonary venous connection with malposition of the atrial septum, and defects in the atrial septum and in the ventricular septum.

Our study suggests that the developmental complex of multiple spleens is closely related to the asplenic syndrome, with the important difference being left-sided symmetry rather than right-sided symmetry.

Additional Indexing Words:

Vena cava | Multiple spleens | Atrial septal defect
Absent spleen | Pulmonary veins | Disorder of body symmetry

SPLENIC anomalies are commonly associated with anomalies of the cardiovascular system and of other organ systems. This phenomenon, as it relates to asplenia, is now commonly recognized.[1-3] In contrast, the association of anomalies with polysplenia has received less attention, and to our knowledge only 19 such cases have been reported.[4-14] It is the purpose of this report to describe our pathological observations in 12 cases in which congenital cardiovascular disease was associated with polysplenia.*

It is also our intention to contrast the anomalies associated with polysplenia, on the one hand, and those associated with asplenia, on the other. In each there is a tendency for "isomerism" or symmetry of body structure.

From the Departments of Pediatrics, Surgery, and Pathology, University of Minnesota, and the Department of Pathology, The Charles T. Miller Hospital, St. Paul, Minnesota.

This investigation was supported by U. S. Public Health Service Research Grant 5 R01 HE-05694 and Research Training Grant 5 T1 HE-5570, from the National Heart Institute.

*Cases 6 and 12 of present report have been previously described.[14, 15]

In asplenia there is a tendency for bilateral "right-sidedness," while in polysplenia there is a trend toward bilateral "left-sidedness." Features of the latter phenomenon include the tendency for the presence of two lobes in each lung, absence of the hepatic segment of the inferior vena cava, and absence of the gallbladder.

As used in this report the term "polysplenia" refers to the state in which the bulk of splenic tissue is divided into two and often more nearly equal-sized splenic masses. This is contrasted to accessory spleen, in which, in addition to a normal-sized spleen, one or more small spleens are present.

From our 12 necropsied cases of polysplenia associated with congenital cardiac disease, it became apparent that when polysplenia is present in association with congenital cardiovascular malformations, the latter tend to be predictable in nature, and the extracardiac organs exhibit characteristic structure.

We shall describe the essential cardiac and visceral malformations observed in our cases of polysplenia according to three subjects as follows: (1) abnormalities of situs, (2) cardiovascular malformations, and (3) noncardiovascular malformations or variations. Where pertinent, comparison will be made with published accounts on polysplenia.

Observations

Among the 12 patients with polysplenia, six were males and six females. The youngest patient died on the day of birth and the oldest patient when 10 years old. Only four of the 12 patients survived the first year of life.

Abnormalities of Situs

Among the 12 cases, abnormalities of the situs of the heart and abdominal organs were frequently observed. Therefore, we divided the cases into three groups according to the relationships of cardiac structures and the position of the major portion of the liver and of the stomach. Certain arbitrary decisions were made in classifying the cases into one of these groups, since partial malrotation of the bowel and hepatic abnormalities were revealed in a number of cases.

The liver tended to be symmetrical but one lobe usually was somewhat larger than the other. For example, in situs solitus under normal conditions the left lobe is distinctly smaller than the right and displays a sharp lower edge. In the cases of polysplenia the lobe which would be anticipated as the smaller tended to be the smaller one, but the difference in size between the two lobes was less distinct than under normal conditions. Also, the lower edge of the smaller lobe was somewhat rounded.

Although the degree of malrotation of the bowel was variable, the relationship between the cardiac structures and the major lobe of the liver was easily determined. Therefore, the following system of classification based principally on the cardiac, hepatic, and gastric positions appeared the easiest to follow.

If the arterial atrium and stomach were on the left side and the venous atrium and the major lobe of the liver were on the right side, *situs solitus* was considered to be present (fig. 1*a*). In *situs inversus*, the arterial atrium and stomach were on the right side, while the venous atrium lay on the left side, as did the major lobe of the liver (fig. 1*b*). In both situs solitus and situs inversus the cardiac apex is generally located on the side opposite the major lobe of the liver, but deviations from this occur. The position of the cardiac apex, however, was of itself not considered in designating the situs of the organs in a given case. Furthermore, these states are considered *concordant* since the relative positions of the heart, liver, and stomach are either normal or the mirror-image of normal. If there were deviations from the relationships basic to determination of situs, the cases were considered to display *discordant* relationships of the organs and the term *mixed situs* was applied. Mixed situs was represented in our cases by certain characteristics. In one the major lobe of the liver and arterial atrium were located on the same side (fig. 1*c*). Another pattern designated as mixed situs was that in which the major lobe of the liver and the stomach were on the same side (fig. 1*d*).

Situs solitus was present in four cases, of

which one revealed dextroversion (right-sided apex) without ventricular inversion (fig. 1*a*, insert). In five other cases situs inversus was present, and in one of these levoversion (left-sided apex) without ventricular inversion (other than that of situs inversus) was present (fig. 1*b*, insert). Three cases were classified as displaying mixed situs and demonstrated two types of discordance between the organs. In two of the cases of mixed situs, the liver and stomach were located as in situs inversus, but the heart was of the situs solitus variety (fig. 1*c*). Both of the cases were associated with continuity of the inferior vena cava with the azygos venous system. The third case displaying mixed situs was basically of situs solitus configuration, but the stomach was located on the right side (fig. 1*d*).

In seven of the 12 cases of polysplenia the cardiac apex was on the left side and in five the apex was on the right side.

Information regarding the relationships and attachments of the mesentery of the small bowel and colon was available in 10 of the 12 cases. Among six of the 10 cases an abnormal mesenteric attachment was observed. The abnormalities varied from the cecum not being retroperitoneal in position to complete malrotation of the bowel. In the latter instances the cecum and ascending colon had mesenteric attachments which permitted considerable mobility of the bowel. In two instances, the malrotation became complicated by intestinal obstruction which required operative relief.

Cardiovascular Malformations

The most consistently occurring malformations of the cardiovascular system involved the pulmonary veins, the venae cavae, and the atrial septum (table 1). Ventricular septal defect, either isolated or as a part of persistent common atrioventricular canal, also was common, as it occurred in nine cases.

Systemic Veins

Abnormalities of the systemic venous system were frequent. In seven of the 12 cases, the hepatic portion of the inferior vena cava was absent, and the abdominal inferior vena cava was continuous with the azygos venous system (so-called interruption of the inferior vena cava). In six of these the inferior vena cava joined the azygos vein while in the seventh case, the hemiazygos vein received the inferior vena cava. In each case the azygos or hemiazygos vein joined the homolateral superior vena cava.

Bilateral superior venae cavae were present in six of the 12 cases, four being cases with interruption of the inferior vena cava, and one of these was the case in which the inferior vena cava joined the hemiazygos vein. In four of these six cases the bilateral superior venae cavae were associated with the developmental complex described by Raghib and co-workers,[16] in which (1) the coronary sinus is absent, (2) each superior vena cava joins its homolateral atrium directly, and (3) an atrial septal defect is present. Connection of the persistent superior vena cava to the left atrium with an intact atrial septum was present in the fifth case. In the remaining case of bilateral superior venae cavae, the persistent left superior vena cava connected with the coronary sinus.

Pulmonary Veins

In 10 of the 12 cases, anomalous pulmonary venous connection existed, six being of the partial variety and four of the total. In each case the anomalous pulmonary venous connection was to the venous atrium. In no case was there anomalous pulmonary venous connection to a systemic vein.

Among the six cases of partial anomalous connection, the form of the anomalous connection was similar. The two pulmonary veins of the lung on the side of the venous atrium (left lung in situs inversus) joined the venous atrium directly (fig. 2). In these cases, the pulmonary veins appeared to connect in a normal location with the posterior atrial wall. The basis for the anomalous termination of pulmonary veins seemed to result from the malposition of the atrial septum toward the arterial atrium. This malposition has two effects: (1) that two pulmonary veins join the

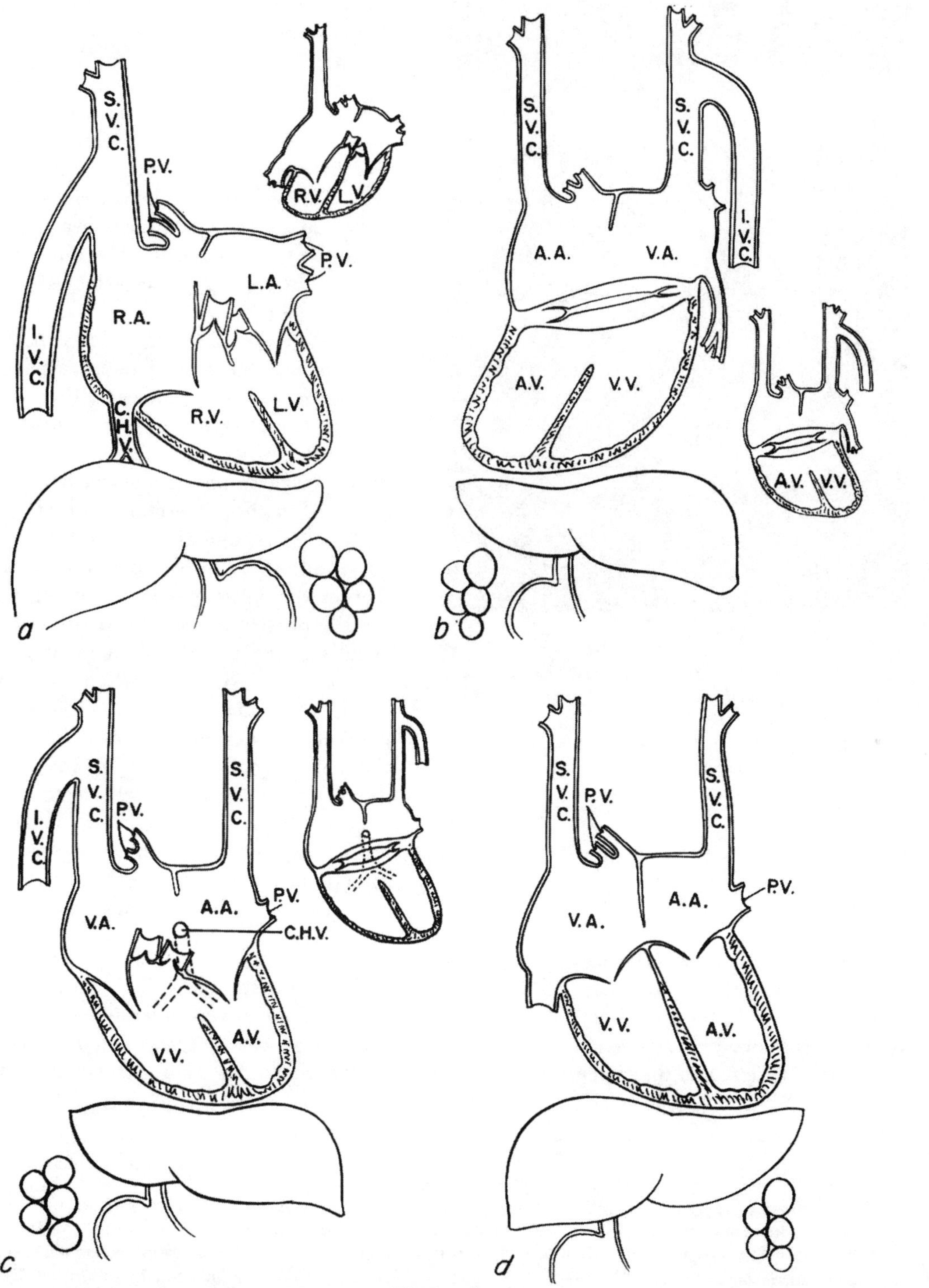

Figure 1

Diagrams of abnormalities of situs with polysplenia. Definition of abbreviations as follows: S.V.C. = superior vena cava; I.V.C. = inferior vena cava; C.H.V. = common hepatic vein; P.V.
(Continued on p. 793.)

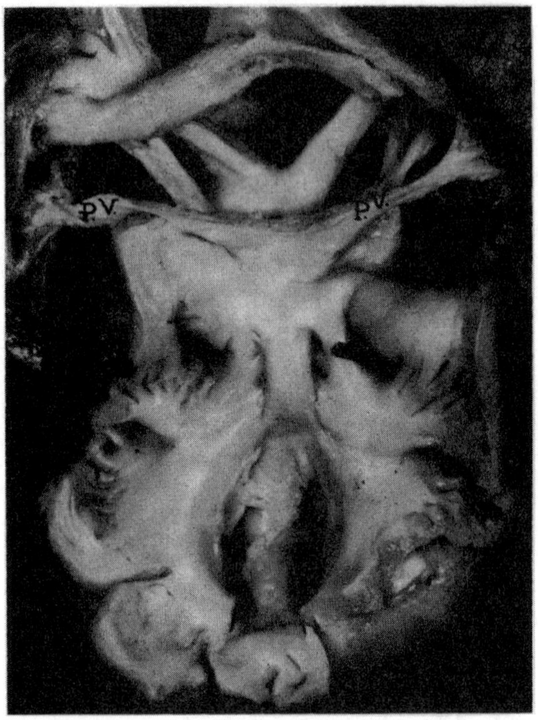

Figure 2

Case 11. Common atrium and persistent common atrioventricular canal from above. Partial anomalous pulmonary venous connection in which pulmonary veins (P.V.) join homolateral side of common atrium. Probes in superior venae cavae.

venous atrium, and (2) that the volume of the arterial atrium is compromised.

In three of the four cases of total anomalous pulmonary venous connection, the four individual pulmonary veins joined the venous atrium directly, and in each the atrial septum was significantly malpositioned toward the arterial atrium. In the fourth case, the pulmonary veins formed a confluence posterior to the venous atrium, and the confluence, in turn, connected with the venous atrium through a single ostium.

Atrial Septum

Several types of abnormalities were noted in the atrial septum. The first, as indicated, was the tendency of the atrial septum to be malpositioned toward the arterial atrium. Secondly, in several cases there was an absence of the fossa ovalis with the only interatrial opening appearing to be ostium II of septum primum (fig. 3).

In 10 of the 12 cases, defects in the atrial septum were present. Among seven of these the atrial septal defect was either in the region of the fossa ovalis or represented by an interatrial ostium II with absence of a fossa ovalis. In three of these seven there was also a defect in the lowermost part of the atrial septum (persistent interatrial ostium primum). In an additional three cases there was a defect in the latter portion, yielding six cases with a defect in the lowermost part of the atrial septum. In four of these six the defect was part of classical persistent common atrioventricular canal with its associated valvular clefts. In the other two cases in both of which the atrial septal defect was of the ostium primum type, no valvular clefts were associated. In one of the four cases with classical persistent common atrioventricular canal, the atrial septum was so rudimentary as to allow a designation of "single atrium."

Ventricular Septum

In nine of the 12 cases reviewed, the ventricular septum was defective. In five of these the defect was of the isolated variety, while in the remaining four the ventricular septal

= pulmonary vein; R.A. = right atrium; L.A. = left atrium; V.A. = venous atrium; A.A. = arterial atrium; R.V. = right ventricle; L.V. = left ventricle; A.V. = arterial ventricle; V.V. = venous ventricle. (a) Case 1. Situs solitus. Major lobe of liver and venous atrium on right; arterial atrium and stomach on left. (Insert) Case 3. Dextroversion of situs solitus heart without ventricular inversion. (b) Case 5. Situs inversus. Major lobe of liver and venous atrium (V.A.) on left; arterial atrium (A.A.) and stomach on right. (Insert) Case 7. Levoversion of situs inversus heart without ventricular inversion. (c) Case 10. Mixed situs. Venous atrium and stomach on right; arterial atrium and major lobe of liver on left. (Insert) Case 11. (d) Case 12. Mixed situs. Situs solitus heart. Stomach and liver in right side of abdomen.

Table 1

*Cardiovascular Malformations in Twelve Cases of Polysplenia Reported**

Case	Position of Cardiac Apex		Associated Cardiovascular Malformations						
	Right	Left	Atrial Sepal Defect	Anomal. Pul. Vein.	"Absent I.V.C."	Bilat. S.V.C.	Vent. Septal Defect	Complete A-V Canal	Other
Situs Solitus									
1		■	■	■	■		■		Double Outlet Rt. Ventricle
2		■	■	■		■	■		Complete Transposition
3	■		■	◩					Patent Ductus Arteriosus
4		■	■						Pulmonary Stenosis
Situs Inversus									
5	■		■	◩	■	■		■	Double Outlet Rt. Ventricle
6	■		■	◩	■		■		Patent Ductus Arteriosus
7		■	■	■	■			■	Patent Ductus Arteriosus
8	■			■	■	■		■	Patent Ductus Arteriosus
9	■				■		■		None
Mixed Situs									
10		■	■	◩	■	■	■		Double Outlet Rt. Ventricle
11		■	■	◩	■	■		■	Subaortic Steno. Pat. Duct. Art.
12		■	■	◩		■			Subaortic Atresia

*Entire shading indicates condition present. Partial shading indicates partial anomalous pulmonary venous connection. Anomal. Pul. Vein = anomalous pulmonary venous connection; "Absent I.V.C." = absence of hepatic segment of inferior vena cava with azygos (or hemiazygos) continuation; Bilat. S.V.C. = bilateral superior venae cavae; Vent. Septal Defect = isolated ventricular septal defect. In cases 10 and 11, liver was on left; stomach on right. In case 12, liver was on right; stomach on right.

defect was a component of the aforementioned cases of persistent common atrioventricular canal.

Other Abnormalities

In three cases, the great arterial vessels were abnormally related. Origin of both great vessels from the right ventricle was present in two of these and, in the third, complete transposition of the great vessels was present.

Subaortic obstruction existed in two cases. In one the anterior leaflet of the mitral valve was fused to the ventricular septum, resulting in subaortic atresia; this case has been reported previously.[15] In the second case of subaortic obstruction, stenosis resulted from

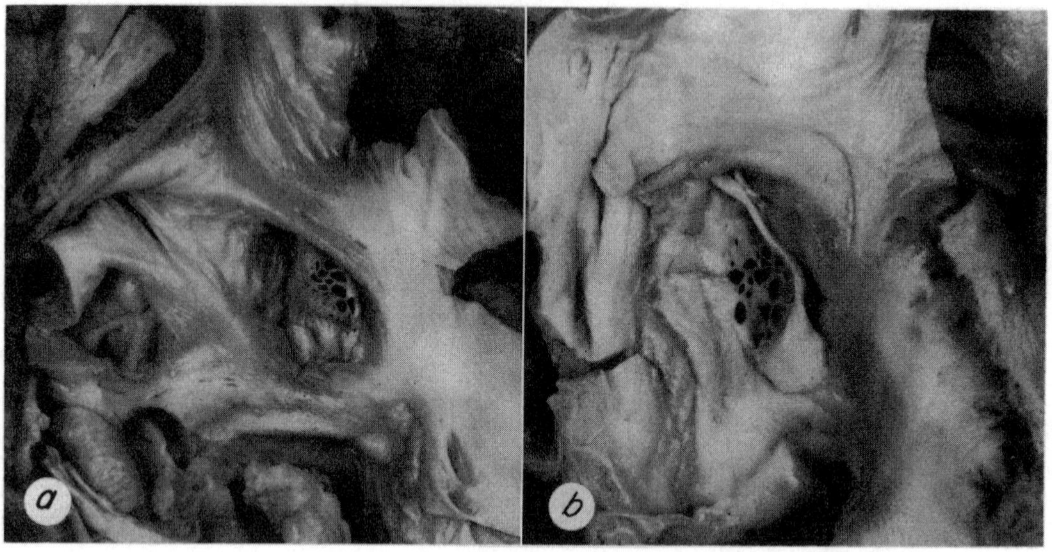

Figure 3

Case 10. Atrial septum characterized by absence of fossa ovalis. (a) Left atrial view. (b) Right atrial view.

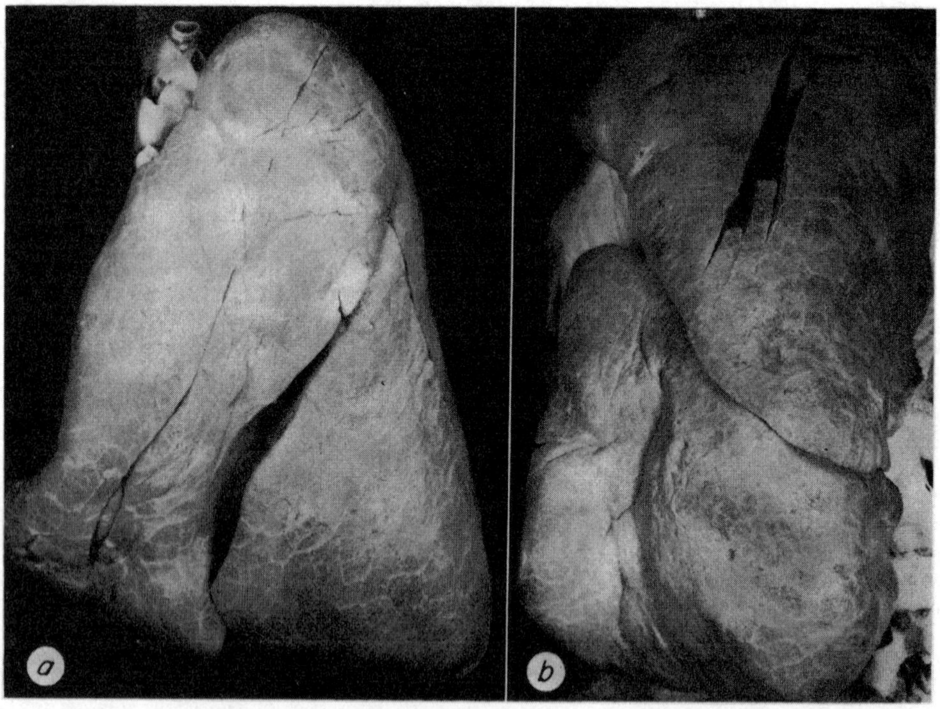

Figure 4

Case 6. Lungs in polysplenia. (a and b) Left and right lungs, respectively. Each has two lobes.

anomalous chordal attachments of the anterior leaflet of the mitral valve to the hypertrophied ventricular septum.

In contrast to asplenia in which pulmonary stenosis is almost universally present, among our 12 cases of polysplenia only a single case

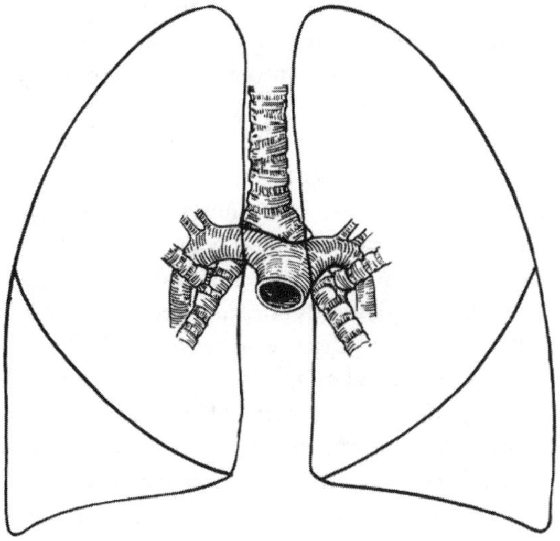

Figure 5

Diagrammatic representation of characteristic relationship between major bronchi and pulmonary arteries in polysplenia. Bilateral hyparterial bronchi.

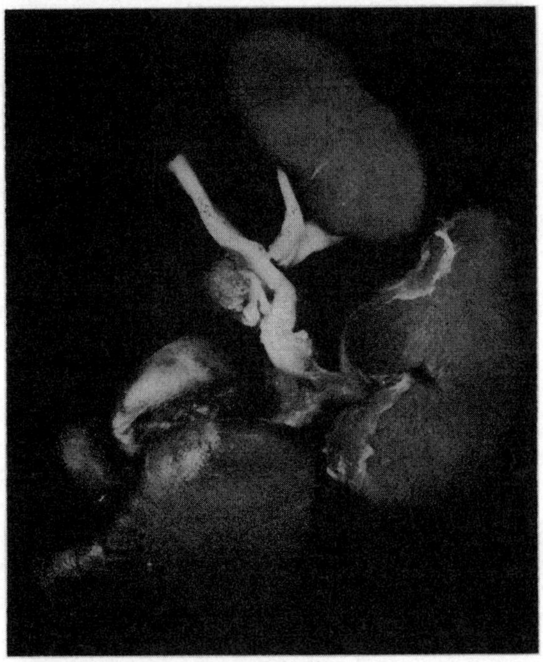

Figure 6

Case 10. Multiple spleens. Six splenic masses located along splenic artery.

of pulmonary stenosis was present. The ductus arteriosus was patent in six patients, each an infant.

Noncardiovascular Anomalies

In eight cases gross specimens of the lungs were available for review. In seven each lung had the fundamental structure of a left lung. In these seven cases, each lung had two lobes (fig. 4). The main stem bronchus to each lung was hyparterial, in that the homolateral pulmonary artery passed over the main stem bronchus and then proceeded behind the bronchus of the upper lobe to descend to the lower lobe (fig. 5). In addition, in each of these cases the distance between the carina and the first division of the major bronchus was identical in both lungs.

In the eighth case, the right lung exhibited rudimentary division into three lobes, and a bronchus suis was present in this lung. The right main stem bronchus was epiarterial. The left lung was normal, and the left main stem bronchus was hyparterial.

The number of multiple spleens varied from two to nine. They were located near the greater curvature of the stomach. The splenic masses were of relatively equal size, and the combined weight was normal (fig. 6).

In a single case the gallbladder was absent (fig. 7).

Comment

A large volume of literature has been accumulated describing the various features of the asplenic syndrome. In contrast, little has

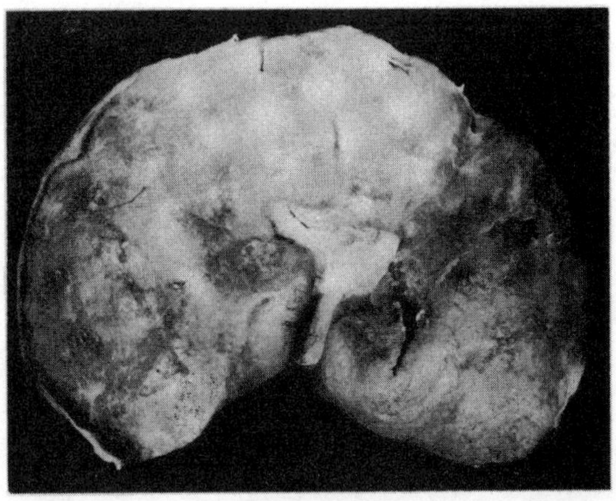

Figure 7

Case 9. Inferior surface of liver. Absence of gallbladder. Both lobes are nearly equal in size.

appeared concerning the cardiovascular anomalies and other malformations associated with the polysplenic state. In most of the reports of cardiac disease associated with polysplenia, the emphasis has been on the nature of the cardiovascular anomalies, and the splenic abnormality has been mentioned only as an incidental necropsy finding. It is, therefore, difficult in reviewing the literature to discover all the cases of polysplenia.

The 17 cases of polysplenia reported from other institutions in general exhibit the same types of cardiovascular abnormalities as we have observed in our cases. Except for one case of Ivemark,[1] in each of the other 16 cases reported in the literature cardiac abnormalities were present which allowed recognition of a tendency for (1) cardiac malposition, (2) interruption of inferior vena cava with azygos continuation, (3) partial or total anomalous pulmonary venous connection to the venous atrium, (4) bilateral superior venae cavae, and (5) defects in the atrial and ventricular septa. The cases described in the literature also exhibited frequent visceral malformations including (1) partial or total abdominal heterotaxy, (2) abnormality of pulmonary lobulation, and (3) symmetrical liver. In one of the cases reported by McLoughlin and associates[9] the gallbladder was absent also, a condition also observed in one of our cases. From the experience with the literature and with our material, it appears that the malformations associated with polysplenia represent a developmental complex. As in the asplenic syndrome certain predictable cardiac and visceral abnormalities are present in polysplenia.

Comparison of the form of the visceral malformations present in these two syndromes discloses certain distinct differences (table 2). In asplenia, the frequent occurrence of three lobes in each lung, symmetrical liver, and absent spleen has suggested to some authors that this developmental complex represents a tendency for duplication of the normal right-sided structures. It is cited that the spleen is the only unilateral mesenchymal organ, and since it is a left-sided structure, its absence is part of "bilateral right-sidedness." The organs in the left side of the body exhibit the appearance of the normal right-

Table 2

Comparison of Features of Asplenia and Polysplenia

Organ system	Features associated with asplenia	Features associated with polysplenia
Cardiac	Corrected transposition of great vessels with ventricular septal defect or single ventricle	Continuity of inferior vena cava with azygos or hemiazygos vein
	Pulmonary atresia or stenosis	Anomalous pulmonary venous connection to venous atrium
	Common atrium	Atrial septal defect or common atrium
	Bilateral superior venae cavae	Ventricular septal defect
	Total anomalous pulmonary venous connection	Bilateral superior venae cavae
	Malposition	Malposition
Pulmonary	Three lobes—each lung	Two lobes—each lung
	Bilateral epiarterial bronchi	Bilateral hyparterial bronchi
Abdominal	Heterotaxy	Heterotaxy
	Complete	Complete
	Situs inversus	Situs inversus
	Partial	Partial
	Horizontal liver	Horizontal liver
	Malrotation of bowel	Malrotation of bowel
	Duodenum—common mesentery	Absent gallbladder
	Midline gallbladder	

sided structures, hence three lobes in the left lung and a symmetrical liver.

In contrast to the tendency for duplication of right-sided structures in the asplenic syndrome are the features of the complex of polysplenia. In the latter there appears to be a tendency for duplication of left-sided structures, with an absence of normal right-sided structures. The evidence to support this belief is the following. The first is the presence of polysplenia. The second is the frequent phenomenon that each lung has but two lobes and has the structure of a left lung. Seven of our eight cases of polysplenia in which the lungs were available for review revealed this anatomic relationship. Brandt and Liebow[12] were the first to describe this feature of the lungs in a case of polysplenia. These authors emphasized the importance of the relationships between the bronchi and arterial branches in identifying whether the structure is that of a right or a left lung. The third feature favoring a concept of bilateral "left-sidedness" is absence of the gallbladder, as occurred in one of our cases and one described in the literature.[9] The fourth is the frequent infrahepatic interruption of the inferior vena cava. This portion of the inferior vena cava normally develops from a right-sided venous structure.

Because of these features, it appears logical to consider that the polysplenic syndrome represents bilateral left-sidedness or levo-isomerism, the opposite form of isomerism from the asplenic developmental complex.

There are, on the other hand, basic similarities between cases with multiple spleens and those with asplenia as indicated by Ivemark, who found more variability of the cardiac malformations in the former group than in the latter. Campbell and Deuchar[17] recently discussed the embryological implications of the malformations associated with asplenia and noted that some of their cases with cardiovascular features of the asplenic syndrome had multiple small spleens. The implications of these observations are important. The asplenic syndrome and the polysplenic syndrome are closely related developmental complexes in that each represents a defect occurring early in embryogenesis, which results in the lack of development of the normal body asymmetry. Furthermore, the types of cardiovascular and noncardiovascular malformations may appear similar. There is, however, one important difference between these two. The asplenic syndrome generally is associated with the tendency for right-sided symmetry, and polysplenia with the trend toward left-sided symmetry.

The cardiovascular and splenic abnormalities of these two developmental complexes have received considerable emphasis because significant cardiovascular malformations are present in the majority of cases. Abnormalities of these two organ systems are not invariably present, however. As indicated by Ivemark's one case of polysplenia without cardiac disease, cardiovascular malformations need not be uniformly present. Ivemark also suggested that the absence of the spleen is not always associated with other features of the asplenic syndrome. This is illustrated by a recently reported case with the typical cardiovascular malformations of asplenia and with three lobes in each lung in which an accessory spleen was present.[18] It is, therefore, probably possible to have each of these syndromes with a normal spleen.

The manifestations of these two developmental complexes are, therefore, variable and are represented by a spectrum of abnormalities with a varying number of structures showing symmetrical development.

The tendency for symmetrical organ structure may involve only one organ system, for example, the lungs. Therefore, it would appear advisable to classify these developmental complexes in a more inclusive fashion, namely, disorders of body symmetry with tendencies to either dextro-isomerism or levo-isomerism and with the extent of symmetry and organ involvement being defined.

Since the cardiac malformations associated with polysplenia follow a relatively uniform pattern, it would be helpful to the clinician to be able to recognize the polysplenia as a basis for anticipating the cardiovascular malformations that might be present in a given case. The asplenic syndrome can be readily recognized by finding Howell-Jolly bodies in a peripheral blood smear. We know of no easy clinical means of identifying polysplenia. The finding of absence of the hepatic segment of the inferior vena cava should suggest this possibility, but it appears that, other than angiographic or radioactive isotopic visualization of the splenic structures, there are no definite means of identifying the presence of polysplenia short of surgical exploration or necropsy.

An important clinical difference between polysplenia and asplenia relates to cyanosis. In asplenia, wherein pulmonary stenosis and defects of the ventricular septum are common, cyanosis and diminished pulmonary blood flow are usually present. In polysplenia, considering the tendency for absence of pulmonary stenosis and for the presence of septal defects, acyanosis with increased pulmonary blood flow forms the usual clinical pattern.

References

1. Ivemark, B. I.: Implications of agenesis of the spleen on the pathogenesis of cono-truncus anomalies in childhood: Analysis of the heart malformations in the splenic agenesis syndrome, with fourteen new cases. Acta Pediat **44** (suppl. 104): 1, 1955.
2. Ruttenberg, H. D., et al.: Syndrome of congenital cardiac disease with asplenia: Distinction from other forms of congenital cyanotic cardiac disease. Amer J Cardiol **13**: 387, 1964.
3. Forde, W. J., and Finby, N.: Roentgenographic features of asplenia, a teratologic syndrome of visceral symmetry. Amer J Roentgen **86**: 523, 1961.
4. Ongley, P. A., Titus, J. L., Khoury, G. H., Rahimtoola, S. H., Marshall, H. J., and Edwards, J. E.: Anomalous connection of pulmonary veins to right atrium associated with anomalous inferior vena cava, situs inversus and multiple spleens: Developmental complex. Mayo Clin Proc **40**: 609, 1965.
5. Hickman: Transposition of viscera: Malformation of heart; pulmonary veins from right lung entering left auricle, and from left lung entering right auricle. Trans Path Soc London **20**: 93, 1869.
6. Royer, B. F., and Wilson, J. D.: Incomplete heterotaxy with unusual heart malformations: Case report. Arch Pediat **25**: 881, 1908.
7. Miller, A. J.: Congenital heart disease with partial situs inversus, absence of inferior vena cava, and other anomalies. Amer J Path **1**: 467, 1925.
8. Campbell, M., Gardner, F., and Reynolds, G.: Cor biloculare. Brit Heart J **14**: 317, 1952.
9. McLoughlin, T. G., Krovetz, L. J., and Scheibler, G. L.: Heart disease in the Laurence-Moon-Biedl-Bardet syndrome: A review and a report of 3 brothers. J Pediat **65**: 388, 1964.
10. Greenburg, S. D.: Multilobulated spleen in association with congenital heart disease: Report of a case. AMA Arch Path **63**: 333, 1957.
11. Grover, R. F., Lanier, R. R., Lowry, J. K., and Blount, S. G., Jr.: Congenital absence of the hepatic portion of the inferior vena cava. Amer Heart J **54**: 794, 1957.
12. Brandt, H. M., and Liebow, A. A.: Right pulmonary isomerism associated with venous, splenic, and other anomalies. Lab Invest **7**: 469, 1958.
13. Muir, C. S.: Splenic agenesis and multilobulate spleen. Arch Dis Child **34**: 431, 1959.
14. Anderson, R. C., Adams, P., Jr., and Burke, Barbara: Anomalous inferior vena cava with azygos continuation (infrahepatic interruption of the inferior vena cava): Report of 15 new cases. J Pediat **59**: 370, 1961.
15. Jue, K. L., and Edwards, J. E.: Anomalous attachment of mitral valve causing subaortic atresia: Observations in a case with other cardiac anomalies and multiple spleens. Circulation **35**: 928, 1967.
16. Raghib, G., Ruttenberg, H. D., Anderson, R. C., Amplatz, K., Adams, P., Jr., and Edwards, J. E.: Termination of left superior vena cava in left atrium, atrial septal defect, and absence of coronary sinus: A developmental complex. Circulation **31**: 906, 1965.
17. Campbell, M., and Deuchar, D. C.: Absent inferior vena cava, symmetrical liver, splenic agenesis, and situs inversus, and their embryology. Brit Heart J **29**: 268, 1967.
18. Layman, T. E., Levine, M. A., Amplatz, K., and Edwards, J. E.: "Asplenic syndrome" in association with rudimentary spleen. Amer J Cardiol. **20**: 136, 1967.

Congenital cardiac disease associated with polysplenia. A developmental complex of bilateral "left-sidedness"

James Moller, M.D.

As Jesse and I worked on the pathologic material resulting in this paper, on congenital cardiac disease associated with polysplenia, we faced a challenge. Since about half of the specimens had dextrocardia and we often had information about abdominal organs and the lungs, we tried to classify them as either situs solitus or situs inversus. We found that we could not classify the same specimen consistently into one of these two categories. As we took a fresh look we recognized the left-sided symmetry of the lungs and the atrial characteristics displayed by the pathologic material, so we termed our complex of findings bilateral left sidedness. This complex was the opposite, but complimentary of the asplenia or bilateral right sidedness described in the previous decade by Ivemark.

The terms that have been subsequently used to describe these two syndromes referred to sidedness, splenic status or broadly as situs ambiguous have been confusing and inadequate to depict them. Robert Anderson has applied his segmental approach to the anatomy of these anomalies and has termed them isomerisms of the atrial appendages. This reflects that the only parts of the heart or viscera, which truly show isomerism, are the atrial appendages. The left and right atrial appendages have distinct anatomic differences. The broad use of the term isomerism of the right or left atrial appendage hopefully will clarify the confusion and result in a more uniform classification.

As more reports have appeared about the range and complexity of the cardiac anatomy associated with the isomerism syndromes, the more common patterns of cardiac malformations have been understood. Freedom wrote that right isomerism is one of the worse forms of congenital heart disease and even those with left isomerism undergoing single ventricle repair had higher operative mortality and decreased survival compared to those with normal situs. Indeed the 50 percent survival for left isomerism is 20 years and for right isomerism is about seven years. Anomalies of other organs also influence morbidity and mortality. Intestinal malrotation, either non-rotation or reverse rotation of the midgut loop is very common, pancreatic and hepatic structural anomalies are found and may influence the patients course.

Since in humans and all other vertebrates, visceral asymmetry is the rule, these isomeric conditions are being actively investigated. One approach has been pedigree analysis, which has found various types of genetic transmission in families with an index case of isomerism. Another approach has been the study of cilia and the embryonic organizer. The motion of cilia during early development is important in the ultimate location of organs. The finding of abnormal dynein filaments in the cilia of patients with Kartageners syndrome (bronchiectasis and dextrocardia) showed a potential cause of cardiac malposition. Subsequently structurally abnormal cilia have been found in patients with isomeric conditions. Several genes, nodal, sonic hedgehog and lefty have been identified as involved in the process of laterality. A knockout model of sonic hedgehog produces left isomerism.

So, in four decades, from describing left isomerism we have progressed to some genetic understanding of the condition. We are moving closer to the dream of Helen Taussig, who said "the great day will come when we can not only treat these conditions, but prevent them."

Proceedings of the

STAFF MEETINGS OF THE MAYO CLINIC

Published Fortnightly for the Information of the Members of the Staff and the Fellows of the Mayo Foundation for Medical Education and Research

Volume 31 ROCHESTER, MINNESOTA, WEDNESDAY, MARCH 21, 1956 Number 6

CONTENTS

Symposium on Total Anomalous Pulmonary Venous Connection

Page

A Classification of Total Anomalous Pulmonary Venous Connection Based on Developmental Considerations *151*
JESSE E. EDWARDS AND H. FRED HELMHOLZ, JR.

Total Anomalous Pulmonary Venous Drainage: Clinical and Physiologic Patterns *161*
HOWARD B. BURCHELL

Total Anomalous Pulmonary Venous Connection: Clinical Aspects *67*
JAMES W. DUSHANE

Roentgenologic Findings in Total Anomalous Pulmonary Venous Connection *171*
ANDRÉ BRUWER

Hemodynamic Findings in Total Anomalous Pulmonary Venous Drainage *177*
H. J. C. SWAN, ELY TOSCANO-BARBOZA AND EARL H. WOOD

Complete Surgical Correction of Total Anomalous Pulmonary Venous Connection: Report of Three Cases *182*
JOHN T. BURROUGHS AND JOHN W. KIRKLIN

End of Symposium

SYMPOSIUM

A CLASSIFICATION OF TOTAL ANOMALOUS PULMONARY VENOUS CONNECTION BASED ON DEVELOPMENTAL CONSIDERATIONS

Jesse E. Edwards, M.D., Section of Pathologic Anatomy, and
H. Fred Helmholz, Jr., M.D., Section of Physiology

In previous communications[1,2] the point was made that the terms *anomalous pulmonary venous connection* and *anomalous pulmonary venous drainage* are not necessarily synonymous. The former is an anatomic designation and the latter a physiologic one. It was indicated that while some patients with anomalous pulmonary venous drainage may have anomalous venous connection as a basis for this functional disturbance, others may have normal anatomic arrangements as regards the pulmonary veins. Moreover, some patients with

1. Edwards, J. E.: Pathologic and Developmental Considerations in Anomalous Pulmonary Venous Connection. Proc. Staff Meet., Mayo Clin. 28:441-452 (Aug. 26) 1953.
2. Swan, H. J. C., Burchell, H. B. and Wood, E. H.: Differential Diagnosis at Cardiac Catheterization of Anomalous Pulmonary Venous Drainage Related to Atrial Septal Defects or Abnormal Venous Connections. Proc. Staff Meet., Mayo Clin. 28:452-462 (Aug. 26) 1953.

anomalous anatomic arrangements of the pulmonary veins may nevertheless deliver all of the pulmonary venous blood to the left atrium.[3]

The position taken in this presentation adheres to the definitions already given and perhaps even goes a step beyond. In this way we would define total anomalous pulmonary venous connection as any condition in which there is a significant anatomic derangement in the pulmonary venous pathway to the heart involving all of the pulmonary venous bed. Among cases so designated anatomically, functionally there are examples with no shunts, shunts of bidirectional nature, left-to-right shunts and right-to-left shunts.

Another approach in definition is to state that any derangement in the structural development of the pulmonary venous supply involving the entire pulmonary bed may be defined as total anomalous pulmonary venous connection. In order for the reader to appreciate fully this definition, it is appropriate to review the story of normal pulmonary venous development.[1]

DEVELOPMENT OF PULMONARY VEINS

The lungs represent a specialized portion of the foregut and in their early stages share their blood supply with the foregut. Two systems of venous drainage exist in the early developing lungs, represented by multiple communications. One of these systems is the cardinal system of veins, from which such structures as the superior vena cava, the azygos vein, and the coronary sinus develop. The other system is the umbilicovitelline system, represented in final stages of development principally by the portal venous system. At this early stage, there is no direct communication between the venous supply of the lungs on one hand and the heart on the other. It is to be remembered that in the early stages of development the blood supply of one lung also communicates with that of the other.

The next important stage of development is the growth of a channel from that portion of the sino-atrial region of the heart which is to become the left atrium. This channel grows toward the developing lungs and eventually establishes communication with the pulmonary venous bed. This channel from the sino-atrial region may be termed the *common pulmonary vein.* After the common pulmonary vein has established communications with the pulmonary venous system, the more primitive connections between the pulmonary venous system and the cardinal and umbilicovitelline veins normally disappear. Functionally, this leaves the definitive normal condition in which all the pulmonary venous system has direct connection with that portion of the heart to become the left atrium.

The final important step is that by a process of differential growth the common pulmonary vein becomes incorporated into the left atrium and disappears as an identifiable structure. This is evidenced by the

3. Becu, L. M., Tauxe, W. N., DuShane, J. W. and Edwards, J. E.: Anomalous Connection of Pulmonary Veins With Normal Pulmonary Venous Drainage: Report of Case Associated With Pulmonary Venous Stenosis and Cor Triatriatum. A.M.A. Arch. Path. 59:463-470 (Apr.) 1955.

adult condition in which two right and two (sometimes one) left pulmonary veins connect directly with the left atrium.

The various forms of total anomalous pulmonary venous connection may be looked on as deviations in the normal process outlined. These deviations are represented principally by retention of primitive stages with or without failure of the heart to make direct connection with the pulmonary venous supply by way of the common pulmonary vein.

From the description of normal pulmonary venous development, we may now go to various types of total anomalous pulmonary venous connection.

CLASSIFICATION OF TOTAL ANOMALOUS PULMONARY VENOUS CONNECTION

A. Anomalous connection only to left atrium
  a. With normal lobular venous pattern (cor triatriatum)
  b. With abnormal lobular venous pattern

B. Connection both to right atrium or tributary veins and to left atrium
  a. With stenotic left atrial connection
  b. With normal left atrial connection
  c. With normal left atrial connection, but with mitral or aortic valvular atresia

C. Connection only to right atrium or tributary veins
  a. Without major intracardiac defects
  b. With major intracardiac defects

D. Connection between a pulmonary artery and the left atrium

A. ANOMALOUS CONNECTION ONLY TO LEFT ATRIUM

a. With Normal Lobular Venous Pattern.—This condition is represented by the condition called *cor triatriatum*. It is characterized by all of the pulmonary veins emanating from the pulmonary lobes in a normal manner and then joining an accessory cardiac chamber which in turn communicates with the left atrium. The frequently narrow diameter of the opening between the accessory left atrial chamber and the true left atrium causes pulmonary venous obstructive phenomena which are similar to those in mitral stenosis. From the point of view of drainage, however, all of the pulmonary venous blood reaches the left atrium and there is no anomalous drainage into the right side of the heart.

The accessory chamber is considered to be the common pulmonary vein, which has failed to become normally incorporated into the heart as an integral part of the left atrium (fig. 1*a* and *b*).

b. With Abnormal Lobular Venous Pattern.—Previously reported from the Clinic was a rare form of anomalous connection of pulmonary veins only to the left atrium which was characterized by an abnormal lobular venous pattern.[3] In this case, the left lower pulmonary vein was atretic near its junction with the heart, and an anomalous channel carried blood from the lower lobe of the left lung to the left upper pulmonary vein. This vein in turn crossed the midline behind the pericardium to form a venous sinus and then to make communication with the right upper pulmonary vein. Neither upper pulmonary vein joined the heart directly. The right upper vein then communicated

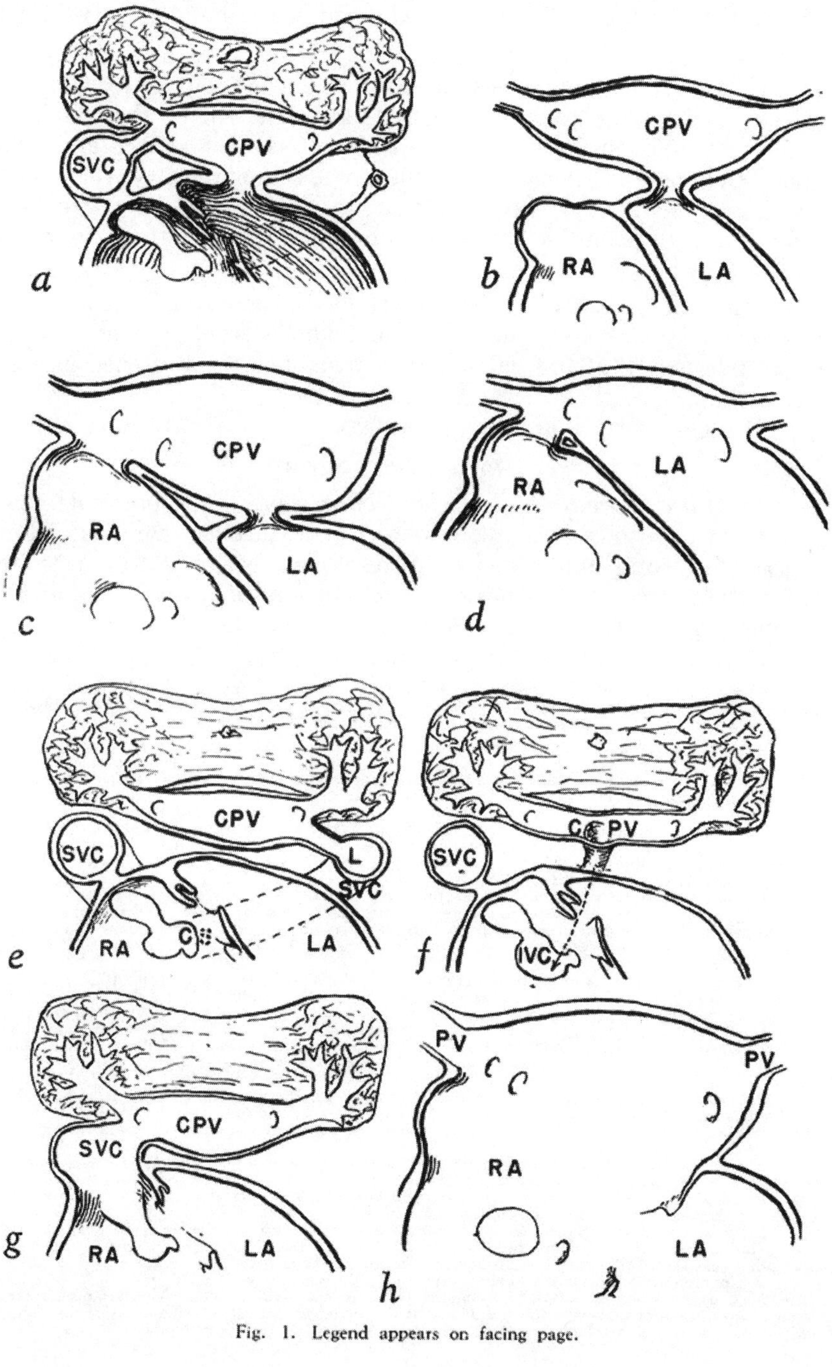

Fig. 1. Legend appears on facing page.

with the right lower pulmonary vein by means of a tortuous channel within the hilar portion of the right lung. The right lower pulmonary vein, therefore, received the blood from the entire pulmonary bed. It then joined an accessory left atrial chamber of the type characteristic of cor triatriatum.* Stenosis of the right lower pulmonary vein also existed.

The developmental basis for the peculiar venous pattern in this case is probably related in part to the obstruction of the left lower pulmonary vein and also to the failure of the left upper and right upper pulmonary veins to join the common pulmonary vein. The anomalous channels between the veins of the various lobes represent elaborations of primitive connections between the venous supply of the two lungs.

Although in this case there must have existed an obstruction to pulmonary venous flow, the anatomic channels were such as to make an avenue for all of the pulmonary venous flow to be carried into the left atrium. No channel for a shunt existed.

B. CONNECTION BOTH TO RIGHT ATRIUM OR TRIBUTARY VEINS AND TO LEFT ATRIUM

a. With Stenotic Left Atrial Connection.—In a particular case which we have observed, there were the features of cor triatriatum, constituting total anomalous pulmonary venous connection with the left atrium, according to our concept. In addition, there was a communication between the accessory cardiac chamber (representing the

*An atretic vascular cord connected the pulmonary venous sinus, which lay behind the pericardium, and the left innominate vein. For this reason, in the strict sense, this case might be classified as having total anomalous connection with both the left and right atria.

Fig. 1. Developmental basis for certain types of anomalous pulmonary venous connection.

a. Representing an early stage in development of the pulmonary veins. The common pulmonary vein (C.P.V.) has joined the pulmonary veins with the left atrium. Incorporation of the common pulmonary vein as an integral part of the left atrium is not yet complete. At this stage, there are still retained connections between the pulmonary venous system and the cardinal and umbilicovitelline system of veins. In this diagram these connections are represented by a communication between the common pulmonary vein and the superior vena cava (S.V.C.).

b. Total anomalous connection of the pulmonary veins to the left atrium with no connection to the right atrium (cor triatriatum). This condition represents an arrest in development at the stage shown in *a*, wherein the common pulmonary vein has not yet become incorporated into the left atrial chamber. The primitive connections with the cardinal and umbilicovitelline systems of veins are lost.

c. Total anomalous connection of the pulmonary veins with the right atrium (R.A.) and with the left atrium (L.A.). The anomalous connection with the left atrium is like that shown in *b*, producing an accessory chamber receiving the pulmonary veins. The connection with the right atrium is explained developmentally by a retention of a communication between the common pulmonary vein and the superior vena cava, as illustrated in *a*, and then by incorporation of the proximal part of the superior vena cava into the right atrium. Such a situation is portrayed by the case illustrated in figure 2.

d. Anomalous connection of the pulmonary veins with the right atrium but with normal left atrial connection. The arrangement illustrated may be considered to have developed like that in the arrangement illustrated in *c*, but with the common pulmonary vein normally becoming incorporated into the left atrium.

e, f, g and *h.* Types of total anomalous connection of the pulmonary veins to the right atrium or tributary veins without connection to the left atrium.

e. Connection of the common pulmonary vein with the left anterior cardinal vein, the proximal end of which normally becomes the coronary sinus (C.S.).

f. Persistence of communication of the pulmonary venous system with an umbilicovitelline vein creates the arrangement in which there is connection between the common pulmonary vein and an abdominal vein leading directly or indirectly into the inferior vena cava.

g. Connection of the common pulmonary vein to the superior vena cava.

h. Connection of the common pulmonary vein to the right atrium. This arrangement may result from a basic anomalous connection like that illustrated in *g*, but with dilatation of the common junction of the common pulmonary vein, superior vena cava, and right atrium.

common pulmonary vein) and the right atrium. Viewed from the right side, this communication appeared as an atrial septal defect in an unusual position lying superior to the region of the fossa ovalis and in close proximity to the superior vena caval junction with the right atrium (fig. 2*a* and *b*). Since this opening on the left side was in communication with a structure which developmentally we consider to be a pulmonary vein, it seems proper to consider that there is, in fact, an anomalous pulmonary venous connection between the entire pulmonary venous system and the right atrium (fig. 1*a* and *c*).

In an early stage of development of the individual there probably existed a connection between the common pulmonary vein and the primordia of the superior vena cava. With progressive development

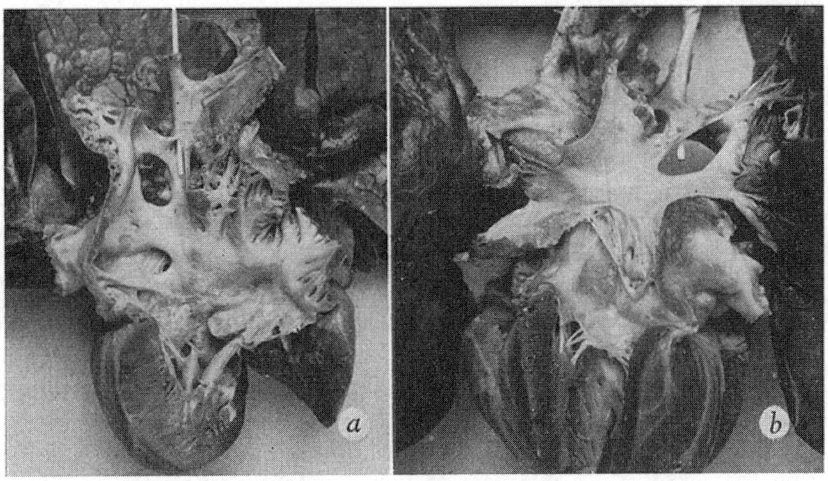

Fig. 2. A case of total anomalous pulmonary venous connection both to the left atrium and to the right atrium in a boy 4 months old.

a. Right side of heart. The region of the fossa ovalis is normally developed except for a tiny patency of the foramen ovale. In the upper part of the atrial septum near the entrance of the superior vena cava (containing probe) is a defect which opens into an accessory left atrial chamber illustrated in *b*.

b. Left side of heart. The left ventricle communicates with the left atrium by way of a normal mitral valve. An accessory left atrial chamber receives the pulmonary veins and communicates by a funnellike opening with the true left atrium. The accessory left atrial chamber has a large opening allowing it to communicate with the right atrium.

and gradual absorption of some of the systemic venous system into the right atrium and with retention of the early connection, there appeared the final picture of a connection between a derivative of the common pulmonary vein and the right atrium.

From a functional point of view it is probable that, while some of the pulmonary venous blood flowed into the left atrium, some escaped into the right atrium through the anomalous connection present. It is possible also that some right atrial blood, especially of superior vena caval origin, flowed in a right-to-left direction through the anomalous connection.

In a functional way this case may be compared to a case with coexistent mitral stenosis and atrial septal defect.

b. With Normal Left Atrial Connection.—A developmental variant of the case described may be represented by those cases in which the left atrium is normally formed, but in which there is an interatrial communication at the upper level of the atrial septum above the fossa ovalis, as illustrated diagrammatically in figure 1*d*. However, such cases may developmentally represent partial anomalous pulmonary venous connection of a right pulmonary vein to the right anterior cardinal vein.

Yet another anatomic picture may represent anomalous pulmonary venous connection to the systemic venous system with normal connection to the left atrium. We refer to the rare cases in which the coronary sinus, while emptying normally into the right atrium, has a large communication with the left atrium. This lesion functions as an interatrial communication.

For the developmental explanation of this malformation, it should be recalled that the coronary sinus represents the proximal end of the left anterior cardinal vein. With this in mind, one can explain the malformation as follows: Anomalous connection between the common pulmonary vein and that part of the left anterior cardinal vein destined to become the coronary sinus results in a communication between the coronary sinus and the left atrium as differential growth takes place, incorporating the communication into the left atrium.

c. With Normal Left Atrial Connection, But With Mitral or Aortic Valvular Atresia.—In the usual instance of mitral or aortic valvular atresia, blood from the left atrium escapes through an interatrial communication at the site of the foramen ovale. In a rare instance, the foramen ovale is sealed, and no interatrial communication is possible. One of such cases was reported by McIntosh[4] and one from the Clinic.[5] In our case, a vein connected the left atrium with the beginning of the left innominate vein. In a previous paper, we referred to this communication as a "levoatrio-cardinal vein." Developmentally such cases may be looked on as retention of a connection between the common pulmonary vein of the embryo on one hand, and the cardinal venous system on the other. In the case of McIntosh the systemic component of the anomalous connection was the superior vena cava. Through such channels left atrial blood finds a route which leads ultimately to the right atrium. In such cases, by virtue of free mixing of pulmonary and systemic venous blood in the right atrium, there are bidirectional shunts.

C. CONNECTION ONLY TO RIGHT ATRIUM OR TRIBUTARY VEINS

The cases of total venous connection of the pulmonary veins only to the right atrium or to its tributary veins, there being no connection with the left atrium, constitute the commonest variety of anomalous

4. McIntosh, C. A.: Cor Biatriatum Triloculare. Am. Heart J. *1*:735-744 (Aug.) 1926.
5. Edwards, J. E. and DuShane, J. W.: Thoracic Venous Anomalies. I. Vascular Connection of the Left Atrium and the Left Innominate Vein (Levoatrio-cardinal vein) Associated With Mitral Atresia and Premature Closure of the Foramen Ovale (Case 1). II. Pulmonary Veins Draining Wholly Into the Ductus Venosus (Case 2). Arch. Path. *49*:517-537 (May) 1950.

pulmonary venous connection. This type of case is the one which forms the major subject of the other papers which follow in this symposium. By definition, there is no communication with the left atrium, the entire pulmonary venous blood being carried into the right atrium directly or into one of its tributary veins. In these cases all the incoming blood is pooled in the right atrium, and bidirectional shunts

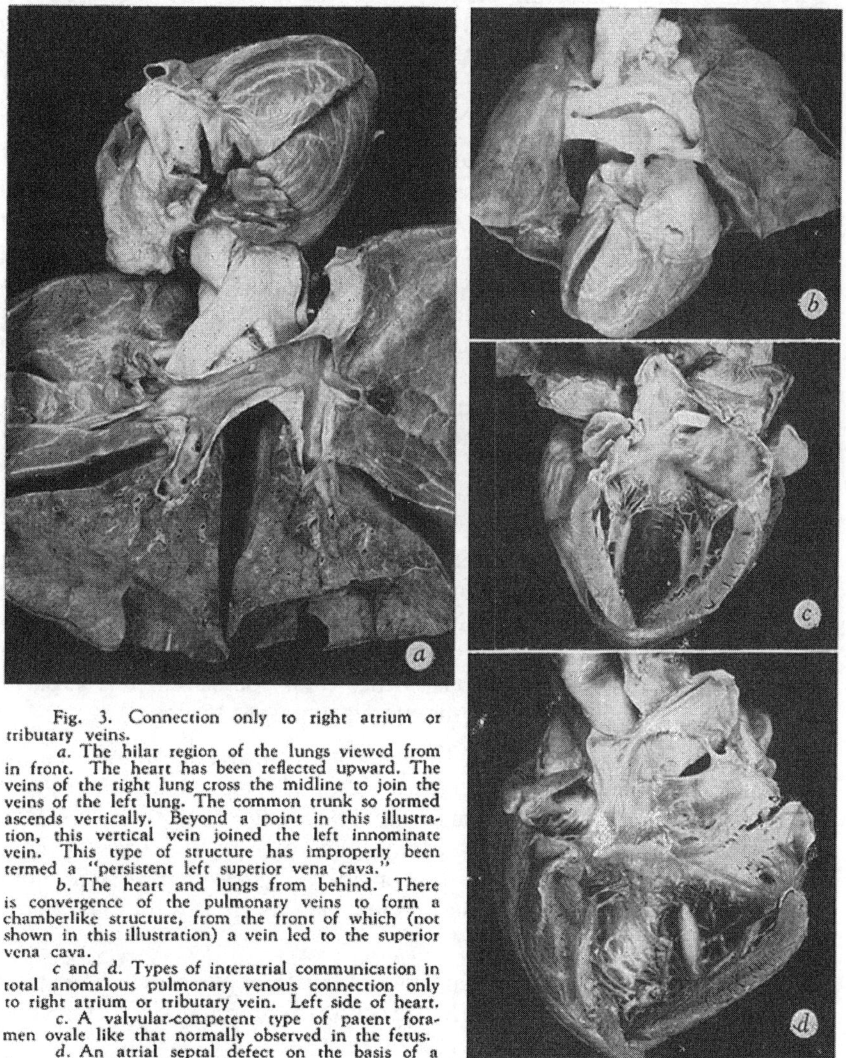

Fig. 3. Connection only to right atrium or tributary veins.
a. The hilar region of the lungs viewed from in front. The heart has been reflected upward. The veins of the right lung cross the midline to join the veins of the left lung. The common trunk so formed ascends vertically. Beyond a point in this illustration, this vertical vein joined the left innominate vein. This type of structure has improperly been termed a "persistent left superior vena cava."
b. The heart and lungs from behind. There is convergence of the pulmonary veins to form a chamberlike structure, from the front of which (not shown in this illustration) a vein led to the superior vena cava.
c and *d*. Types of interatrial communication in total anomalous pulmonary venous connection only to right atrium or tributary vein. Left side of heart.
c. A valvular-competent type of patent foramen ovale like that normally observed in the fetus.
d. An atrial septal defect on the basis of a short valve of the foramen ovale.

exist. The developmental basis for this type of anomaly resides either in failure of the common pulmonary vein of the embryo to join the venous plexus of the developing lungs, or, if such connection is made, it is secondarily obliterated. A secondary obliteration would occur at an early time, before the primitive connections between the pulmonary vessels and the cardinal and umbilicovitelline systems of veins are lost.

Retention of one of these channels represents the anomalous connection existing in any particular case (fig. 1*e* and *f*).

When all of the pulmonary veins join the right atrium or a tributary vein, there are two types of anatomic features in the pulmonary venous system. There is either a simple junction of veins without formation of a chamberlike structure, or the veins may converge into a sinus or chamber (fig. 3*a* and *b*). From this, a venous channel runs to the site of connection with the systemic venous system or the right atrium. In any event, the pulmonary veins do not perforate the pericardium and usually converge posterior to it.

One particular type of connection deserves special mention because it is relatively common, and it has been given a misnomer. We refer to the situation wherein all the pulmonary venous blood is carried to a vein that runs vertically, usually anterior to the aortic arch, and terminates in the beginning of the left innominate vein (fig. 3*a*). This structure does not make junction with the heart, but it has been referred to as a "persistent left superior vena cava." The structure that is a true persistent left superior vena cava represents the left anterior cardinal vein of the embryo and has, as one of its characteristics, a communication with the heart in its becoming the coronary sinus at its proximal end. In the absence of a connection with the heart the vertical vein which receives all of the pulmonary veins cannot be considered as a persistent left superior vena cava. On developmental grounds, it may represent a persistent left superior vena cava, which has lost its connection with the coronary sinus. However, it is considered more probable that it represents a separate persisting channel. Dr. Burchell and we have been of the opinion that this vein should be designated by some term other than "persistent left superior vena cava," possibly "vertical anomalous pulmonary vein."

It is pertinent to consider the anatomic arrangement wherein all the pulmonary veins join the right atrium. In an earlier paper,[1] one of us (Edwards) considered this type of arrangement to result from faulty placement of the atrial septum. There is an alternate explanation for this condition. It may be considered as resulting from anomalous connection of the entire pulmonary venous supply to the superior vena cava (fig. 1*g* and *h*).

By differential growth a part of the superior vena cava is carried into the right atrium and by this process the anomalously connected pulmonary veins are likewise brought into the right atrium.

Whatever the details of anatomic arrangement, when all the pulmonary veins join the right atrial system and the left atrium fails to have pulmonary venous connection, the functional disturbances depend to a great extent on details in cardiac structure. This consideration makes it pertinent to subdivide cases of total anomalous connection of the pulmonary veins only to the right atrium as follows:

a. Without Major Intracardiac Defects.—Of particular importance with regard to potential in therapy are the cases in which basically there is a normally developed heart. Here the left atrium and the systemic circulation depend for their blood on an interatrial communication. This may be a valvular-competent foramen ovale of varying size or a true atrial septal defect (fig. 3*c* and *d*).

b. With Major Intracardiac Defects.—Among the major intracardiac malformations are examples of serious defects in the cardiac septa. Usually such cases are represented by cor biloculare. Considering the presence of such a type of intracardiac malformation, the anatomic site of termination of the pulmonary veins is of secondary importance, since there is free mixing of blood in the cardiac chambers.

Among cases of this type are examples of the syndrome associated with congenital absence of the spleen. In the latter there is usually a common atrioventricular valve, often an absent atrial or ventricular septum or both, situs inversus of the abdominal organs, and anomalies of the major blood vessels. Total anomalous pulmonary venous connection may in some cases be numbered among the latter.[6,7]

D. CONNECTION BETWEEN A PULMONARY ARTERY AND THE LEFT ATRIUM

We have not observed an example of the very rare condition wherein a pulmonary artery connects with the superior aspect of the the left atrium.[8,9] In such instances, a right-to-left shunt is possible through the connection. Developmentally it is pertinent to place these cases among examples of total anomalous pulmonary venous connection. They may represent a congenital pulmonary arteriovenous fistula between a pulmonary artery and the common pulmonary vein. As this is retained, and as the common pulmonary vein is carried into the left atrium, the condition under discussion would result.

SUMMARY

"Total anomalous pulmonary venous connection" is an anatomic term used to designate any major deviation in development affecting the entire pulmonary venous system. It is particularly important to understand the nature of these anomalies when surgical correction is being contemplated.

From relatively simple differences in details of development, diverse gross anatomic pictures may result. Depending, in part, on differences in the final anatomic picture, there results a wide spectrum of functional disturbances in total anomalous pulmonary venous connection. Only one of these disturbances is total anomalous pulmonary venous drainage.

6. Polhemus, D. W. and Schafer, W. B.: Congenital Absence of the Spleen; Syndrome With Atrioventricularis and Situs Inversus. Pediatrics 9:696-708 (June) 1952.
7. Ivemark, B. I.: Implications of Agenesis of the Spleen on the Pathogenesis of Cono-truncus Anomalies in Childhood: An Analysis of the Heart Malformations in the Splenic Agenesis Syndrome, With Fourteen New Cases. Acta Paediatrica Suppl. 104, vol. 44, (Nov.) 1955, 110 pp.
8. Friedlich, A. L., Bing, R. J. and Blount, S. G., Jr.: Physiological Studies in Congenital Heart Disease; Circulatory Dynamics in the Anomalies of Venous Return to the Heart Including Pulmonary Arteriovenous Fistula. Bull. Johns Hopkins Hosp. 86:20-57 (Jan.) 1950.
9. Mack, J. and McNie, A.: Unpublished data from Massachusetts General Hospital.

A Classification of Total Anomalous Pulmonary Venous Connection Based on Developmental Considerations.

Fouad Butto, M.D.

Total anomalous pulmonary venous connection is a rare congenital heart defect accounting for 1.5 percent of all heart defects. Since its first description by Wilson in the 17th century and its classification in the early 1950s, major strides have been made in the diagnosis and therapy of this potentially highly fatal type of heart defect. There is still controversy in the interpretation of the developmental embryology of the defect. Jesse Edwards was a pioneer and a leader in explaining the development of the fetal pulmonary circulation and the classification of total anomalous pulmonary venous connection while making a point of distinguishing between anomalous connection and anomalous drainage. The former is an anatomic designation, and the later a physiologic one.

The lungs in the fetus represent a specialized portion of the foregut, and in the early stages they share their blood supply with the foregut. Two systems of venous drainage exist in the early developing lungs, represented by multiple communications: One is the anterior cardinal system of veins that eventually develops into the superior vena cava, the azygos vein and the coronary sinus. The other is the umbilicovitelline system, which develops into the IVC, portal venous system and ductus venosus.

A further venous channel then develops from a mid-line strand formed within the mediastinal tissues. This channel, when canalized, drains the developing intrapulmonary venous plexuses from both lungs, and joins the heart at the site of the persisting part of the dorsal mesocardium, to be later cannibalized and incorporated in the left atrium. At this stage the more primitive connections between the pulmonary venous system and the cardinal and umbilcovitelline systems disappear.

There has been controversy as to the relationship between this newly formed pulmonary venous confluence and the tributaries of the systemic venous sinus. Anderson and colleagues believe that from the stance of the morphology, and the lineage of the cells forming the pulmonary vein, that during normal development the pulmonary venous structure has never had any connection with the systemic venous tributaries. It forms as a new structure within the mediastinum, and opens within the mediastinal myocardium to the left atrium. As such, it is positioned to the left of the site of appearance of the primary atrial septum, which is also derived from mediastinal myocardium. The pulmonary venous structures are also recognizable from the outset as being derived from mediastinal myocardium, whereas the systemic venous tributaries initially possess a primary myocardial lineage. They have shown that the systemic venous tributaries can be identified in molecular terms by their expression of the transcription factor Tbx18. The pulmonary veins, in contrast, do not contain this protein.

Jesse Edwards defines TAPVC as any condition in which there is significant anatomic derangement in the pulmonary venous pathway to the heart involving all of the pulmonary venous bed, or any derangement in the structural development of the pulmonary venous supply involving the entire pulmonary bed.

Anderson defines TAPVC as the consequence of failure of canalization of the pulmonary venous channel in the mediastinum. An anastomosis with the anterior cardinal systemic venous system then results in supracardiac anomalous connection. Anastomosis with the systemic venous sinus, or the left sinus horn, produces cardiac connection, while infradiaphragmatic connection is the consequence of anastomosis with the omphalomesenteric system. A mixed type of TAPVC may also occur. If the common pulmonary vein fails to incorporate into the dorsal left atrial wall, pulmonary vein stenosis/atresia or cor triatriatum will occur.

The etiology of TAPVC is multi-factorial. TAPVC is known to be part of the Holt-Oram, Klippel-Feil, phocomelia, and Schachermann syndromes. There are some examples of familial clustering, with one report suggesting autosomal dominant inheritance. The gene locus for familial TAPVC was localized to chromosome 4p13-q12. TAPVC in association with cat eye syndrome is inherited as trisomy of the centromeric portion of chromosome 22q. Another study suggested that dysregulation of the PDGFRA gene causes inflow tract anomalies including TAPVC. Some evidence suggested that maternal exposure during the first 3 months of pregnancy to teratogens like lead may result in TAPVC. Isomerism of the atrial appendages, especially the right one is very highly associated with TAPVC.

Management of patients with TAPVC has evolved and improved significantly over time. Medical therapy is considered supportive but may include balloon dilatation and stenting of an obstructed pulmonary vein or placing the patient on ECMO support for temporary stabilization of the morbidly sick patient prior to surgical repair. Results of surgical repair have also improved even in the very sick baby with obstructed TAPVC, with mortality rates varying between 5 to 15 percent at different institutions.

I had the honor and privilege to work and learn from Jesse Edwards, and join him for what he called "archeological journey" to "dig in" and discover.

Lesions of the Atrioventricular Conduction System after Repair of Ventricular Septal Defect

Relation to Heart Block

By JACK L. TITUS, M.D., GUY W. DAUGHERTY, M.D., JOHN W. KIRKLIN, M.D., AND JESSE E. EDWARDS, M.D.

DURING the repair of congenital defects of the ventricular septum, various disturbances of cardiac function may occur.[1-5] Permanent complete heart block has been the most serious of these disturbances. Right bundle-branch block seems benign. Increased knowledge of the anatomic features of the atrioventricular (AV) conduction system has resulted in surgical technics that have nearly eliminated complete heart block.[5] These technics are based on the assumption that trauma to the AV conduction system occurring during surgical repair of a ventricular septal defect is the cause of postoperative functional disturbances. However, studies documenting an anatomic cause for heart block are few; Reemtsma and associates[6] investigated the lesions responsible for fatal postoperative complete heart block in three cases—one of isolated ventricular septal defect, one of tetralogy of Fallot, and one of common AV canal.

There is general agreement that permanent complete heart block is almost always associated with a lesion in the proximal portion of the AV conduction system.[7, 8] There is not such general agreement concerning the morphology of the conduction system of hearts with right bundle-branch block.[7]

The present study of cases operated upon during a period when heart block was not rare (1955 to 1960) was undertaken to determine whether postoperative interference with AV conduction can be correlated with lesions in the conduction system.

Materials and Methods

In 13 of the 21 human hearts with congenital ventricular septal defects, in which we previously described[9] the location and course of the AV conduction system, surgical closure of ventricular septal defects had been performed. We reviewed these 13 cases in order (1) to establish the presence or absence of injury to the AV conduction system as a result of surgical repair of ventricular septal defects and (2) to correlate morphologic findings with the postoperative functional status of the conduction system.

Since the location and course of the conduction system of the 13 cases under consideration have been previously reported,[9] we have retained in this report the case numbers assigned to the specimens previously. The 13 cases were grouped, according to the situation of the ventricular septal defect, into the following divisions:

1. High ventricular septal defect (immediately beneath aortic cusps) (cases 7 to 15).
2. Multiple defects (cases 18 and 19).
3. Tetralogy of Fallot (cases 20 and 21).

Serial histologic sections of the appropriate areas had already been prepared.[9] These were reviewed, seeking lesions within the conduction system presumed to have resulted from surgical repair of the defect. Since all the patients had died in the immediate postoperative period, the lesions encountered were acute. They included (1) hemorrhage, (2) infarction, and (3) traumatic disruption. Edema was not considered a specific lesion in this study, because its morphologic appearance could not be satisfactorily defined. Lesions were graded 1 to 4, grade 1 representing minimal definite involvement and grade 4 representing involvement of all fibers in any cross section.

The functional status of cardiac conduction after operation was determined from the postoperative electrocardiograms, if available. In some

From the Mayo Clinic and the Mayo Foundation, Rochester, Minnesota.

Abridgment of portion of thesis submitted by Dr. Titus to the Faculty of the Graduate School of the University of Minnesota in partial fulfillment of the requirements for the degree of Doctor of Philosophy in Pathology.

Supported in part by Research Grant H-4014 from the National Heart Institute, U. S. Public Health Service.

cases an electrocardiogram had not been made in the immediate antemortem period. In such situations the most recent observation of the physician who cared for the patient was used as the basis for categorizing the type of cardiac rhythm present. The postoperative functional status of the conduction system was considered in one of the following four categories: (1) sinus rhythm, (2) right bundle-branch block, (3) complete heart block, and (4) postoperative functional status of conduction system not established.

In the 13 cases discussed herein the anomalies were surgically repaired during the years 1955 through 1959.

Results

Type of Lesion

1. High Ventricular Septal Defect (Cases 7 through 15). In these nine specimens, it had been previously found that the AV node was normally located and that the common bundle (bundle of His), or either of its main branches, passed posterior and inferior to the defect. Lesions within some part of the major divisions were found in all specimens except that from case 8. The lesions are listed in table 1 and representative examples are illustrated in figures 1 and 2.

2. Multiple Defects (Cases 18 and 19). The common bundle was related to the anterior rim of a large posterior-basal ventricular septal defect in case 18, but not to a smaller midseptal defect. The bundle and both its branches were hemorrhagic where they lay near the repaired basal defect (fig. 3).

In case 19 (fig. 4) the common bundle passed through the valvular ring in the region of intact ventricular septal myocardium separating the two defects and then lay in the remnant of membranous septum forming the posterior limit of the anterior defect. Hemorrhages were found in the bundle and the bundle branches, and a suture had been placed adjacent to the right branch.

3. Tetralogy of Fallot (Cases 20 and 21). In each specimen, a flame-shaped hemorrhage in the floor of the right atrium emanated from

Table 1

Histopathologic Findings in High Ventricular Septal Defect

Case	AV node	Histopathologic findings Common bundle	Left bundle branch	Right bundle branch
7	Normal	Hemorrhage—grade 3	Hemorrhage—grade 2	Hemorrhage—grade 3
8	Normal	Normal	Normal	Normal
9	Normal	(1) Hemorrhage—grade 4 (2) Injury from suture	(1) Hemorrhage—grade 4 (2) Injury from suture	(1) Hemorrhage—grade 4 (2) Injury from suture
10	Normal	Hemorrhage—grade 1	Not determined	Hemorrhage—grade 3
11	Normal	Not determined	Not determined	(1) Hemorrhage—grade 4 (2) Infarction
12	Normal	(1) Hemorrhage—grade 3 (2) Infarction	(1) Hemorrhage—grade 2 to 3 (2) Infarction	(1) Hemorrhage—grade 4 (2) Infarction
13	Normal	(1) Hemorrhage—grade 4 (2) Infarction	(1) Hemorrhage—grade 4 (2) Infarction	(1) Hemorrhage—grade 4 (2) Infarction
14	Normal	(1) Hemorrhage—grade 3	Hemorrhage—grade 1	(1) Hemorrhage—grade 1
15	Normal	(1) Hemorrhage—grade 4 (2) Infarction (3) Injury from suture	(1) Hemorrhage—grade 2 to 3 (2) Infarction	(1) Hemorrhage—grade 2 to 3 (2) Infarction

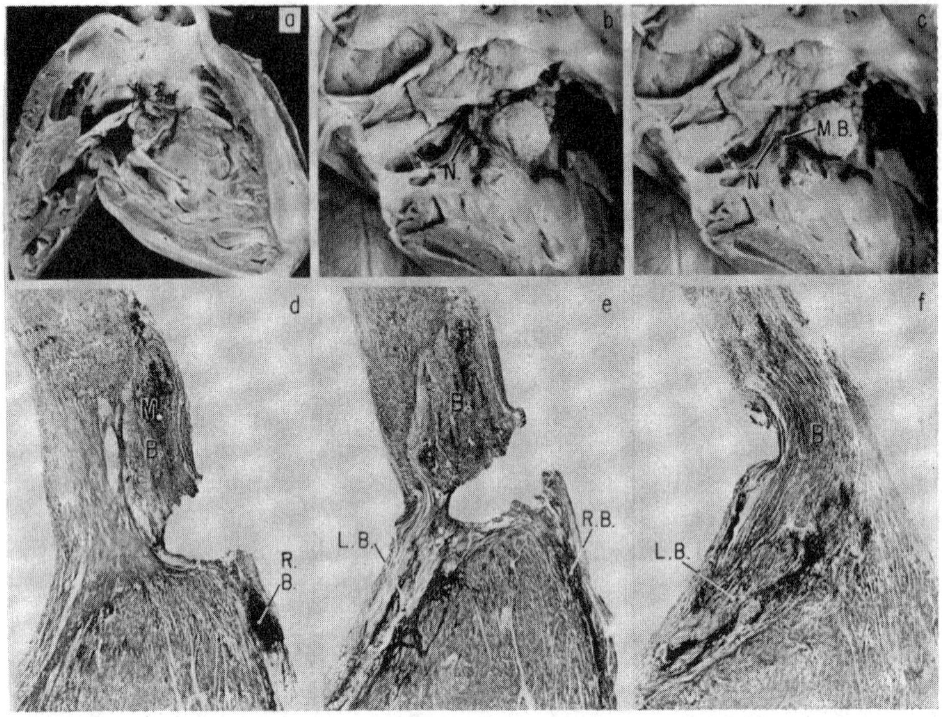

Figure 1

Lesions in conduction system following surgical repair of high ventricular septal defect (case 9). a. *Right ventricle and pulmonary valve. Defect posterior and inferior to crista supraventricularis has been repaired with Ivalon patch.* b. *Right atrium and right ventricle. AV conduction system has been dissected. Suture lies across junction of the AV node (N) and main (common) bundle.* c. *Suture crossing conduction tissue* (b) *removed to better show AV node and main bundle (M.B.), both of which appear hemorrhagic.* d. *Histologic section through remnant of membranous septum forming posterior edge of ventricular septal defect (V.S.D.). Common bundle (M.B.) is hemorrhagic (dark areas) and interrupted in its lower part by defect made with suture. The right bundle branch (R.B.) is hemorrhagic [Mallory-Heidenhain (M-H); × 15].* e. *Branching of common bundle (B) in remnant of membranous septum forming posterior edge of V.S.D. Bundle nearly transected by a suture (defect) and both left bundle branch (L.B.) and right bundle branch (R.B.) are hemorrhagic (Mallory-Heidenhain; × 15).* f. *Common bundle and left bundle branch at posterior-inferior angle of V.S.D. are hemorrhagic (Mallory-Heidenhain; × 15).*

a sutured area in the region of the AV node (fig. 5), and histologically, hemorrhages were seen in the AV node of each heart (fig. 6*a*). In each specimen, the common bundle lay close to the posterior rim of the septal defect, where, in each instance, trauma to the bundle had occurred (fig. 6*b,c,d*).

Correlation of Morphologic Findings with Antemortem Functional Status of AV Conduction System (Fig. 7)

1. Sinus Rhythm. A sinus rhythm was present at the end of the operation in case 8, and no lesions were found in the conduction system.

2. Right Bundle-Branch Block. Three patients manifested right bundle-branch block.

Postoperative electrocardiograms in case 11 demonstrated right bundle-branch block; also, varying degrees of AV block occurred at times, suggesting disturbances (electrocardiographically) in both nodal and bundle areas. A large part of the bundle was not conclusively demonstrated in the specimen, presumably because it lay in an area of infarction in the ventricular septum. The only demonstrably abnormal part of the conduction system was the right bundle branch, which was infarcted and hemorrhagic.

The postoperative electrocardiograms of cases 12 and 18 showed right bundle-branch block. In each specimen, large areas of hemorrhage and infarction were present in the right bundle branch, and lesser degrees of hemorrhage and infarction were found in the common bundle and in the left bundle branch.

3. Complete Heart Block. Complete heart block was proved in six cases (cases 13 to 15 and 19 to 21) and was probable in two others (cases 9 and 10).

In case 9, although a sinus rhythm had been observed at the end of the surgical procedure, a sudden arrhythmia or acute heart

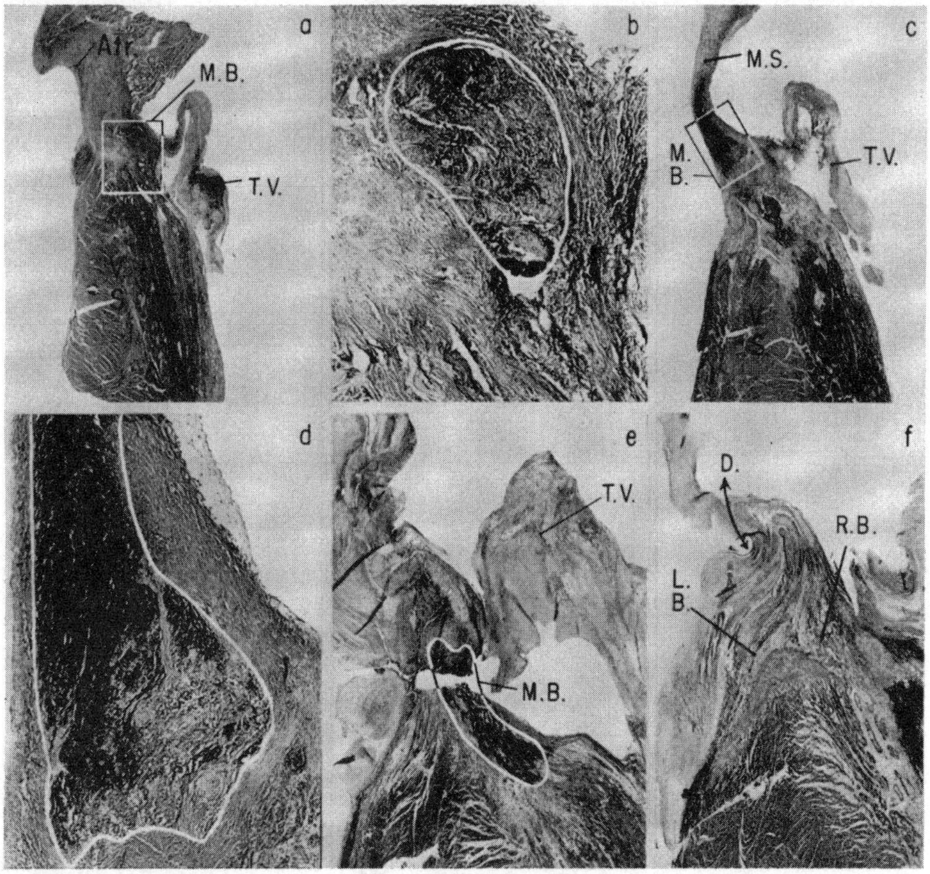

Figure 2

Lesions in conduction system associated with postoperative complete heart block (case 15). a. *Main bundle (dark oval area within rectangle) penetrating fibrous valvular ring is hemorrhagic, as are portions of septal leaflet of tricuspid valve (T.V.) and ventricular septum (V.S.). Portion of atrium (Atr.) is also shown (Mallory-Heidenhain; × 7).* b. *Higher magnification of area enclosed by rectangle in* a *shows hemorrhage in main bundle (outlined) (Mallory-Heidenhain; × 40).* c. *Main bundle (within rectangle M.B.) in remnant of membranous septum (M.S.) forming the posterior edge of V.S.D. is hemorrhagic (Mallory-Heidenhain; × 7).* d. *Higher magnification of area enclosed by rectangle in* c *shows hemorrhage in main bundle (Mallory-Heidenhain; × 40).* e. *Main bundle (outlined) has been transected by a suture. This section is near the posterior-inferior angle of V.S.D. (Mallory-Heidenhain; × 12).* f. *Main bundle branching into left and right branches at the posterior-inferior angle of the surgically closed V.S.D. (D). Dark areas within conduction tissues are hemorrhages (Mallory-Heidenhain; × 12).*

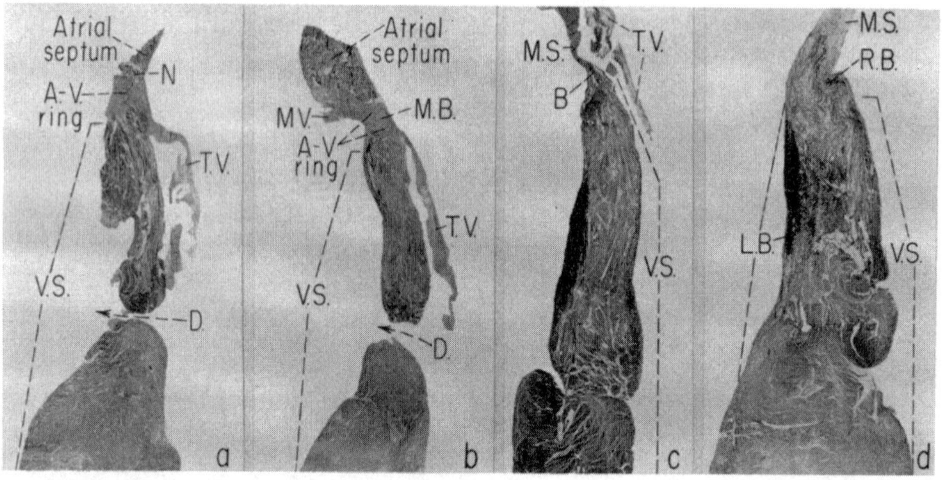

Figure 3

Postoperative right bundle-branch block in case of repaired, large posterior-basal V.S.D. (case 18). a. *Normal AV node is in plane of defect in ventricular septum (Mallory-Heidenhain; × 4).* b. *Normal main bundle passes through fibrous AV ring in plane of defect. "M.V." indicates portion of mitral valve (Mallory-Heidenhain; × 4).* c. *Main bundle (B) branches in lower portion of intact membranous septum just anterior to large, posteriorly situated V.S.D. Dark area along the left endocardial surface is hemorrhage (Mallory-Heidenhain; × 7).* d. *Right and left bundle branches are hemorrhagic just distal to origin from common bundle. Section represents area approximately 3 mm. anterior to section shown in c. (Mallory-Heidenhain; × 7).*

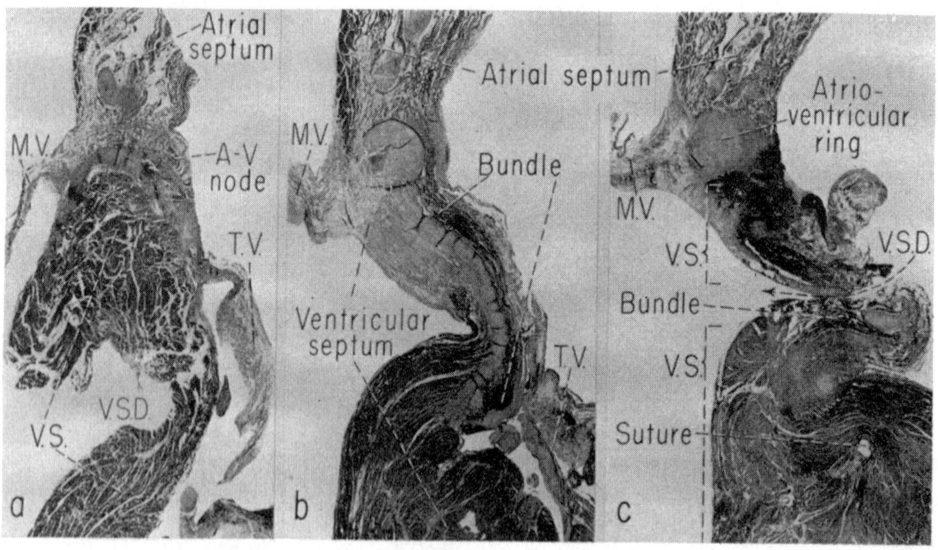

Figure 4

Postoperative complete heart block in case of repaired V.S.D. (case 19). Two defects were present: unrepaired posterior defect just below tricuspid ring and sutured defect posterior and inferior to the crista supraventricularis. a. *Normal AV node is in same plane as anterior extremity of more posterior V.S.D. "M.V." and "T.V." indicate mitral and tricuspid valves, respectively (Mallory-Heidenhain; × 8).* b. *Common bundle near posterior rim of more anterior V.S.D. is hemorrhagic (Mallory-Heidenhain; × 8).* c. *Hemorrhagic disrupted common bundle immediately subjacent to posterior-inferior extremity of V.S.D. (Mallory-Heidenhain; × 8).*

block was thought to have occurred terminally. Hemorrhages and a suture involved the common bundle and both bundle branches.

Another patient (case 10) had temporary complete heart block during part of the operation. Asystole, refractory to an electric pacemaker, occurred 12 hours after the operation. The bundle of His was hemorrhagic (grade 2).

In cases 13, 14, 15, and 19 complete heart block was present at the end of the operative procedure. Hemorrhages or areas of infarction or both were found in the common bundle in each specimen. In cases 13, 15, and 19 the bundle branches were similarly involved.

During operative correction of the tetralogy of Fallot (cases 20 and 21), complete heart block developed and persisted. In each instance, hemorrhage (grade 1 or 2) involved the AV node, and marked traumatic disruption of the bundle and both bundle branches was present.

4. Functional Status of the Conduction System Not Determined. In case 7, postoperative electrocardiograms were not available; therefore, this case was not classifiable according to the antemortem functional status. Histologically, hemorrhages were found in the common bundle, the right branch and, to a lesser degree, in the left branch.

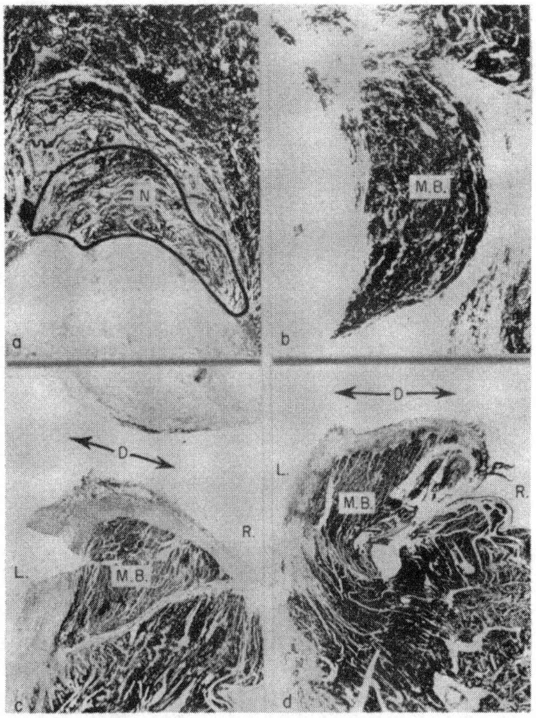

Figure 6

Postoperative, complete heart block in case of tetralogy of Fallot (case 20). a. *Hemorrhage in AV node (outlined) and surrounding atrial myocardium (Mallory-Heidenhain; × 50).* b. *Main bundle in fibrous valvular ring is hemorrhagic (Mallory-Heidenhain; × 50).* c. *Main bundle in posterior rim of V.S.D. is hemorrhagic. The split in septal endocardium on left (L) is an artifact. (Mallory-Heidenhain; × 20).* d. *Main bundle subjacent to endocardial lining of posterior-inferior rim of defect is hemorrhagic and disrupted by suture. "L." and "R." designate left and right sides of ventricular septum (Mallory-Heidenhain; × 20).*

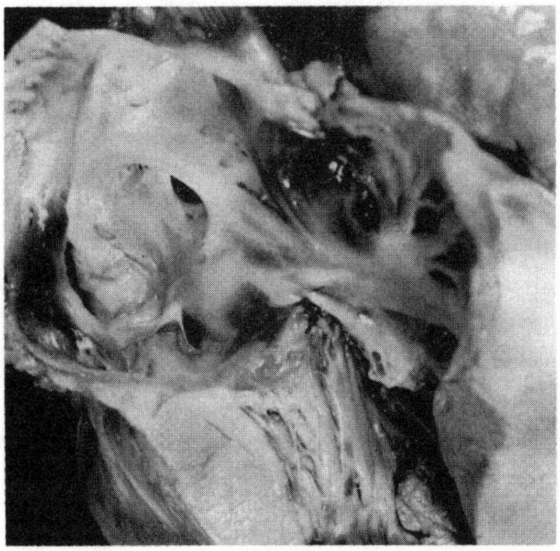

Figure 5

Floor of right atrium in repaired tetralogy of Fallot (case 21). A flame-shaped hemorrhage (dark area) in region of AV node emanates from a suture. Complete heart block occurred postoperatively.

Summary and Conclusions

Lesions of the atrioventricular (AV) conduction system related to the surgical repair of ventricular septal defects were sought in 13 human hearts from patients who were operated on from 1955 through 1959 and who died in the postoperative period. Lesions were found in 12 of the 13 cases (fig. 8).

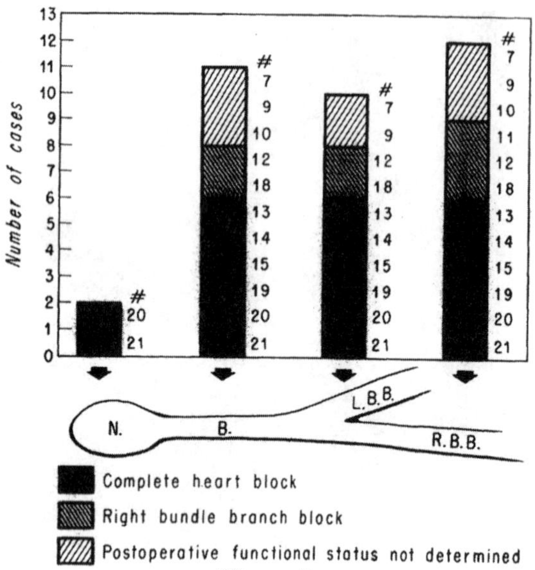

Figure 7

Correlation of postoperative functional status and location of lesions within AV conduction system is schematically represented. "L.B.B." represents left bundle branch; and "R.B.B.," right bundle branch. Numbers beside each column refer to case numbers (see text).

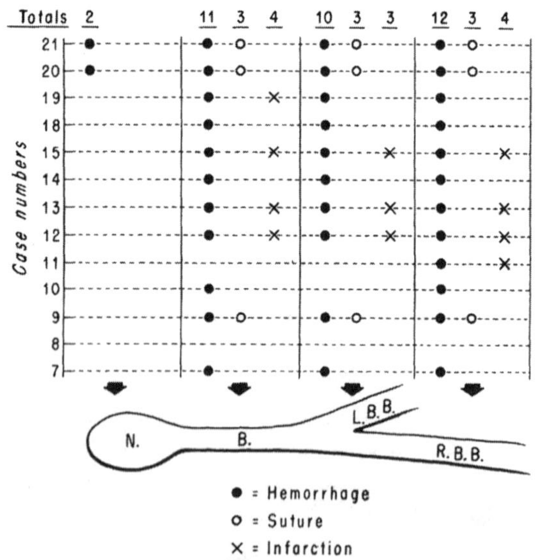

Figure 8

Types of lesions with locations in conduction system are indicated. No such lesions were found in case 8.

Complete heart block was demonstrated postoperatively in six of nine patients whose hearts showed major lesions in the AV node or the main bundle of His, or both. In two of the nine, available evidence suggested that complete heart block had been present. In the other case, records were insufficient to permit evaluation of the functional status of the conduction tissue.

Three patients had right bundle-branch block. In each of their hearts, lesions were observed in the right branch; in two, lesions also were observed in the common bundle.

We conclude that, in patients operated on for closure of ventricular septal defects, postoperative interference with AV conduction may be correlated with lesions in the conduction system.

References

1. KIRKLIN, J. W., HARSHBARGER, H. G., DONALD, D. E., AND EDWARDS, J. E.: Surgical correction of ventricular septal defect: Anatomic and technical considerations. J. Thoracic Surg. **33:** 45, 1957.
2. LILLEHEI, C. W.: Discussion. J. Thoracic Surg. **33:** 57, 1957.
3. LAUER, R. M., ONGLEY, P. A., DUSHANE, J. W., AND KIRKLIN, J. W.: Heart block after repair of ventricular septal defect in children. Circulation **22:** 526, 1960.
4. BRISTOW, J. D., KASSEBAUM, D. G., STARR, A., AND GRISWOLD, H. E.: Observations on the occurrence of right bundle-branch block following open repair of ventricular septal defects. Circulation **22:** 896, 1960.
5. KIRKLIN, J. W., MCGOON, D. C., AND DUSHANE, J. W.: Surgical treatment of ventricular septal defect. J. Thoracic Surg. **40:** 763, 1960.
6. REEMTSMA, K., DELGADO, J. P., AND CREECH, O. JR.: Heart block following intracardiac surgery: Localization of conduction tissue injury. J. Thoracic Surg. **39:** 688, 1960.
7. LEV, M.: The conduction system. *In* Gould, S. E.: Pathology of the Heart. Ed. 2. Springfield, Illinois, Charles C Thomas, Publisher, 1960, p. 156.
8. LEV, M.: The anatomic basis for disturbances in conduction and cardiac arrhythmias. Prog. Cardiovasc. Dis. **2:** 360, 1960.
9. TITUS, J. L., DAUGHERTY, G. W., AND EDWARDS, J. E.: Anatomy of the atrioventricular conduction system in ventricular septal defect. Circulation **28:** 72, 1963.

Anatomy of the Atrioventricular Conduction System in Ventricular Septal Defect

By JACK L. TITUS, M.D., GUY W. DAUGHERTY, M.D., AND JESSE E. EDWARDS, M.D.

IT IS important to know the location, in relation to congenital ventricular septal defects, of the atrioventricular (AV) conduction system of the heart, in order to avoid damaging conduction tissue during surgical correction of such defects.[1, 2] Furthermore, knowledge of the anatomic relationship of the ventricular septal defect to the conduction system may cast light on the embryology of various types of defects. Therefore, having familiarized ourselves with the gross anatomic and histologic features of the proximal portions of the AV conduction system in normal human hearts,[3] we undertook an investigation of the location and course of these structures in hearts having congenital ventricular septal defects. Interest centered on the AV node (node of Tawara), AV bundle (common bundle or bundle of His), and the proximal portions of the right and left bundle branches.

In the normal heart, the AV node is situated in the floor of the right atrium on the fibrous AV ring, at or just anterior to the coronary sinus ostium; the AV bundle extends anteriorly and inferiorly from the node through the fibrous valvular ring into the inferior part of the membranous septum; the left bundle branches are usually given off as discrete muscular fascicles over a broad extent of the common bundle, usually beginning at a point just distal to the fibrous valvular ring and ending at the posterior-inferior angle of the membranous septum; and the right bundle branch, usually forming a continuation of the common bundle, passes obliquely anteriorly and inferiorly through the upper part of the ventricular septum toward the crista supraventricularis.[3]

From the Mayo Clinic and the Mayo Foundation, Rochester, Minnesota.

Abridgment of portion of thesis submitted by Dr. Titus to the Faculty of the Graduate School of the University of Minnesota in partial fulfillment of the requirements for the degree of Doctor of Philosophy in Pathology.

Supported in part by Research Grant H-4014 of the National Heart Institute, U. S. Public Health Service.

Historical Notes

Mönckeberg,[4] Keith,[5] Abbott,[6] Yater and co-workers,[7] and Yater[8] all found that AV bundles were situated along the lower rims of ventricular septal defects. Kirklin and coauthors,[1] Lillehei,[2] and Rodriguez and Wofford[9] concluded from their surgical experiences that the bundle is situated at or near the posterior-inferior margin of the defect when the defect is inferior to the crista supraventricularis. Morris[10] pointed out that in the fetus the bundle lies along the posterior and inferior margins of the foramen of the unclosed septum. Reemtsma and Copenhaver[11] found the bundle along the posterior-inferior aspect of a "membranous" ventricular septal defect, but not closely related to a more posterior defect. In a study of the conduction systems in 15 malformed hearts, Truex and Bishof[12] found the common bundles and their branches along the posterior-inferior margins of septal defects in 13 specimens. The bundle and its branches passed anterior to a lower defect in one specimen and close to the anterior margin of the defect in another. Reemtsma, Copenhaver, and Creech[13] found the bundles in the posterior-inferior margins of "membranous" ventricular septal defects, but not closely related to high muscular defects.

Lev studied the conduction system in hearts with persistent common atrioventricular canal[14] and, later, in hearts with tetralogy of Fallot.[15] In these studies, he found the following variations from the usual situations:

1. The common bundle was on the left side of the septum below the defect. (It may also occur on the left in normal hearts.) 2. The right bundle often divided into two or more parts. 3. The left bundle was more compact than usual. 4. The AV node deviated "horizontally" from its usual location, if a persistent left superior vena cava entered the coronary sinus. In hearts with ventricular septal defects, Lev[16, 17] found the bundles to be close to the posterior margins of the defects, except when the defects were situated posteriorly.

Materials and Methods

Specimens

Beginning in 1957, we selected 21 hearts for this study. Each heart had a ventricular septal defect, either as the only anomaly or as part of a recognized complex, and each had been obtained at necropsy during the years 1954 through 1959 and had been preserved in formalin for up to 3 years. Specimens were selected without regard to location of the defect, presence of other cardiac anomalies, or age or sex of the deceased patient.

Eight hearts came from patients who had not been operated on and 13 from patients whose ventricular septal defect had been closed surgically.

Methods of Examination

In 12 instances, gross dissection of the conduction system preceded histologic examination of serial sections, while, in nine instances, only histologic examination of serial sections was done.

When the heart was viewed from the right side, the area included in the block cut for histologic study extended approximately from the level of the coronary sinus ostium posteriorly to the crista supraventricularis anteriorly. The anterior portion of the block included the posterior-inferior rim of the defect. The block also included a portion (approximately 1 cm.) of the atrial septum above the AV groove. Below the AV groove, the full thickness of the interventricular septum to approximately 0.5 cm. below the inferiormost limit of the ventricular septal defect was included. The blocks were cut serially so that individual sections were approximately 7 μ thick. Then every twentieth section (every tenth in the case of small hearts) was stained with hematoxylin and eosin. The next succeeding section to the hematoxylin and eosin-stained section was stained with the Mallory-Heidenhain stain.

Sections were studied at magnifications of 35 to 400 and, occasionally, of 1000. The number of sections of each specimen examined varied considerably, but usually ranged from 250 to 350. (From previous studies,[3] it was known that examination of every section was not necessary for a "geographic" study of the conduction system.)

Classification of Defects Studied

The classification of ventricular septal defects proposed by Becu and co-workers[18] was modified to give the following groupings of the 21 specimens examined:

Group 1 (cases 1 through 14). Defect in right ventricular outflow tract, posterior and inferior to crista supraventricularis.

Group 2 (case 15). Defect not in right ventricular outflow tract.

Group 3 (cases 16 through 19). Multiple defects.

Group 4 (cases 20 and 21). Tetralogy of Fallot.

Clinical and General Pathologic Features of Cases Studied

The ages of the patients from whom the specimens were obtained ranged from 2 days to 37 years. The specimens included the hearts of 12 males and eight females. (The sex and other clinical features of the patient represented by one specimen could not be obtained.)

The factors responsible for death in these cases were most often cardiac, either related to the congenital anomaly (most cases) or a complication of it (for example, one patient died of brain abscess secondary to subacute bacterial endocarditis). In a few instances, death was related to the presence of associated noncardiac congenital anomalies.

Many surgically repaired specimens represented an early period in intracardiac surgery when closure of the defect frequently was accomplished by using an Ivalon sponge, a procedure less commonly employed in current reparative procedures.

Results

Group 1

The location of the conduction system and its relation to the ventricular septal defect were similar in the 14 cases in this group. Therefore, the generally prevailing circumstances will be described and illustrated (figs. 1 to 5), and exceptions will be noted.

The AV node usually occupied its normal position in the base of the right atrium. In two instances (cases 1 and 2), it was situated slightly posterior to the usual location. No morphologic abnormalities of nodal structure were noted.

The common bundle penetrated the fibrous

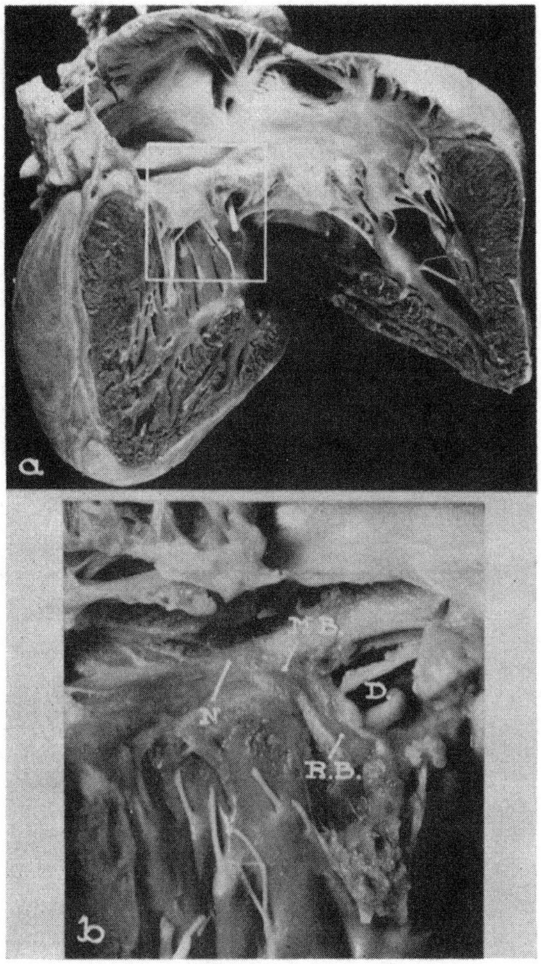

Figure 1

AV conduction system in usual type of ventricular septal defect (case 3). a. *Open heart, showing right ventricle and right atrium, has probe in ventricular septal defect. Outline includes area illustrated in* b. b. *"N" is AV node; "MB" is main (common) bundle; "D" is ventricular septal defect; "RB" is right bundle branch.*

valvular ring and then entered the remnant of membranous septum that usually formed the posterior rim of the ventricular septal defect. In this location, conduction tissue was intimately related to the margin of the defect. Along the posterior or posterior-inferior aspect of the ventricular septal defect, the bundle gave off left bundle branches.

The left bundle branches promptly fanned out over the left ventricular septal surface so that the bulk of these fibers was not intimately related to the defect. Generally, all the left bundle-branch fibers had been given off from the common bundle before it reached the level of the posterior-inferior angle of the defect.

The right bundle branch pursued its usual anterior-inferior course. In some instances it was intimately associated with the inferior margin of the defect, while in other cases it was inferior to the margin.

In 13 of these 14 cases, some part of the conduction system was close to the posterior

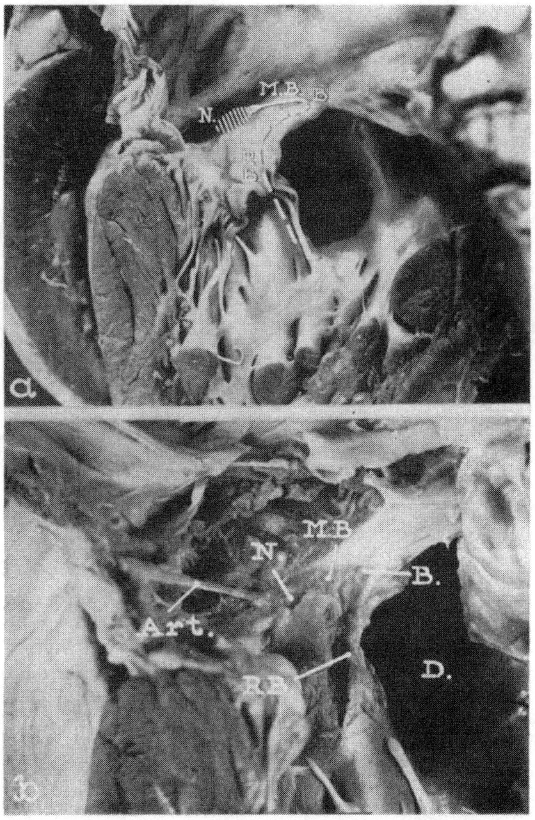

Figure 2

AV conduction system in large ventricular septal defect of persistent-common-AV-canal type (case 4). a. *Course of AV conduction system superimposed on right ventricular view of ventricular septal defect. (Reproduced with permission from Neufeld, H. N., Titus, J. L., DuShane, J. W., Burchell, H. B., and Edwards, J. E.: Isolated ventricular septal defect of the persistent common atrioventricular canal type.* Circulation **23:** *685, 1961).* b. *Dissection of conduction system. "Art." is artery to node; "B." is branching bundle.*

or inferior margin of the defect, or both. In the single instance in which no such relationship prevailed (case 5), the defect was small, relative to the large size of the heart. In one instance (case 9), the left bundle branch lay close to the posterior-inferior rim of the defect, and the right bundle branch originated posterior to the defect. In three cases (4, 6, and 12), the bundle fibers bordered the posterior-superior angle of the defect (figs. 2 and 5), and then coursed inferiorly in the curved posterior rim of the defect, forming an arc. Two of the hearts manifesting this relationship (cases 4 and 6) had large defects of the sort referred to as "persistent common atrioventricular canal type" of ventricular septal defect.[19]

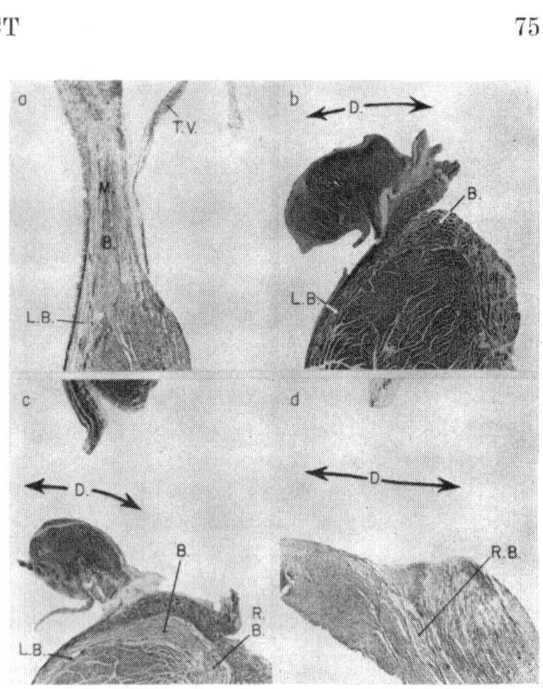

Figure 4

Continuation of figure 3. a. *Left bundle branch (L.B.) shown originating from main bundle in remnant of membranous septum forming posterior limit of ventricular septal defect (Mallory-Heidenhain; × 30).* b. *Bundle beginning to branch near posterior-inferior angle of ventricular septal defect (Mallory-Heidenhain; × 15).* c. *Bundle (B) branching into left and right branches at posterior-inferior angle of ventricular septal defect (Mallory-Heidenhain; × 15).* d. *Right bundle branch in midseptum along inferior edge of ventricular septal defect (Mallory-Heidenhain; × 30).*

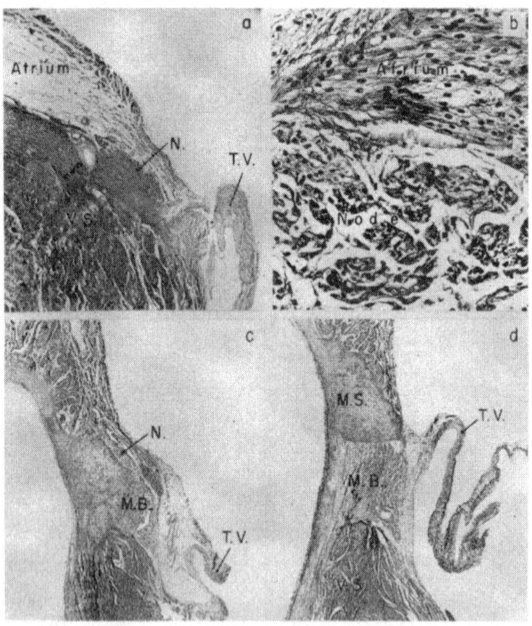

Figure 3

Representative serial histologic sections of conduction system in usual type of ventricular septal defect. a. *AV node lies in floor of right atrium. "T.V." is tricuspid valve (septal leaflet); "V.S." is ventricular septum (Mallory-Heidenhain; × 20).* b. *AV node and adjacent atrial myocardium (hematoxylin and eosin; × 300).* c. *Origin of main bundle from AV node (Mallory-Heidenhain; × 30).* d. *Main bundle in inferior portion of remnant of membranous septum (M.S.) (Mallory-Heidenhain; × 30).*

Group 2

In one specimen (case 15), the ventricular septal defect was situated not in the ventricular outflow tract but in the region of the AV valve. The defect measured 7 mm. in diameter and involved the membranous portion of the septum just above the septal leaflet of the tricuspid valve, resulting in a communication between the right atrium and left ventricle (fig. 6).

Histologic examination revealed that the AV node was normally situated and that the more distal part of the common bundle lay within remnants of the membranous septum close to the posterior edge of the defect. The bundle coursed along the posterior-inferior rim of the defect and gave off its main branches in the region of the inferior edge of the defect (fig. 6).

Group 3

Four hearts with multiple ventricular septal defects were investigated.

Case 16. The more anterior of two ventricular septal defects was located in the common position of such defects with a portion of the membranous septum forming its posterior rim. Posterior to this defect (to the left in figure 7*a*), a column of apparently normal ventricular muscle separated the anterior defect from a second defect, fairly close to the AV valvular ring, but separated from it by a rim of muscular tissue.

The AV node was situated somewhat posterior to its usual site (fig. 7*b*). The common bundle originated in the normal way; and its anatomic relations appeared to be normal (fig. 7*c*), except that, at the posterior-inferior angle of the anterior ventricular septal defect, it was situated closer to the left ventricular endocardial surface than to the right (fig. 7*d*). The bundle remained intimately related to the endocardial lining along the posterior and inferior edges of the defect for nearly 2 mm. The main part of the left bundle branched off while the common bundle was under the ventricular septal defect (fig. 7*e*). The continuation of the common bundle, as the right bundle branch, turned more apexward at approximately the level of the midplane of the defect; it thus quickly lost its intimate relationship to the defect. However,

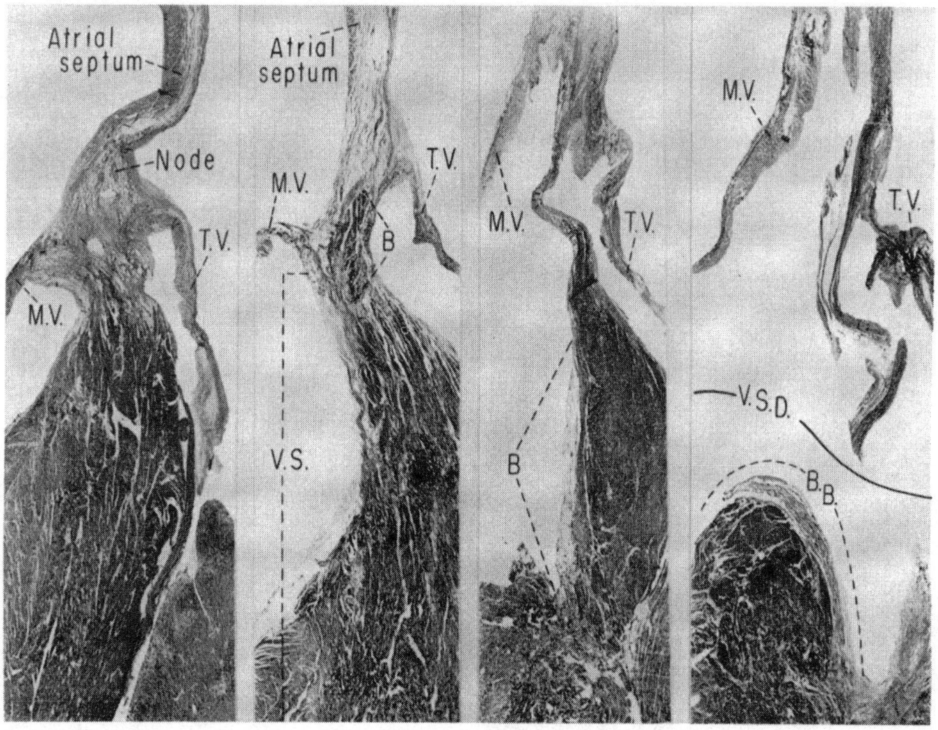

Figure 5

Histologic sections representative of large ventricular septal defect (case 6). The AV node and first part of common bundle (B) are normally situated. Bundle descends on left side of septum (V.S.) in posterior rim of defect, and branches (B.B.) at posterior-inferior angle of defect. "M.V." is mitral valve leaflet, and "T.V." is tricuspid valve leaflet (Mallory-Heidenhain; × 5). (Reproduced with permission from Neufeld, H. N., Titus, J. L., DuShane, J. W., Burchell, H. B., and Edwards, J. E.: Isolated ventricular septal defect of the persistent common atrioventricular canal type. Circulation **23:** *685, 1961.)*

left bundle branches were still close to the margin of the defect.

Case 17. Examination of the heart of a 4-day-old girl revealed two ventricular septal defects. The more posterior one was situated under the septal leaflet of the tricuspid valve, close to the tricuspid ring and on a level with the ostium of the coronary sinus. It measured 4 mm. in diameter. The more anterior defect was located under the area of the commissure between the anterior and septal leaflets of the tricuspid valve and between the tricuspid ring and the crista supraventricularis. It measured 5 mm. in diameter. The ventricular septum intervening between the defects was not remarkable.

Histologic examination disclosed that the AV node, the common bundle, and the bundle branches were normally situated and constructed. None of these structures was closely related to either defect.

Case 18. This heart, from a 6-year-old boy, had multiple ventricular septal defects. Situated in the posterior part of the ventricular septum, inferior to the septal leaflet of the

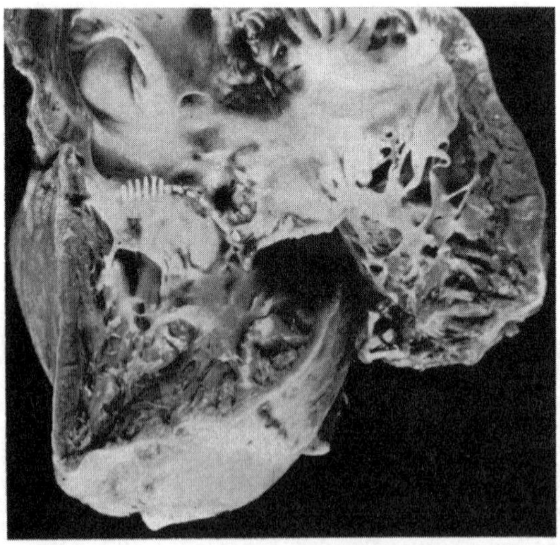

Figure 6

Open right heart of case 15 shows ventricular septal defect forming right-atrial-left-ventricular communication; location of conduction system is superimposed. Hatched oval represents the AV node; short lines represent course of common bundle; longer lines represent right bundle branch.

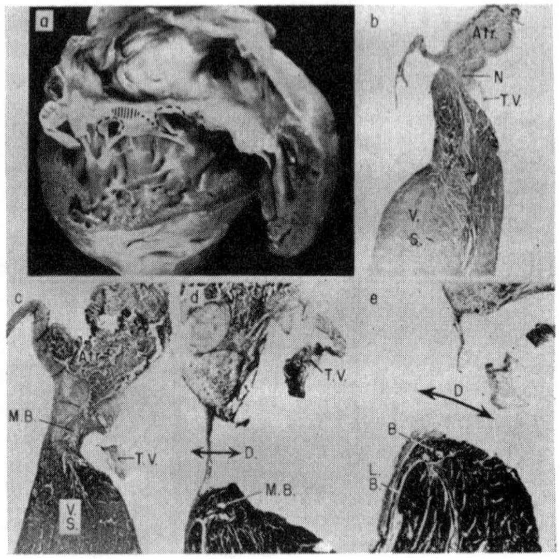

Figure 7

Conduction system of heart with two ventricular septal defects (case 16). a. *Rims of defects, hidden by the tricuspid valve, are outlined as in figure 6.* b. *Relation of node to atrium ("Atr."), tricuspid valve, and ventricular septum is shown (Mallory-Heidenhain; × 10).* c. *Main bundle in remnant of membranous septum which forms posterior rim or more anterior ventricular septal defect (Mallory-Heidenhain; × 10).* d. *Main bundle in lower posterior rim of ventricular septal defect (Mallory-Heidenhain; × 15).* e. *Bundle branching under posterior-inferior angle of ventricular septal defect (Mallory-Heidenhain; × 15).*

tricuspid valve, was a large, fan-shaped defect measuring approximately 3.3 by 2.5 cm., which had been closed by suturing (fig. 8). The posterior (dorsal) margin of this defect was 0.8 cm. below the tricuspid ring, and the anterior (ventral) margin was 1.5 cm. below the ring. In addition to this large repaired deficiency, there was a 1-cm.-in-diameter defect near the middle of the septum, which had been sutured. Lower and more anterior in the septum were two small (probe-patent only) defects in the muscle.

Histologically, the AV node was essentially normal in all respects. Because of the anterior extent of the posterobasal defect, the common bundle and its penetrating portions lay in the same plane and the bundle branched on a plane immediately anterior to the most anterior extent of this defect (fig. 9). The duction system of the specimen from a 3½-year-old boy revealed the following: The AV node was in its normal location. The bundle of His penetrated the fibrous valvular ring and came into intimate relation with the mid-posterior edge of the defect. The bundle followed the curved posterior rim of the defect and continued subendocardially along the posterior rim of the defect. It branched into its right and left branches at approximately the level of the posterior-inferior angle of the defect.

Case 21. Histologic examination of this specimen from a 6-year-old girl with tetralogy of Fallot showed that the AV node was in a normal location. At the level where the common bundle was just completing its penetration of the valvular ring, it was beneath the endocardium of the posterior rim of the defect close to the defect's posterior-superior angle. The bundle tissue, remaining subendocardial, then followed the curved posterior rim inferiorly. The main left bundle branched off, over a broad area, along the posterior edge of the defect. As the bundle (mainly right bundle-branch fibers) neared the posterior-inferior angle of the defect, it was situated more toward the left side of the apex of the intact septal tissue under the defect. It remained just under the endocardial lining of the defect; it could not be traced satisfactorily beyond the level corresponding, approximately, to the posterior-inferior angle of the defect, because of marked disruption of all tissue by sutures and hemorrhage resulting from the surgical procedure.

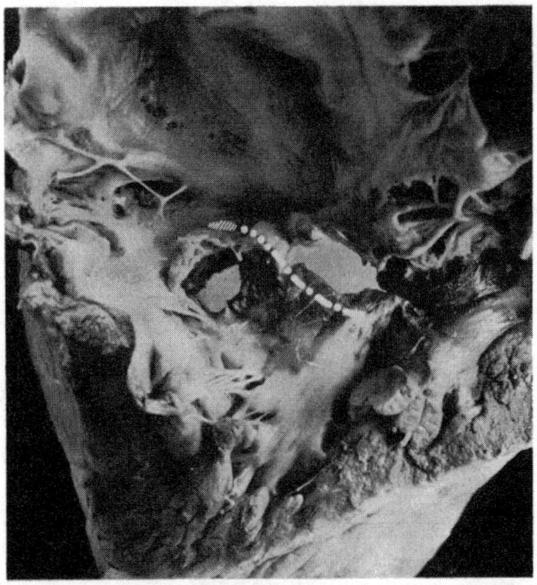

Figure 10

Conduction system between two ventricular septal defects (case 19). The broken line is the branching bundle and its continuation as the right bundle branch. (Reproduced with permission from Neufeld, H. M., Titus, J. L., DuShane, J. W., Burchell, H. B., and Edwards, J. E.: Isolated ventricular septal defect of the persistent common atrioventricular canal type. Circulation **23**: *685, 1961.)*

Discussion

Types of Defects Studied

Fourteen of the 21 specimens had isolated ventricular septal defects posterior and inferior to the crista supraventricularis, which is in accord with the incidences of different types of defects as determined by surveys of surgically treated cases.[1, 20] No defects superior to the crista supraventricularis were studied; however, Edwards[21] has pointed out that such defects would not be closely related to the conduction system.

Although our classification differed somewhat from others proposed in the literature,[18] especially concerning classification of tetralogy of Fallot,[15] we intended only that it serve as a basis for grouping our material. Arguments relative to its embryologic or functional soundness are, therefore, irrelevant.

Location of Conduction System in Ventricular Septal Defect

In this study of 21 hearts with various types of ventricular septal defects, the following generalization regarding the location of the AV conduction system evolved: The course of the conduction tissue follows a normal pattern, except when a ventricular septal defect is interposed. In that circumstance, the conduction tissue follows a deviated course as close to normal as the defect will allow.

Defect Posterior and Inferior to the Crista Supraventricularis. In this type of defect our findings relative to the conduction system agreed with those previously described in the literature.[4, 5, 7, 11–13, 16] Variations from the normal situation[3] included slight posterior displacement of the AV node, in two specimens, and origination of the right bundle branch from the common bundle before that of left bundle branches, in one instance (case 9).

The position of the bundle within the septum was central in five of the hearts, closer to the left in six, closer to the right in one, and not accurately determined in two.

Mahaim fibers were noted in most of these cases.

In none of these cases were any parts of the proximal divisions of the AV conduction system related to superior-anterior edges of the septal defect.

Defect Not in the Ventricular Outflow Tract (case 15). The conduction system was related to this defect in essentially the same manner as in the usual type of defect.

Multiple Defects. Truex and Bishof[12] studied two specimens with two defects each; however, since the exact location of the defects was not specified for either, comparison of their findings with ours was not possible.

In hearts with both a posterior septal defect and an anterior defect in the membranous septum (cases 16 and 19), the conduction system was not closely related to the more posterior defect, but had an intimate relationship to the posterior and inferior edges of the more anterior defect.

In a heart (case 17) with a small anterior defect of the common type and a small posterior defect, no part of the conduction system was intimately related to either defect, apparently because both defects were too small to impinge on the tissues normally carrying conduction fibers.

The location of the posterior defect of the specimen representing case 18 was basically similar to that of case 16; however, because of its large size, its anterior margin was closely related to the common bundle and its branches as these traversed the intact septum. A similar situation in specimens with posterior defects had been reported previously in the description of two of the specimens examined by Truex and Bishof,[12] and Lev[17] speculated that such a relationship might occur in defects in this location.

Defect of Tetralogy of Fallot. Specimen 4 of Truex and Bishof,[12] though not labeled as such, seemed to be an example of Fallot's tetralogy, according to their description. In it, an aberrant fascicle of the right bundle branch passed above the defect and then descended in the anterior edge of the defect. The bulk of the bundle tissue, however, came into close relation with the defect at its posterior-superior angle and followed the posterior, then inferior, edges of the deficiency. Lev[15] did not observe any such aberrant branches in the four cases of tetralogy of Fallot that he studied, in each of which the bundle was situated on the left side of the septum below the defect.

No aberrant branch of the right bundle was found in either of the examples of the tetralogy of Fallot studied in the present series. Otherwise, our study of the two cases in the present series confirmed the essential parts of the works previously mentioned. The relationship of the AV conduction system to the defect was the same as in those hearts with the usual type of ventricular septal defect.

Summary

The major parts of the atrioventricular conduction system of the human heart were traced in 21 instances of ventricular septal defect: 19 were examples of variously located uncomplicated ventricular septal defects and two of the tetralogy of Fallot.

In the presence of a ventricular septal defect, the conduction system was found to have a normal course, except when the ventricular septal defect lay in a position normally occupied by the conduction system. In each specimen with a defect posterior and inferior to the crista supraventricularis, the conduction system occupied a position posterior and inferior to the defect. In no instance did the conduction system occupy a position superior to a defect of this type. Defects located in the posterobasal portion of the muscular part of the ventricular septum sometimes were posterior to the main parts of the conduction system, so that the conduction tissue was related to the anterior edge of the defect. No example of a defect lying superior to the crista supraventricularis was studied. In our two examples of tetralogy of Fallot, the position of the conduction system was essentially similar to that occurring in the usual variety of ventricular septal defect, that is, posterior and inferior to the crista supraventricularis.

References

1. KIRKLIN, J. W., HARSHBARGER, H. G., DONALD, D. E., AND EDWARDS, J. E.: Surgical correction of ventricular septal defect: Anatomic and technical consideration. J. Thoracic Surg. 33: 45, 1957.
2. LILLEHEI, C. W.: Discussion. J. Thoracic Surg. 33: 57, 1957.
3. TITUS, J. L., DAUGHERTY, G. W., AND EDWARDS, J. E.: Anatomy of the normal human atrioventricular conduction system. Unpublished data.
4. MÖNCKEBERG, J. G.: Die Missbildunges des Herzens. *In* Henke, F., and Lubarsh, O.: Handbuch der Speziellen pathologischen Anatomie und Histologie. Berlin, Verlag von Julius Springer, 1924, Bd. 2, pp. 183.
5. KEITH, A.: Malformations of the heart. Lancet 2: 519, 1909.
6. ABBOTT, M. E.: Quoted by Yater, W. M., Lyon, J. A., and McNabb. P. E.[7]
7. YATER, W. M., LYON, J. A., AND MCNABB, P. E.: Congenital heart block: Review and report of second case of complete heart block studied by serial sections through the conduction system. J.A.M.A. 100: 1831, 1933.
8. YATER, W. M.: Congenital heart-block: Review of the literature; report of a case with incomplete heterotoxy; the electrocardiogram in dextrocardia. Am. J. Dis. Child. 38: 112, 1929.
9. RODRIGUEZ, J. A., AND WOFFORD, J. L.: Surgical anatomy of the cardiac septa. S. Forum 8: 274, 1957.
10. MORRIS, E. W.: The interventricular septum. Thorax 12: 304, 1957.
11. REEMTSMA, K., AND COPENHAVER, W. M.: Anatomic studies of the cardiac conduction system in congenital malformations of the heart. Circulation 17: 271, 1958.
12. TRUEX, R. C., AND BISHOF, J. K.: Conduction system in human hearts with interventricular septal defects. J. Thoracic Surg. 35: 421, 1958.
13. REEMTSMA, K., COPENHAVER, W. M., AND CREECH, O., JR.: The cardiac conduction system in congenital anomalies of the heart: Studies on its embryology, anatomy, and function. Surgery 44: 99, 1958.
14. LEV, M.: The architecture of the conduction system in congenital heart disease. I. Common atrioventricular orifice. Arch. Path. 65: 174, 1958.
15. LEV, M.: The architecture of the conduction system in congenital heart disease. II. Tetralogy of Fallot. Arch. Path. 67: 572, 1959.
16. LEV, M.: The architecture of the conduction system in congenital heart disease. III. Ventricular septal defect. Arch. Path. 70: 529, 1960.
17. LEV, M.: The pathologic anatomy of ventricular septal defects. Dis. Chest 35: 533, 1959.
18. BECU, L. M., FONTANA, R. S., DUSHANE, J. W., KIRKLIN, J. W., BURCHELL, H. B., AND EDWARDS, J. E.: Anatomic and pathologic studies in ventricular septal defect. Circulation 14: 349, 1956.
19. NEUFELD, H. N., TITUS, J. L., DUSHANE, J. W., BURCHELL, H. B., AND EDWARDS, J. E.: Isolated ventricular septal defect of the persistent common atrioventricular canal type. Circulation 23: 685, 1961.
20. WARDEN, H. E., DEWALL, R. A., COHEN, M., VARCO, R. L., AND LILLEHEI, C. W.: A surgical-pathologic classification for isolated ventricular septal defects and for those observed in Fallot's tetralogy based on observations made on 120 patients during repair under direct vision. J. Thoracic Surg. 33: 21, 1957.
21. EDWARDS, J. E.: Malformations of the ventricular septal complex. *In* Gould, S. E.: Pathology of the Heart. Ed. 2, Springfield, Illinois, Charles C Thomas, Publisher, 1960, p. 303.

Lesions of the Atrioventricular Conduction System After Repair of Ventricular Septal Defect.
Relation to Heart Block.

Anatomy of the Atrioventricular Conduction System in Ventricular Septal Defect.

James K. Kirklin, M.D.

The prevention of heart block following repair of congenital heart malformations stands as one of the cornerstones of successful cardiac operations. A major barrier to successful cardiac surgery was the acquisition of necessary knowledge in several vital areas: techniques for accurate reconstruction/repair of congenital malformations, effective support of the circulation, preservation of myocardial function during the repair, and control of bleeding associated with cardiac surgery. Beyond these challenges, preservation of atrio-ventricular (AV) conduction was perhaps the most critical initial obstacle to the surgical therapy of congenital heart disease.

My father, John W. Kirklin, often remarked publically that Maurice Lev and Jesse Edwards, through their intellect and rigorous, accurate anatomic and histologic studies had a direct and monumental impact on the rapid early improvements in survival following open cardiac surgery. Their combined impact in defining and refining the location of critical components of the conduction system stands as a sentinel contribution to the achievement of safe reconstructive cardiac operations with the expectation of nearly uniform survival and the probability of a nearly normal quality of life thereafter.

In these two companion papers in *Circulation*, Edwards and his colleagues refined existing knowledge about the location of the AV node, bundle of His, and bundle branches in hearts with ventricular septal defects. The first paper examined 21 hearts with ventricular septal defects (VSD) to elucidate anatomic details of the conduction system, and the second paper focused on the 13 hearts in which the VSD had been closed surgically. This paper exemplified early clinico-pathologic correlations in cardiac surgery by relating the functional status of cardiac conduction after operation to the histologic examination of areas of surgical "activity" near the conduction system. Edwards and his colleagues provided elegant evidence that actual surgical injury to the conduction system was responsible for AV block. Of particular importance was the revelation that not only actual suture injury (one of six cases of complete heart block) but also the collateral damage of hemorrhage and infarction secondary to sutures in proximity to the AV node or His bundle was a major factor in the development of heart block.

As we view the evolution of open cardiac surgery from its nascent period to the current era more than 50 years later, surgical practice has gradually transitioned away from the necessarily hurried, less accurate repair of cardiac defects (imposed by lack of scientific/anatomic knowledge and less effective support systems) to a demand for efficient operations that embrace an unhurried, accurate reconstruction. Adherence to principles of gentle tissue handling is emphasized to minimize the inimical effects of "tissue hemorrhage" described by Edwards and colleagues that is so easy to induce with our surgical "invasion." Indeed, every congenital heart surgeon "relives" the salient points of each of these papers when (s)he enters the domain of a small infant's heart with a hole that needs closing.

The scientific value of exhaustive analyses of individual cases remains a vital component, even today, in advancing the field of cardiac surgery. With the exponential increase in the "n" of cases for analysis in ensuing years, the contributions of Berkson (the prominent Mayo Clinic statistician of the 1950s) and Kirklin in the analytic research process would become evident. But by any assessment, the exquisitely accurate anatomic studies that characterized the work of Jesse Edwards helped set the standard for future cardiac surgical investigations.

The beauty, elegance, and painstaking accuracy of these two papers embody an entire culture that developed at the Mayo Clinic in those early days. Their mantra of intellectual honesty and clarity of thought set the tone for future cardiac surgeons, physicians, and pathologists whose life's work "emanates from the heart."

Pathologic Spectrum of Dysplasia of the Tricuspid Valve

Features in Common With Ebstein's Malformation

Anton E. Becker, MD; Mies J. Becker, MD; and Jesse E. Edwards, MD, Minneapolis

Congenitally malformed tricuspid valves may show (1) downward displacement of the basal attachments of the leaflets, as seen in classical Ebstein's malformation, and (2) a variety of conditions involving the leaflets, chordae, and papillary muscles, collectively called dysplasia. A study of the anatomic tricuspid valve in 36 specimens of heart evaluated the relationship between downward displacement and valvular dysplasia. Twenty-four showed coexistent valvular dysplasia and downward displacement, classified as Ebstein's malformation. One case, in the group of corrected transposition, showed downward displacement without features of valvular dysplasia. In 11 of 36 cases, valvular dysplasia without downward displacement was present. The malformed tricuspid valve may show a gradation of changes which range from the feature of downward displacement only, through combinations of downward displacement and dysplasia, to dysplasia only.

AMONG congenitally malformed tricuspid valves, faulty development of chordae and papillary muscles and thickening or focal agenesis of valvular tissue may be present. These processes, collectively, may be termed "tricuspid valvular dysplasia."

The characteristics of dysplasia vary from case to case, both as to nature and degree. Also, in the presence of tricuspid valvular dysplasia there may be variation as to the basal attachments of the tricuspid leaflets. In some cases, these are normally attached. Other cases show downward displacement of the basal attachment and, on this basis, are classified as Ebstein's malformation. In view of these variations, an anatomic study was done of 36 hearts for the following purposes: (1) to define the spectrum of the structural features of tricuspid valvular dysplasia; (2) to evaluate the relationship between the features of downward displacement and those of tricuspid valvular dysplasia; (3) to determine whether or not tricuspid valvular dysplasia has a tendency to be associated with malformations of other cardiac valves.

Our observations suggest that there may be a gradation of tricuspid valvular malformations which range from downward displacement as the sole anomalous feature, through a variety of cases showing downward displacement associated with valvular dysplasia, into an entity in which the tricuspid valve apparatus shows intrinsic malformations. The basal attachments, however, remain normal.

Accepted for publication Aug 6, 1970.

From the departments of pathology of the Charles T. Miller Hospital, St. Paul, Minn, and of the University of Minnesota, Minneapolis.

Reprint requests to Department of Pathology, the Charles T. Miller Hospital, 125 W College Ave, St. Paul, Minn 55102 (Dr. Edwards).

Definition of Terms

The terms used to evaluate the abnormalities of the tricuspid valve observed were the following: dysplasia and downward displacement.

Dysplasia.—The characteristics of dysplasia include (*a*) focal or diffuse thickening of the valve leaflets, (*b*) deficient development of chordae and papillary muscles, (*c*) improper separation of valve components from the ventricular wall, and (*d*) focal agenesis of valvular tissue.

Dysplasia, when present, was divided into three grades according to the following criteria.

Grade 1.—The papillary muscles and chordae tendineae supporting the valve were normal. The involved valve leaflets showed slight, partially nodular thickening comprised of mucoid fibrous tissue (Fig 1 and 2).

Grade 2.—The papillary muscles and chordae tendineae were involved in the developmental disorder, as well as the leaflets (Fig 3 and 4). The valve leaflets were longer than normal, often irregularly shaped with an edematous

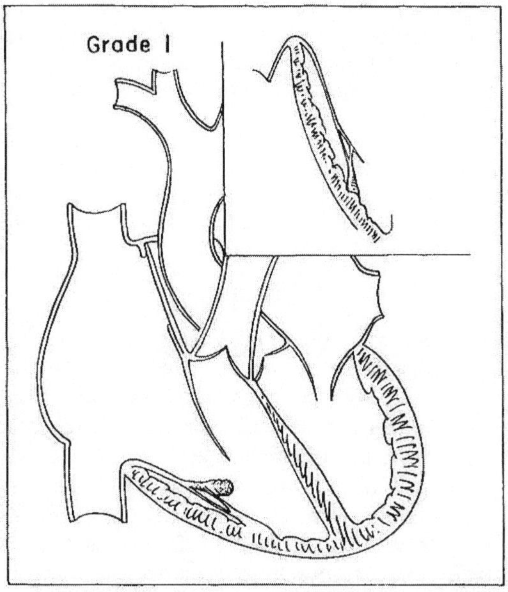

Fig 1.—Diagrammatic portrayal of tricuspid valvular dysplasia, grade 1, characterized by thickening of the free aspect of the leaflet. Chordae and papillary muscles normal. Inset shows normal tricuspid valve leaflet, chordae, and papillary muscles in relation to right ventricular wall.

appearance and thickening by mucoid fibrous tissue. The chordae tendineae showed fibrous thickening and shortening and they were often abnormally inserted, both at the valvular and muscular aspects. In addition to anomalous chordal attachments, the valve leaflets, in part, were attached directly either (1) to the papillary muscles (which themselves were often underdeveloped) or (2) to unspecialized parts of the right ventricle. In grade 2, although anomalous attachments of leaflets occurred, there remained wide spaces between the leaflets and the ventricular wall.

Grade 3.—Grade 3 was characterized by a wide variety of changes including focal agenesis of valvular tissue, as well as a variety of highly abnormal features in recognizable valvular tissue.

In general, the leaflets were thickened and elongated in a curtain-like fashion, often containing multiple irregular fenestrations. A common finding was abnormally close adhesion of valvular tissue to the right ventricular wall (Fig 5 and 6). Often, broad areas of involved leaflets were adherent to the right ventricular wall so that, in some areas, no space was present between the leaflet and the wall. In other areas, small spaces were present between anomalous attachments of the valvular tissue to the ventricular mural endocardium.

Inferior to zones of extensive direct adhesion of valvular tissue to the ventricular wall, the lowermost part of the leaflet tissue might extend into the right ventricular cavity as a rudimentary, at times nodular, flap. The valve leaflets might contain varying amounts of myocardial tissue in their ventricular aspects. Included in the grade 3 category was the state in which the only detectable valvular tissue was represented merely by a ridge of mucoid fibrous tissue with or without haphazardly distributed "supporting" chordal strands.

Agenesis of the tricuspid valve refers to the state in which the tricuspid orifice is partially or totally devoid of guarding valvular tissue. When present, the agenesis is designated as a form of grade 3 dysplasia. Agenesis of the valve should be differentiated from the condition in which leaflet tissue is present but adherent to the endocardial aspect of the right ventricle.

For each case, a designation of "maximal dysplasia" was given to indicate the severest form of this abnormality present at some part of the tricuspid valve.

Downward Displacement.—In normal hearts, attachment of the septal leaflet of the tricuspid valve to the ventricular septum lies a few millimeters below the annulus. This finding, which is most pronounced in hearts with left ventricular hypertrophy, is normal. In the case of the septal leaflet, only when the basal attachment was lower than normal was the term "downward displacement" applied. For the posterior and anterior leaflets, the term was applied when the basal attachment of either one or both was below the annulus.

The degree of downward displacement was determined as follows. The distance between the anticipated normal basal attachment and the right ventricular apex was determined. The degree of deviation downward of the involved leaflet or leaflets from the anticipated normal was used to indicate three grades of displacement (Fig 7).

Grade 1 was represented by downward displacement less than 10% of the distance from the anticipated basal attachment and the apex.

Grade 2 constituted a lower attachment from 10% to 50% of the distance involved and grade 3, more than 50%.

The greatest degree of downward displacement found at some point in the tricuspid valve was designated as the "maximal downward displacement" for that case.

Material and Methods

Included in this study were 36 specimens of the heart in which the tricuspid valve showed either dysplasia or downward displacement or both. Twenty-eight of the hearts were with normally related great vessels, while eight were examples of corrected transposition of the great vessels in which the anatomic tricuspid valve is located on the left side of the heart. In corrected transposition it is known that Ebstein-like abnormalities may occur in the inverted tricuspid valve.[1,2]

Cases with pulmonary valvular atresia and intact ventricular septum associated with major hypoplasia of the right ventricle and tricuspid orifice were excluded from this study, since with the methods used in this study, it would be difficult to determine with accuracy the degrees of downward displacement and of valvular dysplasia. Ebstein-like tricuspid malformations, however, may occur among such cases.[3] Cases of pulmonary atresia or stenosis with Ebstein's malformation and a normal-sized or enlarged right ventricle were included. In each of the 36 cases studied, death had been considered to have resulted from cardiac disease.

In each, the tricuspid valve was studied for the presence or absence of dysplasia and downward displacement. When present, each condition was graded according to the foregoing definitions.

In addition, a tabulation was done of associated anomalies which were present, with special reference to the condition of the other cardiac valves and the occurrence of septal defects.

Results

The results obtained with hearts showing normal orientation of the great vessels and ventricles will be considered in a separate section from cases with corrected transposition of the great vessels.

Hearts With Normally Related Great Vessels.—There were 28 specimens with normally related great vessels. Fifteen cases were from males, nine from females and four in which the sex was unknown to us. The ages

Fig 2.—Histologic representation of grade 1 tricuspid valvular dysplasia in two cases. In each case, the adjacent portions of the right atrium (**RA**) and right ventricle (**RV**) and the related tricuspid leaflet are shown. Free aspect of the leaflet shows nodular thickening by mucoid fibrous tissue. The supporting chordae are normal. The leaflet is normally attached at the annulus (elastic tissue stain, slightly reduced from × 8 [**left**] and × 12 [**right**]).

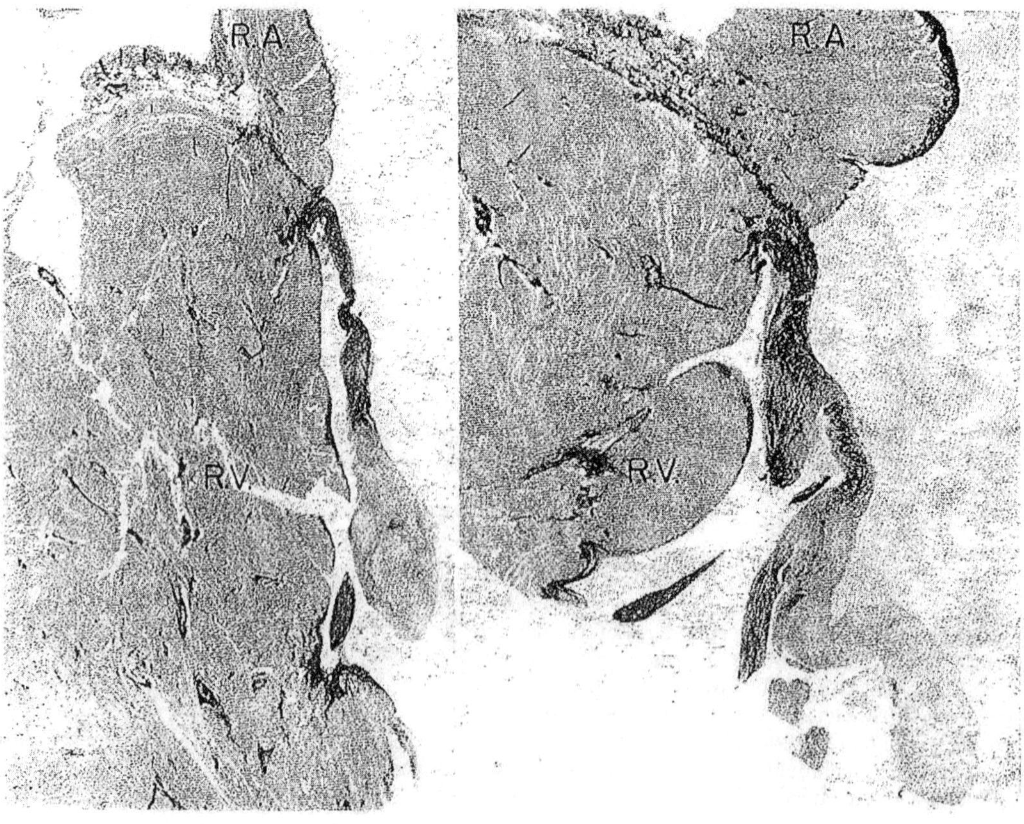

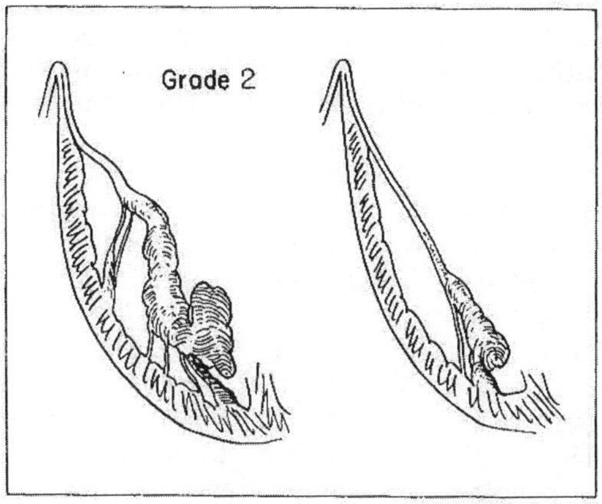

Fig 3.—Diagrammatic portrayal of tricuspid valvular dysplasia, grade 2. In addition to thickening of leaflets, chordae and papillary muscles show abnormalities in the form of thickening and abnormal orientation of the chordae and direct attachment of papillary muscles to leaflets. Wide spaces remain between the leaflets and the right ventricular wall.

ranged from newborn to 39 years of age, with the following distribution: under 1 week of age, five cases; from 1 week to 1 year, 14 cases (including seven cases in which the exact age was known and seven other cases of unknown age which appeared to belong to this age group); 1 to 9 years, one case (aged 2 years); 10 to 19 years, four cases; 20 to 29 years, one case (aged 28 years); 20 to 39 years, three cases.

The cases were placed into two groups depending upon whether downward displacement was present (group 1) or absent (group 2).

Group 1 (Normally Related Great Vessels With Downward Displacement).—Eighteen of the 28 cases with normally related great vessels showed downward displacement and were designated as group 1 (Fig 8). Dysplasia was also present in each and, in three,

Fig 4.—Histologic representation of grade 2 tricuspid valvular dysplasia from three cases. Orientation as in Fig 3. The leaflets are larger than normal and irregularly shaped. In addition to normal basal attachments, there are abnormalities of attachments of the leaflets. At **left** and **center**, leaflets make secondary attachments to ventricular wall (**arrows**). At right, there is direct attachment of papillary muscles to leaflet. Right atrium, **RA**; right ventrice, **RV** (elastic tissue stain, slightly reduced from × 4 [**left**], × 2.5 [**center**], and × 2.8 [**right**]).

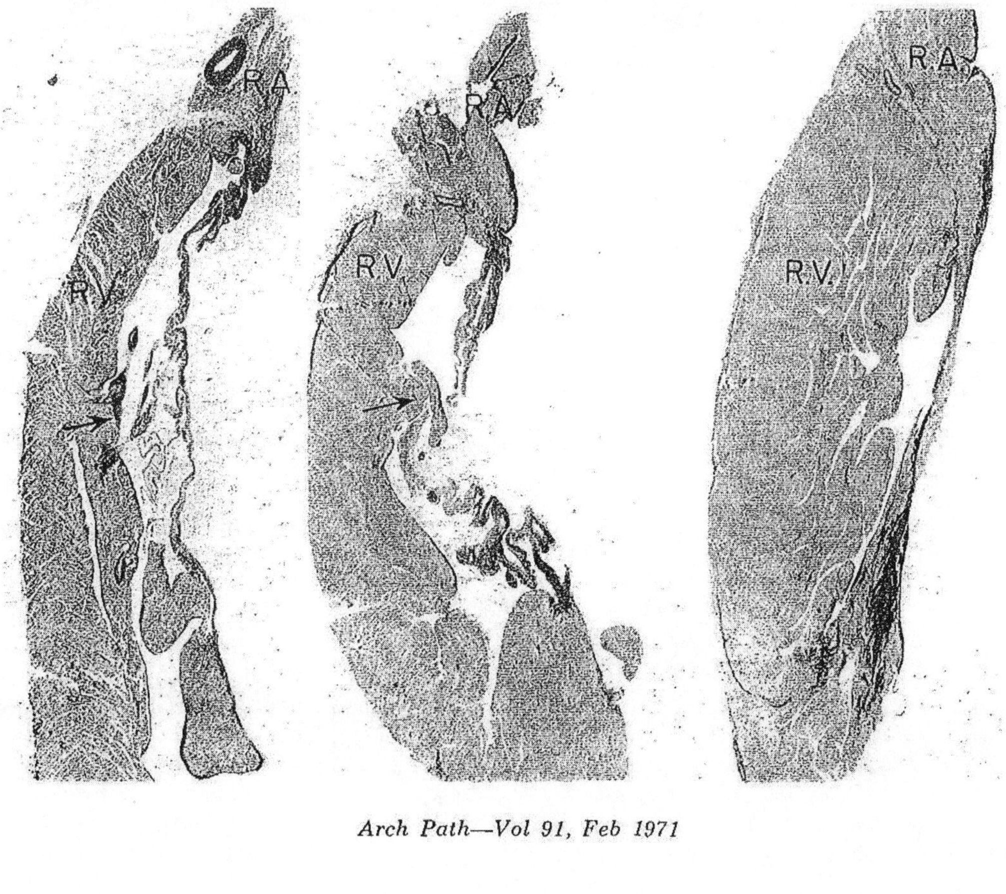

focal agenesis of the valve was displayed.

Among the 18 cases with downward displacement of the tricuspid valve, pulmonary valvular anomalies causing obstruction were present in six cases (33%), five with intact ventricular septa. Four of these were young infants, three with pulmonary atresia and one with dome-shaped pulmonary stenosis. Each of the remaining two cases with pulmonary valvular obstruction was an adult, aged 28 and 38 years, respectively. In each, the stenotic pulmonary valve was bicuspid. In one case, a ventricular septal defect was present. Regarding the alterations in the tricuspid valve, there was no apparent difference between the cases with and without obstruction at the pulmonary valve.

In 14 of the 18 cases of group 1, the process of downward displacement involved both the septal and posterior leaflets, while in the remaining four cases, this process was limited to the septal leaflet. In no case of this series was the anterior leaflet involved in the process of downward displacement. As stated, each of the 18 cases with downward displacement showed dysplasia of the tricuspid valve apparatus but the parts involved in downward displacement and in dysplasia did not coincide in each case. In general, a greater portion of the valve was involved by dysplasia than by downward displacement.

Eleven of the 18 cases with downward displacement showed dysplasia involving each of the three leaflets, while downward displacement in these cases was restricted to the septal leaflet in two and to the septal and posterior leaflets in nine.

In six of the seven remaining cases, the process of dysplasia was confined to the leaflet involved in downward displacement. Among these, there were two in which only the septal leaflet was involved and four in which downward displacement and dysplasia involved both the septal and posterior leaflets.

In the 18th specimen, both the septal and posterior leaflets were displaced downward, while dysplasia was limited to the septal leaflet.

From a quantitative point of view, it was apparent that the maximal grades of dysplasia did not, in all cases, coincide with the maximal grades of downward displacement (Fig 9), although in seven of the 18 cases the two coincided, each being grade 3.

In three of the 18 specimens of group 1, there was focal agenesis of the tricuspid valve. In each case, the septal region was so involved (Fig 8, *bottom left*).

Associated cardiac anomalies, exclusive of those involving the pulmonary valve and the atrial septum, were observed in six cases.

Two cases, each with a

Presence or Absence of Downward Displacement of Tricuspid Valve and Nature of Pulmonary Valve*

Downward Displacement	Total	Pulmonary Valve		
		Normal	Stenosis	Atresia
Present (group 1)	18	12	3	3
Absent (group 2)	10	2	4	4

* Among 28 subjects with normally related great vessels.

Fig 5.—Diagrammatic portrayal of tricuspid valvular dysplasia, grade 3. One feature is adhesion of leaflet tissue to the right ventricular wall over broad areas at left and center. Also, there is gross thickening of the free aspects of the leaflets. The latter change, combined with downward displacement, is illustrated at right.

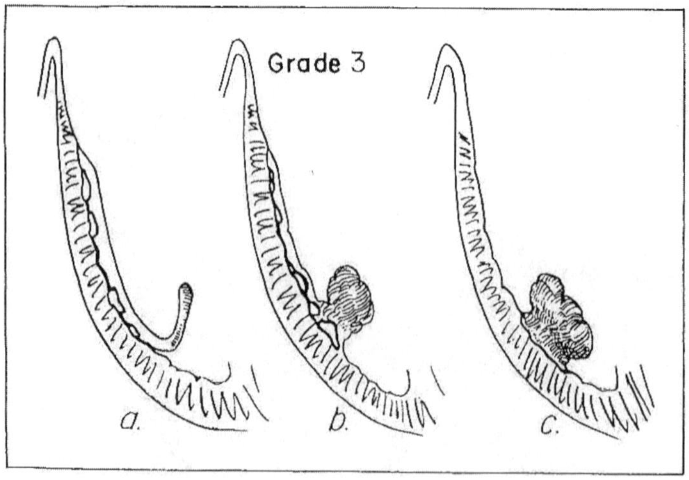

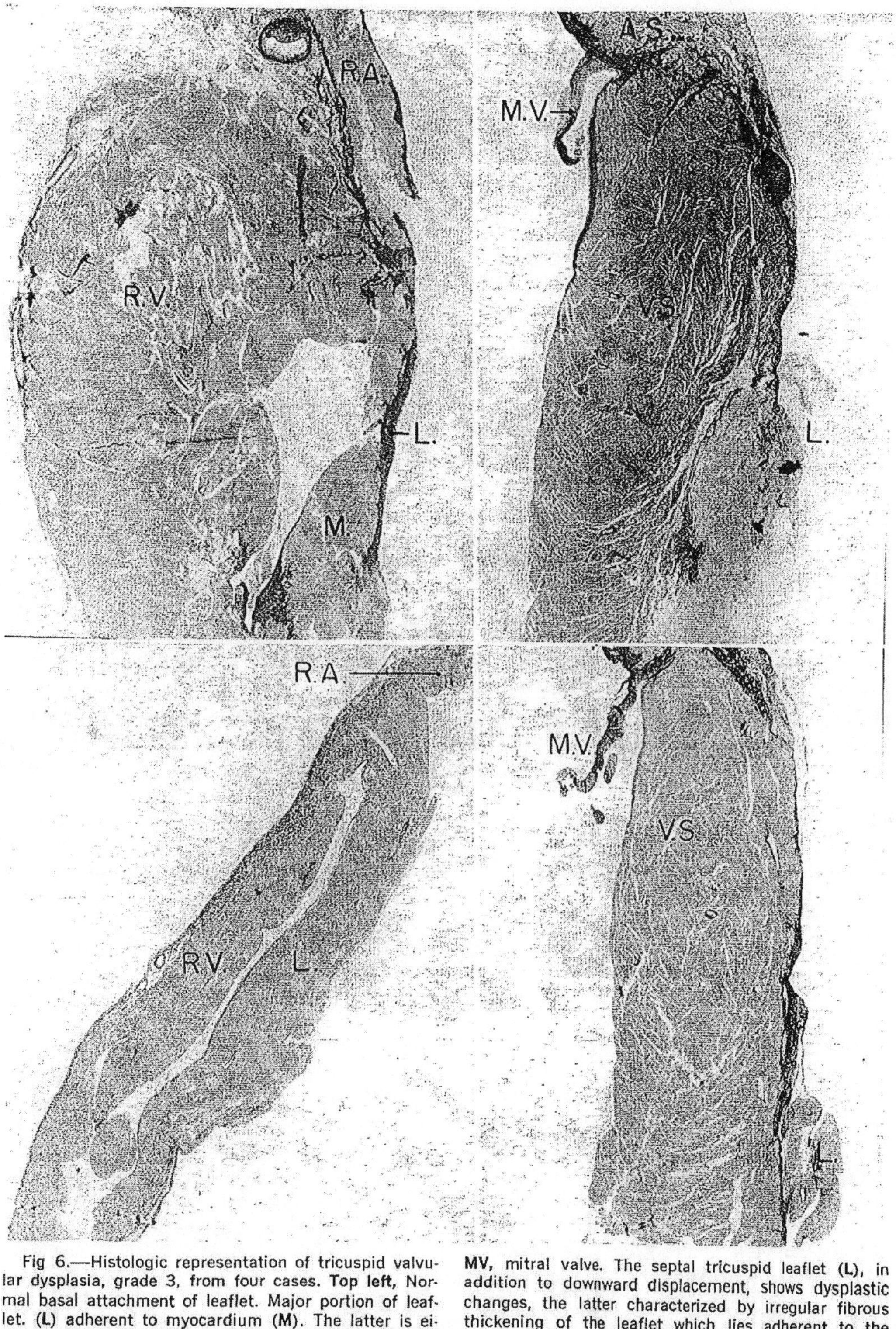

Fig 6.—Histologic representation of tricuspid valvular dysplasia, grade 3, from four cases. **Top left,** Normal basal attachment of leaflet. Major portion of leaflet. (**L**) adherent to myocardium (**M**). The latter is either an abnormal papillary muscle or a columna carna (elastic tissue stain, slightly reduced from × 5.2). **Bottom left,** Leaflet (**L**) hardly recognizable as such, since it is composed primarily of myocardial tissue (elastic tissue stain, slightly reduced from × 2.5). Top right, Section through ventricular (**VS**) and atrial (**AS**) septa. **MV,** mitral valve. The septal tricuspid leaflet (**L**), in addition to downward displacement, shows dysplastic changes, the latter characterized by irregular fibrous thickening of the leaflet which lies adherent to the septum. Right atrium, **RA**; right ventricle, **RV** (elastic tissue stain, slightly reduced from × 9). **Bottom right,** Orientation as in **top right.** Major degree of downward displacement and dysplasia. The latter is characterized by irregular fibrous thickening of leaflet (elastic tissue stain, slightly reduced from × 8).

Arch Path—Vol 91, Feb 1971

normal pulmonary valve, showed a congenital bicuspid aortic valve.

A ventricular septal defect was found in three of the 18 cases in group 1. In one of these, a case with a stenotic bicuspid pulmonary valve, the defect appeared to be occluded by accessory dysplastic tissue of the tricuspid valve. The two remaining cases, each without pulmonary valvular obstruction, showed a small ventricular septal defect. The opening lay proximal to the displaced tricuspid valve, yielding a functional left ventricular-right atrial communication.

An interatrial communication at the fossa ovalis was present in each of the 18 cases of group 1. In three, this took the form of a valvular competent foramen ovale, while in the remaining 15 cases, disproportion between the size of the foramen ovale and its valve yielded a persistent interatrial opening but usually of small size.

When the spread of ages in group 1 was viewed in relation to the presence or absence of pulmonary valvular obstruction, the following data were obtained. Twelve cases without pulmonary valvular obstruction showed a range of ages from four days to 39 years, with half of the cases being under one year of age, while in the remaining half, the ages ranged from 13 to 39 years. The six cases in which pulmonary valvular obstruction was present showed a range of ages from newborn to 38 years. Four of these cases were under one year of age, while two cases were 28 and 38 years, respectively. In each of the latter two cases, the pulmonary obstruction took the form of pulmonary stenosis.

Group 2 (Normally Related Great Vessels Without Downward Displacement).—The ten cases with normally oriented great arteries and ventricles in group 2 showed, by selection, absence of downward displacement, only dysplastic changes being present (Fig 9 and 10). In none of these cases was there agenesis of the tricuspid valve. Pulmonary valvula obstruction was present in eight of the ten cases (80%). Four showed domeshaped pulmonary valvular stenosis and four, pulmonary valvular atresia.

Regarding the alterations in the tricuspid valve, there was no apparent difference between the cases with and without obstruction at the pulmonary valve.

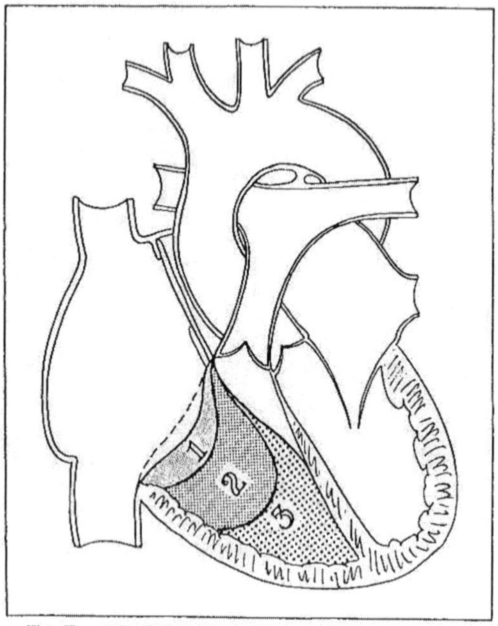

Fig 7.—Diagrammatic portrayal of the three grades of downward displacement of the basal attachment of the tricuspid valve. Basal attachment within the identified zones is graded accordingly.

In each of the cases in group 2, dysplasia involved each of the three tricuspid leaflets and the maximal grade was uniform, being grade 2 in each leaflet of each case (Fig 9).

Associated cardiac anomalies, exclusive of those involving the pulmonary valve and atrial septum, were observed in one case. In this particular case with a dome-shaped pulmonary valvular stenosis, a small ventricular septal defect was present, although the defect appears to be occluded by accessory dysplastic tissue of the tricuspid valve.

An interatrial communication at the fossa ovalis was present in each of the ten cases of group 2. In eight, this took the form of a valvular competent foramen ovale, while in the remaining two cases, disproportion between the size of the foramen ovale and its valve yielded a persistent interatrial opening of small size in each.

None of the specimens in group 2 showed anomalies of the mitral or aortic valves.

In group 2, the ages ranged from newborn to 2 years, with nine of the ten subjects being under 1 year of age. In seven of the nine cases under 1 year of age, pulmonary valvular obstruction was present (three with stenosis and four with atresia). The 2-year-old subject exhibited pulmonary stenosis.

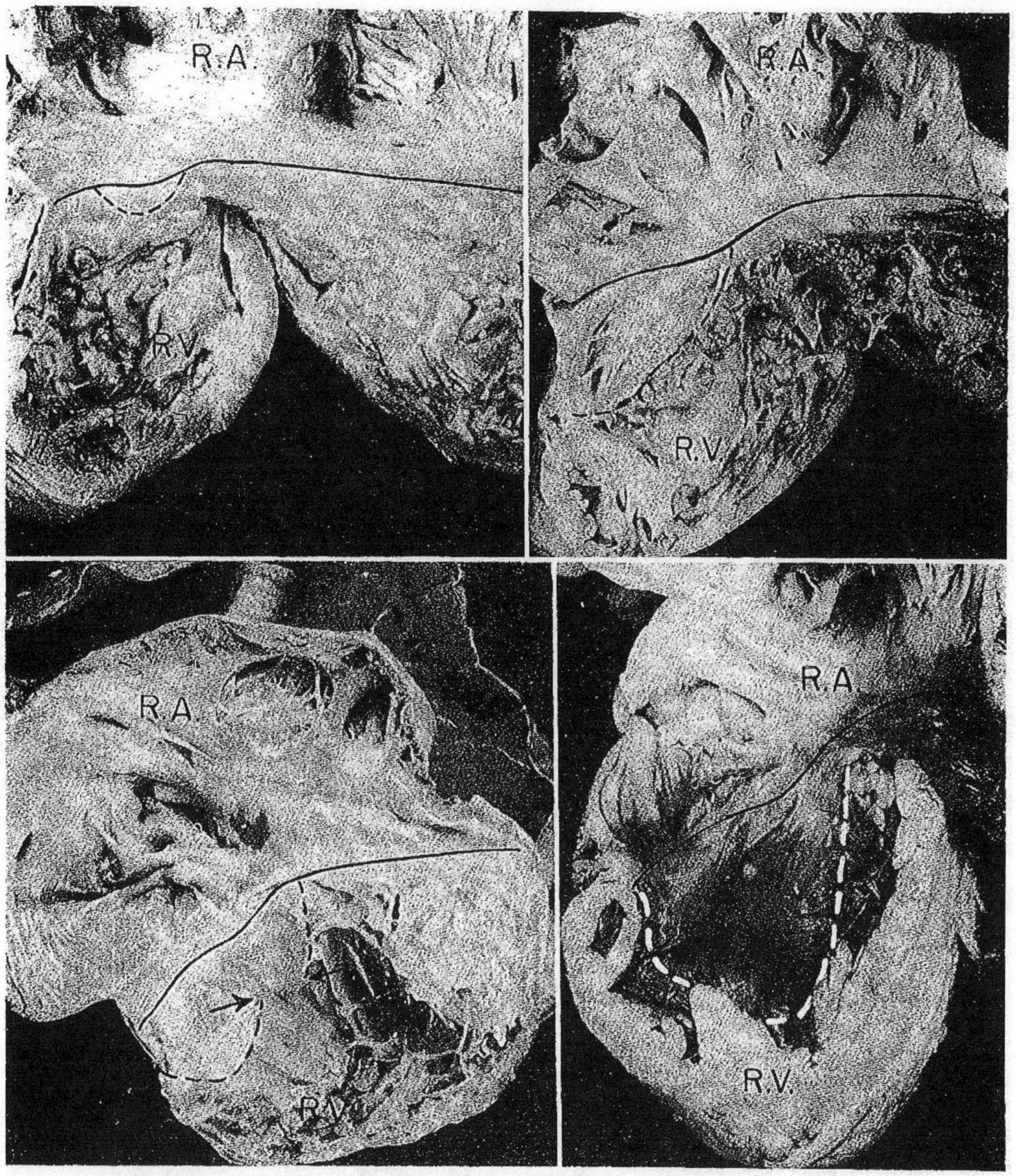

Fig 8.—Right atrial (**RA**) and right ventricular (**RV**) views of four hearts with downward displacement of the tricuspid valve. In each, **solid line** indicates line of anticipated normal basal attachments. **Dotted line** indicates actual basal attachment of downwardly displaced segments. In one of the cases (**bottom left**), the pulmonary valve was atretic. **Top left,** Grade 1 downward displacement of the septal leaflet and a grade 2 dysplasia involving all three leaflets. **Top right,** Grade 2 downward displacement of the septal and posterior leaflets, associated with a grade 3 dysplasia of these leaflets. Grade 2 dysplasia of anterior leaflet. **Bottom left,** Grade 2 downward displacement of septal and posterior leaflets. There is an area of focal agenesis (between **arrows** [grade 3 dysplasia]) in the territory of the septal leaflet, while the remainder of the downwardly displaced leaflets is represented by a ridge of valvular tissue only (grade 3 dysplasia). The anterior leaflet is normally attached but shows a grade 2 dysplasia. **Bottom right,** Grade 3 downward displacement of septal and posterior leaflets associated with a grade 2 dysplasia of each of the three leaflets.

Relationship Between Pulmonary Valvular Obstruction and Tricuspid Anomalies.—According to our method of including material in this study, only cases with anomalies of the tricuspid valve were included (Table). In spite of this element of selection, it was of interest to relate the types of tricuspid anomalies to the nature of the pulmonary valve. As stated earlier, each case, whether or not pulmonary valvular disease was present, exhibited tricuspid valvular dysplasia.

Regarding downward displacement, it was observed that of the 14 cases without pulmonary valvular obstruction, 12 cases showed downward displacement (86%), while two cases failed to show this abnormality.

Among the 14 cases with pulmonary valvular obstruction, there were six cases (43%) with downward displacement of the tricuspid valve.

Hearts With Corrected Transposition of Great Vessels.—There were eight specimens with classical corrected transposition of the great vessels and abnormalities of the left-sided atrioventricular valve. In corrected transposition, this valve has the morphologic characteristics of a tricuspid valve. There were five males and three females in this group.

It will be recalled that the cases of corrected transposition included in this study showed abnormalities in the left-sided tricuspid valve.

Each of the eight specimens of corrected transposition was placed into one of two groups: group 3, comprising cases with downward displacement, consisted of seven cases; group 4, was comprised of one case in which downward displacement was not present.

Group 3 (Corrected Transposition With Downward Displacement).—Group 3 consisted of seven cases, each of which showed downward displacement. In six of these, valvular dysplasia was present including one with focal agenesis of the valve.

In four of the seven cases, the process of downward displacement was limited to the septal leaflet, while three showed involvement of both the septal and posterior leaflets. None of the specimens showed downward displacement of the anterior leaflet.

In only one case with downward displace-

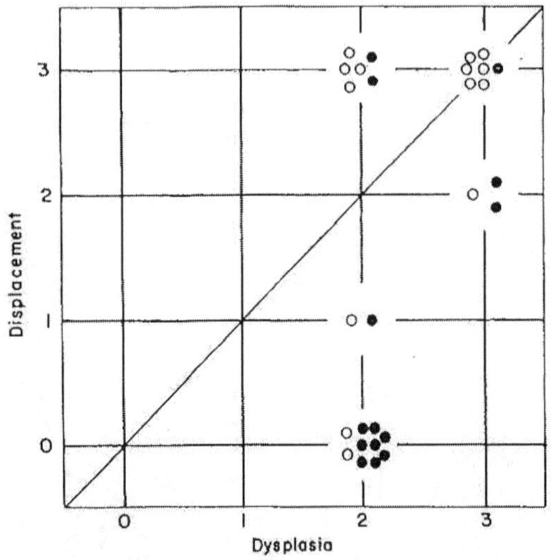

Fig 9.—Scattergram of the degrees of maximal downward displacement and maximal valvular dysplasia for each of the 28 cases with normally related great vessels. Common deviation from line of identity is evident. Cases without downward displacement are classified as tricuspid valvular dysplasia, while those with displacement are classified as Ebstein's malformation. Normal pulmonary valve, **open circle**; pulmonary stenosis or atresia, **solid circle.**

Fig 10.—Right atrium (**RA**) and right ventricle (**RV**) in case with pulmonary valvular atresia. Grade 2 dysplasia involves each of the three valve leaflets, while the basal attachments are normal. The malformation of the tricuspid valve is classified as tricuspid valvular dysplasia.

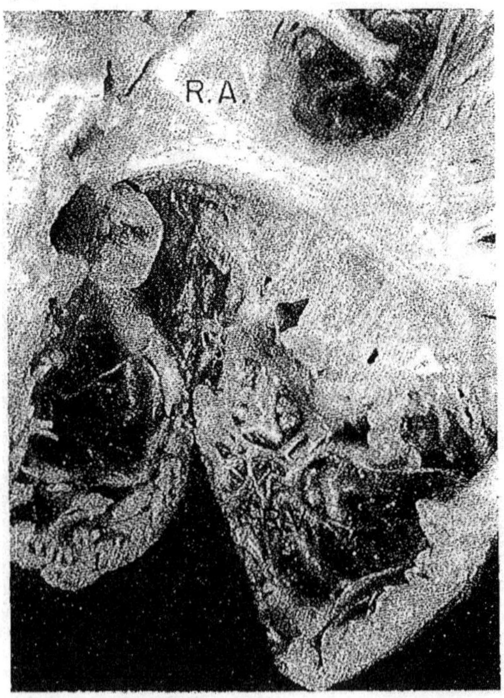

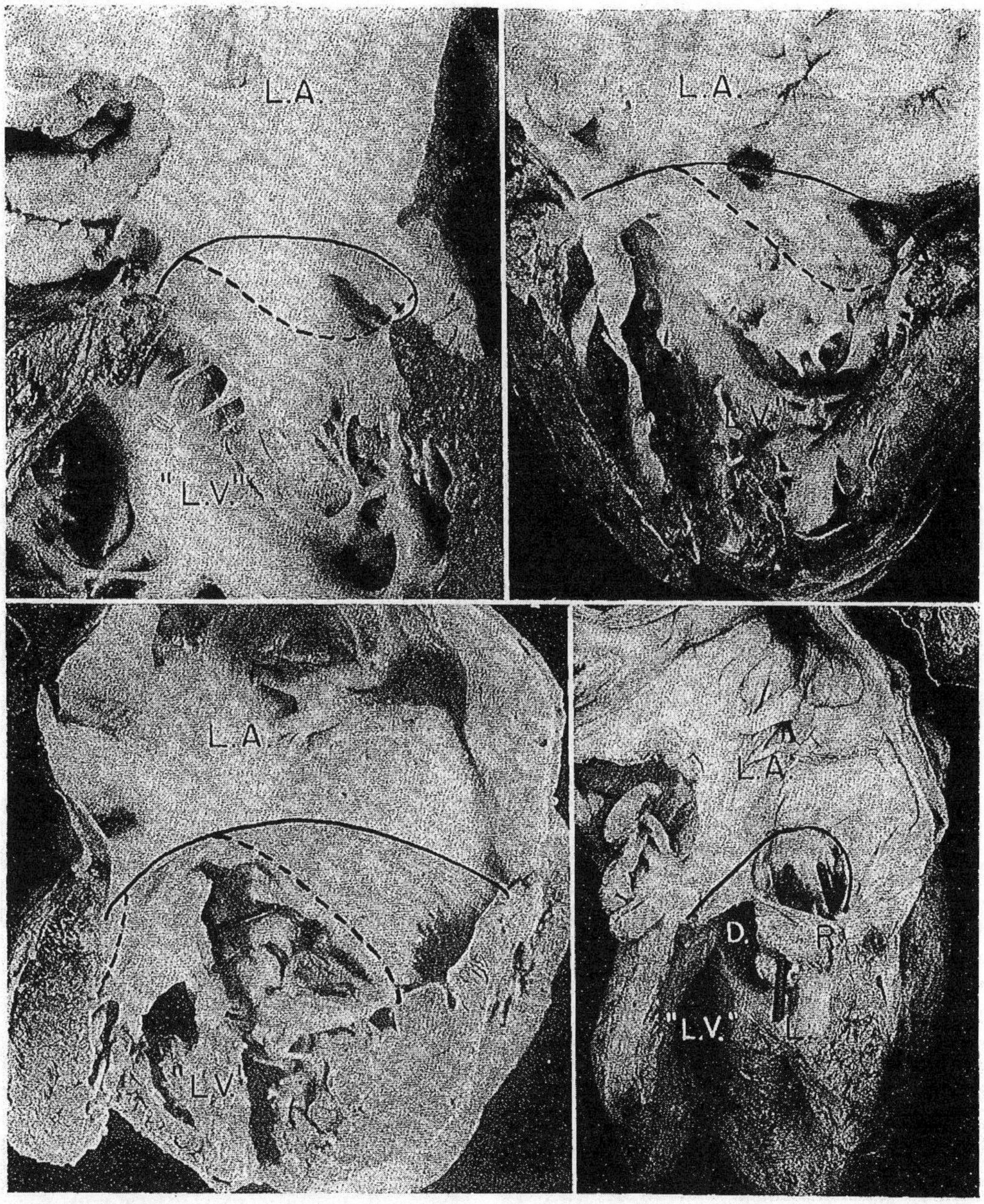

Fig 11.—Left side of heart in four cases of corrected transposition. Each illustration shows left atrium (**LA**), the left-sided ventricle ("**LV**") and the left-sided anatomic tricuspid valve. **Solid** and **dotted** lines as in Fig 8. The specimens at **top** and **bottom left** each show downward displacement, while that at **bottom right** shows valvular dysplasia without downward displacement. **Top left,** Grade 2 downward displacement of the septal leaflet with no valvular dysplasia (dysplasia grade 0). **Top right,** Grade 2 downward displacement and grade 1 restricted to septal leaflet. **Bottom left,** Grade 2 downward displacement of septal and posterior leaflets associated with grade 2 dysplasia of these leaflets. **Bottom right,** Grade 2 dysplasia of each of the three leaflets, while downward displacement is absent. The ventricular chamber is small and a ventricular septal defect (**D**) is present. The dysplastic valve opens, in part, through a narrow orifice into the left-sided ventricle (probe **L**). The valve also communicated with the right-sided ventricle (probe **R**).

ment (involving the septal leaflet) was dysplasia absent (Fig 11, *top left*). In three of the six cases showing both conditions, downward displacement and dysplasia were limited to the septal leaflet (Fig 11, *top right*), while two other cases showed simultaneous involvement of both the septal and posterior leaflets (Fig 11, *bottom left*). In one case, in which downward displacement was limited to two leaflets (septal and posterior), dysplasia involved the three leaflets.

Although the parts of the tricuspid valve involved in downward displacement and dysplasia did not coincide in each case, there was a general tendency for both conditions to affect the same leaflets. From a quantitative point of view, however, it was apparent that the maximal grades of downward displacement and dysplasia did not usually coincide (Fig 12). In one of the seven cases of group 2, there was partial agenesis of the tricuspid valve involving the septal region. This condition was associated with a grade 2 downward displacement of the identifiable portion of the involved leaflet.

In group 3, the ages ranged from newborn to 42 years, four of the seven subjects being under 1 year of age. The other three patients were 2, 21, and 42 years old, respectively.

Except for one specimen with a bicuspid pulmonary valve, none of the remaining valves was abnormal. In six of the seven cases, the patients presented with a ventricular septal defect. An atrial septal defect was found in one instance, the defect being of the fossa ovalis type.

Subaortic stenosis was observed in two cases. In one, this resulted from anomalous muscle bundle of the left-sided anatomic right ventricle. In the second case, the obstruction resulted from accessory tissue of the right atrioventricular valve herniating through a ventricular septal defect.

Group 4 (Corrected Transposition Without Downward Displacement).—There was one specimen in the series of hearts with corrected transposition of the great arteries in which the left-sided tricuspid valve showed a normal basal attachment but with dysplastic features (Fig 11, *bottom right*). The latter process involved each of the three leaflets of grade 2 degree. The heart, from an infant, showed a ventricular septal defect as the sole additional major anomaly.

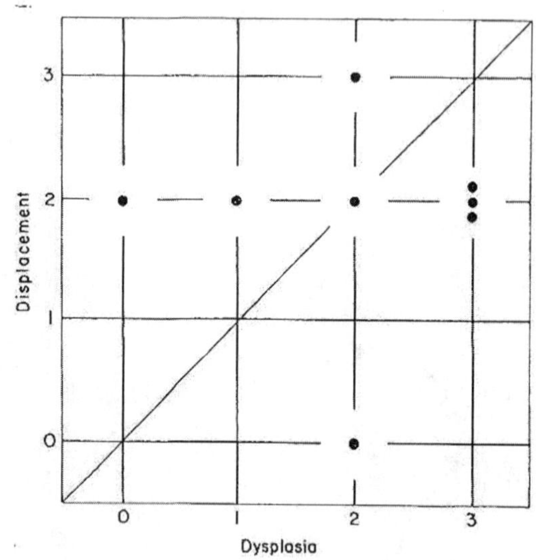

Fig 12.—Scattergram of the degrees of maximal downward displacement and maximal valvular dysplasia of the anatomic tricuspid valve for each of the eight cases with corrected transposition of the great vessels in which the tricuspid valve is situated in the left side of the heart.

Comment

This study on the tricuspid valve identified changes in the tricuspid valve which collectively are called dysplasia of the valve. The anatomic ramifications are wide, including a number of elements. Faulty development of papillary muscles is characterized by incomplete development of these structures. Poorly or incompletely developed chordae are common, yielding a state in which leaflet tissue attaches directly either to malformed papillary muscles or the right ventricular wall. Changes in the leaflets are characterized by absence of part of the leaflet tissue and by thickening of existing leaflets.

These studies showed that if one uses tricuspid dysplasia as a point of departure the cases fall into two groups, those with downward displacement and others without. Cases with downward displacement are, by definition, examples of Ebstein's malformation. Yet, this study emphasizes, as did the original report of Ebstein,[4] that in the condition now named after him, dysplasia is an almost universal feature. Nevertheless, the phenomenon of downward displacement is commonly given as the sole feature of this condition. In only one case of our series was dysplasia absent when downward displacement was present.

The reverse, however, is common in that valvular dysplasia may occur in the absence of downward displacement. This phenomenon has been mentioned by others also.[5,6] The common thread of dysplasia occurring with or without downward displacement suggests that whatever the developmental basis for Ebstein's malformation, a similar mechanism may apply to hearts with dysplasia only. In spite of this apparent relationship, we would propose that the term "Ebstein's malformation" be retained and restricted to cases with downward displacement, whether or not such cases display features of valvular dysplasia, while cases with dysplasia but *without* downward displacement may be considered an anatomic entity which we would propose calling "tricuspid valvular dysplasia."

It is beyond the scope of this communication to consider the complex hemodynamics of the various forms of congenitally malformed tricuspid valve. Yet it is pertinent to emphasize that the category designated as "tricuspid valvular dysplasia" may be associated with signs of tricuspid insufficiency and, thus, is to be recognized as one of the forms of congenital tricuspid insufficiency.

A further link between classical Ebstein's malformation and tricuspid valvular dysplasia is that the pulmonary atresia or stenosis may be associated with either condition.

The incidence of pulmonary valvular obstruction, however, was markedly higher among cases with tricuspid valvular dysplasia (80%) than among cases with Ebstein's malformation (33%).

In our series, there was a difference in the range in age of patients with Ebstein's malformation, on the one hand, and those with tricuspid valvular dysplasia, on the other. In the cases with Ebstein's malformation, individual patients lived to be adults, while each of the cases of tricuspid valvular dysplasia had died while under 2 years of age. This difference may perhaps be explained by the relatively high incidence of pulmonary valvular obstruction in the dysplasia group.

Agenesis which, according to our definition, represents an element of dysplasia involving part of the tricuspid valve was observed in three cases, each with downward displacement of part of the remaining elements. This condition, in association with downward displacement, is a recognized phenomenon[7] and may be included among the various features that may be present in Ebstein's malformation. In our series, there was no case with agenesis of the entire valve. Such a case, however, was reported from this laboratory by Kanjuh and associates.[8] In that case, the tricuspid orifice was unguarded, as no valvular tissue was present. The pulmonary valve was atretic.

It is of interest that the left-sided tricuspid valve of corrected transposition is subject to the same conditions as seen in the tricuspid valve of the normally oriented hearts. In one of the eight cases with corrected transposition, downward displacement without dysplasia was seen. In another case, only dysplasia was observed, while in the remaining six cases, the two conditions coexisted.

This study was supported by Public Health Service research grant 5 R01 HE05694 and research training grant 5 T01 HE05570 from the National Heart and Lung Institute and by the Netherlands Organization for the Advancement of Pure Research (Zuiver Wetenschappelijk Onderzoek).

References

1. Edwards JE: Differential diagnosis of mitral stenosis: A clinicopathologic review of simulating conditions. *Lab Invest* 3:89-115, 1954.

2. Schiebler GL, Edwards JE, Burchell HB, et al: Congenital corrected transposition of the great vessels: A study of 33 cases. *Pediatrics* 27(pt 2):851-888, 1961.

3. Elliott LP, Adams P Jr, Edwards JE: Pulmonary atresia with intact ventricular septum. *Brit Heart J* 25:489-501, 1963.

4. Ebstein W: Ueber einen sehr seltenen Fall von Insufficienz der Valvula tricuspidalis, bedingt durch eine angeborene hochgradige Missbildung derselben. *Arch Anat Physiol Wissensch Med,* pp 283-254, 1866.

5. Bahnson HT, Bauersfeld SR, Smith JW: Pathological anatomy and surgical correction of Ebstein's anomaly. *Circulation* 31(suppl 1):3-8, 1965.

6. Genton E, Blount SG Jr: The spectrum of Ebstein's anomaly. *Amer Heart J* 73:395-425, 1967.

7. Pechstein J: Beitrag zur Ebsteinschen Anomalie der Valvula tricuspidalis. *Arch Kreislaufforsch* 26:282-337, 1957.

8. Kanjuh VI, Stevenson JE, Amplatz K, et al: Congenitally unguarded tricuspid orifice with coexistent pulmonary atresia. *Circulation* 30:911-917, 1964.

Pathologic Spectrum of Dysplasia of the Tricuspid Valve. Features in Common With Ebstein's Malformation.

Joseph A. Dearani, M.D.

This paper reviews anatomic abnormalities of the tricuspid valve collectively referred to as "dysplasia." It correctly and accurately points out changes that may occur with the leaflets and subvalvar apparatus (chordae tendineae and papillary muscles). These anatomic studies demonstrated two categories of tricuspid valve dysplasia... those with and those without downward displacement. Cases with downward displacement, which is due to failure of delamination of valve leaflets from underlying myocardium, are by definition Ebstein's malformation (EM). Although downward displacement is often given as the sole feature of EM, dysplasia of the leaflets and subvalvar apparatus are almost universal features as well. This paper concludes by making a recommendation that EM be retained and restricted to cases with downward displacement, whether or not features of dysplasia are present. Furthermore, when downward displacement is absent, then the anatomic entity should be referred to as "tricuspid valvular dysplasia." In addition to these anatomic issues related to the tricuspid valve, the authors also recognized that concomitant pulmonary valve atresia or stenosis may coexist, although it was more likely to be present with tricuspid valve dysplasia compared to EM.

While hemodynamic issues were not the focus of this review, regurgitation was the exceedingly predominant clinical finding for both lesions. Finally, the authors noted an important difference in the age range of patients between these two entities. In cases of EM, survival into adulthood without intervention was common, whereas many cases of tricuspid dysplasia died by 2 years of age or required intervention early in life. This difference may be explained in part by the high incidence of pulmonary valve obstruction in the dysplasia group.

In this review, the teachings and pearls of Dr. Edwards, a detail-oriented, highly intelligent pathologist and human being extraordinaire, stand true to this day. The wide and infinite variability of anatomic abnormality with EM and congenital tricuspid valve dysplasia will forever be present. The congenital abnormalities of the tricuspid valve as described in this comprehensive review, document that every valve is a little different and no two hearts are alike...illustrating why this lesion continues to be one, if not the most challenging valve lesion for the surgeon. There have been more reports in the literature of tricuspid valvuloplasty techniques for EM and congenital tricuspid dysplasia than any other lesion in the cardiac arena. While the ability to obtain a competent, durable anatomic-like tricuspid repair has improved in recent years, the surgical treatment of the congenitally abnormal tricuspid valve is still considered palliative since the majority of patients will require more than one operation in their lifetime.

Circulation

JUNE 1968
VOL. XXXVII NO. 6
SUPPLEMENT NO. IV

AN OFFICIAL JOURNAL of the AMERICAN HEART ASSOCIATION

Diagrammatic Portrayal of Variations in Cardiac Structure

Reference to Transposition, Dextrocardia and the Concept of Four Normal Hearts

By PAUL STANGER, M.D., ROBERT C. BENASSI, M.S., MICHAEL E. KORNS, M.D., KENNETH L. JUE, M.D., AND JESSE E. EDWARDS, M.D.

SUMMARY

A system of loose leaf diagrams is presented for the purpose of portraying the various types of cardiac structure. Appropriate assembly of the diagrams may be used to define the anatomic details in a given case of which a permanent machine-copy may be made and the basic diagrams re-used.

The diagrams may be used as teaching devices to illustrate the interrelationships between (1) transposition of the great vessels, (2) inversion of the various cardiac chambers and great vessels, and (3) dextrocardia.

The material lends itself to illustration of the concept of "four normal hearts;" that is, the fact that although structurally different, there are four anatomic patterns of heart which allow a normal route for the flow of blood.

The diagrams also may be used to illustrate certain features about potential cardiac transplantation. These include the point that for the recipient with a certain body type (situs solitus or situs inversus), normal channels for the flow of blood may be obtained from a donor with one of three types of cardiac structure. These are either the normal or that of corrected transposition of the same body type as the recipient or complete transposition in a donor with the opposite body type from that of the recipient.

Additional Indexing Words:
Cardiac structure Transposition Situs solitus Corrected transposition
Situs inversus Visceral inversion Dextrocardia Ventricular inversion
Levocardia Cardiac transplantation

CONSIDERABLE has been written on the variations of intrinsic cardiac structure, variations in relationships between the great arteries and the ventricles and on the significance of a right-sided cardiac apex. To the student of congenital heart disease the accumulation has not necessarily led to a clear understanding of these conditions and of their interrelationships. This results, in part, from two conditions. The first is that in some instances authors have failed to emphasize that splenic anomalies have a strong tendency to be associated with generally specific patterns of structure which vary from those ob-

From the Department of Pathology, The Charles T. Miller Hospital, St. Paul, Minnesota and the Departments of Pediatrics and Pathology, University of Minnesota, Minneapolis, Minnesota.

This study was supported by Public Health Service Research Grant 5 RO1 HE05694 and Research Training Grant 2 T1 HE05570 from the National Heart Institute.

served when the spleen is normally formed. The second condition is that verbal descriptions of complicated cardiac structures fall short of conveying clearly to the reader the essential meaning of that described.

To overcome the latter reason a series of diagrams was devised. These are presented in this communication as its main purpose.

When a heart is analyzed, either angiocardiographically or by direct examination, as to its anatomic characteristics, the first step is to define the type of body structure present; then the basic anatomic structure of the heart and its vascular connections is defined. In some cases the basic anatomic structure of the heart will serve to explain identified functional abnormalities of the circulation. In other circumstances, although the structure of one heart may vary from that of another, in neither does the basic anatomic structure explain a functional abnormality. In such a circumstance associated conditions, such as septal defects, valvular abnormalities and so forth, underlie the functional abnormality present. When an analysis is made of the basic anatomic structure of a heart a certain orderly pattern should be followed. If this is done, the significance of seemingly complex phenomena such as an unusual relationship between the great vessels (transposition or inversion), ventricular inversion or a right-sided cardiac apex (dextrocardia) become easily apparent.

The diagrams (Figs. 1-10) presented herein (**in sleeve at end of text**) were devised to be useful in portraying in graphic form the body type and the basic anatomic structure concerning a given heart that is examined. The diagrams may also be used to show how the course of the circulation may be similar in hearts with different anatomic structures. They are also useful as teaching devices dealing with variations in cardiac structure.

Definition of Terms

Splenic Anomalies

A strong tendency for malformations of the spleen to be associated with cardiovascular malformations is recognized. In general, the splenic anomalies fall into two groups, namely (1) that characterized by asplenia and (2) that by *polysplenia.* In polysplenia the splenic tissue is normal in amount and is represented by an aggregation of multiple varying-sized nodules of splenic tissue. Each type of splenic anomaly has a tendency to be associated with cardiovascular malformations peculiar in itself and of additional interest is the fact that each tends to be associated with a peculiar structural pattern of the extracardiac organs. In asplenia "bilateral right-sidedness"[1] and in polysplenia "bilateral left-sidedness"[2] are strong tendencies. In a subsequent section of this communication further consideration will be given to cardiovascular patterns associated with splenic anomalies.

The Cardiac Chambers and Valves

As used in this presentation the name given to a chamber will be derived from its anatomic characteristics. Thus, naming a chamber will not imply the side of the heart in which the chamber lies and in the case of the ventricles the name will not imply whether the chamber carries venous or arterial blood.

For example, use of the term *right ventricle* is synonymous with the term "morphologic right ventricle" and depends upon the chamber's exhibiting those internal features which characterize it anatomically. For convenience the word "morphologic" usually will not be used to qualify the type of chamber although when a cardiac chamber is named it may be implied that this word qualifies it.

Right Ventricle

Each ventricle has certain intrinsic anatomic characteristics which allow it to be identified regardless of its position relative to the other ventricle and regardless of its atrial and arterial connections.

The valve guarding the inlet of a given ventricle is peculiar to that ventricle. The right ventricle is equipped with a tricuspid valve and the left ventricle with a bicuspid (mitral) valve. Among the other features of the right ventricle are a highly trabeculated septal wall and the presence of an infundibulum. The latter lies between the tricuspid valve and the semilunar valve at the outlet of the ventricle. Within the infundibulum are identifiable the crista supraventricularis with its parietal and septal limbs, and the papillary muscle of the conus. The membranous portion of the ventricular septum lies hidden under the septal leaflet of the tricuspid valve. A most important point in understanding the arterial connections with the ventricles is that *the outlet of the infundibulum is the most anterior* and the most cephalad of the ventricular structures. Thus, the infundibulum of the right ventricle lies anterior to and extends in a cephalic direction beyond the outlet of the left ventricle. This phenomenon underlies the principle that *the morphologic right ventricle connects with whichever of the two great arteries is the more anterior.*

Left Ventricle

Among the characteristic features of the left ventricle, in addition to a mitral valve guarding its inlet, is a smooth character to its septal wall. The outlet is short, compared to that of the right ventricle, and lies posterior to the right ventricular infundibulum. Another important feature of the left ventricle is that the anterior leaflet of its atrioventricular valve is in continuity with elements of that semilunar valve (through the mitral-aortic intervalvular fibrosa) which guards its outlet. Still another feature is that the left ventricle usually (but not universally) forms the cardiac apex.

Right Atrium

The atria exhibit a strong tendency to conform to the general orientation of the organs so that the right atrium lies on the same side of the body as the trilobed lung and opposite from the position of the stomach and spleen (Figs. 1 and 2). Similarly, the morphologic left atrium tends to lie on the same side as the stomach, spleen and bilobed lung.

The right atrium, as here defined, is the venous atrium and it may lie in either side of the heart. The superior and inferior venae cavae connect with this chamber, as does the coronary sinus. Its atrial appendage possesses the pectinate muscles. The fossa ovalis lies within the septal wall of this chamber. The atrioventricular node is in that part of the atrial septum which is oriented toward this chamber.

Left Atrium

The left atrium is the arterial atrium. It lies on the contralateral side of the heart to the position of the right atrium and somewhat superior to it. Its superior wall is overhung by the tracheal bifurcation. The septal wall is characterized by the presence of interatrial ostium II.

The Valves

Each atrioventricular valve is closely identified with a ventricle peculiar to itself. The *tricuspid valve* with its septal, anterior and posterior leaflets may be considered a part of the inflow portion of the right ventricle. By the same token, *the mitral valve*, a bicuspid structure with clearly defined anterior and posterior leaflets, is part of the inlet of the left ventricle. The relationships between each atrioventricular valve and its ventricle is so consistent that it is appropriate to say, "As go the ventricles, so go the A-V valves."

The two semilunar valves are so similar in appearance that the determination as to whether a given semilunar valve is an aortic or a pulmonary valve depends upon which vessel the valve guards.

Inversion; Non-inversion

The organs of the body, including the components of the heart, have a strong tendency to be oriented in a way commonly defined as "the normal." For example, (1) the stomach and spleen lie on the left, (2) the major lobe of the liver lies on the right and (3) the right lung possesses three lobes and the left, two lobes. Moreover, the morphologic right atrium lies on the right and the morphologic left atrium lies on the left. An important rule is that the positions of the atria conform to the positions of the non-cardiac organs; for example, the left atrium is on the left when the stomach is on the left. Any interchange of a structure from this usual position to the opposite side of the body is called *inversion* of that structure. *It is important to recognize that inversion indicates a "left-and-right" (frontal plane) interchange but does not imply any differences from the usual with regard to anteroposterior relationships* (Fig. 11). Using this definition of inversion, it is appropriate to use the term *non-inversion* when an organ is in the usual ("normal") position.

When all of the organs are inverted the term *total situs inversus* (or situs inversus) is applicable. When all of the organs lie disposed as they are in the overwhelming proportion of the population, the term *total non-inversion* could be applied but by common usage this condition is called *situs solitus*. It is possible that, in an individual with a situs solitus-orientation of the majority of the organs ("situs solitus body type"), only one or two anatomic elements (as the ventricles and/or the great arteries) may show inversion. By the same token it is possible in the face of a situs inversus-orientation of the majority of the organs ("situs inversus body type") that only one or two anatomic elements (as the ventricles and/or great arteries) are oriented as in the "normal," and so defined as showing *non-inversion.*

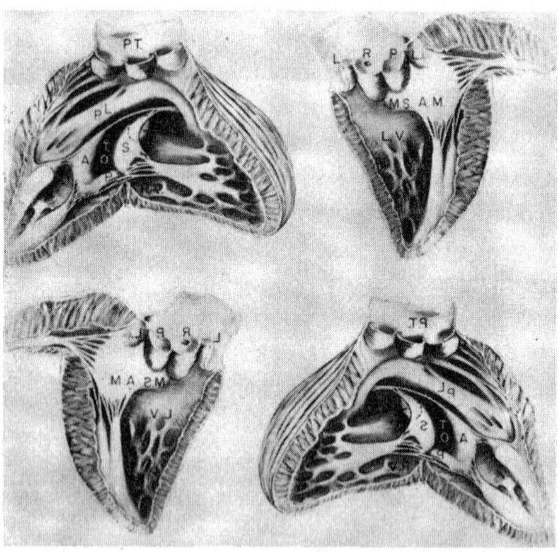

Figure 11

Upper Panel: *Drawing of right ventricle (left) and left ventricle (right) in the usual normal heart. (From Edwards: Seminars in Roentgenol. 1: 2, 1966. Reproduced with permission.)* Lower Panel: *Photographic negative of illustrations shown in Upper Panel printed "backwards" to illustrate inversion of ventricles: "Left and rights" are interchanged in inversion as compared to "the normal" but anterior-posterior relationships are not disturbed.*

Transposition

The term transposition as used here does not identify a specific type of congenital malformation. It simply indicates that there is a different relationship between origins of the great arteries (the ascending aorta and the pulmonary trunk) than is usually found. Depending upon the basic structure of the heart, there are circumstances wherein the direction of the flow of blood may be normal even though transposition is present.

In the overwhelming number of the population a certain relationship exists between the origins of the aorta and pulmonary trunk. This is characterized by the fact that the origin of the pulmonary trunk lies at a level anterior to the origin of the aorta. This relationship, usually called "the normal," may be defined as *non-transposition* of the great arteries. When the reverse is the case and the aortic origin lies anterior to that of the pulmonary trunk, the great arteries may be defined as *transposed.*

The terms *transposition* and *non-transposition* refer to anteroposterior interrelationships between the great arteries. Lateral or side-to-side ("left-and-right") relationships (inversion or non-inversion) vary and play important roles in determining the ventricular-arterial connections.

In the overwhelming proportion of the population (the so-called normal) the ascending aorta sweeps toward the right side of the body and to the right of the pulmonary trunk. This feature of the great vessels, whether or not they are transposed, may be called *non-inversion.* There is an inverted form of this relationship so that regardless as to whether transposition or non-transposition of the great vessels is present, the great vessels may be *inverted;* that is, the ascending aorta bends toward the subject's left and to the left of the pulmonary trunk.

It is vital to an understanding of the various basic cardiac anatomic patterns that the great vessels be defined *both* as to their antero-posterior relationships (transposition or non-transposition) and as to their side-to-side relationships (inversion or non-inversion). There are, therefore, four possible definitions for the great arteries as given in Table I.

Table I

Four Possible Definitions of Great Arteries

- A. Non-transposition
  - 1. Non-inversion
  - 2. Inversion
- B. Transposition
  - 1. Non-inversion
  - 2. Inversion

Dextrocardia; Levocardia

The position of the apex of the heart has received considerable attention in the evaluation of malformed hearts. While this forms an interesting subject, it does not in itself represent a basis either for deciphering the route of the flow of blood or of establishing the anatomic details of the heart.

Two principles should be recognized with regard to the cardiac apex. These are: (1) The morphologic left ventricle usually forms the cardiac apex and (2) under unusual circumstances the morphologic right ventricle forms the cardiac apex.

Using these principles it is appropriate to state that when the apex is on a given side the morphologic left ventricle lies on that side *but exceptions must be recognized under all anatomic circumstances.* Even in cases where the dominant situation applies (homolateral left ventricle and apex), knowledge of the position of the cardiac apex, without knowing other factors such as the state of the atria and of the great arteries, does not define the route of the flow of blood.

A right-sided apex may be termed *dextrocardia,* while a left-sided apex may be termed *levocardia.*

Use of the Diagrams in the Absence of Splenic Anomalies (Figs. 1-6)

Since certain cardiac structures tend to be associated with splenic anomalies (asplenia; polysplenia), this section will deal with those patterns that may occur when the spleen is normally formed. It should be recognized that under certain circumstances both arteries may arise from the morphologic right ventricle while in others the two arteries are not separated, representing persistent truncus arteriosus. Under each of these two circumstances the diagrams presented here are not applicable to the great vessels but do apply to the atria and ventricles. In yet other circumstances the ventricular or atrial septum is absent.

Of the seven loose leaf sheets of diagrams presented in this communication, **(see sleeve at end of text)** four are applicable when the spleen is normally formed. Two of these are opaque (Figs. 1 and 2). The other two are transparent and each may be viewed from one side or the other; thus, with reversal these transparencies constitute four figures (Figs. 3-6).

Figures 1 and 2 portray the body type (Fig. 1, situs solitus; Fig. 2, situs inversus) and the positions of the morphologic right and left atria. In each opaque diagram, except for the atria, the heart is not shown, the aorta having been transected at the beginning of the arch and the pulmonary arteries separated at the hilus of each lung.

Each of the two transparent photographs (represented by Figs. 3-6) illustrates patterns of the ventricles and great arteries and may be viewed from either side. One side shows a given pattern and the opposite side, its inverted form.

One transparent sheet is identified on one side as Figure 3 and on the other side as Figure 4. In Figure 3 the ventricles are shown as non-inverted and the great arteries as non-transposed and non-inverted. The opposite side (Fig. 4) shows the ventricles to be inverted, while the great arteries are non-transposed but inverted.

The second transparent sheet is identified on one side as Figure 5 and on the other as Figure 6. In Figure 5, the ventricular pattern is that of non-inversion while the great arteries are transposed and non-inverted. The opposite side (Fig. 6) portrays the ventricles as inverted while the great arteries are transposed and inverted.

In using the diagrams a portrayal of the basic structure encountered is made as follows. The first step is to identify the positions of the two atria. From this information one is led to select either Figure 1 or Figure 2 as the background. Upon this is overlain Figure 3, 4, 5 or 6 to portray the positions of the ventricles and the nature of the great arteries. After the appropriate diagrammatic assembly is made, a permanent copy of the condition encountered may be obtained with a copying machine. Upon the resulting copy, associated anomalies may be indicated as well as information identifying the case. Additional copies, as desired, may be made of this derived portrayal of the anatomic details observed. The basic diagrams (Figs. 1-6) are reusable.

Using the diagrams supplied (Figs. 1-6) there are eight possible anatomic patterns of cardiac structure to be derived (Table II) of which four allow a normal route for the flow of blood, while in the other four patterns venous blood is delivered to the aorta. Considering that there are four patterns of cardiovascular structure, each with a different structural design but with the capability of supplying normal cardiac function (in the absence of associated anomalies), one is allowed to think, from the functional point of view that *four functionally normal hearts,* may be defined, each with a different anatomic structure

Table II

The Four Normal Hearts and the Four Types of "Complete Transposition"

Diagrammatic Assembly (Figure)	Inversion" Atria	Inversion" Ventricles	Inversion" Great Arteries	Transposition of Great Arteries	Anticipated Location of Cardiac Apex	Name of Entity
THE FOUR NORMAL HEARTS						
SITUS SOLITUS						
1, 3					Left	Usual Normal
1, 6		Present	Present	Present	Right	Corrected transposition in Situs Solitus
SITUS INVERSUS						
2, 4	Present	Present	Present		Right	Normal heart in Situs Inversus
2, 5	Present			Present	Left	Corrected transposition in Situs Inversus
FOUR TYPES OF "COMPLETE TRANSPOSITION"						
SITUS SOLITUS						
1, 5				Present	Left	Classical complete transposition
1, 4		Present	Present		Right	Clinical complete transposition in Situs Solitus
SITUS INVERSUS						
2, 6	Present	Present	Present	Present	Right	Complete transposition in Situs Inversus
2, 3	Present				Left	Clinical complete transposition in Situs Inversus

☐ Absent ▨ Present

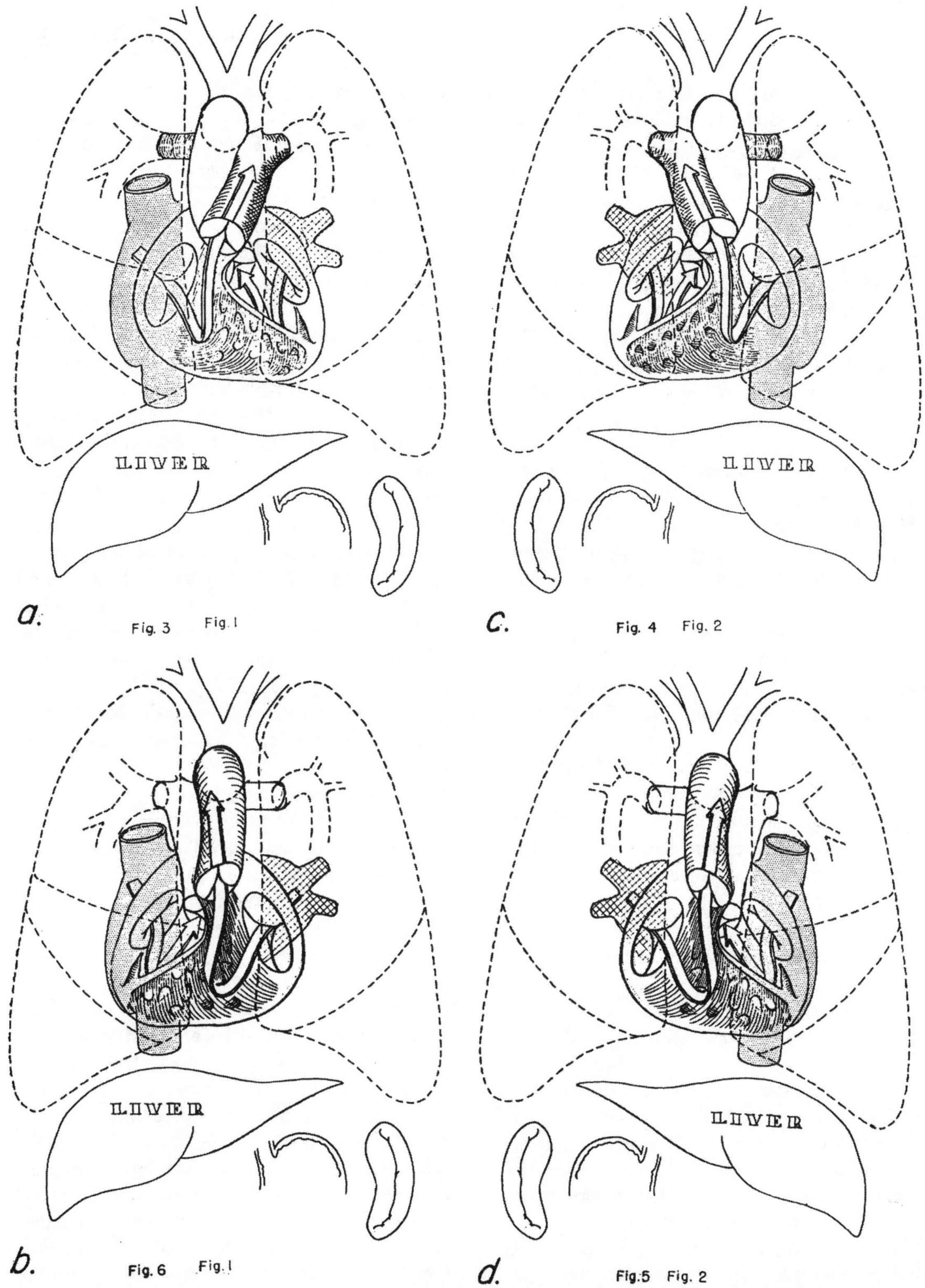

Figure 12

The four normal hearts illustrated diagrammatically by assembly of diagrams as indicated in text. a. *The usual normal.* b. *Corrected transposition in situs solitus.* c. *Normal heart of situs inversus.* d. *Corrected transposition in situs inversus.* a *and* c *are mirror images of each other;* b *and* d *are mirror images of each other.*

(Fig. 12). There are also four anatomic types of "complete transposition" (Table II; Fig. 13).

The Four Normal Hearts (Table II; Fig. 12)

Proper assembly of units of the diagrams will portray four patterns of anatomic structure of the heart and great vessels each of which has been observed in man and in each of which the route of the flow of blood is normal. Among hearts bearing any one of the four basic structures to be described, abnormalities in circulation result not from the basic cardiac structure but from associated conditions, such as valvular abnormalities or septal defects.

1. *"The Usual Normal."* (Diagrammatic Assembly: Figs. 1 and 3. Body Type: Situs solitus. Anatomic Definition: Atrial non-inversion; ventricular non-inversion; non-transposition and non-inversion of great arteries.) (Fig. 12*a*)

This is the prevailing pattern in present-day man and in other mammals. It is called "the normal" but three other anatomic forms may yield a normal route for the flow of blood.

2. *"Corrected Transposition in Situs Solitus."* (Diagrammatic Assembly: Figs. 1 and 6. Body Type: Situs solitus. Anatomic Definition: Atrial non-inversion; ventricular inversion; transposition and inversion of great arteries.) (Fig. 12*b*)

In this pattern, functional abnormality of the circulation results from commonly associated malformations such as ventricular septal defect and/or incompetence of the inverted morphologic tricuspid valve, the latter condition yielding "mitral" insufficiency, clinically. Without associated malformations the basic anatomic structure allows the circulation to be normal. As the morphologic left ventricle lies on the right, the apex would be expected to lie on the right but exceptions to this rule are common in this condition.

The term *isolated dextrocardia* has been used to name the disparity between the right-sided cardiac apex and the left-sided stomach. Among subjects with corrected transposition in situs solitus some represent the exceptional phenomenon that the right ventricle forms the cardiac apex, the apex thus pointing toward the left.

3. *"The Normal Heart of Situs Inversus."* (Diagrammatic Assembly: Figs. 2 and 4. Body Type: Situs inversus. Anatomic Definition: Atrial inversion; ventricular inversion; non-transposition with inversion of the great arteries.) (Fig. 12*c*)

This pattern represents total inversion of "the usual normal" heart and is the usual pattern among individuals with total situs inversus. As the morphologic left ventricle lies on the right side, the apex lies on the right. In this particular situation wherein the dextrocardia is part of the total body inversion, a synonym for this cardiac pattern is *"mirror image dextrocardia."*

4. *"Corrected Transposition in Situs Inversus."* (Diagrammatic Assembly: Figs. 2 and 5. Body Type: Situs inversus. Anatomic Definition: Atrial inversion; non-inversion of ventricles; transposition without inversion of great arteries.) (Fig. 12*d*)

This is the fourth pattern of the four normal hearts and is the least prevalent of the group. In essence, it is the inverted form of corrected transposition in situs solitus (Fig. 12*b*). The greatest variety of terms has been applied to this pattern of normal heart mainly on the basis that the ventricles (and their atrioventricular valves) are not inverted. If, incorrectly, primary attention is given to this point and not to the atria, we observe such expressions as, "The ventricles and the AV valves are normal but the rest of the heart is abnormal."

If, however, the atria are first defined, it becomes immediately apparent that situs inversus is the basic condition. Under this circumstance it would be expected that the morphologic left ventricle would lie on the right side, rather than on the left. The presence on the left of the morphologic left ventricle is an inversion of the anticipated "normal of situs inversus" and the cardiac structure represents a mirror image to the situation in corrected transposition of situs solitus.

In corrected transposition of situs inversus, as the morphologic left ventricle lies on the

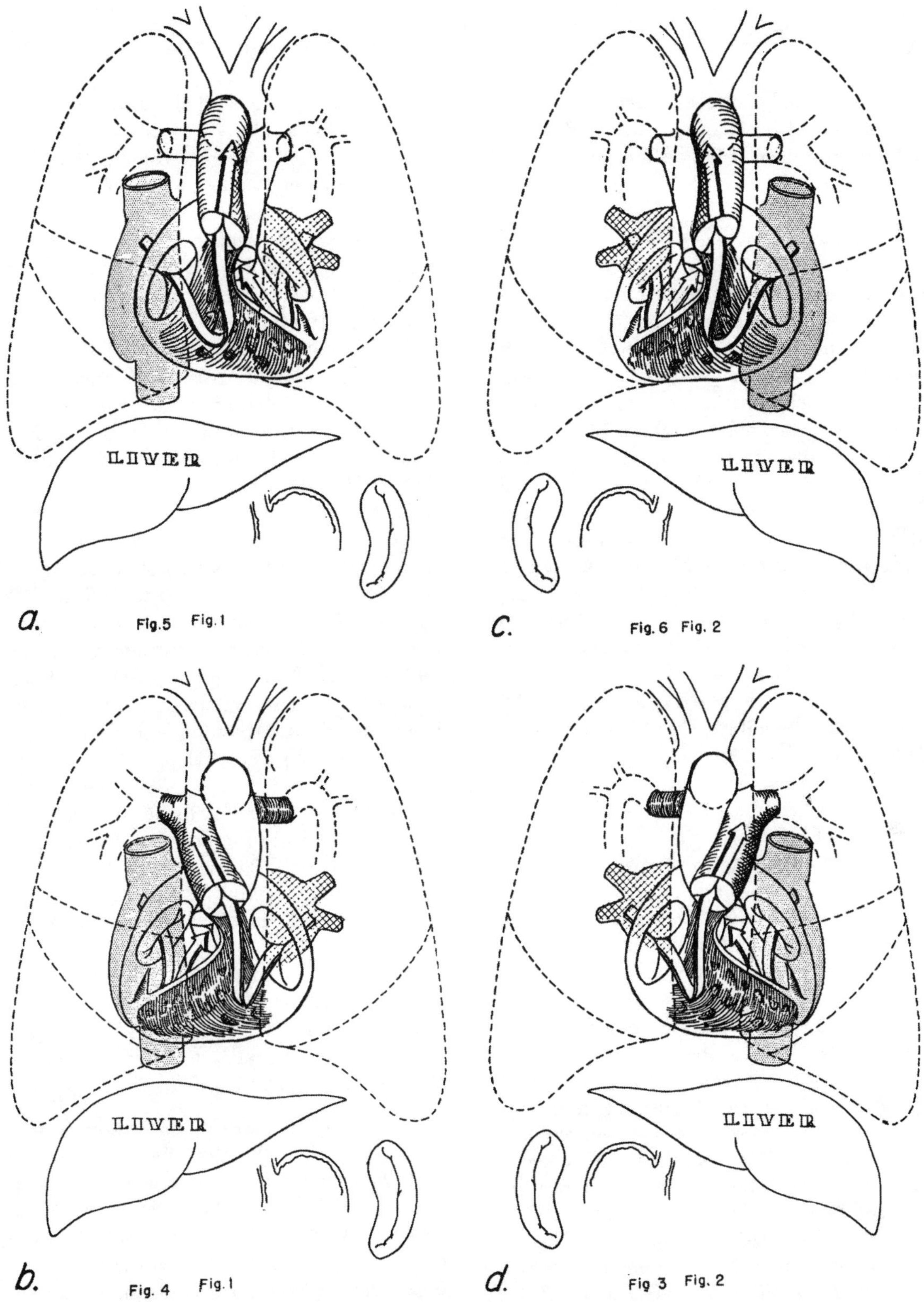

Figure 13

Four types of "complete transposition." a. *Classical complete transposition.* b. *Clinical complete transposition in situs solitus.* c. *Complete transposition in situs inversus.* d. *Clinical complete tranposition in situs inversus.* a *and* c *are mirror images of each other;* b *and* d *are mirror images of each other.*

left side of the heart, the cardiac apex would be anticipated on the left. Such a deviation in total situs inversus has been called *"isolated levocardia."*

The Four Forms of "Complete Transposition" (Table II; Fig. 13)

It has been shown that there are four normal hearts in the sense that certain hearts with different anatomic structures allow a normal route for the flow of blood. There are, in addition, four anatomic patterns of heart, each of which functionally conforms to the definition for complete transposition in the sense that the venous blood is delivered to the aorta and the arterialized blood to the pulmonary trunk. In two of the forms the great arteries anatomically are not transposed but since the circulation is like that in classical complete transposition, they will be specially designated as "clinical complete transposition" and could be called "functional complete transposition."

1. *"Classical Complete Transposition."* (Diagrammatic Assembly: Figs. 1 and 5. Body Type: Situs solitus. Anatomic Definition: Atrial non-inversion; ventricular non-inversion; transposition and non-inversion of the great arteries.) (Fig. 13*a*)

This is the well-known pattern usually called complete transposition.

2. *"Clinical Complete Transposition in Situs Solitus."* (Diagrammatic Assembly: Figs. 1 and 4. Body Type: Situs solitus. Anatomic Definition: Atrial non-inversion; ventricular inversion; inversion without transposition of great arteries.) (Fig. 13*b*)

This rare form exhibits two features in common with corrected transposition in situs solitus, namely inversion of the ventricles and great arteries. The important difference is that in this condition the great arteries are not transposed, while they are transposed in corrected transposition. In the condition under consideration the anterior of the two great arteries is the pulmonary trunk and this joins the morphologic right ventricle. As the latter is inverted, it lies on the left side and receives arterialized blood from the left atrium. The posteriorly lying nontransposed aorta joins the right-sided morphologic left ventricle. The resulting circulation is like that in classical complete transposition. It is anticipated, although situs solitus is the body type, that the cardiac apex, formed by the morphologic left ventricle, will lie on the right side. Under this circumstance this cardiac pattern would be yet another example of *isolated dextrocardia.*

3. *"Complete Transposition in Situs Inversus."* (Diagrammatic Assembly: Figs. 2 and 6. Body Type: Situs inversus. Anatomic Definition: Atrial inversion; ventricular inversion; transposition and inversion of the great arteries.) (Fig. 13*c*)

This cardiac pattern, as indicated by its name, is seen in situs inversus and represents total inversion of the pattern of classical complete transposition as seen in situs solitus.

4. *"Clinical Complete Transposition in Situs Inversus."* (Diagrammatic Assembly: Figs. 2 and 3. Body Type: Situs inversus. Anatomic Definition: Atrial inversion; ventricular non-inversion; non-transposition and non-inversion of great vessels.) (Fig. 13*d*)

This interesting pattern might be described as "normal heart but with atrial inversion." To do so overlooks the fact that the atrial inversion is part of situs inversus. In this circumstance the positions of the ventricles and the great vessels are obviously abnormal for situs inversus.

The anatomic connections determine that the circulation is like that in classical complete transposition. The pattern is the inverted form of that designated as "clinical complete transposition in situs solitus."

Use of the Diagrams in the Presence of Splenic Anomalies

It is recognized that asplenia and polysplenia each have a peculiar tendency for association with specific cardiac anomalies and certain body types. In asplenia there is a tendency for "bilateral right-sidedness" and in polysplenia, "bilateral left-sidedness." In polysplenia the great vessels are usually not transposed and pulmonary stenosis is usually absent. Inversion of the entire heart, as part of total situs inversus, occurs in about one-third of the cases. In asplenia, transposition of the great vessels with or without inversion and with pulmonary stenosis are characteristics.

Polysplenia (Fig. 14)

The diagram illustrating the body type in polysplenia is shown as Figure 7. It is apparent from this that variations in the disposition of the organs is common, some cases showing typical features of situs solitus, others situs inversus and still others no strong tendency for one type of orientation or the other. Use of this diagram requires masking out those features which do not apply for the given case. Among the strong tendencies in this condition is that of "bilateral left-sidedness" of the two lungs. In this, each lung possesses two lobes and the basic arterial and bronchial patterns of the usual left lung. Characteristically, the great vessels are not transposed (although inversion is common) and, in contrast to asplenia, pulmonary stenosis is usually absent. There is a strong tendency for persistence of two superior venae cavae, each of these vessels inserting into the homolateral atrium, although in some cases one superior vena cava joins the coronary sinus. It is also common that the pulmonary veins show anomalous connection to the venous atrium. This may involve either all of the pulmonary veins or only those on the side homolateral with the venous atrium.

Also, it is frequently observed, though not universally, that the inferior vena cava fails to pass through the liver and instead is continuous either with the azygos or hemiazygos vein (so-called interruption of the inferior vena cava).

Diagrammatic construction of the patterns seen in polysplenia makes use of Figure 7 as the body type and combining this either with

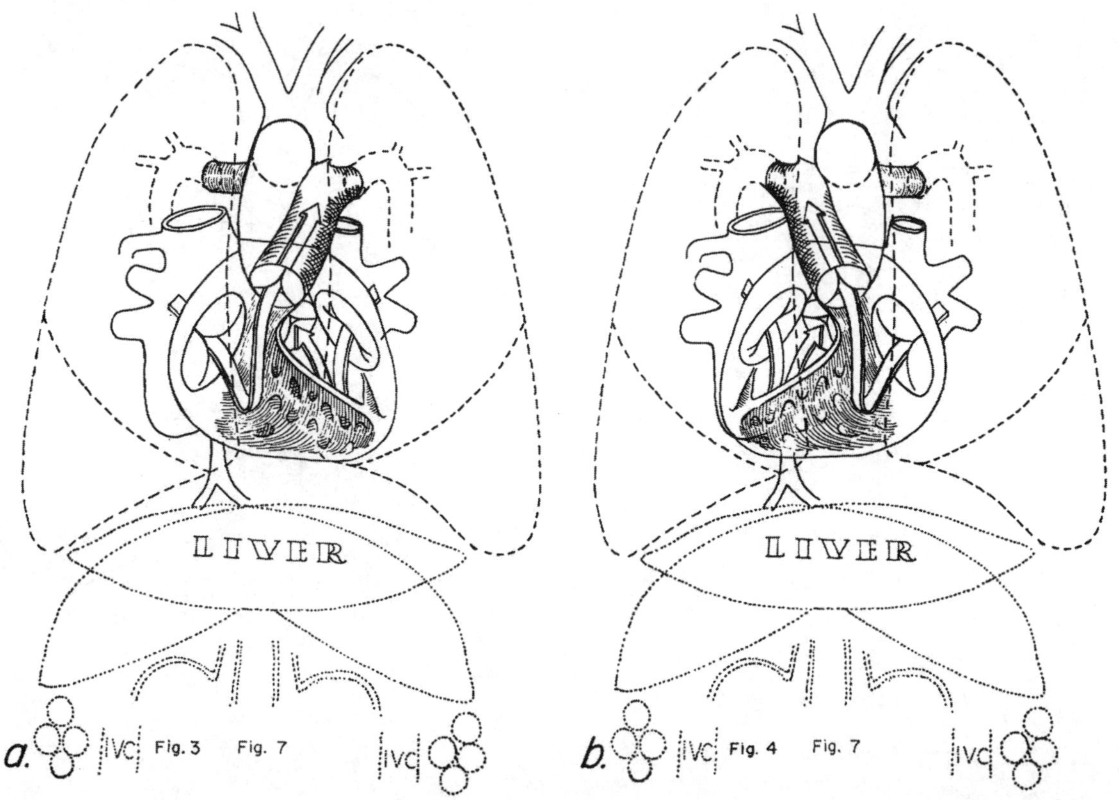

Figure 14

Anatomic patterns observed in polysplenia. Final preparation of diagram for a given case requires masking out non-pertinent material in upper abdomen.

Figure 3 or 4, yielding (before masking of inappropriate structures) the composite illustrations shown in Figure 14. To portray the features in a given case variations in pulmonary venous and in inferior vena caval connections as well as the positions of the upper abdominal organs need to be indicated upon the machine-copied result.

Asplenia (Fig. 15)

Usually, in asplenia the body type may be portrayed by Figure 8. This shows the common phenomenon of bilateral superior venae cavae, each vessel joining the homolateral side of the frequently present common atrium. The usual cardiac structures are shown in Figures 9 and 10. Uncommonly, the basic structure of the heart resembles that in Figures 5 or 6.

The cardiac pattern usually present may be portrayed by that shown in Figure 15*a* or its inverted form which is Figure 15*b*. Each diagram shows the usually present common atrioventricular valve. These diagrams also show two ventricles although some cases, with the basic relationships between the heart and great vessels as portrayed, display a single ventricle.

Among cases of asplenia the stomach may be found in the left or the right side of the abdomen. When a permanent copy is made of the appropriate assembly of diagrams, the position of the stomach may be indicated by masking out that indication of stomach which does not apply.

Comment

Recognizing the occurrence of such entities as single ventricle, persistent truncus arteriosus and origin of both great vessels from the right ventricle and cardiovascular anomalies associated with the maldevelopment of the

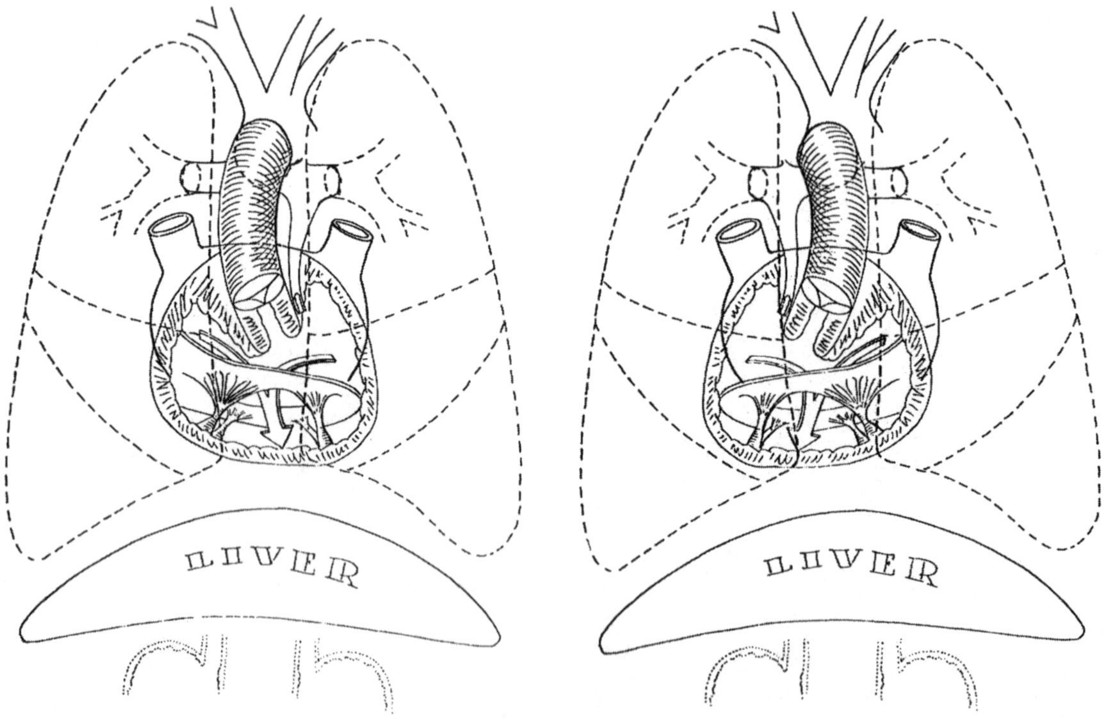

a. Fig. 8 Fig. 9 b. Fig. 8 Fig.10

Figure 15

Anatomic patterns observed in asplenia. Final preparation of diagram for a given case requires masking out non-pertinent material in upper abdomen.

spleen, the diagrams presented have been found useful by the authors in demonstrating the cardiac structure in a given case. By appropriate use of the diagrams one may not only record the basic structure in a given heart, but also anticipate associations in cardiac structure given one anatomic point from which to work such as body situs, the presence or absence of transposition of the great arteries and the position of the cardiac apex. The original concept in constructing the diagram was based on the following question and answer.

"In a recipient with a given type of heart, is it possible to transplant another type of heart and obtain a normal route for the flow of blood?" The answer, supported by the diagrams is, "It is possible, if the arterial connections are made sufficiently distant from the heart." In keeping with this answer, it will be noted that the hypothetical transections of the arteries were made at the beginning of the aortic arch and at the proximal part of each pulmonary artery. Consideration to detailed answers to the question posed will be given in a later part of this communication.

Body Situs

Given a certain type of body structure and in the absence of splenic anomalies, it is apparent (Table III) that four types of cardiac structure may be anticipated, two with a normal route for the flow of blood (the patterns of the usual normal and that of corrected transposition for that body situs; Figs. 12*a* and *b* for situs solitus and Figs. 12*c* and *d* for situs inversus). Also for each body situs two patterns are possible in which venous blood is delivered into the aorta (classical complete transposition and so-called clinical complete transposition for that body situs;

Table III

Types of Heart in Situs Solitus and in Situs Inversus

TYPES OF HEART IN SITUS SOLITUS AND IN SITUS INVERSUS						
Diagrammatic Assembly (Figure)	Inversion			Transposition of Great Arteries	Anticipated Location of Cardiac Apex	Name of Entity
	Atria	Ventricles	Great Arteries			
SITUS SOLITUS						
1, 3					Left	Usual Normal
1, 5				Present	Left	Classical complete transposition in Situs Solitus
1, 4		Present	Present		Right	Clinical complete transposition in Situs Solitus
1, 6		Present	Present	Present	Right	Corrected transposition in Situs Solitus
SITUS INVERSUS						
2, 4	Present	Present	Present		Right	Normal heart in Situs Inversus
2, 6	Present	Present	Present	Present	Right	Complete transposition in Situs Inversus
2, 3	Present				Left	Clinical complete transposition in Situs Inversus
2, 5	Present			Present	Left	Corrected transposition in Situs Inversus

☐ Absent ▨ Present

Figs. 13*a* and *b* for situs solitus and Figs. 13*c* and *d* for situs inversus.)

Transposition of Great Arteries

In considering the positions of the great arteries to each other it is important to re-emphasize that these must be defined from two points of view, the lateral relationship between the vessels (inversion or non-inversion) and the anteroposterior relationship (transposition or non-transposition). Transposition refers to the state in which the aortic origin lies anterior to the pulmonary trunk in contrast to non-transposition in which the reverse is true. In understanding the basis for the connections between the great arteries and the ventricles, it is important to recognize two principles: (1) *the outlet of the morphologic right ventricle lies anterior to the outlet of the morphologic left ventricle* and (2) *the anterior of the two arteries connects with the morphologic right ventricle.* While these two principles are important in understanding the ventricular-arterial relationships, they do not by themselves define the route for the flow of blood, since these additionally depend upon the atrial-ventricular connections. It thus becomes apparent (Table IV) that in the presence of transposition there are circumstances in which the route of the flow of blood may be normal (Figs. 12*b* and *d*) while in other circumstances in the absence of transposition, venous blood may be delivered to the aorta (Figs. 13*b* and *d*). It is evident that without knowing the lateral relationships of the great vessels (inversion or

Table IV

Types of Heart According to Presence or Absence of Transposition of Great Arteries

TYPES OF HEART ACCORDING TO PRESENCE OR ABSENCE OF TRANSPOSITION OF GREAT ARTERIES

Diagrammatic Assembly (Figure)	Inversion			Transposition of Great Arteries	Anticipated Location of Cardiac Apex	Name of Entity
	Atria	Ventricles	Great Arteries			
TRANSPOSITION ABSENT						
SITUS SOLITUS						
1, 3					Left	Usual Normal
1, 4		Present	Present		Right	Clinical complete transposition in Situs Solitus
SITUS INVERSUS						
2, 4	Present	Present	Present		Right	Normal heart in Situs Inversus
2, 3	Present				Left	Clinical complete transposition Situs Inversus
TRANSPOSITION PRESENT						
SITUS SOLITUS						
1, 5				Present	Left	Classical complete transposition
1, 6		Present	Present	Present	Right	Corrected transposition in Situs Solitus
SITUS INVERSUS						
2, 6	Present	Present	Present	Present	Right	Complete transposition in Situs Inversus
2, 5	Present			Present	Left	Corrected transposition in Situs Inversus

☐ Absent ▨ Present

non-inversion) or the relationships between the ventricles and the atria, knowledge of the anteroposterior relationship between the great vessels does not yield definitive information as to normality or abnormality concerning the route of the flow of blood.

Position of the Cardiac Apex

The literature contains considerable reference to the position of the cardiac apex as a point of departure in the anatomic classification of cardiac structure. When the apex lies on the right side, rather than the left, it is correct to use this as an index for suspicion as to a deviation from normal structure but this does not represent a specific entity.

First, it is to be recognized that the cardiac malformations associated either with polysplenia (Fig. 14) or with asplenia (Fig. 15) frequently show a right-sided apex. Consideration to these possibilities should be given early in the analysis of the case, especially when the cardiac apex lies on a side contralateral to that of the stomach.

In the absence of splenic anomalies, a right-sided cardiac apex may be indicative of total inversion of the organs (so-called mirror image dextrocardia; Table V; Figs. 12*c* and 13*c*), or it may represent some other condition. It is to be recognized that the morphologic left ventricle tends to form the cardiac apex but in uncommon situations an otherwise normal heart may display a right-sided apex, formed by the right ventricle. Thus, the position of the cardiac apex is not an absolute indication of the position of the

Table V

Anatomic Types of Heart According to Side of Apex

ANATOMIC TYPES OF HEART ACCORDING TO SIDE OF APEX						
Diagrammatic Assembly (Figure)	Inversion			Transposition of Great Arteries	Anticipated Location of Cardiac Apex	Name of Entity
	Atria	Ventricles	Great Arteries			
LEFT APEX (LEVOCARDIA)						
SITUS SOLITUS						
1, 3					Left	Usual Normal
1, 5				Present	Left	Classical complete transposition
SITUS INVERSUS						
2, 3	Present				Left	Clinical complete transposition in Situs Inversus
2, 5	Present			Present	Left	Corrected transposition in Situs Inversus
RIGHT APEX (DEXTROCARDIA)						
SITUS INVERSUS						
2, 4	Present	Present	Present		Right	Normal heart in Situs Inversus
2, 6	Present	Present	Present	Present	Right	Complete transposition in Situs Inversus
SITUS SOLITUS						
1, 4		Present	Present		Right	Clinical complete transposition in Situs Solitus
1, 6		Present	Present	Present	Right	Corrected transposition in Situs Solitus

☐ Absent ▨ Present

morphologic left ventricle. One recognizes cases in which the cardiac apex lies on the right, while the stomach is on the left (so-called isolated dextrocardia). In such cases, using the point that the left ventricle *tends* to form the apex of the heart, one can assume as an initial step that the ventricles are inverted. Such an assumption (Table V) would lead to a suspicion of corrected transposition in situs solitus (Fig. 12*b*). This usually turns out to be the case. Nevertheless, this is not universally supported. It might represent clinical complete transposition in situs solitus (Fig. 13*b*). Also, the right ventricle may uncommonly form the cardiac apex. The latter point is portrayed in certain cases, particularly of corrected transposition in situs solitus in which the morphologic right ventricle lying on the left may point to the left.

In situs inversus the apex is expected to point to the right but in this body type the apex may point to the left (Figs. 12*d* and 13*d*). As the counterpart of those unusual situations in situs solitus in which the morphologic right ventricle forms the cardiac apex, the cardiac apex may lie on the side opposite to that anticipated.

Types of Heart Potentially Transplantable

Reference to Figures 1-6 indicate that in considering transplantation of the heart, the anatomic state in the donor need not be the same as in the recipient for the resulting route of the flow of blood to be normal. In Table VI the various types of cardiac structure in donors which are applicable to potential recipients are given. In essence, for the recipient with a given body type, the donor's cardiac structure may be the usual normal or corrected transposition of the same body type as in the recipient or complete transposition of the opposite body type.

Table VI

Types of Heart Potentially Transplantable to Accomplish a Normal Route for the Flow of Blood

TYPES OF HEART POTENTIALLY TRANSPLANTABLE	
Type of Body and Heart of Donor	Anatomic Result of Transplantation
SITUS SOLITUS IN RECIPIENT	
Usual Normal Heart in Situs Solitus (1,3)	Usual Normal Heart in Situs Solitus (1,3)
Corrected Transposition in Situs Solitus (1,6)	Corrected Transposition in Situs Solitus (1,6)
Complete Transposition in Situs Inversus (2,6)	Corrected Transposition in Situs Solitus (1,6)
SITUS INVERSUS IN RECIPIENT	
Normal Heart in Situs Inversus (2,4)	Normal Heart in Situs Inversus (2,4)
Corrected Transposition in Situs Inversus (2,5)	Corrected Transposition in Situs Inversus (2,5)
Complete Transposition in Situs Solitus (1,5)	Corrected Transposition in Situs Inversus (2,5)

References

1. PUTSCHAR, W. G. J., AND MANION, W. C.: Congenital absence of the spleen and associated abnormalities. Am. J. Clin. Path. **26:** 429, 1956.
2. MOLLER, J. H., NAKIB, A., ANDERSON, R. C., AND EDWARDS, J. E.: Congenital cardiac disease associated with polysplenia. A developmental complex of bilateral "left-sidedness." Circulation **36:** 789, 1967.

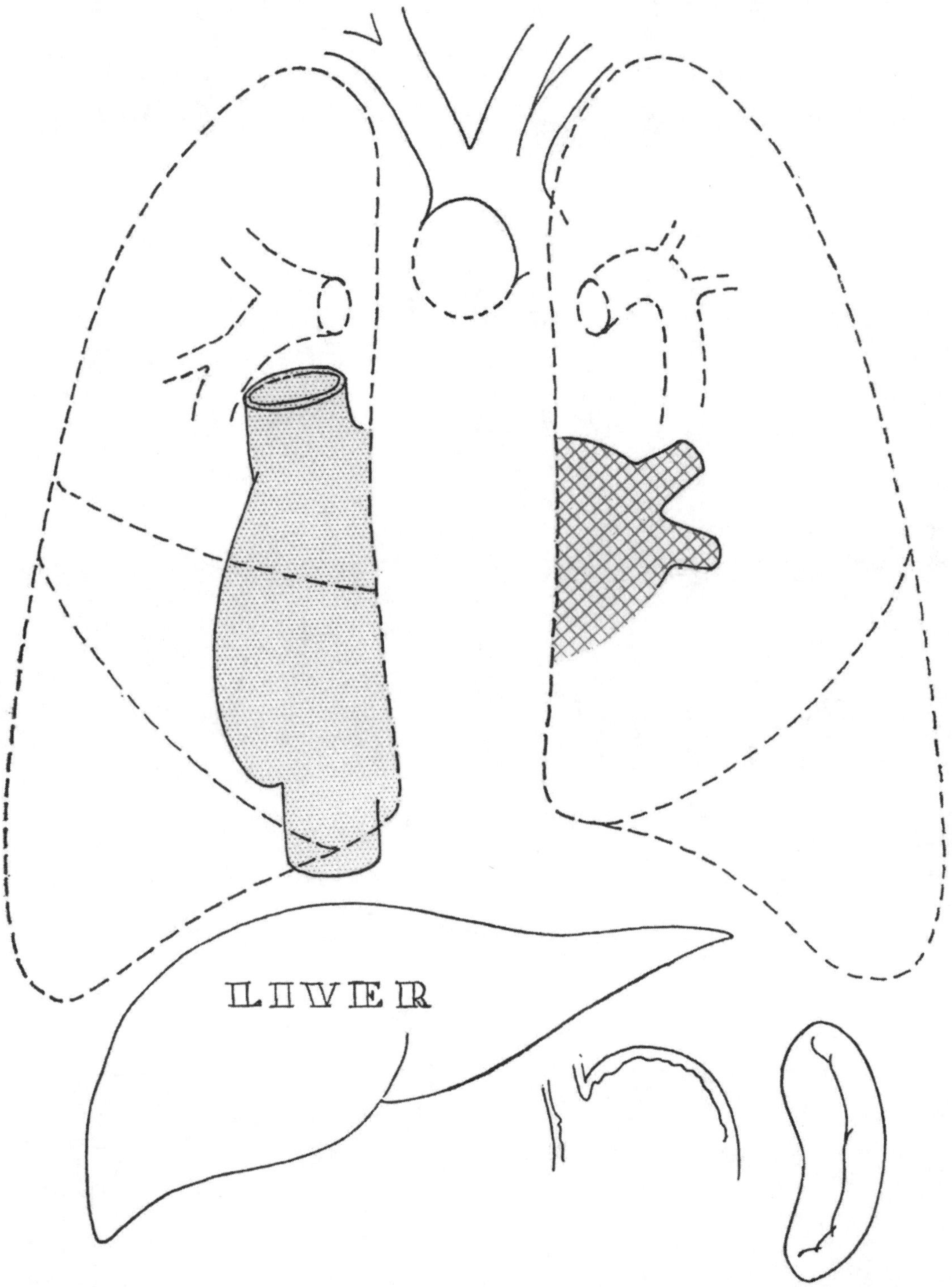

Figure 1

Body type in situs solitus. The morphologic right and left atria lie in the right and left sides of the heart, respectively.

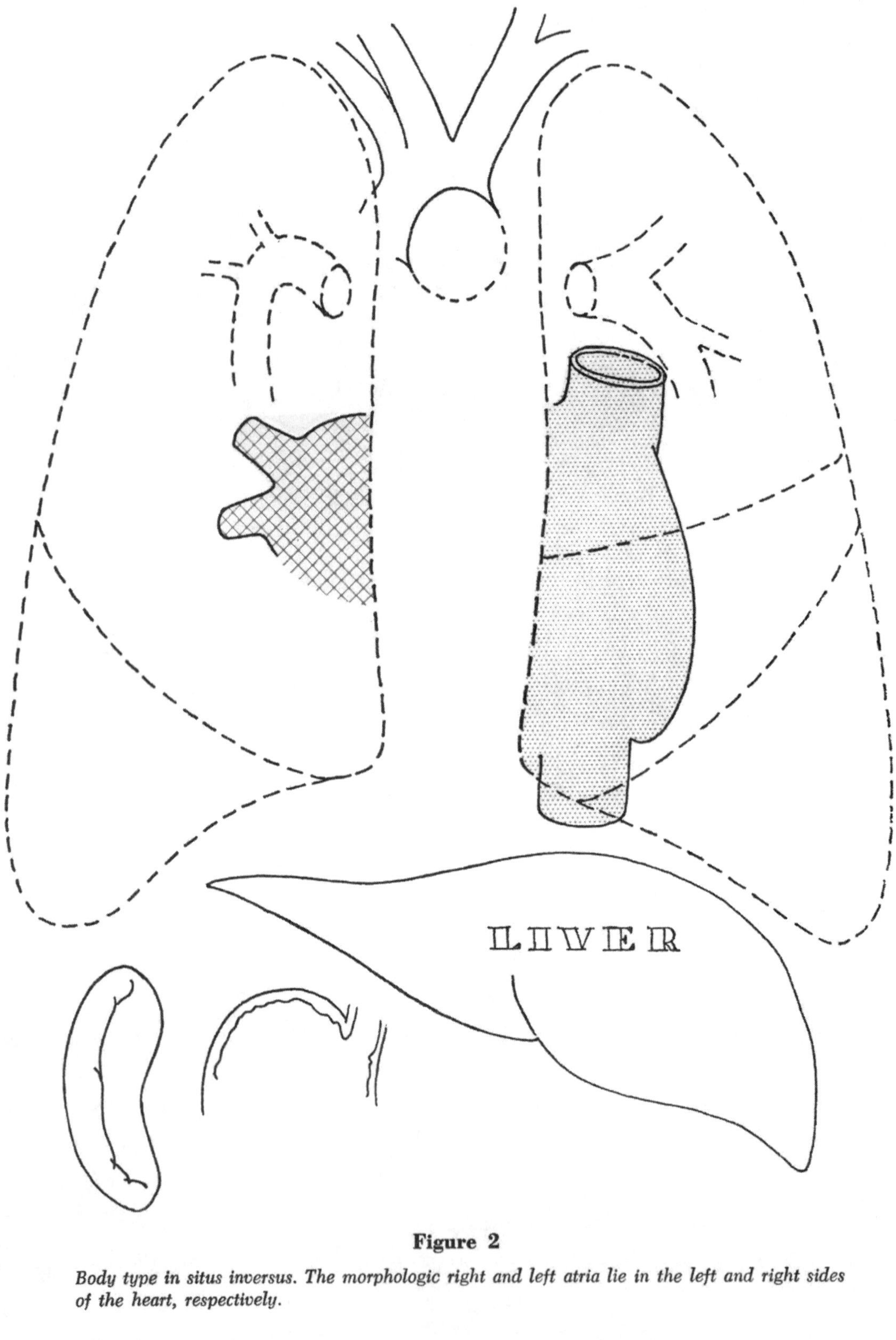

Figure 2

Body type in situs inversus. The morphologic right and left atria lie in the left and right sides of the heart, respectively.

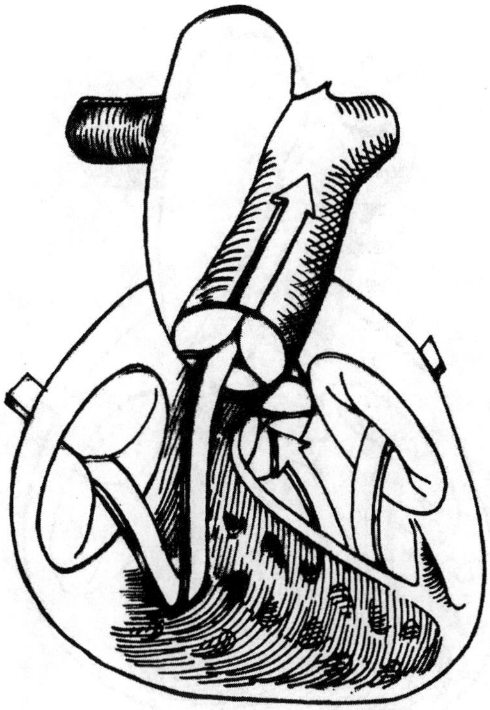

Figure 3

Non-inversion of ventricles: non-inversion and non-transposition of great arteries.

Supplement IV to Circulation, Vols. XXXVII and XXXVIII, June 1968

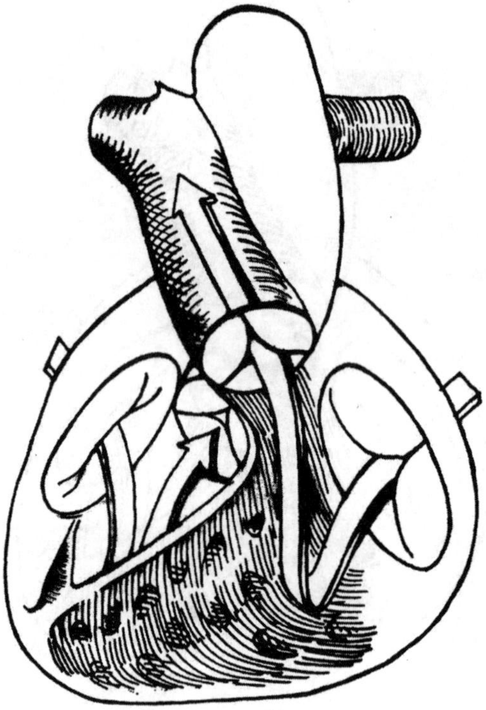

Figure 4

Inversion of ventricles; inversion without transposition of great arteries.

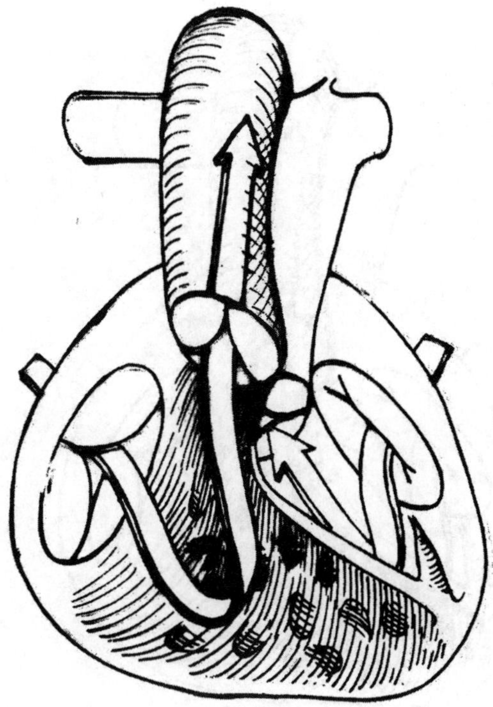

Figure 5

Non-inversion of ventricles; transposition without inversion of great arteries.

Supplement IV to Circulation, Vols. XXXVII and XXXVIII, June 1968

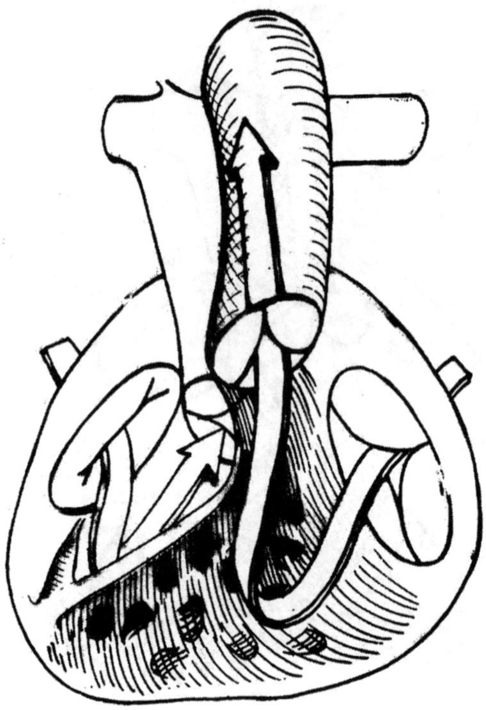

Figure 6

Inversion of ventricles; transposition with inversion of great arteries.

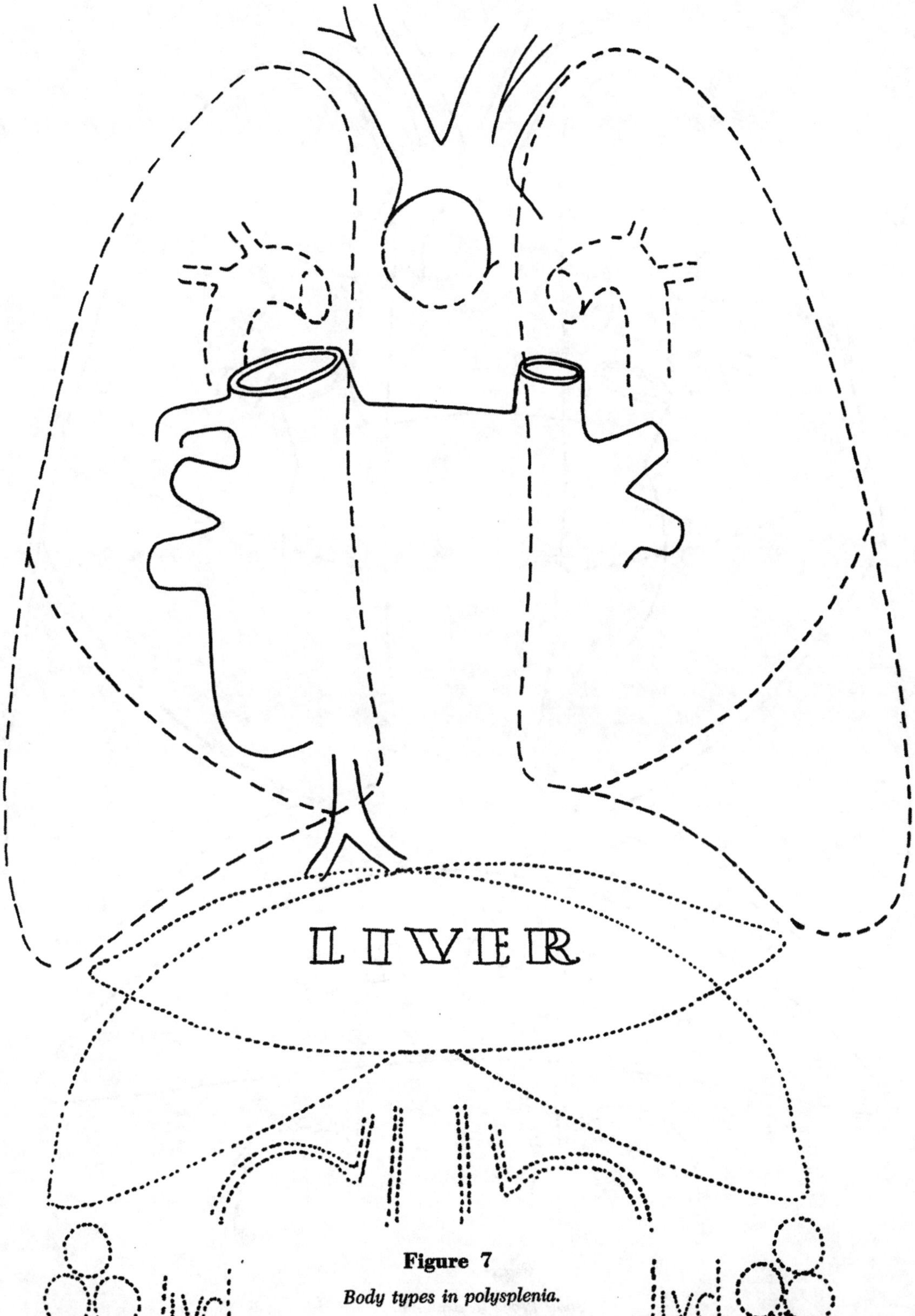

Figure 7

Body types in polysplenia.

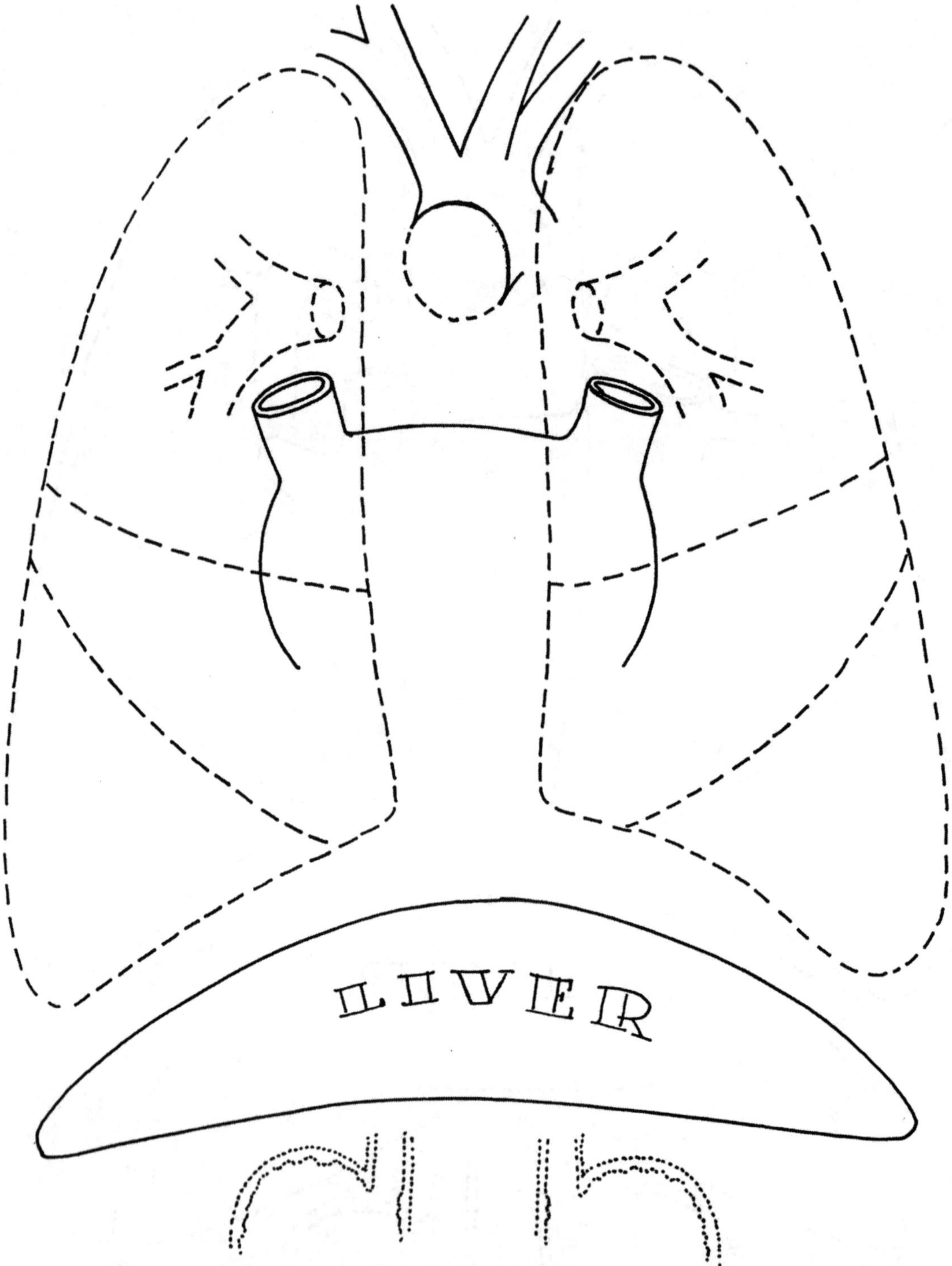

Figure 8
Body types in asplenia.

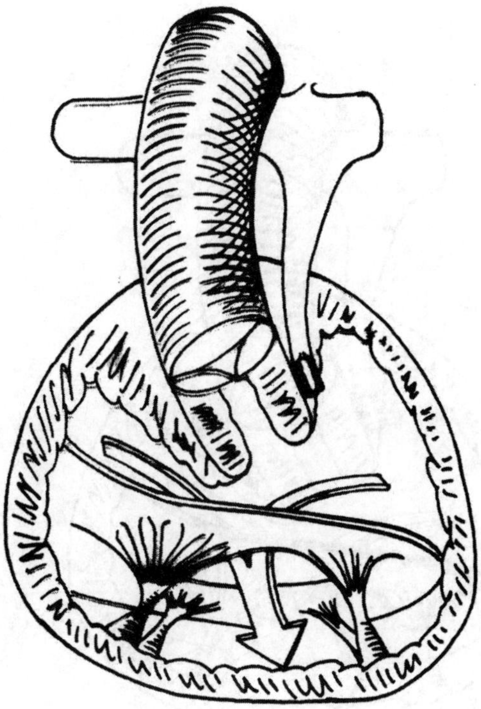

Figure 9

A condition observed in asplenia. Single ventricle; common atrioventricular valve; transposition of great arteries without inversion; pulmonary stenosis.

Supplement IV to Circulation, Vols. XXXVII and XXXVIII, June 1968

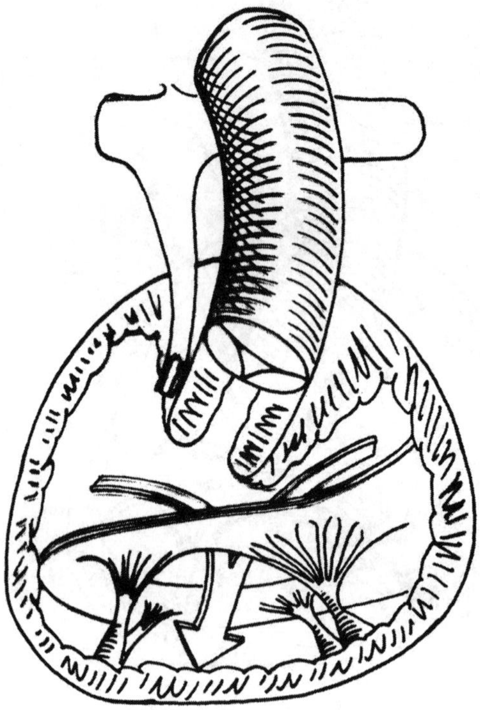

Figure 10

A condition observed in asplenia. Single ventricle; common atrioventricular valve; transposition of great arteries with inversion; pulmonary stenosis.

Diagrammatic Portrayal of Variations in Cardiac Structure.

Reference to Transposition, Dextrocardia and the Concept of Four Normal Hearts.

William D. Edwards, M.D.

Within the realm of congenital heart disease, perhaps no cases are quite as complicated as those associated with the asplenia or polysplenia syndrome. These, in turn, are generally characterized by abnormalities in body sidedness that affect not only the cardiovascular system but also the respiratory and digestive systems. Add dextrocardia (right-sided cardiac apex) to the mix, and it becomes clear why such cases are considered to represent *complex* congenital heart disease.

By the mid 1960's, after a decade of open-heart surgery, movement was afoot to better organize and standardize the existing knowledge of the morphology of congenital cardiac malformations. At this time, Dr. Richard Van Praagh described the segmental approach to the evaluation and diagnosis of congenital heart disease. It is in this context that the article by Stanger et al was produced from the pathology laboratory of Dr. Jesse E. Edwards.

Its strength lay in the clarity of its descriptions (a hallmark of the writings of Dr. Jesse Edwards), and its popularity lay in the power of its illustrations. This article was unique because it provided the reader with clear plastic overlays that could be used to construct schematic diagrams of the four normal hearts, as well as diagrams of hearts with variations in sidedness (normal or inverted), apical direction (levocardia or dextrocardia), and transposition. Thus, the overlays were useful for illustrating hearts with or without splenic anomalies.

The importance of this landmark article lies in its ability to make sense of a complex topic and to organize it in such a way even those who are "three-dimensionally challenged" could readily conceptualize the anatomy. Part of the genius of the article was Jess's astute use of multiple clear plastic overlays, each of which contained only a selected portion of the whole heart diagram.

The reader was no longer a passive learner, but rather an active one who could compile various combinations of overlays to construct and create a wide variety of malformed hearts of progressively increasing complexity. This was an example of a self-teaching module well before such educational methods had been commonly applied to medical education.

The innovative article from Dr. Edwards' laboratory served not only to enlighten those who read it at the time but also to form the foundation for the publications of his successors. In this regard, the later works of Dr. Robert Anderson and his colleagues in London on the topics of nomenclature, apical direction, sidedness, and complex congenital heart disease all have their roots in the pioneering studies and publications of such giants in the field as Dr. Jesse E. Edwards.

Clinical communications

Dissecting aneurysm complicating Marfan's syndrome (arachnodactyly) in a mother and son

Claude M. Grondin, M.D.
Charles L. Steinberg, M.D.
Jesse E. Edwards, M.D.
Minneapolis, Minn.

A hereditary tendency in Marfan's syndrome (arachnodactyly) is recognized, but relatively few cases have been documented with necropsy. This phenomenon was represented by the occurrence of this syndrome in a mother and son which came to our attention. In each, dissecting aneurysm of the aorta was demonstrated pathologically as a major complication. In the son, deformities of the atrioventricular valves were of additional interest. As far as we are aware, there is only one other report in which close relatives with Marfan's syndrome each suffered from dissecting aneurysm of the aorta as supported by necropsy findings.

This phenomenon was described by Whittaker and Sheehan[1] in 1954. A father suffered from dissecting aneurysm at the age of 46 years and his son experienced the same condition when he was 27 years old.

The purpose of this report is to place on record a second family with Marfan's syndrome in which dissecting aneurysm occurred in close relatives.

Case reports

*Case 1.**

CLINICAL FEATURES. A 30-year-old housewife in the twenty-second week of her third pregnancy was admitted to The Charles T. Miller Hospital in October, 1955, with a 48 hour history of substernal pain radiating to the jaws and to the interscapular region.

Physical examination revealed dolichostenomelia, arachnodactyly, scoliosis of the thoracic spine, and pectus carinatum. There were no ocular symptoms or abnormal signs. A loud systolic murmur was heard loudest over the left sternal border at the level of the third intercostal space and it radiated to the neck. No diastolic murmur could be heard. The pulse rate was 60 per minute and regular. The right arm and hand were cool and clammy.

The blood pressure averaged 140 mm. Hg systolic and 55 mm. Hg diastolic in the left arm. In the right arm, the pressure, at first unobtainable, leveled to 70 mm. Hg and this discrepancy persisted throughout the remainder of her life.

The patient's condition stabilized within the next 10 days. Three months later, a cesarean section and tubal ligation were performed. Congestive cardiac failure developed 6 months later, and the patient was rehospitalized. At that time, a Grade II/IV diastolic murmur over the left sternal border and a muffled systolic murmur were heard, the latter radiating to the left axilla.

While in a state of congestive cardiac failure,

From the Department of Pathology, The Charles T. Miller and The Children's Hospitals, St. Paul, Minn., and the Departments of Surgery and Pathology, University of Minnesota, Minneapolis, Minn.

This study was supported by Public Health Service Research Grant 5 RO1 HE05694 and Research Training Grant 2 T1 HE05570 from the National Heart Institute.
Received for publication Dec. 21, 1967.

*Details of this case were reported by Husebye and associates.[2]

the patient died suddenly at home in December, 1956, nearly 14 months after the first admission.

Roentgenograms taken during both hospital admissions had confirmed the clinical diagnosis of dilatation of the ascending aorta and progressive cardiac enlargement. The electrocardiographic tracings showed left axis deviation and left ventricular hypertrophy.

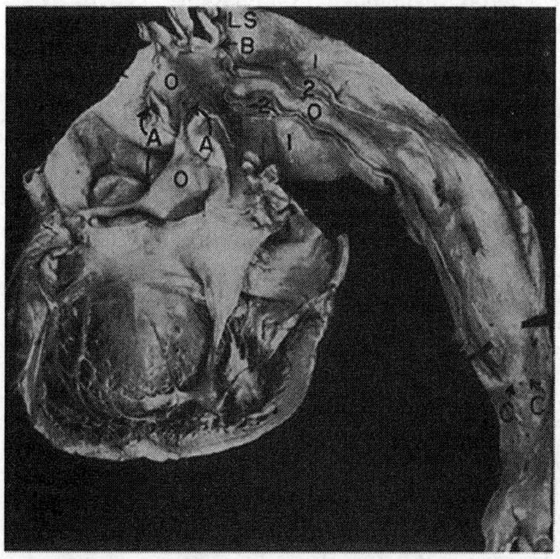

Fig. *1*. Case 1. Gross specimen showing large left ventricular cavity and dissecting aneurysms of the ascending aorta. The intimal tear (*A, A*) in the ascending aorta leads to the first dissecting channel (*1*). Near the left subclavian artery (*LS*) a second tear (*B, B*) leads to a second dissecting channel (*2*). Both re-enter the original aortic lumen (*O*) at a point (*C, C*) above the renal arteries.

FAMILY HISTORY. The patient was the youngest member of a family of 4. Her sister, 41 years of age, has been in a mental hospital since the age of 10 with a diagnosis of Mongolism; according to the institutional records, she has no physical deformities, cardiac murmur, or ocular malformations. Two brothers, now 50 and 42 years of age, are living and well, with no physical deformities or cardiac murmurs. The father died at the age of 65 of unknown cause and the mother is alive and well at the age of 80. Neither parent exhibited physical deformities, ocular malformations, or cardiac diseases.

Of the patient's three children, each of whom are boys, only the oldest, now 16 years old, is normal. The youngest, now 11 years old, exhibits typical features of Marfan's syndrome and a pectus excavatum type of deformity of the sternum. In this sibling since the age of five years the ascending aorta has been noticeably enlarged and mitral insufficiency is currently present. The second sibling represents Case 2 of this report and will be described in a forthcoming section.

PATHOLOGIC FEATURES. The major pathologic findings were limited to the cardiovascular system. Marked enlargement of the left ventricular cavity was present. The left atrium and right ventricle were moderately enlarged. In the ascending aorta, 3 cm. above the posterior and right aortic cusps, was a 6 cm. transverse tear which led to a large false passage within the aortic wall. This channel proceeded distally to encompass the brachiocephalic vessels. It then descended on the left side posteriorly in the descending thoracic aorta and re-entered the original lumen of the aorta just above the level of the renal arteries. A small vertical tear was noted in the posterior wall of the false passage near the left subclavian artery and, from this tear, a second dissecting aneurysm proceeded downward to the level of the renal arteries, where it re-entered the first described and larger false channel (Figs. 1 and 2, *a*). The walls of both dissecting aneurysms ap-

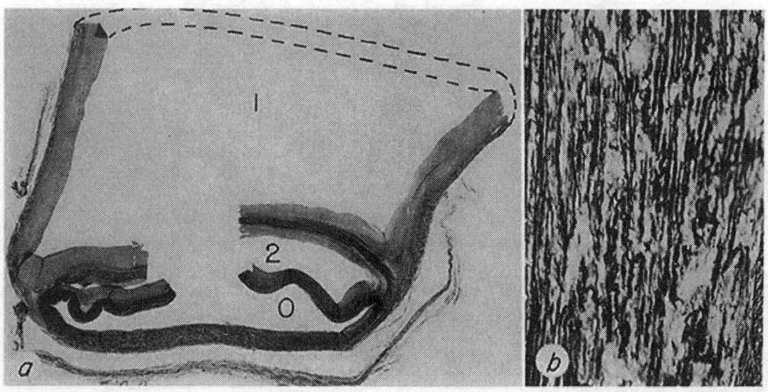

Fig. *2*. Case 1. *a*, Photomicrograph of cross-section of thoracic aorta showing the 3 channels. *0*, Natural lumen of aorta; *1*, major false passage; *2*, false passage within wall of first false passage. ELVG ×3. *b*, Photomicrograph of media of ascending aorta showing multiple cystic spaces and loss of elastic laminae. Elastic tissue stain ×100.

peared old and partly "endothelialized." The larger false channel exhibited retrograde dissection near the right aortic cusp but the ostium of the right coronary artery was not narrowed. Most of the intercostal arteries had been severed from the main aortic channel but none of the abdominal vessels was involved.

The aortic cusps were elongated and tended to prolapse. The pulmonary trunk, pulmonary valve, and tricuspid valve were normal. The leaflets of the mitral valve were thick, rubbery, and somewhat redundant. The left ventricle was huge. The left ventricular wall measured 1.7 cm. in thickness. The papillary muscles appeared flattened, thin, and gray. The chordae tendineae were thin and free of adhesions. The left atrium was large and thick-walled. No jet lesions were seen but that mitral insufficiency had been present during life could not be excluded.

Histologic examination of representative sections from the ascending and descending portions of the aorta showed multiple foci of classical cystic medial necrosis (Fig. 2, *b*). Such foci were represented by pools of basophilic material replacing elements of the aortic media.

Case 2.

CLINICAL FEATURES. The patient was the second son of the patient in Case 1. At 6 years of age, he underwent correction of a severe pectus excavatum. He remained asymptomatic until the age of 10 years when he was admitted to a hospital for precordial pain and low grade fever. A clinical diagnosis of pericarditis was made and was substantiated by the electrocardiographic findings. Recovery was uneventful. At the age of 12 years, in 1963, a second episode of precordial pain prompted a more detailed cardiovascular investigation. The blood pressure on this second admission was 115 mm. Hg systolic and 80 mm. Hg diastolic in each arm. A loud, Grade III/IV, late, systolic murmur, which was heard at the apex, radiated to the left axilla.

Physical examination revealed arachnodactyly, a high arched palate, and moderate thoracic scoliosis. The ophthalmologic examination failed to disclose any abnormality. The electrocardiogram revealed signs of left axis deviation, left ventricular hypertrophy, and left atrial hypertrophy.

A retrograde aortogram (Fig. 3, *a*) disclosed marked dilatation of the ascending aorta beginning at the level of the aortic sinuses and tapering at the arch. The rest of the thoracic aorta was of normal caliber but was tortuous, so that above the diaphragm a pronounced kink of almost 90 degress was present. The abdominal aorta and its major branches were also unusually long. The aortic valve was competent. A left ventriculogram disclosed left ventricular enlargement and Grade II-III/IV mitral insufficiency. A peculiar configuration of the mitral leaflets was apparent (Fig. 3, *b*). When reviewed in the light of the necropsy findings, it became evident that this represented an unusual and probably pathognomonic picture. The mitral leaflets were divided into several large serrations which bulged into the left atrium.

The patient's clinical condition was not judged

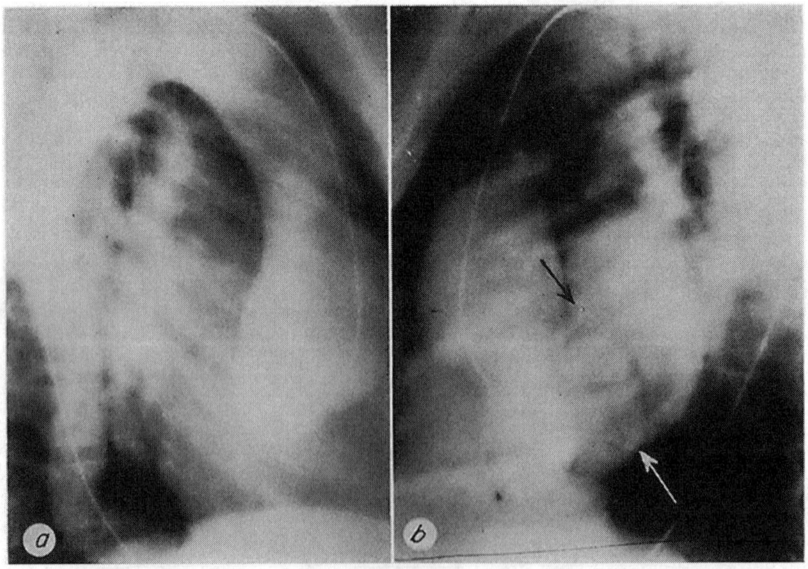

Fig. 3. Case 2. *a*, Lateral view of retrograde aortogram showing the dilated ascending aorta, the competent aortic valve, and the unusually tortuous descending thoracic aorta. *b*, Lateral view of left ventriculogram showing the severe mitral regurgitation and the large serrations (between arrows) in the leaflets of the mitral valve.

serious enough to warrant mitral valvular replacement or resection of the dilated ascending aorta.

One year later, at the age of 13 years, the patient experienced sudden onset of severe pain in the back while lying in bed. He rapidly became dyspneic and died within a few minutes.

PATHOLOGIC FEATURES. At necropsy, 500 ml. of blood were found in the pericardial cavity. The ascending aorta was dilated. Examination of the interior of the aorta revealed a large right-angled tear 4 cm. above the posterior aortic sinus. This led into a false channel within the medial layer of the aorta (Fig. 4), a picture classical for dissecting aneurysm. The dissection had progressed in a retrograde fashion to encircle and obstruct the proximal 2 cm. of the right coronary artery. Distally, the false channel continued to a level just distal to the origin of the left subclavian artery where it reentered the natural aortic lumen. In the adventitial layer of the ascending aorta below the pericardial reflection, there was a 2 cm. vertical tear that served as a tract through which bleeding into the pericardium had occurred.

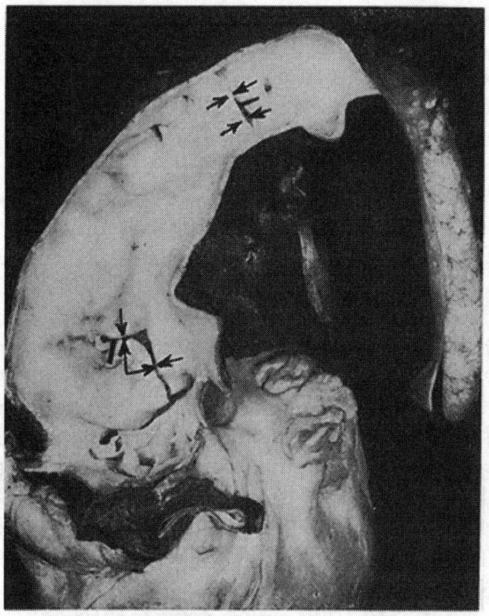

Fig. 4. Case 2. Gross specimen showing right angled tear (between proximal arrows) in dilated ascending aorta and re-entry (between distal arrows) of dissecting aneurysm just below the left subclavian artery.

The aortic cusps were large and downwardly elongated. The coronary ostia lay at a level higher than usual.

The left ventricular cavity was of normal size. The left ventricle was hypertrophied, measuring 1.8 mm. in the free wall. There were no jet lesions in the left ventricular outflow tract. The right atrium and right ventricle were moderately dilated. The pulmonary trunk and pulmonary valve were normal. The atrioventricular valves showed unusual changes more marked in the mitral than the tricuspid valve. From above, each valve showed numerous protrusions toward the related atrium (Fig. 5). These were represented by upward protrusion of the valvular units between the insertions of chordae (Fig. 6). The individual chordae were thin but did not seem unusually long. Incompetence of the mitral valve observed clinically and angiocardiographically appeared to have resulted from "overshoot" of the individual protrusions of the leaflets.

Sections of the ascending and descending aorta and of the brachiocephalic arteries showed cystic medial necrosis. The leaflets of the atrioventricular valve were markedly thickened. When stained for acid mucopolysaccharides, they showed uniform accumulation of chondroitin sulfate as evidenced by the disappearance of the blue stain when testicu-

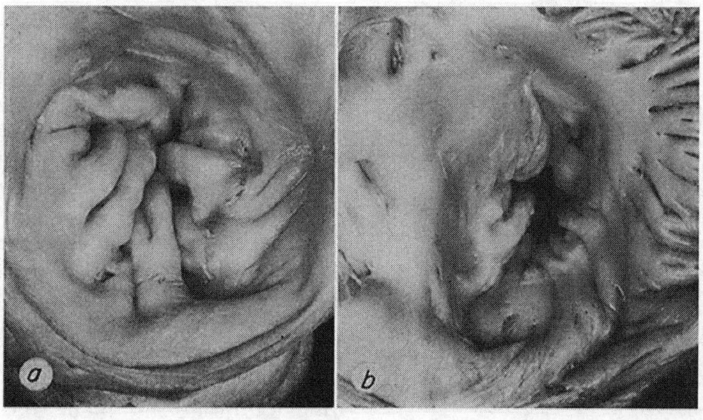

Fig. 5. Case 2. *a*, Mitral valve and *b*, tricuspid valve, each from above. In each, interchordal protrusions of the leaflets present toward the related atrium.

lar hyaluronidase was utilized prior to the colloidal iron solution.

Comment

A hereditary trait in a patient with arachnodactyly was first reported in 1902.[3] In a recent review, McKusick,[4] stating that the disease is autosomal dominant, estimated that de novo mutation is seen in only 15 per cent of the cases. Although arachnodactyly may be present at birth, a period of latency is usually seen before outward manifestations become apparent. The penetrance and expressivity may vary. The skeletal, cardiac, or ocular manifestations may, therefore, be partial or complete. Ectopia of the lenses is present in 50 to 70 per cent of patients. Cardiovascular complications may be expected to occur in 30 to 60 per cent of the cases.[5] The skeletal deformities constitute the most frequent manifestations of the disease.

Aneurysmal dilatation of the ascending aorta, with or without dissecting aneurysm, is the cardiovascular lesion most frequently encountered. It should be pointed out that the diagnosis of Marfan's syndrome in a "tall" patient presenting with aneurysm of the ascending aorta becomes doubtful if the family history is negative or when no skeletal deformities are present.

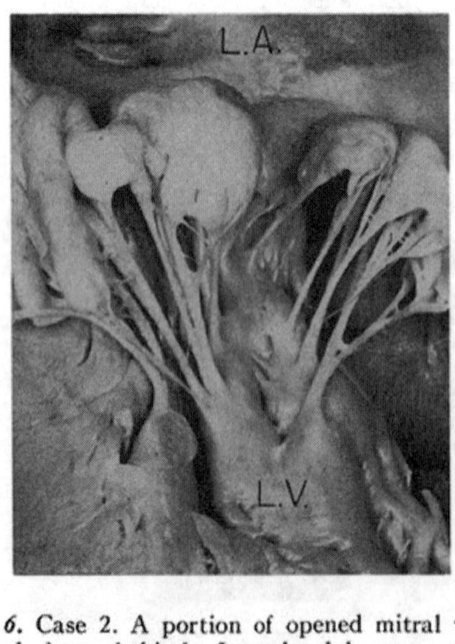

Fig. 6. Case 2. A portion of opened mitral valve viewed from behind. Interchordal segments of leaflet tissue conspicuously bulge upward toward left atrium (*L.A.*). *L.V.*, Left ventricle.

It is generally agreed[4] that atrial or ventricular septal defects, which were given emphasis in the early reports as related to Marfan's syndrome, are probably coincidental. Moreover, in most instances wherein atrial septal defect was claimed, the process was a patent foramen ovale.

Lesions of the atrioventricular valves seem to occur more often than indicated in the literature.[6] There is evidence that the lesions affecting the aorta and the atrioventricular valves have histochemical similarities.[6] In the aortic media, mucopolysaccharides accumulate in pools between elastic laminae or in place of elastic laminae. The relationship between this accumulation of mucoid material and loss of elastic tissue is still unclear.

Erdheim[7] was of the opinion that the mucoid material which normally lay between elastic fibers gradually enlarges to effect loss both of elastic and muscular fibers. As the latter disappear, the small foci become confluent and form cystic spaces. Others[8,9] consider this mucoid material a product of disintegration of the elastic fibers. Hurley[10] expressed the view that the loss of elastic and muscular fibers is similar to that which occurs with aging.

Increase in acid mucopolysaccharides which has been found in the aortic media of patients with Marfan's syndrome has also been observed in the atrioventricular valves.[6]

As in the aortic media, it is presumed that the connective tissue defect manifested histochemically by accumulation of acid mucopolysaccharides is responsible for elongation, stretching, and redundancy of leaflet tissue. The lesions of the atrioventricular valves, like those affecting the great vessels, tend to occur more commonly on the left side, a phenomenon believed to be largely dependent on hemodynamic stresses.

Other factors such as sex, pregnancy, and hypertension may also be pertinent to the location and development of the cardiovascular lesions. While the aortic lesions are seen more often in men,[4] the mitral lesion tends to occur in young women.[6] A predilection for dissecting aneurysm during pregnancy has been observed by several authors.[11-13] In 70 cases of dissecting aneurysm occurring in women under the age of 40 years reviewed by Mandel and associates,[14] 36 (51 per cent) occurred in association with pregnancy. An analogy to the effects of the hormone relaxin on the connective tissue has been postulated,[13] but experimental induction of dissecting aneurysm in animals injected with relaxin and rendered hypertensive has not been successful.[4] There is little information available on histochemical changes of the aortic media during pregnancy. In one reported series of 7 patients who died during pregnancy of causes other than dissecting aneurysm, accumulation of mucoid material in the media of the ascending aorta was found in 6.[13]

Hirst and associates[13] observed among pregnant women that more than half with dissecting aneurysm were hypertensive and postulated that the histochemical changes which occur in the aorta during pregnancy favor the occurrence of dissecting aneurysm rather than precipitate it. Only a small proportion of the reported cases of dissecting aneurysm during pregnancy was associated with arachnodactyly.[2] This may represent the fact that the diagnosis of Marfan's syndrome was not entertained in many of the earlier reports.

Summary

Few reports of dissecting aneurysm of the ascending aorta among close relatives have appeared in the literature and in only one previous report was this described in association with Marfan's syndrome.

Reported are the cases of a mother and son, each with Marfan's syndrome (arachnodactyly) and dissecting aneurysm of the aorta. In the mother, dissecting aneurysm occurred when she was 30 years old and pregnant with her third offspring. Death occurred at the age of 31 years after aortic insufficiency and congestive cardiac failure had developed.

The son was the second offspring and died of acute dissecting aneurysm when he was 13 years old. In the son, interchordal protrusions of the leaflets of the tricuspid and mitral valves were considered manifestations of Marfan's syndrome. Mitral insufficiency had been identified clinically.

REFERENCES

1. Whittaker, S. R. F., and Sheehan, J. D.: Dissecting aortic aneurysm in Marfan's syndrome, Lancet **2**:791, 1954.
2. Husebye, K. O., Wolff, H. J., and Freidman, L. L.: Aortic dissection in pregnancy: A case of Marfan's syndrome, AM. HEART J. **55**:662, 1958.
3. Achard, M. C.: Arachnodactylie, Bull. mém. Soc. méd. hôp. Paris **19**:834, 1902.
4. McKusick, V. A.: Heritable disorders of connective tissue, ed. 2, St. Louis, 1960, The C. V. Mosby Company.
5. Goyette, E. M., and Palmer, P. W.: Cardiovascular lesions in arachnodactyly, Circulation **7**:373, 1953.
6. Grondin, C. M., and Edwards, J. E.: The mitral valve in the Marfan syndrome. Unpublished data.
7. Erdheim, J.: Medionecrosis aortae idiopathica cystica, Virchows Arch. Path. Anat. **276**:187, 1930.
8. Cellina, M.: Medionecrosis disseminata aortae, Virchows Arch. Path. Anat. **280**:65, 1931.
9. Rottino, A.: Medial degeneration of aorta as seen in 12 cases of dissecting aneurysm, Arch. Path. **28**:1, 1939.
10. Hurley, J. V.: Marfan's syndrome: The nature of the aortic defect, Australasian Ann. Med. **8**:45, 1959.
11. Schnitker, M. A., and Bayer, C. A.: Dissecting aneurysm of aorta in young individuals, particularly in association with pregnancy, with report of case, Ann. Int. Med. **20**:486, 1944.
12. Sheehan, H. L.: Pathology of obstetric shock, J. Obst. & Gynaec. Brit. Emp. **46**:218, 1939.
13. Hirst, A. E., Johns, V. J., Jr., and Kime, S. W., Jr.: Dissecting aneurysm of the aorta: A review of 505 cases, Medicine **37**:217, 1958.
14. Mandel, W., Evans, E. W., and Walford, R. L.: Dissecting aortic aneurysm during pregnancy, New England J. Med. **251**:1059, 1954.

Dissecting Aneurysm Complicating Marfan's Syndrome (arachnodactyly) in a Mother and Son

Heidi M. Connolly, M.D.

In 1896, French pediatrician Antoine Marfan first described features he observed in a 5-year-old female, which later came to be known as Marfan syndrome. Since that time there have been a few seminal articles that greatly advanced our understanding of the condition and changed forever, and for better, the diagnosis and treatment of this challenging malady.

"Dissecting Aneurysm Complicating Marfan Syndrome (arachnodactyly) in a Mother and Son" is a report that set a cornerstone for building our current knowledge base on Marfan syndrome. It describes the physical features, devastating aortic complications and cardiovascular pathology found in two family members with aortic dissection related to Marfan syndrome. The clinical and pathologic features meticulously described more than forty years ago by Dr. Jesse Edwards and colleagues in this tragic mother and son case series are still included today in the 2010 updated Ghent criteria for the diagnosis of Marfan syndrome. Current diagnostic components include: 1) proximal aortic dilatation, 2) family history, 3) ectopia lentis, 4) systemic features (skeletal, pulmonary, skin, minor ocular, and minor cardiovascular features), and now, with the availability of genetic testing, 5) presence of the fibrillin-1 mutation.

Dr. Edwards was one of the first to describe aortic dissection in first-degree relatives with Marfan syndrome, and in doing so emphasized the significance of this life-threatening association. A family history of aortic dissection is now recognized as an important risk factor for recurrent dissection among affected family members and is considered an indication for early and aggressive surgical intervention.

The critical observations outlined by Dr. Edwards also awakened the curiosity of subsequent investigators to help build our current knowledge of the genetic mechanisms of this inherited connective tissue disorder. He questioned early on the relationship between the accumulation of mucoid material and loss of elastic tissue. In doing so, he introduced the critical concept of a potential mechanistic bond between the loss of elastic tissue causing aortic dilatation, and myxomatous atrioventricular valve disease in Marfan syndrome. Despite progress in the understanding of the genetic basis of this multisystem disorder, the pathophysiologic mechanism linking the fibrillin mutation with diverse organ involvement such as dilatation of the aorta, elongation of atrioventricular valves and overgrowth of long bones remained unclear until recently. It is now recognized that excessive transforming growth factor beta signaling is responsible for many of the pathologic changes that occur in Marfan syndrome. With this discovery, exciting therapeutic opportunities have emerged. Angiotensin receptor blockers which target the angiotensin receptor and reduce transforming growth factor beta activity have been shown in both animal and early human trials to significantly impact aortic dilatation.

Nevertheless, despite striking diagnostic and therapeutic advances in the care of patients with Marfan syndrome, premature death related to complications of aortic dissection still haunts affected patients, their relatives and health care providers today. Tragically, aortic dissection may occur even before the diagnosis of Marfan syndrome has been considered or in medically treated patients who are being carefully followed by experienced health care providers but have not yet met the criteria in established guidelines for elective aortic replacement. Thus, even though clinical risk factors for aortic dissection have been identified, aortic dissection remains an unpredictable and devastating cardiovascular catastrophe. The search for improved diagnostic and predictive methods continues today.

The important pathologic description and the call to action by Dr. Edwards more than forty years ago impacted progress in the diagnosis and management of patients with Marfan syndrome and allowed improved recognition as well as early therapeutic intervention. Despite this progress, Dr. Edwards' series of dissection described at necropsy continues to serve as a historical alarm calling scientists, health care providers and patients to action.

MAY 1, 1978

The American Journal of CARDIOLOGY®

VOLUME 41

NUMBER 5

CLINICAL STUDIES

Sudden Death in Patients with Hypertrophic Cardiomyopathy: Characterization of 26 Patients Without Functional Limitation

BARRY J. MARON, MD*
WILLIAM C. ROBERTS, MD, FACC*
JESSE E. EDWARDS, MD, FACC†
HUGH A. McALLISTER, Jr., MD, FACC‡
DANIEL D. FOLEY, MD†
STEPHEN E. EPSTEIN, MD, FACC*

Bethesda, Maryland
St. Paul and Minneapolis, Minnesota
Washington, DC

Sudden death is a recognized complication in symptomatic patients with hypertrophic cardiomyopathy. However, its occurrence in patients with no or transient previous cardiac symptoms presents a particularly challenging diagnostic and therapeutic dilemma. Therefore, 26 patients with hypertrophic cardiomyopathy whose death was the first definitive manifestation of cardiac disease were evaluated. Their ages ranged from 8 to 49 years (mean 18) and 23 were less than 25 years of age; 19 were male and 7 female. Of the 26 patients, 13 died during or immediately after moderate or severe physical exertion. Of 12 patients with previous cardiac catheterization, 6 had no or a small left ventricular outflow tract gradient under basal conditions and 6 had an outflow gradient of 50 mm Hg or greater. Left ventricular end-diastolic pressure was elevated in nine patients, and the ventricular septum was moderately to severely thickened (17 mm or more) in all patients. The electrocardiogram was abnormal in all 19 patients studied before death. Thus, sudden death may be the first definitive manifestation of cardiac disease in some patients with hypertrophic cardiomyopathy. Although the effects of patient selection in this study group cannot be excluded, sudden death was common in children and young adults and was often related to physical exertion; each patient showed a distinctly abnormal electrocardiogram and moderate to severe ventricular septal thickening.

Hypertrophic cardiomyopathy is a genetically transmitted disease of cardiac muscle characterized by disproportionate thickening of the ventricular septum.[1-7] Sudden and unexpected death is a recognized complication in symptomatic adults and children with this disease.[8-13] Patients with hypertrophic cardiomyopathy who were asymptomatic or experienced only rare transient symptoms before death have been described occasionally[8,10-15] but not in detail or in a manner permitting proper characterization of this subgroup. Nevertheless, identification and subsequent management of such patients with hypertrophic cardiomyopathy presents particularly difficult problems. Therefore, to define and characterize more clearly this subgroup, we analyzed the clinical and morphologic features of 26 patients with hypertrophic cardiomyopathy whose first definitive symptomatic manifestation of cardiac disease was death.

From the Cardiology Branch and Pathology Branch, National Heart, Lung, and Blood Institute, National Institutes of Health, Bethesda, Maryland*; Department of Pathology, United Hospitals—Miller Division, St. Paul, Minnesota; Department of Pathology, University of Minnesota, Minneapolis, Minnesota†; and Department of Cardiovascular Pathology, Armed Forces Institute of Pathology, Washington, D.C.‡ This work was supported in part by U. S. Public Health Service Research Grant 5R01 HL 05694 and Research Training Grant 5T01 HL 05570 from the National Heart, Lung, and Blood Institute, Bethesda, Maryland; and the Bremer Foundation, St. Paul, Minnesota. Manuscript received July 29, 1977; revised manuscript received November 15, 1977, accepted November 16, 1977.

Address for reprints: Barry J. Maron, MD, National Heart, Lung, and Blood Institute, Cardiology Branch, Bldg. 10, Room 7B-15, Bethesda, Maryland 20014.

TABLE I

Clinical, Hemodynamic and Pathologic Data in 26 Cases

Case no.	Age (yr) & Sex	Electro-cardiogram	Hemodynamics: LVOT Gradient Basal	Hemodynamics: LVOT Gradient Provo-cation	Hemodynamics: LV Pressure	Hemodynamics: RVOT Gradient	Hemodynamics: CI	Circumstances of Death	Family History SD	Necropsy: Heart Weight (g)	Necropsy: VS	Necropsy: PW	Necropsy: VS/PW	Necropsy: Disorga-nized Cells in VS	Possible Cardiac Symptoms
1	8M	—	—	—	—	—	—	After hiking	0	350	25	13	1.9	+	0
2	10M	LVH	—	—	—	—	—	Stepped out of school bus*	+	—	Marked VS hypertrophy[d]			+	0
3	11F	—	—	—	—	—	—	After mild calisthenics	0	400	17	9	1.9	+	1 episode syncope 3 wk before death
4	11M	LAD; probable LVH; LAE; ST-T changes	5	35	92/29	0	3.9	After light play	0	—	—	—	—	—	0
5	12M	ST-T changes‡	—	—	—	6	—	Jogging**	+	270	18	10	1.8	+	0
6	13M	—	—	—	—	—	—	After recreational ball game	+	375	25	17	1.5	—	0
7	14M	LVH with "strain"§; diffuse T wave inversion; Q wave in leads II, III, aVF, V_6	13	—	110/24	0	3.0	After walking up steep hill	+	360	20	10	2.0	+	0
8	15F	LVH; Q waves in leads I, aVL, V_5V_6; S-T depressed in I, aVL	—	—	—	—	—	Sedentary activity	0	320	22	11	2.0	+	Lightheaded-ness
9	15F	LVH; marked LAD; Q waves in leads I, II, III, aVF, V_5, V_6; S-T elevated in II, III, aVF, V_6	50	95	157/20	—	6.0	Stepping out of car	0	550	34	20	1.7	—	0
10	15F	LVH with "strain"; Q waves in lead aVL; LAD; LAE; ST-T changes[a]	10-55	115	110-155/30	15	3.7	Running	+	400	38	16	2.4	+	1 episode dyspnea, lightheaded-ness during running 5 mo before death
11	15F	LVH[φ]; ST-T changes; poor progression of precordial R waves; LAE	100	—	200/24	—	3.0	Running	+	550 (est)	36	14	2.6	+	0
12	15M	—	—	—	—	—	—	During recreational basketball	+	475	—	—	—[e]	—	0

Table I (continued)

			Hemodynamics							Necropsy					
			LVOT Gradient												
Case no.	Age (yr) & Sex	Electrocardiogram	Basal	Provocation	LV Pressure	RVOT Gradient	CI	Circumstances of Death	Family History SD	Heart Weight (g)	VS	PW	VS/PW	Disorganized Cells in VS	Possible Cardiac Symptoms
13	16M	LVH; LAE; Q wave in lead V_6; T wave inversion in leads II, III, aVF; P-R = 0.10	75	—	175/20	0	4.4	After light play	0	520	—	—	—	—	1 episode syncope 1 yr before death
14	16F	Deep Q wave in leads III, aVF; possible RVH	—	—	—	—	—	Jogging	+	310	21	8	2.6	+	0
15	17M	LVH[g]; LAD; T wave inversion in leads I, aVL; S-T elevated in V_1V_2	60	—	140/16	0	4.7	Sedentary	0	—	27[f]	17	1.6	—	0
16	17M	—	—	—	—	—	—	Jogging	0	530	21	12	1.8	+	0
17	17M	—	—	—	—	—	—	During competitive basketball game	0	740	—	—	—[b]	+	Lightheadedness
18	19M	LVH with "strain"[δ]; Q wave in lead V_6; S-T elevated in V_1-V_3	15	50	136/12	8	4.2	Running	0	900	55	30	1.8	—	Lightheadedness
19	21F	T wave inversion in leads III, aVF; LAE; possible LVH	—	—	—	—	—	Walking[θ]	0	400	24	9	2.7	+	1 episode syncope 3 yr before death; lightheadedness: paroxysmal AF and other SVT + PVCs
20[c]	21M	LVH; LAD; poor progression of precordial R waves; QS waves in leads III, aVF, V_1; S-T elevated in V_1-V_3; LAE	65	—	185/16	10	3.3	Mild exertion; throwing football	0	—	—	—	—	—	0
21	22M	LAD; possible LVH; Q waves in leads II, III, aVF[†]	—	—	—	—	—	Running up a grade	+	610	35	21	1.7	+	0

Table I (continued)

Case no.	Age (yr) & Sex	Electro-cardiogram	Hemodynamics: LVOT Gradient Basal	Hemodynamics: LVOT Gradient Provo-cation	Hemodynamics: LV Pressure	Hemodynamics: RVOT Gradient	Hemodynamics: CI	Circumstances of Death	Family History SD	Necropsy: Heart Weight (g)	Necropsy: VS	Necropsy: PW	Necropsy: VS/PW	Necropsy: Disorga-nized Cells in VS	Possible Cardiac Symptoms
22	23M	LVH; deep T wave inversion; VT with exertion	0	—	130/5	0	3.3	During recreational basketball game	0	500	20	15	1.3	0	0
23	23M	—	—	—	—	—	—	Sedentary activity	0	750	30	15	2.0	+	0
24	29M	Probable LVH; LAD;IVCD; 1° AVB (P-R =) 0.24)	0	0	110/12	0	3.7	Dived in ocean surf^Δ	0	450	25	12	2.1	+	Lightheadedness; occasional palpitations
25	31M	RBBB; Q waves in lead aVL	—	—	—	—	—	During mild calisthenics	0	450	24	12	2.0	+	0
26	49M	LVH with "strain"; LAD; ST-T changes; Q waves in leads I, aVL	20	30	130/15	15	3.3	Watching television	0	—	—	—	—	—	A Fl (2:1 block) with diaphoresis and pallor 3 mo before death

Case numbers in boldface italics indicate siblings from two families; that is, Patients 2, 6 and 12 and Cases 5 and 7 are siblings.

AF = atrial fibrillation; A Fl = atrial flutter; CI = cardiac index (liters/min per m^2); est = estimated; 1°AVB = first degree atrioventricular block; IVCD = intraventricular conduction defect; LAD = left axis deviation; LAE = left atrial enlargement; LV Pressure = left ventricular pressure (systolic/diastolic) (mm Hg); LVH = left ventricular hypertrophy; LVOT gradient = left ventricular outflow tract pressure gradient (mm Hg); MV = mitral valve; PVC = premature ventricular complexes; PW = posterior left ventricular free wall (mm); RAD = right axis deviation; RBBB = right bundle branch block; RVH = right ventricular hypertrophy; RVOT gradient = right ventricular outflow tract pressure gradient (mm Hg); SD = sudden death; SVT = supraventricular tachycardia; VS = ventricular septum (mm); VS/PW = ventricular septal to posterobasal left ventricular free wall ratio; VT = ventricular tachycardia.

* Previous cardiac arrest after mild exertion, 20 months before death; this patient died 8 days after his brother (Case 6).

† Electrocardiograms obtained at age 14 to 20 years showed right axis deviation and right ventricular hypertrophy.

‡ Electrocardiogram obtained 5 weeks after cardiac arrest; no tracing recorded before arrest.

** Ventricular fibrillation documented after collapse; patient survived in coma for 5 weeks with evidence of cerebral anoxia; transmural ventricular septal infarct present at necropsy.

Δ Previous cardiac arrest while running, 8 months before death; ventricular fibrillation documented after collapse; atrial flutter after syncopal spell, 1 month before death.

§ Appearance of "strain pattern" (left ventricular hypertrophy with secondary ST-T abnormalities) 7 months before death.

δ Appearance of "strain pattern" (left ventricular hypertrophy with secondary ST-T abnormalities) 3 1/2 years before death.

φ RAD present at age 12 years; normal QRS axis present at age 13 and subsequently.

θ Ventricular fibrillation documented after collapse; patient survived 2 hours.

[a] Electrocardiogram normal at age 10 years, abnormal at age 12 and subsequently.

[b] Although ventricular wall thickness data were not available in this patient, the presence of echocardiographically determined asymmetric septal hypertrophy in his mother and brother and the presence of disorganized cardiac muscle cells in his ventricular septum provide strong presumptive evidence that he had hypertrophic cardiomyopathy.

[c] Patient had documented cardiac arrest (ventricular fibrillation), was successfully resuscitated and has survived with evidence of severe cerebral anoxia.

[d] Exact wall thickness measurements not available.

[e] Wall thickness measurements not available; diagnosis of hypertrophic cardiomyopathy is a presumptive one, based on the presence of cardiac hypertrophy and a strong family history of hypertrophic cardiomyopathy.

[f] Measurements of ventricular septal and posterobasal left ventricular wall thicknesses made with echocardiography[15] 5 months before death; measurements of ventricular septal thickness with echocardiography and subsequently at necropsy usually agree closely.[20]

[g] RAD, RVH present at age 5 years; normal QRS axis, poor R wave progression and deep Q wave in lead aVL at age 9 years; normal electrocardiogram except for Q wave in lead aVL at age 10 years; left ventricular hypertrophy at age 14 and subsequently.

— Data not available.
\+ Present.
0 Absent.

Methods

Selection of patients: The study group was divided into two subgroups: Group I, 17 patients with hypertrophic cardiomyopathy who had no cardiac symptoms before death, and Group II, 9 patients who were asymptomatic except for rare transient symptoms that may have been due to hypertrophic cardiomyopathy. Group II included three patients with a single syncopal episode, one patient with an episode of mild dyspnea and lightheadedness while running, one patient with one episode of atrial flutter (2:1 block; ventricular rate 150/min) and four patients with lightheadedness. None of these nine patients were evaluated initially because of their symptoms.

Two patients in Group I had ventricular fibrillation and cardiac arrest from which they were successfully resuscitated before death; another patient in Group I experienced ventricular fibrillation. For convenience, we have equated ventricular fibrillation with actual cardiac death in these three patients.

Patients were selected from the case records of the following sources: National Heart, Lung, and Blood Institute (16 patients), Armed Forces Institute of Pathology Cardiovascular Registry (2 patients), United Hospitals-Miller Division Cardiovascular Registry (4 patients) and Children's Hospital of Pittsburgh (4 patients). The diagnosis of hypertrophic cardiomyopathy was confirmed in 23 patients at necropsy or with echocardiography (ventricular septal to left ventricular free wall thickness ratio of 1.3 or more) or on the basis of the typical clinical and hemodynamic features of hypertrophic cardiomyopathy. In the remaining three patients the diagnosis of hypertrophic cardiomyopathy was made presumptively, on the basis of presence of cardiac hypertrophy and a confirmed family history of hypertrophic cardiomyopathy.

Description of patients: The patients ranged in age from 8 to 49 years (mean 18); 23 of the 26 patients were less than 25 years old at death. Nineteen patients were male and 7 female; 24 were white and 2 black. Nineteen of the 26 patients had a cardiac evaluation before death. Right and left heart hemodynamic studies were performed in 12 of these patients from 6 months to 11 years (median 2 1/2 years) before death, usually because of the presence of a heart murmur, abnormal electrocardiogram or family history of heart disease or sudden death. Five patients were competitive athletes, including one who had competed on his varsity college basketball team for 4 years without evidence of limitation. There were two sets of siblings, two patients from one family and three from another. Four other patients had at least one first degree relative who died suddenly of hypertrophic cardiomyopathy.

Results

No differences in any of the following variables were found between the two patient groups. The clinical, hemodynamic and pathologic findings in each of the study patients are summarized in Table I.

Physical findings: Four patients had not had an adequate cardiac physical examination before death. Heart murmurs were present in 16 of the remaining 22 patients. These murmurs, first identified from birth to age 28 years, were usually grade 2 to 3/6 systolic ejection murmurs heard loudest at the lower left sternal border or apex. In the other six patients no murmur had been identified.

Chest radiographic findings: Heart size was normal in 14 of the 17 patients who had a chest radiograph taken; the remaining three patients had a cardiothoracic ratio of 0.55 to 0.60. No patient had abnormal pulmonary arterial or venous markings on X-ray examination.

TABLE II

Electrocardiographic Abnormalities in 19 Patients

	Patients (no.)	
Left ventricular hypertrophy	15	
Probable		10
Possible		2
With "strain" pattern*		4
S-T segment and T wave abnormalities	14	
Abnormal Q or QS†	10	
Left axis deviation	8	
Left atrial enlargement	5	
Right bundle branch block	1	
First degree atrioventricular block	1	
Intraventricular conduction defect	1	
Marked diffuse T wave inversion (ventricular tachycardia with exercise)	1	
Possible right ventricular hypertrophy	1	

* Tall voltages in the left precordial leads associated with secondary S-T segment and T wave changes.

† 4 or more mm in depth or 0.04 second in duration, in one or more leads.

Electrocardiographic findings: Electrocardiograms were obtained in 19 of the 26 patients and were abnormal in each (Table II). Although no electrocardiographic pattern was entirely characteristic of the study group, the most common abnormalities were left ventricular hypertrophy, S-T segment and T wave changes and deep, wide Q waves.

In six patients the electrocardiographic pattern changed 7 months to 4 years before death. A left ventricular "strain" pattern developed in three of these patients, including one with a previously normal electrocardiogram. In three other patients the electrocardiograms initially revealed right ventricular hypertrophy or right axis deviation, or both, but later were consistent with left ventricular hypertrophy.

Only one patient demonstrated premature complexes in the routine electrocardiogram; however, one other patient (Case 22) did show ventricular tachycardia (6 seconds' duration) and frequent premature ventricular complexes during the course of a routine treadmill stress test. In five patients ventricular fibrillation was documented after the patient's sudden collapse. One of these patients (Case 24) also had atrial flutter with variable block (3:1 to 6:1) after a severe syncopal episode 7 months after his initial cardiac arrest and 1 month before death. Another patient (Case 26) also demonstrated atrial flutter (with 2:1 block), associated with diaphoresis and pallor, 3 months before death.

Hemodynamic and angiographic data: *Right and left heart hemodynamic studies* were performed in 12 cases. In 6 of the 12 patients peak systolic left ventricular outflow tract pressure gradients of 50 mm Hg or greater were present under basal conditions (Fig. 1). In the remaining six patients, either no outflow gradient (two patients) or a small gradient of 20 mm Hg or less (four patients) was present. One patient with a 5 mm Hg

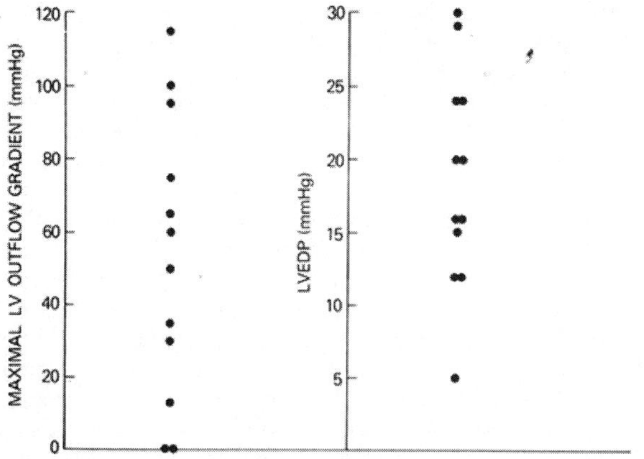

FIGURE 1. Left ventricular (LV) outflow gradients (maximal under basal conditions or with provocation) and left ventricular end-diastolic pressures (LVEDP) in the 12 patients with such measurements.

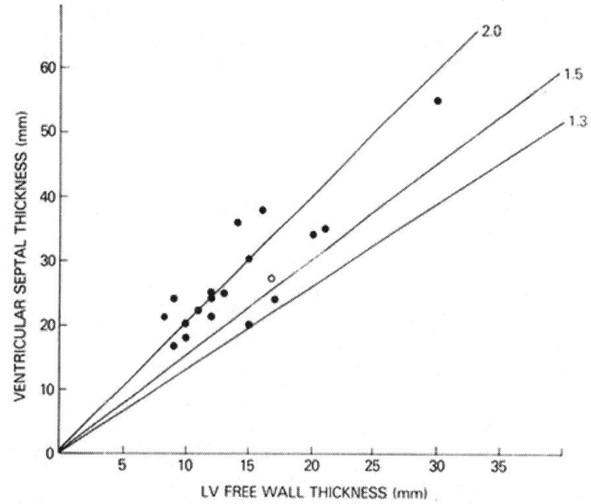

FIGURE 2. Ventricular septal and left ventricular (LV) free wall thicknesses in the 19 patients in whom such measurements were obtained. **Identity lines** define septal/free wall ratios of 1.3, 1.5 and 2.0. **Open symbol** denotes a patient whose ventricular septal and left ventricular free wall thicknesses were measured with echocardiography during diastole 5 months before death.

gradient under basal conditions had a 35 mm Hg gradient with provocation with isoproterenol infusion, and another with a 15 mm Hg gradient under basal conditions had a 50 mm Hg gradient with provocation. Five of the 12 patients had a relatively small peak systolic gradient of 6 to 15 mm Hg between the right ventricle and pulmonary artery. Left ventricular end-diastolic pressure ranged from 5 to 30 mm Hg and was elevated (more than 12 mm Hg) in 9 of the 12 patients (Fig. 1).

Left ventricular angiography was performed in nine patients. In five of these patients, the study showed obliteration of the left ventricular apex during systole, a finding considered characteristic of hypertrophic cardiomyopathy. Two other patients showed severe narrowing of the mid left ventricular cavity during systole that appeared to be due to papillary muscle encroachment. In the remaining two patients, left ventricular contraction was considered normal although deformities in the contour of the left ventricle suggested bulging of a hypertrophied ventricular septum into the left ventricular cavity.

Circumstances of death: Cardiac arrest was sudden and occurred without warning in each of the 26 patients. In 23 patients death occurred instantaneously or within a few minutes. Of the other three patients, one (Case 5) was resuscitated and survived 5 weeks after cardiac arrest with evidence of severe cerebral anoxia, and another (Case 19) survived 2 hours after cardiac arrest; the remaining patient (Case 20) had an episode of ventricular fibrillation, was successfully resuscitated and has survived to date. In 2 of the 26 patients the fatal cardiac arrest was preceded by an initial cardiac arrest that occurred 20 (Case 2) and 8 (Case 24) months earlier. None of the 26 patients were hospitalized at the time of the initial cardiac arrest.

Death occurred during sedentary or normal activities in 6 patients, during or just after mild exertion in 7 and during or just after moderate or severe exertion in 13. No patient died during sleep.

Necropsy findings: Heart weight ranged from 270 to 900 g (median 450) and was increased with respect to age in each patient.[16] In 18 patients either the heart was in suitable condition for detailed examination or sufficient pathologic information was available to assign a septal/free wall ratio. In one other patient (Case 15), in whom necropsy was not performed, measurements of ventricular septal and posterobasal left ventricular wall thicknesses were obtained with echocardiography[2] 5 months before death. Each of these 19 hearts showed disproportionate thickening of the ventricular septum with respect to the left ventricular free wall (septal/free wall ratio 1.3 or more[2,17]) (Fig. 2). Septal/free wall ratios ranged from 1.3 to 2.7 (median 1.9). Absolute ventricular septal thickness ranged from 17 to 55 mm (median 25); in all but two patients septal thickness was 20 mm or greater. The two patients in this study with a septal thickness of less than 20 mm (17 and 18 mm) were only 11 and 12 years of age, respectively (Cases 3 and 5). One patient (Case 5), who survived for 5 weeks after cardiac arrest, had a large transmural ventricular septal infarct despite widely patent extramural coronary arteries; none of the other hearts had areas of transmural scarring or evidence of coronary artery disease (more than 50 percent cross-sectional narrowing of a coronary arterial lumen).

Of the 17 hearts in which the mitral valve and endocardial surface of the left ventricular outflow tract could be studied, 8 showed an endocardial contact plaque on the ventricular septum adjacent to a thickened anterior mitral leaflet. One patient had only an endocardial plaque, one only a thickened anterior mitral leaflet and seven patients had neither an endocardial plaque nor a thickened mitral leaflet.

In 16 of the 17 patients with histologic studies, numerous cardiac muscle cells in the ventricular septum showed a disorganized arrangement characteristic of hypertrophic cardiomyopathy.[15,18,19] In another patient disorganization was only minimal. Microscopy in the remaining patient, who demonstrated the typical gross anatomic features of hypertrophic cardiomyopathy, revolved normally arranged cardiac muscle cells in the ventricular septum.

Morphologic observations regarding arrangement of cardiac muscle cells in the left ventricular free wall were made in 15 of the 17 patients. Six of the 15 had numerous disorganized cardiac muscle cells in the left ventricular free wall, 2 had mild disorganization and 7 had a normal arrangement of virtually all cardiac muscle cells in the left ventricular free wall.

Therapy: Seven of the 26 patients had been treated with propranolol. Each of these patients was under treatment at the time of death and had been taking propranolol for 3 months to 2 1/2 years. The dose of propranolol was considered adequate (2 or more mg/kg per day) in three patients and inadequate in the other four. Six of these patients were given propranolol in the hope of arresting progression of disease; the seventh was given propranolol because of an episode of atrial flutter.

Discussion

Our results indicate that sudden death is not rare in patients with hypertrophic cardiomyopathy who previously did not manifest functional limitation. Moreover, children and young adults appear to be particularly susceptible to sudden death: 23 of our 26 patients were less than 25 years of age at death.

Characteristic clinical features: Two clinical features were characteristic of this unique population of patients: (1) a distinctly abnormal electrocardiogram, and (2) a moderately to severely thickened ventricular septum. Although this latter finding is based on necropsy measurements, we have previously shown a relatively close correlation between measurements of ventricular septal thickness obtained with echocardiography and subsequently at necropsy in patients with disproportionate septal thickening.[20] Our finding of moderate to severe ventricular septal thickening in the patients in our study group has potentially important clinical implications, but one must be aware of the possible influence of patient selection. For example, it may be less likely that patients with hypertrophic cardiomyopathy and only a mildly hypertrophied septum would be systematically identified as having this disease at necropsy. Therefore, such patients may not have been referred to us. Nevertheless, our findings that a distinctly abnormal electrocardiogram and moderate to severe ventricular septal thickening were characteristic of our study group are highly relevant to any future prospective studies designed to identify the risk factors for sudden death in patients with hypertrophic cardiomyopathy.

No clinical or hemodynamic variable was an entirely reliable predictor of death in our patients. These variables included radiographically determined heart size, specific electrocardiographic abnormality and left ventricular end-diastolic pressure. Although previous investigators[12] have suggested that elevated left ventricular end-diastolic pressure is a poor prognostic sign in patients with hypertrophic cardiomyopathy, this was not true in the present study group or in our previous study[13] of children with hypertrophic cardiomyopathy. Although 6 of the 12 patients had markedly elevated left ventricular end-diastolic pressure (20 mm Hg or greater), 3 had only mildly elevated pressure (15 to 16 mm Hg) and 3 had a normal pressure (12 mm Hg or less). However, 6 of our 25 patients showed electrocardiographic evidence of increasing left ventricular overload within 4 years of the time of death. Hence, such an evolution in the electrocardiographic pattern may be an early sign of impending sudden death in some patients with hypertrophic cardiomyopathy even though there may be no symptomatic evidence of disease.

Therapeutic implications: Treatment with propranolol did not appear to be entirely protective against sudden death in our patients. Seven patients had been taking propranolol before and at the time of death; but the dosage could be considered adequate (2 or more mg/kg per day) in only three. Moreover, we do not know the role that patient selection played in these data, that is, how many patients at risk of sudden death did not die *because* they were taking propranolol. Hence, the available data are inconclusive regarding the potential efficacy of propranolol administered prophylactically in asymptomatic or mildly symptomatic patients with hypertrophic cardiomyopathy.

Mechanisms of sudden death: Although the exact mechanism of sudden death in patients with hypertrophic cardiomyopathy is not known, ventricular arrhythmias have been suggested as the terminal event.[13] Our finding that four patients had ventricular fibrillation immediately after their collapse supports this contention. It also is not uncommon to observe frequent ventricular premature complexes in such patients.[21] However, our data also raise the possibility that atrial arrhythmias play an etiologic role in the precipitation of ventricular fibrillation in some patients with hypertrophic cardiomyopathy. For example, one patient (Case 26) was completely asymptomatic until age 49 years, when he experienced an episode of atrial flutter; he died suddenly 3 months later. Another patient (Case 24), who experienced two cardiac arrests, had atrial flutter documented immediately after a syncopal spell 1 month before his death. Thus, it is possible (but purely speculative) that rapid supraventricular tachycardias lead to inadequate ventricular filling (particularly in hearts with diminished compliance) that then results in hypotension and subsequent cardiac arrest. Alternatively, it is possible that abnormally rapid atrioventricular transmission can occur in patients with hypertrophic cardiomyopathy through accessory conduction pathways and that the extremely rapid ventricular response may ultimately deteriorate into ventricular fibrillation.

Family history: About one third of our 26 patients had a family history of sudden cardiac death in a first degree relative (including siblings in two instances). This finding suggests that sudden death is more prevalent in some families with hypertrophic cardiomyopathy and that a history of sudden death in a closely related relative may be a poor prognostic factor for patients with hypertrophic cardiomyopathy. Although about 75 percent of our study patients were male, this prevalence rate does not differ significantly from that of male subjects in the overall population of patients with hypertrophic cardiomyopathy (67 percent).[10]

Acknowledgments

We thank Drs. J. R. Zuberbuhler and Frank Sherman of Children's Hospital of Pittsburgh, Dr. Robert A. Miller of Children's Memorial Hospital, Chicago and Dr. David Bialostozky, Mexico City, for providing some of the clinical and pathologic data.

References

1. **Clark CE, Henry WL, Epstein SE:** Familial prevalence and genetic transmission of idiopathic hypertrophic subaortic stenosis. N Engl J Med 289:709–714, 1973
2. **Henry WL, Clark CE, Epstein SE:** Asymmetric septal hypertrophy (ASH): echocardiographic identification of the pathognomonic anatomic abnormality of IHSS. Circulation 47:225–233, 1973
3. **Epstein SE, Henry, WL, Clark CE, et al:** Asymmetric septal hypertrophy. Ann Intern Med 81:650–680, 1974
4. **Abbasi AS, MacAlpin RN, Eber LM, et al:** Left ventricular hypertrophy diagnosed by echocardiography. N Engl J Med 289:118–121, 1973
5. **Menges H, Brandenburg RO, Brown AL:** The clinical, hemodynamic and pathologic diagnosis of muscular subvalvular aortic stenosis. Circulation 24:1126–1136, 1961
6. **Roberts WC:** Valvular, subvalvular and supravalvular aortic stenosis: morphologic features. Cardiovasc Clin 5: 104–126, 1973
7. **Abbasi AS, MacAlpin RN, Eber LM, et al:** Echocardiographic diagnosis of idiopathic hypertrophic cardiomyopathy without outflow obstruction. Circulation 46:897–904, 1972
8. **Hardarson T, De La Calzada CS, Curiel R, et al:** Prognosis and mortality of hypertrophic obstructive cardiomyopathy. Lancet 2: 1462–1467, 1973
9. **Shah PM, Adelman AG, Wigle ED, et al:** The natural (and unnatural) course of hypertrophic obstructive cardiomyopathy. A multicenter study. Circ Res 34, 35:Suppl II:II-179–II-195, 1973
10. **Frank S, Braunwald E:** Idiopathic hypertrophic subaortic stenosis. Clinical analysis of 126 patients with emphasis on the natural history. Circulation 37:759–788, 1968
11. **Adelman AG, Wigle ED, Ranganathan N, et al:** The clinical course in muscular subaortic stenosis. A retrospective and prospective study of 60 hemodynamically proved cases. Ann Intern Med 77: 515–525, 1972
12. **Swan DA, Bell B, Oakley CM, et al:** Analysis of the symptomatic course and prognosis and treatment of hypertrophic obstructive cardiomyopathy. Br Heart J 33:671–685, 1971
13. **Maron BJ, Henry WL, Clark CE, et al:** Asymmetric septal hypertrophy in childhood. Circulation 53:9–18, 1976
14. **Folger GM, Harper DT, Mehrizi A:** Asymmetrical hypertrophy of the heart in childhood. J Pediatr 67:204–213, 1965
15. **Teare D:** Asymmetrical hypertrophy of the heart in young patients. Br Heart J 20:1–18, 1958
16. **Gould SE:** Pathology of the Heart and Blood Vessels, third edition. Springfield, IL, Charles C Thomas, 1968, p 1139
17. **Henry WL, Clark CE, Roberts WC, et al:** Differences in distribution of myocardial abnormalities in patients with obstructive and nonobstructive asymmetric septal hypertrophy (ASH): echocardiographic and gross anatomic findings. Circulation 40:447–455, 1974
18. **Ferrans VJ, Morrow AG, Roberts WC:** Myocardial ultrastructure in idiopathic hypertrophic subaortic stenosis. A study of operatively excised left ventricular outflow tract muscle in 14 patients. Circulation 45:769–792, 1972
19. **Maron BJ, Ferrans VJ, Henry WL, et al:** Differences in distribution of myocardial abnormalities in patients with obstructive and nonobstructive asymmetric septal hypertrophy (ASH): light and electron microscopic findings. Circulation 50:436–446, 1974
20. **Maron BJ, Henry WL, Roberts WC, et al:** Comparison of echocardiographic and necropsy measurements of ventricular wall thicknesses in patients with and without disproportionate septal thickening. Circulation 55:341–345, 1977
21. **Lever HM, Shah PM, Reeves WC, et al:** The relation of left ventricular outflow obstruction to ventricular arrhythmias in hypertrophic subaortic stenosis (abstr). Circulation 53, 54:Suppl II:II-105, 1976

Sudden Death in Patients With Hypertrophic Cardiomyopathy:

Characterization of 26 Patients Without Functional Limitation.

Barry Maron, M.D.

Early in my career at the National Institutes of Health, I became interested in hypertrophic cardiomyopathy (HCM). At that time (early 1970s), there was a considerable focus on the now obsolete thickness ratio of ventricular septum to the LV free wall, as a diagnostic marker for HCM, as that was the early era of M-mode echocardiography. However, we became convinced that the septal:free wall ratio principle required extensive measurements and data in large numbers of hearts with HCM and other cardiac diseases. Therefore, I arranged a collaborative relationship with Dr. Edwards (I was never able to bring myself to refer to him with the less formal Jesse or Jess) to utilize his extensive and unique registry of heart specimens to better understand ventricular asymmetry in a variety of cardiac diseases, including HCM. I made several short trips to St. Paul to visit Dr. Edwards between 1973 – 1977, and during the day endlessly sectioned hearts in the basement of (old) Miller Hospital, which no longer exists but was located on the bluff overlooking the Minnesota State Capitol. Dr. Edwards was gracious and at night frequently brought me to his home or to St. Paul restaurants. I recall meeting Brooks (now a Mayo Clinic cardiologist) on occasion although he probably doesn't recall. Miller Hospital was a nice facility but not an impressive physical structure. However, we came to Miller because that is where Jesse Edwards worked and built the massive and unique heart registry.

My collaboration with Dr. Edwards was very productive, and we wrote nine papers together, including six published in Circulation. At that time, Dr. Edwards probably did not have an overwhelming personal interest in HCM, but he warmed to the task leading to collaboration on papers specifically related to the disease, such as the one selected for this compendium, *Maron BJ, Roberts WC, Edwards JE, McAllister HA, Foley DD, Epstein SE. Sudden Death in Patients with Hypertrophic Cardiomyopathy: Characterization of 26 Patients without Functional Limitation. Am J Cardiol 1978;41:803-810.* This clinicopathologic study was one of the first "contemporary" reports defining segments of the HCM clinical profile for the first time with 3 major findings: 1) that sudden death can be the first clinical manifestation of HCM, a principle now well accepted and particularly relevant to strategies for prophylactic defibrillator implants for sudden death prevention; and 2) such deaths are often related to physical exertion, now a recognized part of the HCM clinical profile, and in fact the basis for disqualifying trained athletes with this disease from competition to reduce their event risk; and 3) about one-third of the hearts in this study had massive left ventricular hypertrophy with a maximum wall thickness ≥ 30 mm (range 30-55), now an accepted independent risk factor for HCM–related sudden death. Such observations may seem obvious and possibly even rudimentary to the current 2010 cardiology trainees, but at the time (32 years ago), these were novel and important insights, which became part of our current understanding regarding this complex disease.

Dr. Edwards was a great man and cardiovascular investigator. He is deserving of this book and more. His contributions to cardiology are immense and too numerous to detail here... and even included important observations related to HCM.

Acquired Diseases of the Heart

PROCEEDINGS
of the Staff Meetings of
THE MAYO CLINIC

Published fortnightly by the Mayo Association for members of the staff of the Mayo Clinic, for fellows of the Mayo Foundation for Medical Education and Research and for other interested physicians

Vol. 33 ROCHESTER, MINN., WED., OCT. 15, 1958 No. 21

CONTENTS

Symposium on Mitral Insufficiency

	Page
Pathologic Anatomy of Mitral Insufficiency JESSE E. EDWARDS AND HOWARD B. BURCHELL	497
Mitral Insufficiency: Clinical Consideration ROBERT O. BRANDENBURG AND HOWARD B. BURCHELL	510
Hemodynamic Considerations in Mitral Regurgitation HIRAM W. MARSHALL AND EARL H. WOOD	517
The Surgical Treatment of Mitral Insufficiency by Mitral Annuloplasty LESLIE D. GUIDRY, JOHN A. CALLAHAN, HIRAM W. MARSHALL AND F. HENRY ELLIS, JR.	523
Prosthetic Replacement of the Mitral Valve. I. Preliminary Experimental Observations F. HENRY ELLIS, JR., AND ARTHUR H. BULBULIAN	532

PATHOLOGIC ANATOMY OF MITRAL INSUFFICIENCY

Jesse E. Edwards, M.D., Section of Pathologic Anatomy
Howard B. Burchell, M.D., Section of Medicine

The anatomic factors which underlie incompetence of the mitral valve are as complex as those which are responsible for competence of this structure. Therefore, in order to present the principles involved in the genesis of mitral insufficiency, it seems appropriate first to define those characteristics of the mitral valve which, in the normal heart, allow it to close during ventricular systole. An understanding of these principles will lead easily to an appreciation of the varied factors which may operate singly or in combination to make the valve incompetent.

It is convenient and imperative to realize that the mitral valve is composed not only of leaflets but also of chordae tendineae (fig. 1*a*). The leaflets are two in number, the anterior (or medial) and the posterior (or lateral). Each leaflet may be said to have a basal, or attached, aspect and a free mobile one. It is commonly stated that the basal aspect of each leaflet is attached to the "mitral ring," the implication being that the general relations of one leaflet to the rest of the heart are similar to those of the other. This is a misconception. The posterior leaflet is attached by fibrous tissue (which may be termed the "mitral ring" or "annulus") to the left ventricular wall, and at the same time the leaflet may be recognized as continuous with the endocardium of the left atrium (fig. 1*b*).

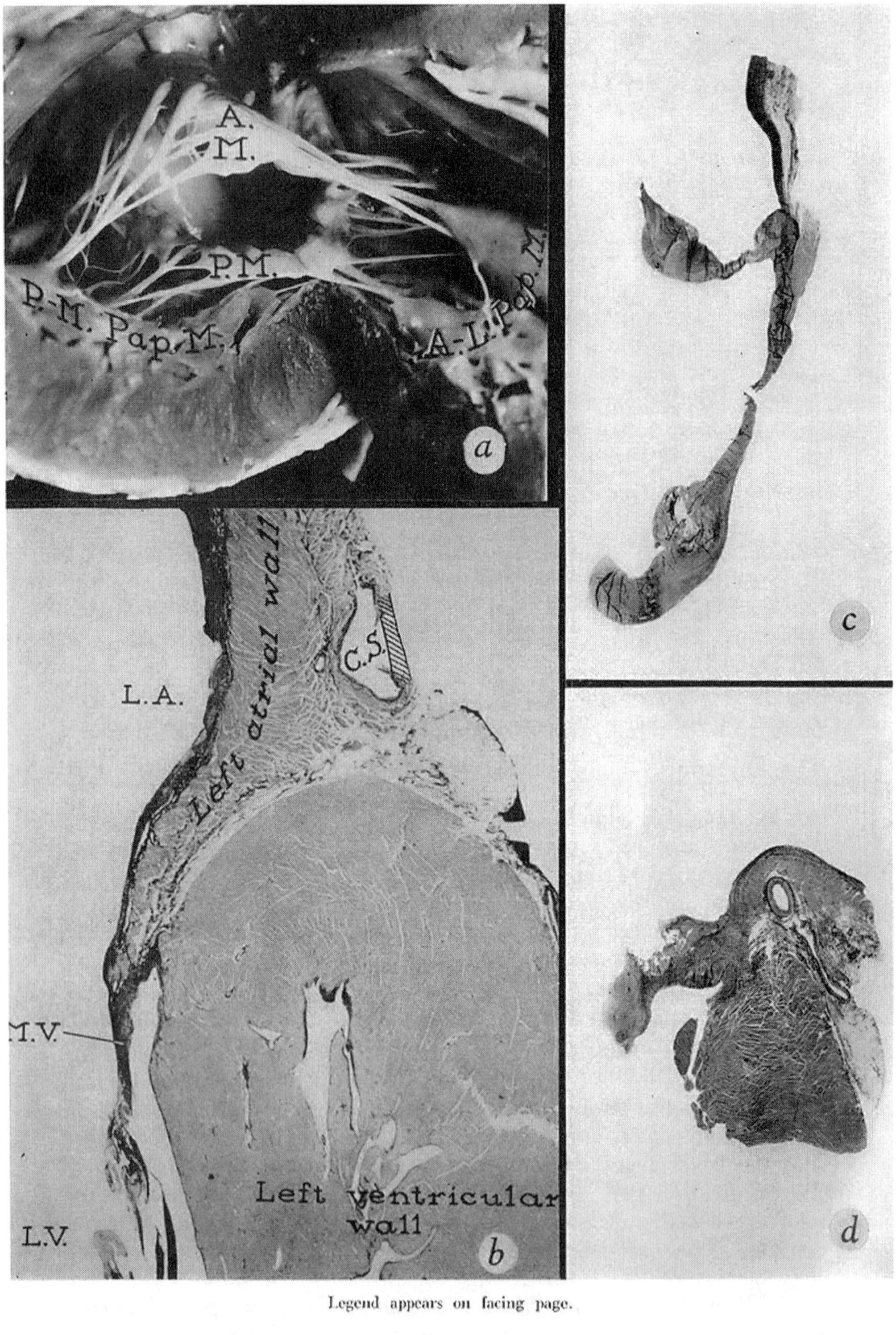

Legend appears on facing page.

The basal aspect of the posterior leaflet has direct attachment with the left ventricular myocardium, but the anterior leaflet does not. The anterior leaflet, while also continuous with the endocardium of the left atrium, makes its firm connection to the aortic root by being continuous with it and portions of the left and posterior cusps of the aortic valve (fig. 1*c*).

During systole the two mitral leaflets are in contact one with the other along their respective "lines" or surfaces of closure. The latter lies somewhat basal to the free edge of the leaflet.

The two angles where the two leaflets approach each other at their basal attachments are the commissures, the anterolateral and the posteromedial. At these regions a small amount of valvular tissue bridges the two leaflets.

The fulcrum on which each valve leaflet moves is its basal attachment. Thus, during ventricular diastole, the two leaflets move away from each other and during systole they move toward each other, not only at the commissures but also along the entire line of contact.

A single papillary muscle or a set of papillary muscles of the left ventricle lies below each commissure and bears the name of the commissure. The chordae tendineae attach to the papillary muscles below and to various parts of the ventricular surfaces of the mitral leaflets above. Usually no chordae attach to the very edge of the free aspects of the leaflets.

It is important to realize that each set of chordae (anterolateral and posteromedial) attaches to that half of *each* leaflet which is related to the particular commissure to which the chordae belong.

For the valve to close properly the following conditions must exist: 1. The leaflets must be intact membranes. 2. The leaflets must be large enough so that together they are larger than the orifice. 3. The leaflets must be sufficiently mobile, by virtue of their intrinsic nature and chordal relationship, to allow unrestrained apposition of one leaflet against the other. 4. When the leaflets have reached a position of apposition, they must be restrained by the chordae tendineae and papillary muscles from everting into the atrium beyond the level of optimal contact for closure.

Fig. 1. *a*. Normal mitral valves viewed from below. The anterior leaflet of the mitral valve (A.M.) and the posterior leaflet (P.M.) join chordae from each set. Chordae related to the anterolateral commissure attach inferiorly to the anterolateral papillary muscle (A.-L. Pap. M.) and those related to the posteromedial commissure insert into the posteromedial papillary muscle (P.-M. Pap. M.).

b. Longitudinal section through the posterior leaflet of a normal mitral valve. The leaflet of a normal mitral valve. The leaflet (M.V.) is continuous with the endocardium of the left atrium (L.A.). The leaflet also joins the left ventricular myocardium at the so-called annulus fibrosus. L.V. = left ventricular cavity; C.S. = coronary sinus.

c. Longitudinal section through anterior leaflet of mitral valve and posterior leaflet of the aortic valve in a case of rheumatic aortic valvular stenosis and mitral insufficiency. Although the anterior mitral leaflet is thickened, it is not appreciably shortened as compared with the posterior leaflet shown in *d* (elastic tissue stain; ×2.5).

d. Longitudinal section through posterior leaflet of mitral valve in the case of rheumatic endocarditis illustrated in figures 1c and 2*a*. The posterior leaflet which is greatly thickened with fibrous tissue and focal calcification shows appreciable shortening (elastic tissue stain; ×2.5).

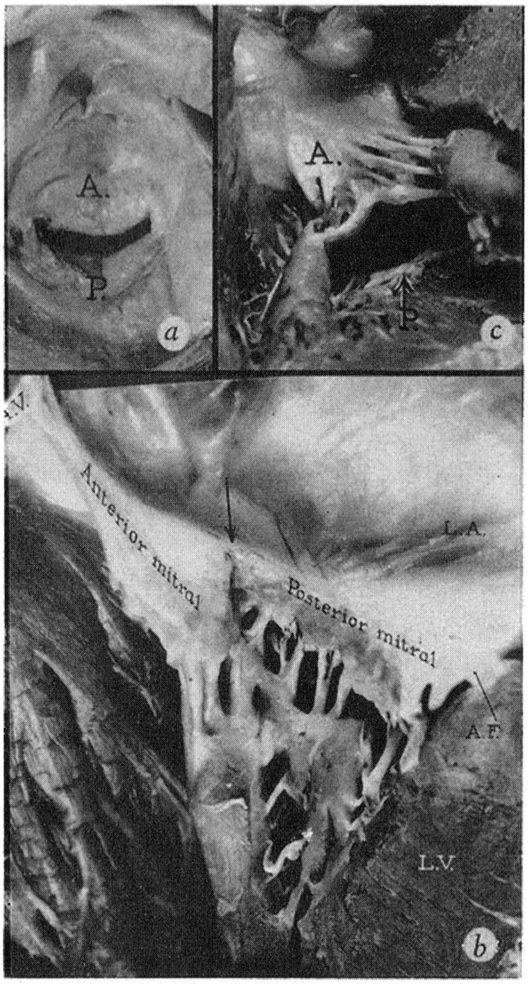

Fig. 2. Rheumatic mitral valvular insufficiency. *a.* Unopened valve viewed from above. The incompetence resulted mainly from shortening of the posterior leaflet (P.). There is only slight fusion of the anterolateral commissure, if any. A. = anterior leaflet of mitral valve. Photomicrographs from this case are illustrated in figures 1*c* and *d*.

b. Opened mitral valve in which shortening of the posterior leaflet and shortening of the chordae contributed significantly to the incompetence of the valve. The former reduced the amount of valvular area and the latter caused restricted mobility of the leaflets.

c. Unopened mitral valve from below. As a result of tension on the posterior leaflet by a dilated left atrium and shortening of the chordae attached to it, the posterior leaflet is held snugly against the posterior wall of the left ventricle as an ineffective valvular structure.

With the conditions for normal closure of the mitral valve presented, it now seems proper to consider the various states in which the mitral valve is incompetent and, at the same time, to define the anatomic basis for the incompetence. In each of these conditions one or several of the conditions required for normal closure of the valve are lacking. These will be considered as the various states are presented.

CHRONIC RHEUMATIC MITRAL DISEASE

Chronic or healed rheumatic valvular disease is often associated with thickening and shortening of the valvular leaflets. Of particular significance with regard to incompetence is shortening, a process which is usually more advanced in the posterior than in the anterior leaflet (fig. 1*c* and *d*). This process alone might account for incompetence on the basis that together the two leaflets are smaller than the orifice (fig. 2*a*). Often the process is more complicated. Additional features include chordal shortening and commissural fusion, often with calcification.

Chordal shortening in itself may be responsible for inadequate mobility of the valve, but in rheumatic disease this factor, when present, usually accentuates the incompetence resulting from a shortened posterior leaflet (fig. 2*b* and *c*).

Fusion of the two leaflets by a bridge of calcified material may cause the adjacent parts of the two leaflets to be held immobile in an open position. Usually when fusion exists only one commissure is involved, while in relation to the other commissure the valvular tissue may approach normal function or may exhibit incompetence on the basis of valvular shortening with or without chordal shortening (fig. 3*a* and *b*). In an occasional case calcific fusion of the two leaflets at each commissure occurs causing the valve to be held open, with little change possible in caliber of the orifice, throughout the cardiac cycle (fig. 3*c*).

It has been mentioned that the left atrial endocardium is continuous with the mitral leaflets. The dilatation of the left atrium resulting from the disturbed dynamics may cause tension on the posterior cusp and may tend to pull it away from the anterior cusp. Two factors tend to interfere with posterior displacement of the posterior cusp by the dilated left atrium: commissural fusion and chordal shortening.

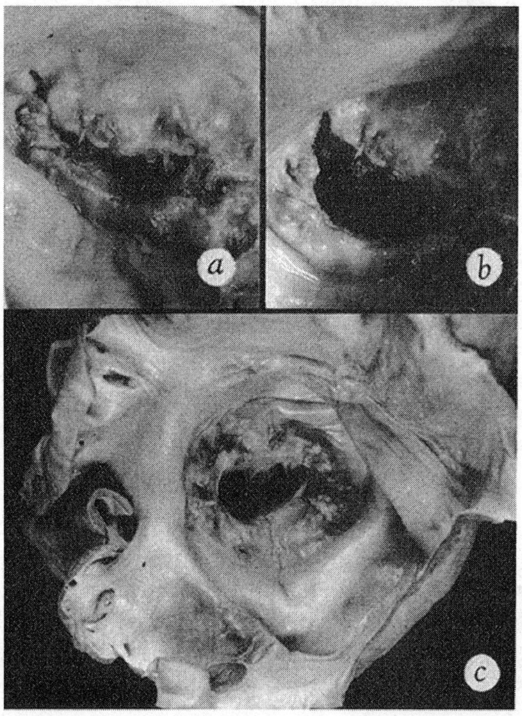

Fig. 3. Rheumatic mitral insufficiency associated with commissural fusion. *a* and *b*. A heart with calcific commissural fusion at the posteromedial commissure. The valve was held open throughout the cardiac cycle in that region. Valve shown from above in a position simulating that during ventricular systole (*a*) and ventricular diastole (*b*). During systole (*a*) at the anterolateral commissure (left portion of illustration) there is relatively good apposition of the two leaflets, while at the posteromedial commissure the two leaflets are held in an open position. During ventricular diastole (*b*) the valve exhibits only mild obstruction.

c. Valve viewed from above. Fusion with calcification at each commissure holds the two leaflets in an open position throughout the cardiac cycle. There appears to have been little possibility of change in the size of the orifice during ventricular systole as compared to diastole.

When commissural fusion is present, posterior retraction of the posterior leaflet inevitably pulls the anterior leaflet with it. This process changes the position of the orifice but does not in itself reduce the capacity of the leaflets.

When chordal shortening is present, the chordae may be viewed as antagonistic to the tension of the dilated left atrium on the posterior leaflet. Tension of each on the posterior leaflet tends to pull the leaflet taut against the posterior wall of the left ventricle. In this way the leaflet is immobilized and becomes a nonfunctional structure (fig. 2 *c*).

BACTERIAL ENDOCARDITIS

Bacterial endocarditis may cause mitral incompetence. During the active phases of the infection the valvular incompetence may exist as one problem among others.

In the bacteriologically healed stage of bacterial endocarditis, mitral incompetence, if it exists, may be the essential problem.

Parenthetically, it is to be emphasized that only among some patients having mitral incompetence as a result of bacterial endocarditis is the antecedent active bacterial endocarditis known. In other patients either no episode of active infection in the past is identified, or a past ill-defined inflammatory disease, possibly confused with rheumatic fever, is recorded.[1]

When healed bacterial endocarditis causes mitral insufficiency, it may do so in one of the following three ways.

1. Organized vegetations in the angle between the posterior leaflet and the left ventricle cause the posterior leaflet to be a fixed structure no longer capable of any mobility. The anterior leaflet is incapable of closing the orifice alone and mitral insufficiency results.

2. Destruction of leaflet tissue may produce deficiencies through which regurgitation of blood may occur. Such destruction may result either from primary bacterial endocarditis of the mitral valve or from mitral endocarditis secondary to aortic valvular endocarditis with aortic regurgitation. The aortic regurgitation may be mild and the secondary effects on the mitral valve may be the dominant problem.

When endocarditis is primary and destruction of valvular tissue occurs, the destructive lesions usually involve the free extremity and the region of the line of closure of either or both leaflets.

When destruction of tissue of the mitral valve occurs secondary to aortic valvular endocarditis, the anterior leaflet only is involved. The site of destruction is usually at the center of the cusp where, as a consequence of the resulting weakness, an aneurysm of the anterior leaflet of the mitral valve occurs. Usually the aneurysm fails to rupture and the lesion is only of incidental interest. If rupture does occur, significant mitral insufficiency may follow (fig. 4*a* and *b*).

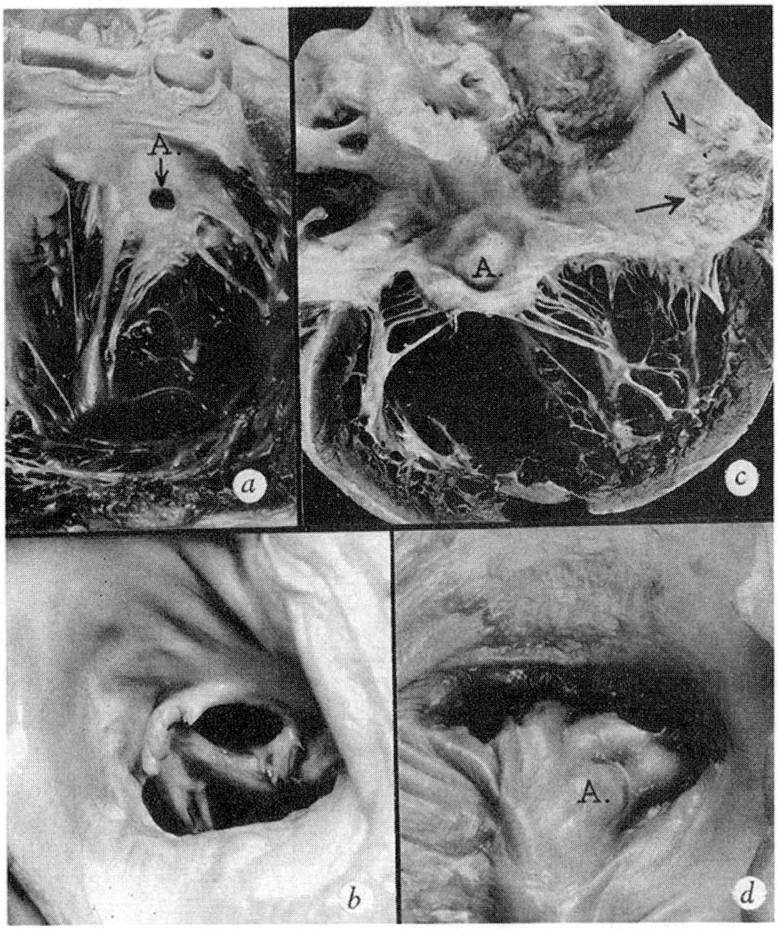

Fig. 4. Mitral insufficiency resulting from bacterial endocarditis. *a*. The aortic valve and ventricular surface of the anterior leaflet of the mitral valve is shown. The aortic valve shows evidence of healed bacterial endocarditis which had left the valve only slightly incompetent. Historically the primary infection occurred 10 years before the patient's death from mitral insufficiency resulting from rupture of chordae attached to the central portion of the anterior leaflet. An unruptured aneurysm involves the central part of the anterior mitral leaflet (A.). This lesion is considered to have resulted from bacterial infection, secondary to aortic regurgitation at the time of active aortic endocarditis. In this instance, in contrast to that case illustrated in *b*, the aneurysm had not ruptured.

b. Ruptured aneurysm of anterior leaflet of mitral valve in a patient who had had aortic bacterial endocarditis 4 years before his death from mitral insufficiency. Unopened mitral valve from above. The pathogenesis of the lesion here is like that in the aneurysm illustrated in *a* and *c*. The difference in function resides in the fact that in this case the aneurysm had ruptured, while the chordae were intact.

c. The left atrium, left ventricle and open mitral valve. In the anterior leaflet of the mitral valve, at the region marked A. is a bulge toward the left atrium, representing the nonruptured aneurysm of the anterior leaflet of the mitral valve which has been illustrated in *a*. The aneurysm here was of incidental significance. Of more importance was the rupture of chordae to the central portion of the anterior leaflet. Tags of these chordae are evident, extending from the free edge of the anterior leaflet. The incompetence of the mitral valve had been responsible for jet lesions in the endocardium of the posterior wall of the left atrium (points of arrows).

d. The mitral valve unopened and viewed from above from the case illustrated in *a* and *c*. As the result of rupture of chordae to the central part of the anterior leaflet of the mitral valve (A.) the leaflet "overshoots" and is responsible for incompetence. The jet lesions illustrated in the open heart in *c* are shown in this perspective also.

3. Rupture of chordae tendineae, although at times occurring as a result of trauma or for idiopathic reasons, probably is most often the result of bacterial endocarditis.[2]

As in the case of destruction of leaflet tissue, so ruptured chordae may result either from primary mitral endocarditis or from mitral endocarditis secondary to aortic valvular endocarditis. Rupture of chordae may occur alone or it may be associated with destruction of tissue of one or both leaflets. When aortic endocarditis results in rupture of chordae, the chordae are usually those inserting into the central part of the anterior leaflet (fig. 4*c* and *d*). Primary mitral endocarditis may cause rupture of chordae in any part of the valve.

Rupture of chordae will allow the involved portion of the leaflet to "overshoot" beyond its opposite member and so deny the chance of proper apposition of the two leaflets (fig. 4*d*). Our experience indicates that the severity and duration of the clinical picture depend on the amount of valvular tissue deprived of chordae. When many chordae rupture, the time of occurrence may be identified by the patient; a severe clinical course soon follows. When only a few chordae rupture, the incompetence of the mitral valve may cause insignificant manifestations for years. After a time the degree of incompetence seems to be compounded of secondary factors. Severe clinical manifestations may then become apparent late. These compounding features will be discussed subsequently under the section on "Mitral insufficiency begets mitral insufficiency."

CONGENITAL MANIFESTATIONS

Various malformations of the mitral valve exist which may cause it to be incompetent. These usually fall into the following two groups: (1) inadequate tissue of a leaflet, and (2) anomalous chordal insertion which either restricts mobility of valvular tissue or allows the leaflets to "overshoot."

Inadequate Tissue.—A cleft of the anterior mitral leaflet is usually present in the complex malformation known as "persistent common atrioventricular canal." This malformation, which has associated septal defects, does not require further consideration here.

In a rare case a cleft of the anterior mitral leaflet occurs similar to that in persistent common atrioventricular canal but without associated septal defects. The functional disturbance therefore is simply incompetence of the mitral valve.

Anomalous Chordal Insertion.—In some hearts without other malformations, but in our experience more commonly in association with ventricular septal defect, there is anomalous insertion of some of the chordae, usually of those connecting with the posterior leaflet. The anomalously inserting chordae are usually unduly short, their lower ends attach more basally than normal and they are associated with accessory commissures (or clefts) in the posterior leaflet (fig.

5). These chordae seem to exert a restraining influence on the leaflet and prevent proper excursion for closure at the accessory commissure.

A special variety of anomalous insertion of chordae occurs in the complex malformation commonly known as "corrected transposition of the great vessels." In such hearts the left atrioventricular valve bears a form that is a mirror image of the tricuspid valve of normally disposed hearts. Some of these hearts contain a ventricular septal defect, but regardless of the absence or presence of this malformation the mitral valve is often grossly incompetent.[3] This results either from the restraining influence on the septal and posterior cusp by stout short chordae (fig. 6*a*) or from the existence of a complex valvular malformation which is the counterpart of Ebstein's malformation of otherwise normally disposed hearts.[4]

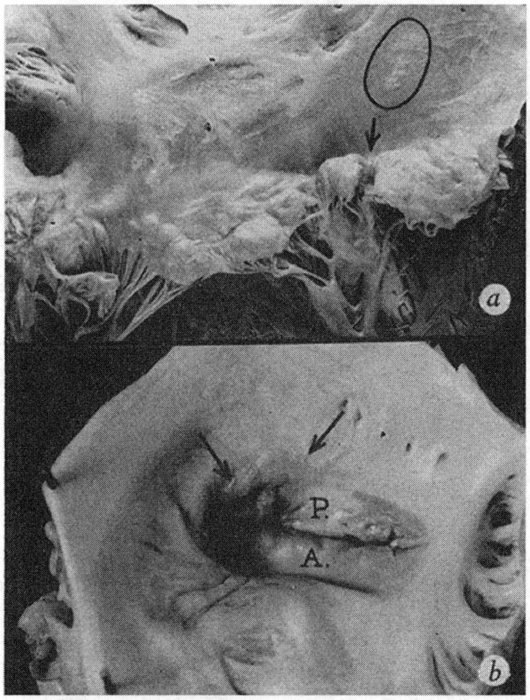

Fig. 5. Congenital causes of mitral insufficiency. *a*. In the posterior leaflet of the mitral valve, there is an accessory commissure (arrow). Attached to this are chordae, of which the ventricular attachment lies considerably more basal than usual. As a result of the anomalous and short chordae and the accessory commissure, there is insufficient mobility of leaflet tissue to overcome a deficiency in tissue. Anatomic evidence for this resides in the jet lesion (circle) which lies in the posterior wall of the left atrium above the accessory commissure.

b. The unopened mitral valve viewed from above in a case of ventricular septal defect with normal disposition of the great vessels. Accessory commissures in the posterior leaflet of the mitral valve. Resulting from the accessory commissures and anomalously attached chordae is incompetence which has been responsible for the creation of jet lesions (between points of arrows) in the posterior wall of the left atrium.

In *endocardial sclerosis* of the left ventricle the chordae may be involved by the process of excess deposit of connective tissue. The resulting retraction of the chordae may present sufficient mobility of the leaflets for closure of the valve during systole.

Double orifice of the mitral valve is usually considered a malformation only of incidental interest and of little functional importance. Usually, in this condition the basic chordal attachments of the two leaflets are normal. An orifice exists in one of the leaflets, and surrounding the edges are accessory chordae whose lower portions converge and attach to a papillary muscle. It is not known

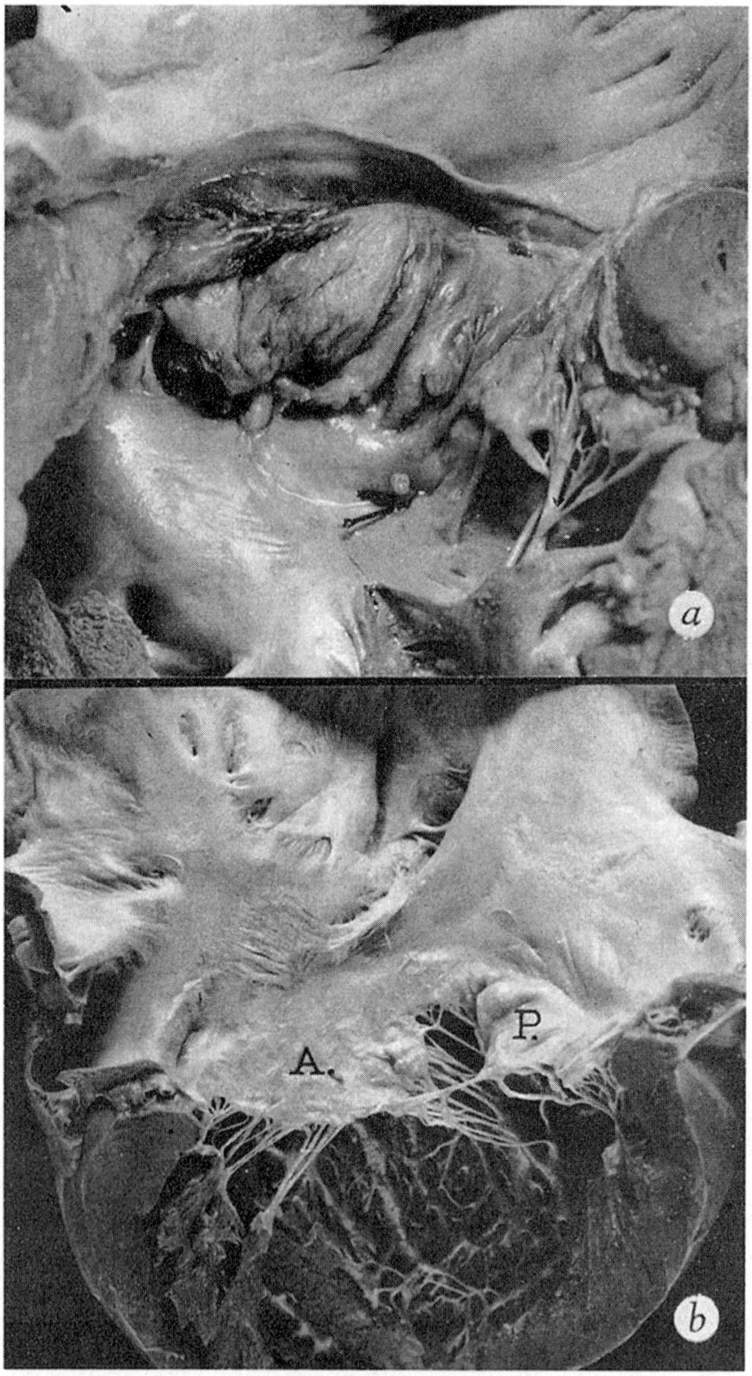

Legend appears on facing page.

whether in the usual case there is or is not some regurgitation through the accessory orifice. The major part of the valve, however, seems competent in the usual instance since each of the leaflets has its basic chordal attachments.

We observed an unusual case in a 45-year-old man with mitral insufficiency in whom the deformed valve could be classified best as "double mitral orifice." The mitral valve was viewed as having two normal leaflets but central chordae did not insert into a papillary muscle. Instead, chordae from the center of the anterior leaflet commerged into a single cord which attached to the center of the posterior leaflet (fig. 6*b*). Thus the center of each leaflet failed to be joined normally to a papillary muscle. That incompetence resulted was supported during life by functional studies. At operation the incompetence seemed to have resulted from the "overshoot" of the two leaflets. One may view the orifice at one side of the anomalous cord as the true mitral orifice and at the other side as an accessory orifice. If this is done the malformation may be placed in an established category.

MITRAL INSUFFICIENCY BEGETS MITRAL INSUFFICIENCY

Observation of established mitral insufficiency reveals two striking phenomena:

First, mitral insufficiency may be present for years and may be well tolerated up to a certain point. Beyond that point clinical evidence for gross mitral incompetence may become apparent, and the disease continues in a severe, unrelenting and possibly accentuating manner.

Second, in some patients with dilated left ventricles, as in ventricular septal defect with a large left-to-right shunt, mitral incompetence may be demonstrated during life. At necropsy in some of these patients no anatomic basis for the incompetence may be demonstrated either in the intrinsic nature of leaflets or chordae.

For an explanation of either of these phenomena one may possibly grasp at and be satisfied with a common concept: as the left ventricle dilates, so does the mitral orifice, and the two mitral leaflets of normal size are now smaller than the enlarged orifice. While part of the explanation probably resides in this concept, perhaps additional factors are in operation.

In observing dilated ventricles one becomes aware of the fact that the two papillary muscles are farther apart than they are normally. This deviation changes the direction of the chordae as they

---

Fig. 6. Congenital causes of mitral insufficiency. *a*. Mitral incompetence in a case with corrected transposition of the great vessels. Incompetence results from unusually short chordae which bind the leaflets to the myocardium in such a way as to restrict their mobility.

b. Mitral incompetence in a 45-year-old man. The left atrium, left ventricle and mitral valve have been opened in a standard manner. In addition to the orifice which has been opened there is a secondary orifice which is separated from the primary one by a strand of chordal tissue extending from the anterior leaflet (A.) to the posterior leaflet (P.). Since this chordal tissue does not connect with the ventricle, it is incapable of exerting a restraining action on the two leaflets. This allows the two leaflets to overshoot.

run between the papillary muscles and the valve leaflets. It changes their direction from a more or less vertical one (with respect to the inflow channel) toward a horizontal direction. Such a change in the direction of the chordae might decrease their capability of holding the two leaflets in an optimal position during ventricular systole and might allow "overshoot" (fig. 7).

If this theory is correct, the dilatation of the left ventricle from a given degree of mitral incompetence would set into operation a vicious cycle conveniently expressed as "mitral insufficiency begets mitral insufficiency."

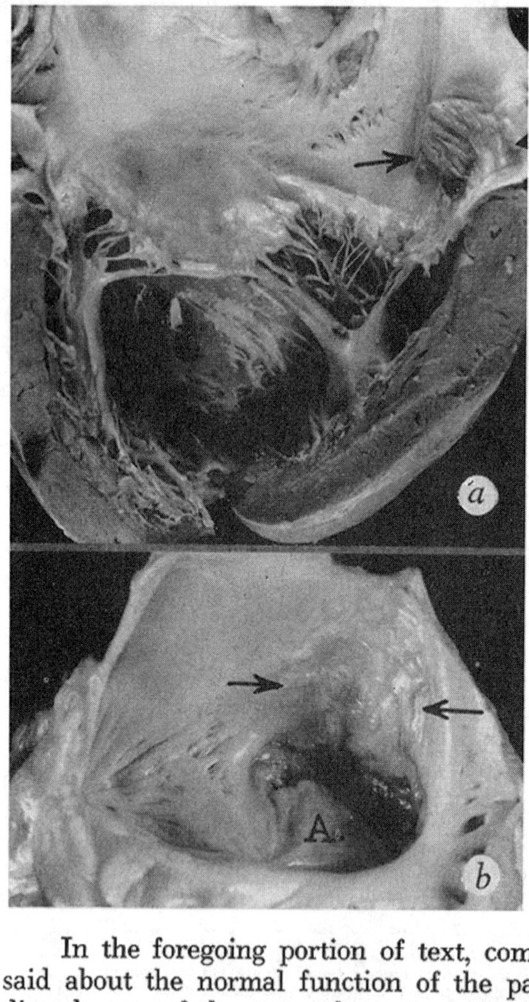

Fig. 7. Mitral insufficiency in a patient having ventricular septal defect and no apparent intrinsic malformation or other disease of the mitral valve. *a.* The left ventricle is moderately dilated; the mitral valve appears normal. On the posterior wall of the left atrium, a patch of jet lesions (arrows) indicates that mitral incompetence had been present, a finding which was supported by the clinical obvservations.

b. The unopened mitral valve from above. The anterior leaflet (A.) overshoots the posterior leaflet. In the left atrium opposite the "overshot" anterior leaflet is the patch of jet lesions (arrows) which is also illustrated in *a.*

In the foregoing portion of text, comparatively little has been said about the normal function of the papillary muscles and how disturbances of these muscles cause mitral incompetence.

Rupture of a papillary muscle, which is usually a complication of myocardial infarction, causes attached chordae tendineae to lose their moorings and thus allows obvious "overshoot" of the leaflets.

In certain instances of healed myocardial infarction wherein tissue of a papillary muscle is lost, we have had the impression that mitral insufficiency resulted. In general, knowledge regarding the specific function of the papillary muscles in closure of the mitral valve is rudimentary. More needs to be learned about the role of the papillary muscles in regard to function of the mitral valve in health and disease.

SUMMARY

Closure of the normal mitral valve depends on the following conditions: (1) the presence of intact leaflets, (2) leaflets which, in the aggregate, are larger than the mitral orifice, (3) leaflets of sufficient mobility to allow apposition, and (4) sufficient restraining action on the part of the chordae tendineae and papillary muscles to prevent "overshoot" of the leaflets.

Mitral insufficiency results primarily from rheumatic fever, bacterial endocarditis and congenital malformations.

Incompetence of the valve by any of these conditions results from loss of one or several of the conditions operative in the normal valve.

Mitral insufficiency may establish a vicious cycle wherein this functional derangement is progressively increased in severity.

REFERENCES

1. Hepper, N. G. G., Burchell, H. B. and Edwards, J. E.: Cardiac Clinics. CXLVI. Mitral Insufficiency in Healed, Unrecognized Bacterial Endocarditis. Proc. Staff Meet., Mayo Clin. *31*:659-664 (Dec. 12) 1956.
2. Osmundson, P. J., Callahan, J. A. and Edwards, J. E.: Mitral Insufficiency From Ruptured Chordae Tendineae Simulating Aortic Stenosis. Proc. Staff Meet., Mayo Clin. *33*:235-244 (Apr. 30) 1958.
3. Helmholz, F. H., Jr., Daugherty, G. W. and Edwards, J. E.: Cardiac Clinics. CXLV. Congenital "Mitral" Insufficiency in Association With Corrected Transposition of the Great Vessels: Report of Probable Clinical Case and Review of Six Cases Studied Pathologically. Proc. Staff Meet., Mayo Clin. *31*:82-91 (Feb. 22) 1956.
4. Becu, L. M., Swan, H. J. C., DuShane, J. W. and Edwards, J. E.: Cardiac Clinics. CXLIV. Ebstein Malformation of the Left Atrioventricular Valve in Corrected Transposition of the Great Vessels With Ventricular Septal Defect. Proc. Staff Meet., Mayo Clin. *30*:483-490 (Oct. 19) 1955.

Pathologic Anatomy of Mitral Insufficiency

Maurice Enriquez-Sarano, M.D.

My encounter with Jesse E. Edwards preceded by far my "physical" encounter with him. It was in the mid-1970s, I had just passed the "Internat des Hopitaux de Paris" the most prestigious medical training program in France, and I was doing my military service as a cooperating physician in Tunisia, as a fellow in the main cardiology service of that country. I learned to love cardiology, to have a profound attraction for understanding the mitral valve and its dysfunctions, to get a lasting friendship with my Tunisian counterparts and to understand the plight that poverty and epidemic rheumatic fever imparted on a young and desperate population. I learned to do what you can with what you have. I also got to connect from afar with Jesse. We (the fellows) took calls and had a cot in the library of the cardiology service where the chief of service had his issues of the cardiology journals available for reading and among them "Circulation," when the journal was still grey and monthly. Around 1 AM, generally work slowed down, and I had time to lie down. However, the window of the call room was open to a flea market called "Melassine," where drums were beating all night for men dancing together and where half-wild dogs barked continuously. At that time of the night, I had an appointment with my friend Jesse. He was a prolific writer on many subjects, but some resonated with me, particularly those that described valvular heart diseases. I did not always stay awake to read the whole article, let alone understand it, but it was my moment of calm and of serene encounter with intelligence, insight and desire to learn. It was my time with Jesse.

Many years later, I pushed the door of my friends Terri and Brooks Edwards, and met a man that I learned later to be my Jesse. Sometimes, it is difficult to encounter a real person who has been a myth for you and one may be disappointed, but the little twinkle in the eye, the pointed questions, the desire to connect were all telling me that this was my Jesse. I probably never told him of this remote connection, but I am sure he knows.

What was known in 1958 about the pathological anatomy of Mitral Insufficiency and what was guessed? We have to remember that very little could be done in living human beings and that most of what was known was through the clinical-pathological correlation. There was no angiography, no echocardiography, and cardiac surgery was only nascent. What is the 2011 value of a 1958 paper? All the incredibly persistent value is in the astute observation of the flaccid heart on the autopsy table coupled with the insights that makes one imagine what the movement of life would be. When one reads the part about the normal mitral valve function, there is very little more that fellows or cardiologists need to know. The comprehension of the role of chordae and papillary muscles position and movement, in preventing the "overshoot" (remember that mitral "prolapse" had not yet been coined) is brilliant. I spend my time in the echocardiography review room explaining it again and again in the never-ending job of teacher. The mitral annulus structure is described in few but precise words that have yet to be understood by the majority. The attachments of the leaflets, to the aortic root for the anterior leaflet and to the left ventricle for the posterior leaflet are luminous guides of what can and cannot be done by surgery and by the new interventional therapies. Whether one directs his career to valve disease or not, this section on the normal mitral valve should be mandatory reading. The keen reflection of what the apposition of leaflets must entail for proper coaptation, based on pathological observation of immobile structures, is human ingenuity at work. We now see by echocardiography the closure and coaptation and have the privilege of observing the movement of life, but there is little that we would change to the imagined coaptation of 1958.

When one looks at the pathological lesions causing mitral regurgitation (it was still called "insufficiency" in 1958), one can only report the prevalent diseases of the time. Rheumatic disease retraction and its necessary combination with leaflet separation in producing regurgitation is not obsolete knowledge. The new diseases, such as post-radiation heart disease, also cause the retraction, immobility, separation and regurgitation that rheumatic disease created. Even more relevant is the sequential understanding, from endocarditis with ruptured chordae to unexplained ruptured chordae, that mitral regurgitation may be the result of an "overshoot of leaflet." Behind this direct observation is the puzzlement caused by the ruptured chordae that are not observed with endocarditis. Are these due to an endocarditis that has been cured, or are they due to something else. The concept of degenerative mitral regurgitation was not defined yet, and only in the early 1960s was the concept of mitral regurgitation due to ruptured chordae gaining wide-ranging acceptance. These unclassified observations are here, offered to the reader to bring a future completion of the explanation. The beauty of medicine is that it is constantly progressing, said one of the Mayo brothers, but to progress the teachers of 1958 and those of today need to offer to the investigators of tomorrow what they do not understand and cannot yet guess.

What is most amazing in that spirit of gaining insight by careful observation coupled with unleashed imagination is the segment on what was not yet called functional mitral regurgitation and the mode of progression of mitral regurgitation ("mitral insufficiency begets mitral insufficiency"). The concept that a disease that does not intrinsically affect the mitral valve may cause mitral regurgitation was not self-evident, and only modern detailed quantitative echocardiography has given us the in-vivo details of the complex mechanisms that may lead to such an oddity. My colleagues and I have been among the few to examine the nature and mechanisms of mitral regurgitation progression. We made complex measurements of regurgitant orifice, volume, multi-chamber size and function. We observed the mitral regurgitation progression or rather confirmed such a progression and tried to delineate its mechanisms. All of that is useful to the understanding of mitral valve diseases, but if we had to summarize it in one sentence, it would be Jesse's "mitral insufficiency begets mitral insufficiency."

My teacher Jesse, you were smiling to me from your Minnesota home to my call room in Tunisia and then also back to the infinite nights of call in France where I continued to read you. I am sure you are still smiling, watching the infinite torch of the teachers being passed from one to the other, over thousands of miles, oceans and continents. I can now tell you what I did not tell you that afternoon in your son's house, of a teacher discovered in its human existence, among a loving and loved family, of all that I owe you like many, many others. We can only teach again and again the same things that we try to enrich by our research and by telling what we do not yet know, hoping that the student of today will be our teacher of tomorrow. Like you, we always need to finish with a wink and a smile.

The Myxomatous Mitral Valve and Sudden Death

ELLIOT CHESLER, M.D., RICHARD A. KING, M.D., AND JESSE E. EDWARDS, M.D.

SUMMARY The clincopathologic features of 14 cases of sudden death attributable to dysrhythmias associated with the myxomatous mitral valve are described. The patients were 14–59 years old (mean 27 ± 11 years). Eleven were female and three male. Of the seven ECGs available, none showed prolongation of the QT interval, but two showed repolarization abnormalities. The material was classified according to the degree of prolapse in the pathologic specimen. When obvious prolapse was found, the expected auscultatory findings had been documented. In three cases there was minimal prolapse, casting some doubt on the hypothesis that traction on the papillary muscles or diastolic dumping of the leaflets may be implicated in the pathogenesis of the dysrhythmias. In one of the cases with minimal prolapse there was a strong family history of sudden death. Endocardial friction lesions were present in 11 cases, including two of the three with minimal prolapse. In five cases there was a thrombotic lesion in the angle between the posterior leaflet and the left atrial wall containing fibrin and platelets. These abnormalities may be important in the pathogenesis of the ventricular dysrhythmias.

SUDDEN DEATH is a very uncommon complication of the mitral valve prolapse–click syndrome. While there is strong clinical evidence that the cause of sudden death is a ventricular tachyarrhythmia, its pathogenesis is not known. One theory is that the voluminous prolapsing leaflets produce abnormal tension on the papillary muscles, resulting in electrocardiographic abnormalities and dysrhythmias. However, mitral valve prolapse may be associated with other conditions, such as congestive cardiomyopathy and hypertrophic subaortic stenosis, which in their own right may be important determinants of prognosis, including a predisposition to fatal dysrhythmias.

We found 39 reported cases of sudden death attributed to mitral valve prolapse,[1–23] including three cases from our laboratory.[7] In only 19 of the reported cases were autopsies performed, but even among these cases the information is, in many instances, sparse, so other pathologic conditions cannot be excluded. Because of the important clinical and forensic implications, we report the clinicopathologic findings in 14 cases of sudden death in whom myxomatous change of the mitral valve was the principal identifiable pathologic abnormality.

Materials and Methods

The 14 specimens were referred from various centers during 1973–1981. Complete autopsies in each case identified the cardiac abnormalities as the only possible causes of sudden death. Two cases emanated from county coroners, and no supplementary clinical information was available. The family history was available in 12 cases, clinical information in 10 and ECGs in seven.

The circumstances surrounding cardiac arrest were determined from paramedic, hospital and county coroner records. From these sources, the interval between the onset of cardiac arrest and the cessation of resuscitative measures was estimated.

The specimens of heart were examined macroscopically for evidence of congenital and other cardiac abnormalities. The coronary arteries were sectioned transversely at 3–5-mm intervals, and representative segments were examined microscopically. Multiple blocks of tissue were taken from the free and septal walls of both ventricles for histologic examination. Particular attention was paid to the histology of the papillary muscles. The atrioventricular node and the proximal portion of the bundle branches were examined in two cases by spot check sections. Serial sections were not made. The mitral valve apparatus was examined for chordal thickening and elongation, and the degree of prolapse of the mitral leaflets was graded from I to III. Friction lesions on the endocardium of the left ventricle adjacent to the chordae were sought.

Definition of Grades of Mitral Valve Prolapse

The degrees of prolapse of the mitral valve leaflets are listed in table 1. Grade I was characterized by mild focal degrees of prolapse or interchordal hooding. Recognizing that some hooding may be present in the normal valve, the cases included under this category were considered to exhibit mild degrees of change but in excess of the normal (fig. 1). Histologic evidence supported the diagnosis of myxomatous change in each case in this category (fig. 2A), and in two there were endocardial friction lesions (fig. 2B), as described by Salazar and Edwards.[24] Grade II was characterized by moderate redundancy and grade III by severe redundancy of the leaflets (fig. 3).

Results

Among the 14 cases, three showed grade I, eight grade II and three grade III mitral valve prolapse. The clinicopathologic features pertaining to the 14 cases are summarized in table 1. There were 11 female and three male patients, ages 14–59 years (mean 27 ± 11 [± SD]). Two patients had a history of chest pain, four had palpitations and one patient had dizziness.

Family History

A family medical history was available in 12 cases and was significant in two. In case 13, the father was found to have a nonejection click.

From the Department of Cardiology, Veterans Administration Medical Center, Minneapolis, the Departments of Medicine and Pathology, University of Minnesota, Minneapolis, and the Department of Pathology, United Hospitals, St. Paul, Minnesota.

Supported by USPHS research grant 5 R01 HL05694, NHLBI.

Address for correspondence: Jesse E. Edwards, M.D., Department of Pathology, United Hospitals, 333 North Smith Avenue, St. Paul, Minnesota 55102.

Received March 18, 1982; revision accepted September 3, 1982.
Circulation 67, No. 3, 1983.

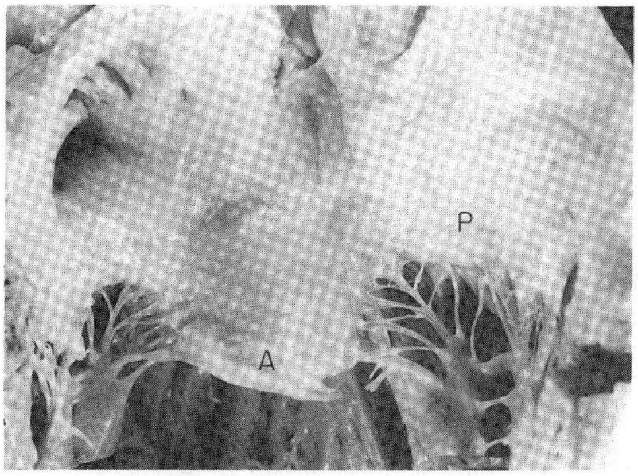

FIGURE 1. *Case 1. Mitral valve showing grade I prolapse. The anterior leaflet (A) is slightly thickened, and there are focal areas of interchordal hooding involving both leaflets. P = posterior leaflet.*

In case 3, a family pedigree was available (fig. 4). Case 3 was a 14-year-old girl whose mother died suddenly at age 36 years. The girl had nine siblings, two of whom died suddenly at the ages of 11 and 12 years, respectively. County coroner reports were available on the mother and these two siblings. No pathologic cause of death was found, but the report on the 12-year-old brother noted thickening of the "septal cusp of the mitral valve." Six of the remaining seven siblings and the father were examined. All six siblings had normal ECGs, but three had echocardiographic evidence of mitral valve prolapse. The father had a normal echocardiogram and ECG. The expression is consistent with an autosomal dominant pattern of inheritance in this family.

Electrocardiogram

Of the seven cases in whom some electrocardiographic study had been done, ventricular premature complexes were documented in six. In two of these there was bigeminy, but in only one case was the dysrhythmia treated aggressively. This was a 25-year-old woman (case 8) who had complained of increasing

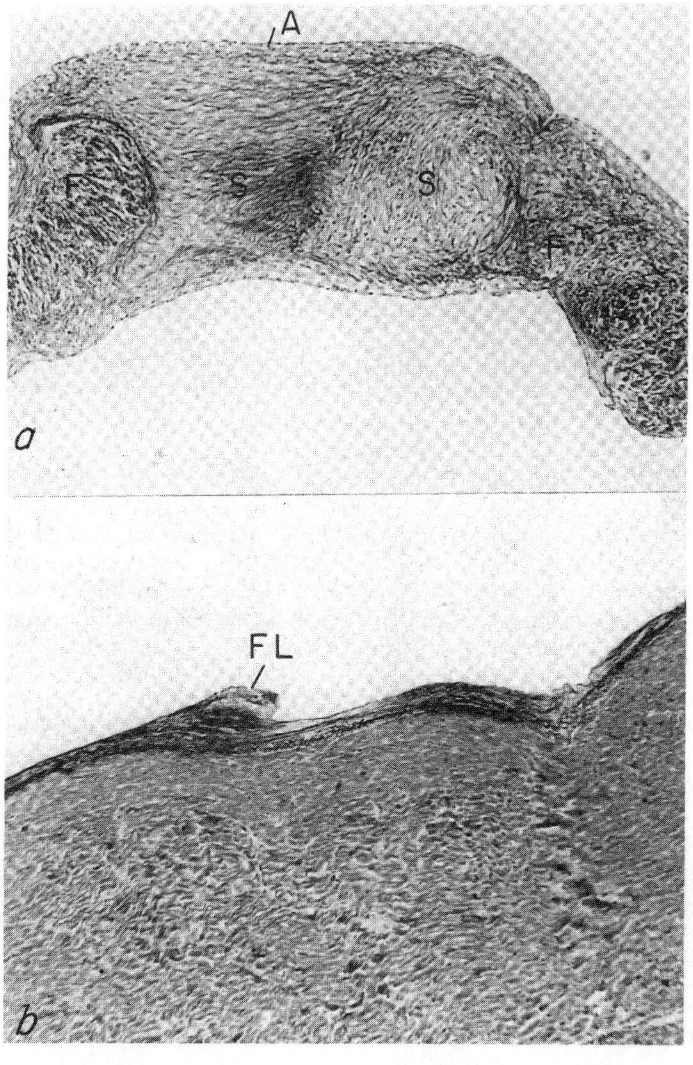

FIGURE 2. *Case 3. Photomicrographs of (A) posterior mitral leaflet and (B) the related endocardium and myocardium of the left ventricle. (A) The spongiosa layer (S) in the leaflet is increased and encroaches on the atrialis (A) and fibrosa (F) layers. Elastic tissue stain; magnification × 40. (B) There is a fibrous friction lesion (FL) of the endocardium adjacent to chordae of the posterior leaflet. Elastic tissue stain; magnification × 40.*

TABLE 1. *Clinicopathologic Features in 14 Cases of Sudden Death and Myxomatous Mitral Valve*

Case	Age (years)	Sex	Symptoms	History of dysrhythmias	Medications	Auscultation	Length of survival after resuscitation
Grade I mitral valve prolapse							
1	39	F	—	VPCs	—	Normal	6 days
2	59	F	—	—	Methyldopa	Not examined	8 days
3*	14	F	—	—	—	Not examined	90 minutes
Grades II and III mitral valve prolapse							
4	24	F	—	—	Primidone	HSM	No resuscitation
5	21	F	—	VPCs; bigeminy	—	MSC	60 minutes
6	19	F	No information	No information	No information	No information	15 minutes
7	26	F	No information	No information	No information	No information	2 days
8	25	F	Palpitations; dizziness; chest pain	VPCs; bigeminy; bradycardia; pacemaker	Propranolol	MSC + LSM	No resuscitation
9	29	M	Palpitations	VPCs; 1 paroxysm, atrial fibrillation	—	HSM	No resuscitation
10	30	M	—	—	—	MSC	90 minutes
11	21	F	Palpitations	VPCs	—	MSC + LSM	60 minutes
12	27	F	—	—	—	HSM	90 minutes
13†	26	F	Chest pain; palpitations	VPCs	Acebutalol; disopyramide	MSC + LSM	No resuscitation
14‡	19	M	—	—	Steroid inhaler	MSC + LSM	No resuscitation

*Family history of sudden death.
†Father with click.
‡Marfan's syndrome.
Abbreviations: VPCs = ventricular premature complexes; MSC = midsystolic click; LSM = late systolic murmur; HSM = holosystolic murmur; — = not present.

lightheadedness, one episode of syncope and periodic substernal pain radiating to the shoulders and arms. Electrocardiographic monitoring demonstrated atrial ectopy and protracted runs of ventricular bigeminy. These persisted despite a therapeutic trial of digoxin and quinidine. Because of persistent symptoms, propranolol, 20 mg twice daily, was administered and quinidine discontinued. This abolished the bigeminy but resulted in symptomatic bradycardia, and a demand pacemaker was implanted. The patient remained well for 6 weeks until she suffered sudden unexpected death. One day before death the pacemaker was found to be functioning perfectly.

One other patient (case 9) had one previous episode of atrial fibrillation, successfully treated with i.v. digoxin and propranolol.

Exercise electrocardiography was performed in cases 5, 9 and 13, each with known ventricular ectopy. In two of these, ventricular ectopy was abolished by exercise, and in one ectopy was aggravated. The remaining patient did not have ectopy immediately before, during or after the exercise test, but bigeminy had been observed on several other occasions. The QT interval was measured in seven available tracings and was 0.4 (upper limit of normal for age and sex[25] 0.432), 0.32 (normal 0.347), 0.36 (normal 0.384), 0.37 (normal 0.405), 0.32 (normal 0.36), 0.28 (normal 0.36), 0.32 (normal 0.395), and 0.32 (normal 0.34) second. ST-T-wave changes in the inferior and left precordial leads were observed in two of these tracings.

Toxicology and Medications

The medications taken immediately before death are

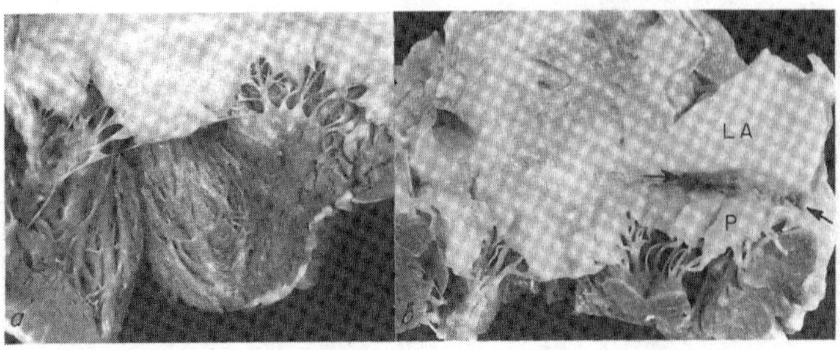

FIGURE 3. *(A) Case 9. Mitral valve demonstrates moderate (grade II) prolapse. (B) Case 12. Mitral valve showing severe (grade III) prolapse. There is a nodular deposit of fibrin (between arrows) in the angle between the posterior mitral leaflet (P) and the left atrial wall (LA). See also figure 5.*

TABLE 1. *(Continued)*

Heart weight (g)	Degree of prolapse: Anterior leaflet	Degree of prolapse: Posterior leaflet	Chordae	Endocardial friction lesions
348	+	+	Normal	–
320	–	+	Thickened	+
230	+	+	Thickened	+
350	+	++	Long	+
260	–	++	Long	–
230	Normal	++	Long	+
340	+	++	Long	+
220	+	++	Long	+
365	+	+++	Long	+
325	+	++	Long	+
290	+	++	Long	+
325	++	++	Long	+
240	+	+++	Long	+
220	++	+++	Long	+

listed in table 1. Toxicologic studies were negative in cases 4, 5, 8, 9, 10 and 13.

Auscultatory Findings

Among the three cases with grade I prolapse, two were asymptomatic and had not sought medical attention. Case 1 had a routine physical examination before operation for a prolapsed lumbar disc. The auscultatory findings were normal.

Among the 11 cases with grades II or III prolapse, in two we had no antemortem information. The remaining nine cases had auscultatory evidence of mitral valve prolapse (four with a midsystolic click and late systolic murmur, three with holosystolic murmurs and two with a midsystolic click only).

Pathologic Findings

The hearts weighed 195–365 g (mean 279 ± 57 g). In none of the specimens was there evidence of cardiomyopathy, myocarditis, significant coronary atherosclerosis or congenital abnormality to account for sudden death.

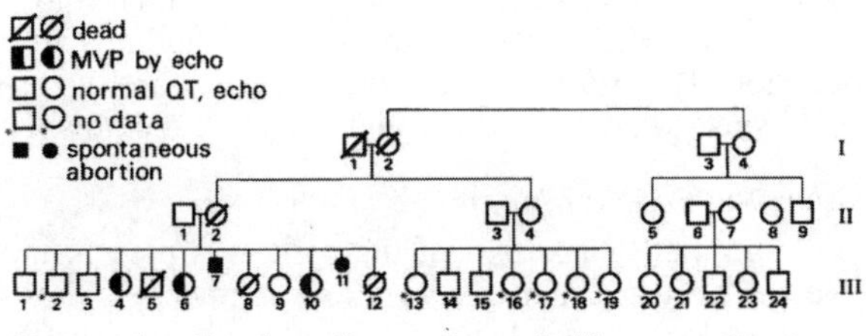

FIGURE 4. *Family pedigree of case 3. The propositus is patient III-12. MVP = mitral valve prolapse.*

Grade I Mitral Valve Prolapse (Three Cases)

Mitral valve apparatus. In two cases, both leaflets of the mitral valve were macroscopically thickened; in the other case, only the posterior leaflet was thickened. The chordae tendineae were intact and of normal length but were thickened in two cases. In case 1, microscopic deposits of fibrin and platelets were present at the junction of the left atrium and posterior mitral leaflet.

Endocardial friction lesions. In two cases there was thickening of the mural endocardium of the left ventricle beneath the posterior leaflet.

Coronary arteries. There was no evidence of atherosclerosis.

Conduction system. The conduction system was examined in case 2 and was normal.

Myocardium. Extensive changes in the myocardium were observed in cases 1 and 2. In case 1, there were multifocal areas of acute necrosis, and interspersed among areas of scarring were lesions of intermediate age, characterized by removal of myocardial fibers. The intramyocardial arteries were normal. These changes were considered to be a result of cardiac arrest and prolonged cardiopulmonary resuscitation. This patient had been in ventricular fibrillation for at least 30 minutes before cardioversion was performed by paramedical personnel. After this, she remained unconscious and was maintained on a respirator for 6 days.

The findings were similar in case 2. Multifocal areas of acute necrosis of muscle were present, and in other areas there were features of muscle removal. Also, there were several arteries within the papillary muscle that showed marked narrowing of the lumen by fibrous intimal thickening. This patient had also been in ventricular fibrillation for at least 15 minutes before cardioversion by paramedical personnel. She did not regain consciousness and died 8 days later despite assisted respiration.

Grades II and III Mitral Valve Prolapse (11 Cases)

Mitral valve apparatus. The leaflets, in particular, the posterior leaflets, were floppy, thickened and redundant with multiple areas of hooding. The chordae were elongated but not ruptured in any instance. Case 12 showed prominent macroscopic abnormalities at the junction of the left atrium and the posterior mitral leaflet. These consisted of a linear array of deposits of fibrin in the angle between the posterior mitral leaflet and the wall of the left atrium (figs. 3B and 5). There were also fibrous nodules just above this angle that involved the left atrial wall and the superior surface of the posterior mitral leaflet at their zone of mutual contact. Sections taken through the posterior mitral leaflet and adjacent portions of the left atrium and left ventricle showed several processes. The base of the mitral valve showed a focus of dense laminated collagen containing elastic tissue deposited along its atrial surface. Opposite this accumulation, the atrial endocardium showed a focus of thickening with collagen in the superficial part in which there were some elastic fibers. On the surface of each of the fibrous nodules there was

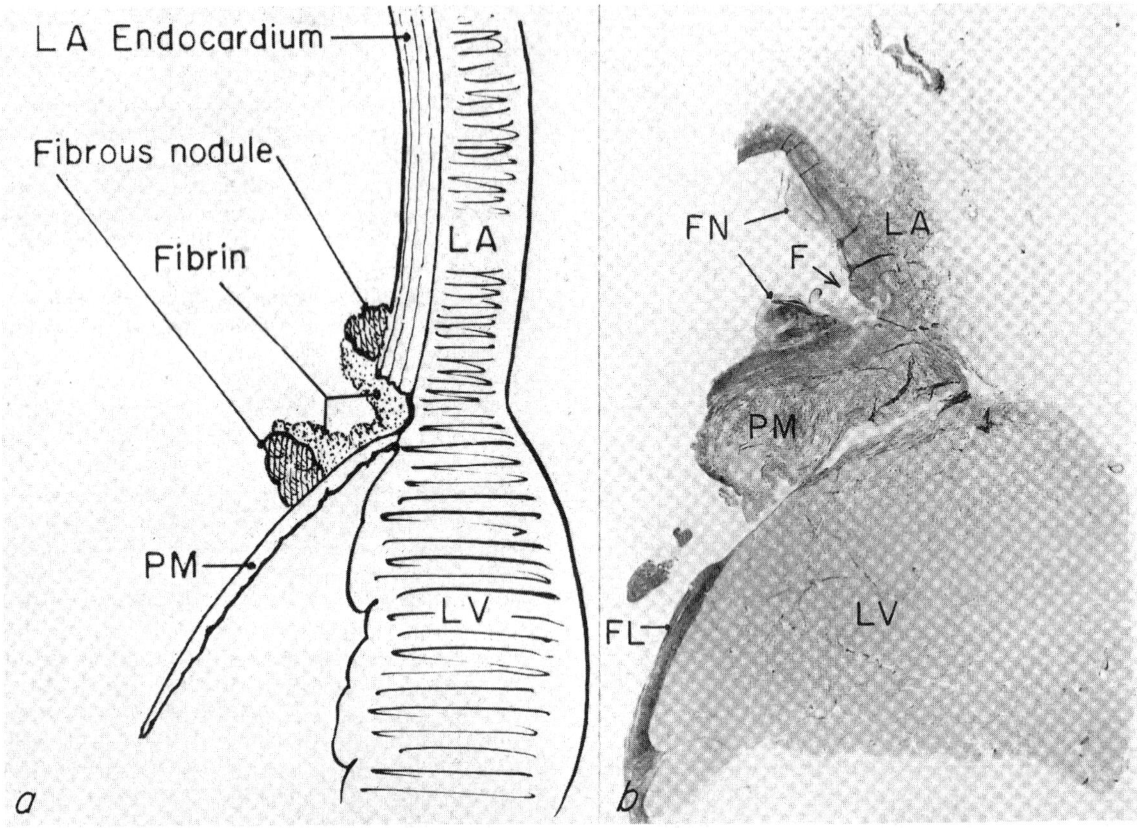

FIGURE 5. *Case 12. (A) Diagram and (B) photomicrograph of the junction of the left atrium (LA) and the posterior mitral leaflet (PM), as well as the related wall of the left ventricle (LV). There is deposition of fibrin (F) in the angle between the posterior mitral leaflet and the left atrial endocardium. Fibrous nodules (FN) are present both above the angle, involving the left atrial wall and below, involving the superior surface of the posterior mitral leaflet. In the photomicrograph, there is also a friction lesion (FL) of the left ventricular endocardium. Elastic tissue stain; magnification × 5.*

fibrin undergoing organization. This extended downward from each nodule toward the angle between the atrium and the base of the mitral leaflet. The actual angle between the base of the mitral leaflet and the left atrium showed destruction of tissue filled in by incompletely organized fibrin. At the very apex of the lesion there was an accumulation of dense collagen with an island of fibroelastic tissue resembling that of the atrial endocardium. No significant leukocytic infiltrate was evident, nor was there any calcification.

In case 13, the macroscopic findings in the angle between the left atrial wall and the posterior leaflet consisted of a linear array of hemorrhagic lesions. Microscopically, this consisted of aggregates of connective tissue, fibrin, platelets, leukocytes and red cells. No bacteria were observed (fig. 6). A similar lesion was present in case 4. In case 7, fibrin deposits were identified by microscopy.

Endocardial friction lesions. Friction lesions were present in nine of the 10 cases.

Coronary arteries. Abnormalities of the coronary arteries were present in case 9 only. This 29-year-old man had a focal 50% narrowing of the left anterior descending coronary artery 0.5 cm from its origin and a focal 25% atherosclerotic narrowing of the intermediate segment of the right coronary artery. The ascending aorta showed minimal atherosclerosis.

Conduction system. The conduction system was examined in case 5 and was normal.

Myocardium. Case 7 had evidence of multifocal acute myocardial necrosis with hypereosinophilia and coagulation necrosis. This 26-year-old woman collapsed because of ventricular fibrillation. After cardiopulmonary resuscitation, she was cardioverted to sinus rhythm and transported to the hospital. She had numerous episodes of ventricular tachycardia and fibrillation requiring repeated cardioversion and died 48 hours later despite assisted respiration.

In cases 8, 9, and 10, some sections showed small focal areas of interstitial fibrosis without cellular infiltrate or loss of myocardial fibers. These findings are occasionally observed in routine autopsies and were considered to be nonspecific and the cause unknown.

Other Pathologic Findings

Cystic medial necrosis of the aorta was present in five cases. In the four cases without stigmata of Marfan's syndrome, the changes were grade II in case 10 and grade I in cases 3, 9 and 12. Case 14 was recognized as having Marfan's syndrome clinically. The

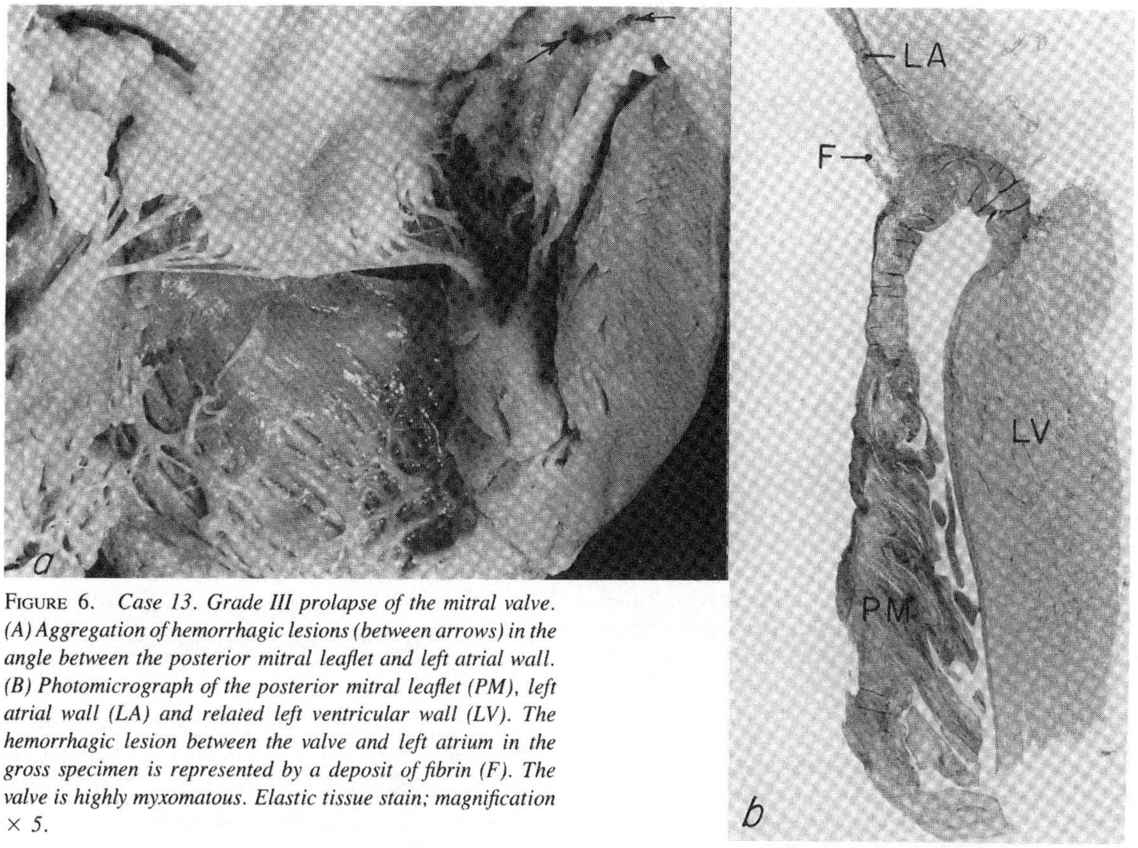

FIGURE 6. *Case 13. Grade III prolapse of the mitral valve. (A) Aggregation of hemorrhagic lesions (between arrows) in the angle between the posterior mitral leaflet and left atrial wall. (B) Photomicrograph of the posterior mitral leaflet (PM), left atrial wall (LA) and related left ventricular wall (LV). The hemorrhagic lesion between the valve and left atrium in the gross specimen is represented by a deposit of fibrin (F). The valve is highly myxomatous. Elastic tissue stain; magnification × 5.*

aortic root was dilated (10 cm in circumference), and there was grade II cystic medial necrosis.

Discussion

Considering the frequency of mitral valve prolapse in the general population, cases of sudden death attributable to this syndrome have attracted disproportionate attention. The possibility has been raised that associated coronary artery disease, left ventricular myopathy, or prolongation of the QT interval may be responsible factors.[26–29] One of the purposes of our study of 14 patients was to ascertain whether some other form of cardiac abnormality may have played a role in the pathogenesis of the fatal cardiac dysrhythmias. In general, most instances of sudden cardiac death can be resolved by pathologic examination into ischemic heart disease, nonatherosclerotic coronary artery disease (e.g., dissecting aneurysms), or left ventricular hypertrophy associated with idiopathic hypertrophic subaortic stenosis or aortic valve stenosis.[30] Other causes, such as congestive cardiomyopathy, severe pulmonary hypertension, myocarditis and sarcoidosis, are also readily identifiable. All of these were excluded from this study. Also, there was no evidence that drug toxicity or medications caused sudden death in our patients. (An additional case of sudden death and mitral valve prolapse in our collection was excluded because of a strong suspicion of quinidine toxicity.)

Three of our cases had evidence of multifocal myocardial necrosis. These changes are attributed to inadequate coronary blood flow as a reult of prolonged circulatory arrest and the protracted resuscitation that followed the dysrhythmia. Experimental studies in dogs have demonstrated lack of coronary blood flow during closed-chest resuscitation.[31] None of the specimens showed evidence of "contraction band necrosis," suggestive of acute myocardial ischemia, as found in sudden coronary death. The myxomatous mitral valve and secondary changes in adjacent structures were thus the only important pathologic abnormalities. Five cases showed evidence of aortic cystic medial necrosis, one of which had all the clinical features of Marfan's syndrome, which is associated with the myxomatous mitral valve.[29]

In his review of 25 cases of sudden death associated with mitral valve prolapse, Jeresaty[32] identified the potential victim as having the following features: A 40-year-old woman with a history of syncope who has a late systolic murmur preceded by a click, or a pansystolic murmur with late systolic accentuation. The ECG shows inferolateral ST-T changes and frequent premature ventricular systoles. Left ventriculography demonstrates obvious mitral valve prolapse and minimal-to-moderate mitral regurgitation. Patients with "silent" mitral valve prolapse or an isolated click do not appear to be susceptible. A family history of sudden death is an added risk factor. Traction on the papillary muscle is favored as the mechanism for the repolarization changes and dysrhythmias.

Our material was classified according to the degree of prolapse of the myxomatous valves in the pathologic specimens. In patients with grade II and III prolapse, the findings conform in general with the clinical description of Jeresaty,[32] in that the expected auscultatory findings were present. However, only two of the seven ECGs showed repolarization changes.

In the patients with grade I prolapse, the findings are of particular interest. Case 1 had been examined before lumbar disc surgery, and no abnormal auscultatory findings were recorded. The ECG was normal except for frequent ventricular ectopy.

The family history of case 3 is germane in that sudden death afflicted a mother and three of her children, none of whom had sought medical attention. The occurrence of sudden death in such asymptomatic patients with minimal prolapse may refute the hypotheses that either traction on the papillary muscle or "diastolic dumping" by voluminous leaflets may produce endocardial or papillary muscle irritability and dysrhythmias.[15, 33] Additionally, the degree of prolapse demonstrated in these patients at autopsy is unlikely to be demonstrable by angiography or echocardiography.

The cause of the dysrhythmias in subjects with the myxomatous mitral valve remains an enigma. Endocardial friction lesions were present in 12 of the 14 cases (86%), including two of the three cases with grade I prolapse. These lesions arise as a result of friction between chordae and the left ventricular mural endocardium which, in some instances, may lead to marked fibrosis of the mural endocardium.[24] Mechanical stimulation of the endocardium by the thickened chordae could be responsible for the ventricular dysrhythmias and the repolarization changes. In those cases wherein repolarization changes are permanent, the endocardial scarring may be responsible. In five other specimens (36%), there was a lesion in the angle between the posterior leaflet of the mitral valve and the left atrial wall.[34] These contained aggregates of platelets and fibrin. Embolism from these deposits could lead to transient cerebral ischemic attacks and, more important relative to sudden death, to small coronary emboli, the latter causing dysrhythmias. Actual emboli were not detected in our material, possibly because of spontaneous lysis. Their sequelae may be difficult to demonstrate microscopically. Such embolism may also perhaps account for electrocardiographic evidence of myocardial infarction reported in patients with mitral valve prolapse in whom the coronary arteries are normal angiocardiographically.[35] In another study from this laboratory, which included 102 cases of myxomatous valves not associated with sudden death, endocardial friction lesions were present in 77 instances (77%) and fibrin deposits between the posterior mitral leaflet and left atrial wall were found in four instances (4%).[36]

Ventricular fibrillation has been reported as a complication in those cases of mitral valve prolapse with prolongation of the electrocardiographic QT interval.[33, 37, 38] The latter abnormality was not evident in this study, and the true frequency of this finding is uncertain.[32] In our material the major portions of the conduction system were examined in only two cases, and there were no abnormalities. Bharati et al.[20, 21] performed a detailed study of the conduction system in three cases of mitral valve prolapse and sudden death. In two cases there was premature aging and sclerosis of the cardiac skeleton, with involvement of the atrioventricular node and trifascicular conduction system; in one of these cases there was also thrombosis of the sinoatrial node artery.[21] In the third case there was fatty infiltration in the approaches to the sinoatrial and atrioventricular nodes and atrial preferential pathways.[20] The role of these findings in the pathogenesis of lethal brady- or tachyarrhythmias is uncertain, since their frequency in hearts without myxomatous mitral valves is unknown. Senges and associates[39] studied three patients electrophysiologically who had mitral valve prolapse, strong family histories of sudden death and high-grade ventricular ectopy. In these, normal intracardiac conduction and refractoriness were demonstrated. These studies provided no evidence for underlying reentrant mechanisms as a potential cause of ventricular ectopy.

References

1. Hancock EW, Cohn K: The syndrome associated with midsystolic click and late systolic murmur. Am J Med **41:** 183, 1966
2. Barlow JB, Bosman CK, Pocock WA, Marchand P: Late systolic murmurs and non-ejection ("mid-late") systolic clicks: an analysis of 90 patients. Br Heart J **30:** 203, 1968
3. Trent JK, Adelman AG, Wigle ED, Silver MD: Morphology of a prolapsed posterior mitral valve leaflet. Am Heart J **79:** 539, 1970
4. Shappell SD, Marshall CE, Brown RE, Bruce TA: Sudden death and the familial occurrence of mid-systolic click, late systolic murmur syndrome. Circulation **48:** 1128, 1973
5. Marshall CE, Shappell SD: Sudden death and the ballooning posterior leaflet syndrome. Detailed anatomic and histochemical investigation. Arch Pathol **98:** 134, 1974
6. Jeresaty RM: Mitral valve prolapse-click syndrome. Prog Cardiovasc Dis **15:** 623, 1973
7. Jeresaty RM: Sudden death in the mitral valve prolapse-click syndrome. Am J Cardiol **37:** 317, 1976
8. Guthrie RB, Edwards JE: Pathology of the myxomatous mitral valve. Nature, secondary changes and complications. Minn Med **59:** 637, 1976
9. Gulotta SJ, Gulco L, Padmanabhan V, Miller S: The syndrome of systolic click, murmur, and mitral valve prolapse — a cardiomyopathy? Circulation **49:** 717, 1974
10. Appelblatt NH, Willis PW III, Lenhart JA, Shulman JI, Walton A Jr: Ten to 40 year follow-up of 69 patients with systolic click with or without apical late systolic murmur. (abstr) Am J Cardiol **35:** 119, 1975
11. Sorensen HD, Smith RF: Lethal cardiac arrhythmias in the prolapsing valve syndrome. (abstr) J Tenn Med Assoc **68:** 667, 1975
12. Rakowski H, Waxman MB, Wald RW, Wigle ED: Mitral valve prolapse and ventricular fibrillation. (abstr) Circulation **52** (suppl II): II-93, 1975
13. Belardi J, Lardani H, Manubens S, Sheldon WC, Moreyra A: Idiopathic prolapse of the mitral valve; a follow up study in 137 patients studied by angiography. (abstr) Am J Cardiol **37:** 120, 1976
14. Koch FH, Hancock EW: Ten year follow-up of forty patients with the mid-systolic click/late systolic murmur syndrome. (abstr) Am J Cardiol **37:** 149, 1976
15. Cobbs BW Jr, King SB III: Ventricular buckling: a factor in the abnormal ventriculogram and peculiar hemodynamics associated with mitral valve prolapse. Am Heart J **93:** 741, 1977
16. Mills P, Rose J, Hollingsworth J, Amara I, Craige E: Long-term prognosis of mitral-valve prolapse. N Engl J Med **297:** 13, 1977
17. Barnett HJM, Jones MW, Boughner DR, Kostuk WJ: Cerebral ischemic events associated with prolapsing mitral valve. Arch Neurol **33:** 777, 1976
18. Davies MJ, Moore BP, Braimbridge MV: The floppy mitral valve.

Study of incidence, pathology, and complications in surgical, necropsy, and forensic material. Br Heart J **40:** 468, 1978

19. Mair WJ: Sudden death in young females with floppy mitral valve syndrome. Aust NZ J Med **10:** 221, 1980
20. Bharati S, Granston AS, Liebson PR, Loeb HS, Rosen KM, Lev M: The conduction system in mitral valve prolapse syndrome with sudden death. Am Heart J **101:** 667, 1981
21. Bharati S, Rosen KM, Miller LB, Strasberg B, Lev M: Sudden death in three teenagers. (abst) Circulation **64** (suppl IV): IV-72, 1981
22. Dupasquier E, Berney JL: Le syndrome du prolapsus valvulaire mitral. Deux complications rares: la mort subite, l'embolie cérébrale. Schweiz Med Wochenschr **111:** 73, 1981
23. Anderson RC: Idiopathic mitral valve prolapse and sudden death. (letter) Am Heart J **100:** 941, 1980
24. Salazar AE, Edwards JE: Friction lesions of ventricular endocardium. Relation to chordae tendineae of mitral valve. Arch Pathol **90:** 364, 1970
25. Ashman R, Hull E: Essentials of Electrocardiography, 2nd ed. New York, MacMillan, 1941
26. Malcolm AD, Čanković-Darracott S, Chayen J, Jenkins BS, Webb-Peploe MM: Biopsy evidence of left ventricular myocardial abnormality in patients with mitral-leaflet prolapse and chest pain. Lancet **1:** 1052, 1979
27. Mason JW, Koch FH, Billingham ME, Winkle RA: Cardiac biopsy evidence for a cardiomyopathy associated with symptomatic mitral valve prolapse. Am J Cardiol **42:** 557, 1978
28. Leatham A, Brigden W: Mild mitral regurgitation and the mitral prolapse fiasco. Am Heart J **99:** 659, 1980
29. Barlow JB, Pocock WA: Mitral valve prolapse, the specific billowing mitral leaflet syndrome, or an insignificant non-ejection systolic click. Am Heart J **97:** 277, 1979
30. Davies MJ, Popple A: Sudden unexpected cardiac death — a practical approach to the forensic problem. Histopathology **3:** 255, 1979
31. Ditchey RV, Winkler JV, Rhodes CA: Lack of coronary blood flow during closed-chest resuscitation. (abstr) Circulation **64** (suppl IV): IV-304, 1981
32. Jeresaty RM: Mitral Valve Prolapse. New York, Raven Press, 1979, p 219
33. Criley JM, Heger J: Prolapsed mitral leaflet syndrome. Cardiovasc Clin **10:** 213, 1979
34. Wigle ED, Rakowski H, Ranganathan N, Silver MD: Mitral valve prolapse. Annu Rev Med **27:** 165, 1976
35. Chesler E, Matisonn RE, Lakier JB, Pocock WA, Obel IWP, Barlow JB: Acute myocardial infarction with normal coronary arteries. A possible manifestation of the billowing mitral leaflet syndrome. Circulation **54:** 203, 1976
36. Lucas RV Jr, Edwards JE: The floppy mitral valve. An anatomic study of 171 autopsied patients. Curr Prob Cardiol **7:** 1, 1982
37. Forbes RB, Morton GH: Ventricular fibrillation in a patient with unsuspected mitral valve prolapse and a prolonged Q-T interval. Can Anaesth Soc J **26:** 424, 1979
38. Swartz MH, Teichholz LE, Donoso E: Mitral valve prolapse. A review of associated arrhythmias. Am J Med **62:** 377, 1977
39. Senges J, Zebe H, Pelzer D, Brachmann J, Krämer B, Kübler W: Nitrates and ectopic ventricular activity in mitral valve prolapse: clinical and experimental data. Z Kardiol **68:** 26, 1979

The Myxomatous Mitral Valve and Sudden Death

Paul A. Friedman, M.D.

The mitral valve, named for its resemblance to a bishop's mitre, functions to prevent retrograde flow from the left ventricle to the left atrium during systole. To accomplish this task, chordae tendineae secure the valve to papillary muscles, which act as shock absorbers and provide counter tension during systole, when left ventricular pressure significantly exceeds left atrial pressure. Each leaflet is composed of distinct tissue layers: the atrialis, fibrosa, and spongiosa. With myxomatous degeneration, excessive connective tissue results in leaflet thickening and chordae tendineae elongation. Mitral valve prolapse occurs when the leaflets of the mitral valve are displaced superiorly by more than 2 mm during systole in a standardized echocardiographic long axis view, with maximal leaflet thickness of the least 5 mm during diastases. A number of medical complications have been attributed to mitral valve prolapse including endocarditis, ischemic central nervous system events, thromboembolism, and the most feared complication sudden cardiac death in an otherwise apparently healthy person.

In 1983, Drs. Chesler, King, and Edwards published "The Myxomatous Mitral Valve in Sudden Death." In this paper, 14 hearts from patients who had died of unexpected sudden death were examined. In all cases, cardiac abnormalities of the myxomatous valve and secondary changes in adjacent structures were the only abnormalities present and the only possible cause of death. Whenever possible, clinical history, ECG findings, family history, and physical exam findings were collected. In a paper that vividly describes the pathologic anomalies present, key observations were made that informed subsequent studies on the topic. First, heterogeneity amongst patients was found, with the majority of patients having grade 2 or grade 3 mitral regurgitation (more extreme prolapse and chordal redundancy). Subsequent population studies by Nishimura et al. would confirm the importance of the degree of regurgitation in leading to complications related to mitral valve prolapse. The observation by the Edwards team of the role of family history has also since borne fruit, in that familial associations in the mitral valve prolapse syndrome have subsequently been well demonstrated. Particularly intriguing was the high prevalence friction lesions seen in the study. Friction lesions occur adjacent to the mitral valve where redundant chordae repetitively make contact with the endocardium of the ventricle. As any trainee who has attempted to manipulate a catheter in the left ventricle will recognize, mechanical contact with the wall of the ventricle leads to ventricular ectopy. Thus, the very high prevalence of friction lesions in the collection of specimens speaks to the importance of mechanical effects and arrhythmia. Indeed, the importance of this concept is seen in other disease states. Patients with otherwise normal hearts and so-called "idiopathic fascicular ventricular tachycardia" frequently have left ventricular bands, fibrous strands that many believe participate in arrhythmogenesis by applying mechanical tension to the endocardium. The pathologic roadmap laid out in 1983 was further expanded in 2006 by Edwards and Edwards in a father and son co-authored atlas of sudden death that photographically detailed the progression of myxomatous degeneration of the mitral valve.

While we now understand that mitral valve prolapse affects 2 to 3 percent of the population, poses the greatest risk to those with significant mitral regurgitation, and is quite often asymptomatic, many questions remain unanswered. What are the genetic and environmental factors that promote excess connective tissue development? Why is the excess regionalized to the mitral valve? The intelligent collection of cardiac specimens with shared phenotypic elements that include detailed clinical backgrounds permits questions regarding the mechanisms of disease to be asked. It is from these carefully culled specimens that Jesse Edwards answered so many of the questions of his day, and it is that same collection, thoughtfully curated and meticulously reviewed, that will answer tomorrow's questions.

Pathologic Changes in Aortic-Coronary Arterial Saphenous Vein Grafts

By ZEEV VLODAVER, M.D., AND JESSE E. EDWARDS, M.D.

SUMMARY

This is a pathologic study of segments of saphenous vein used as a graft between the aorta and a coronary artery in the surgical treatment of coronary atherosclerosis. Except for an occasional case with thrombotic occlusion of the graft, no lesions were observed in grafts which had been in place for less than 1 month. In each of two grafts in place for 1 month, mild fibrous thickening of the intima was present. Eight grafts which had been in place for 3½ months or longer consistently showed lesions, either organized thrombi (two grafts) or intimal fibrotic proliferative lesion (six grafts). In this group, five of the six grafts with intimal fibrous proliferation showed near or complete occlusion of the lumen.

The intimal fibrous proliferative lesion appears primarily to be a response to arterial pressure within the segment of vein. Obstructive atherosclerosis in the artery beyond the anastomosis with the graft may favor the development of the intimal lesion. The intimal lesion may progress rapidly according to the data in one of the cases. In this, patency of the graft demonstrated angiographically 3½ months after the operation was followed by near-complete occlusion of the lumen by the proliferative lesion 3 weeks following demonstration of patency.

Additional Indexing Words:
Coronary surgery Angina pectoris Coronary atherosclerosis
Myocardial infarction

RECENT INTEREST in the use of saphenous veins as grafts between the aorta and coronary arteries in the treatment of atherosclerosis makes the long-range character of the vein graft of considerable practical importance.[1-7] With this in mind, a pathologic study was done on 21 patients who had had this operation, yielding a total of 29 vein grafts. The operations had been done in various hospitals in the Twin Cities of Minnesota, but most of the cases were either from the Charles T. Miller or University of Minnesota hospital.

Among the cases studied, each was a classic example of coronary atherosclerosis, often with involvement of each of the three coronary arteries. In each instance, healed myocardial infarction in one or more than one area of the left ventricle was present.

From the Departments of Pathology of the Charles T. Miller Hospital, St. Paul, Minnesota and of the University of Minnesota, Minneapolis, Minnesota.

Supported by U. S. Public Health Service Research Grant 5 R01 HE05694 and Research Training Grant 5T01 HE05570 from the National Heart and Lung Institute and by the Otto Bremer Foundation.

Address for reprints: Jesse E. Edwards, M.D., Department of Pathology, The Charles T. Miller Hospital, 125 West College Avenue, Saint Paul, Minnesota 55102.

Received June 8, 1971; accepted for publication July 1, 1971.

Method

Each case was placed into one of four groups according to length of survival after operation as follows. Group I consisted of 15 grafts from 10 patients who died either during the operation or in the early postoperative hours. In group II, there were four grafts from three patients. The patients lived 1 day, 4 days, and 7 days, respectively. Group III consisted of two grafts from two patients, each patient living 1 month. Group IV consisted of eight grafts from six patients who survived from 3½ to 9 months after the operation. In each instance, except one, the entire specimen of heart and graft (or grafts) was available for study. In one case (6½ months) only histologic segments of the vein grafts were available to us.* Each of the patients in group IV had died suddenly.

Obstructive lesions were observed in seven of the eight grafts which had been in place for 3½ months or longer. These consisted either of intimal fibrous proliferation or organized thrombi.

Before describing the details of these changes, a review will be made of the histologic character of the normal greater saphenous vein in the adult and the observations made among the four groups representing different time intervals after insertion of the grafts.

*We are indebted to Dr. Allen S. Judd of St. Mary's Hospital, Minneapolis, Minnesota, for material from this case.

The Normal Saphenous Vein

The normal greater saphenous vein exhibits a thin, relatively acellular, fibrous intima which may show irregular minimal dense collagenous thickening. The media is relatively thick and varies in structure depending upon the relationship to the venous valves. In segments between valves, the muscle of the media is oriented, for the most part, in a circular fashion (fig. 1*a*). In contrast to arteries in which the circular medial muscle is a continuous layer, the circular muscle of the saphenous vein, as in other veins, is made up of interlacing bundles of smooth muscle, on the one hand, and of collagen and elastic tissue, on the other. In the vicinity of the

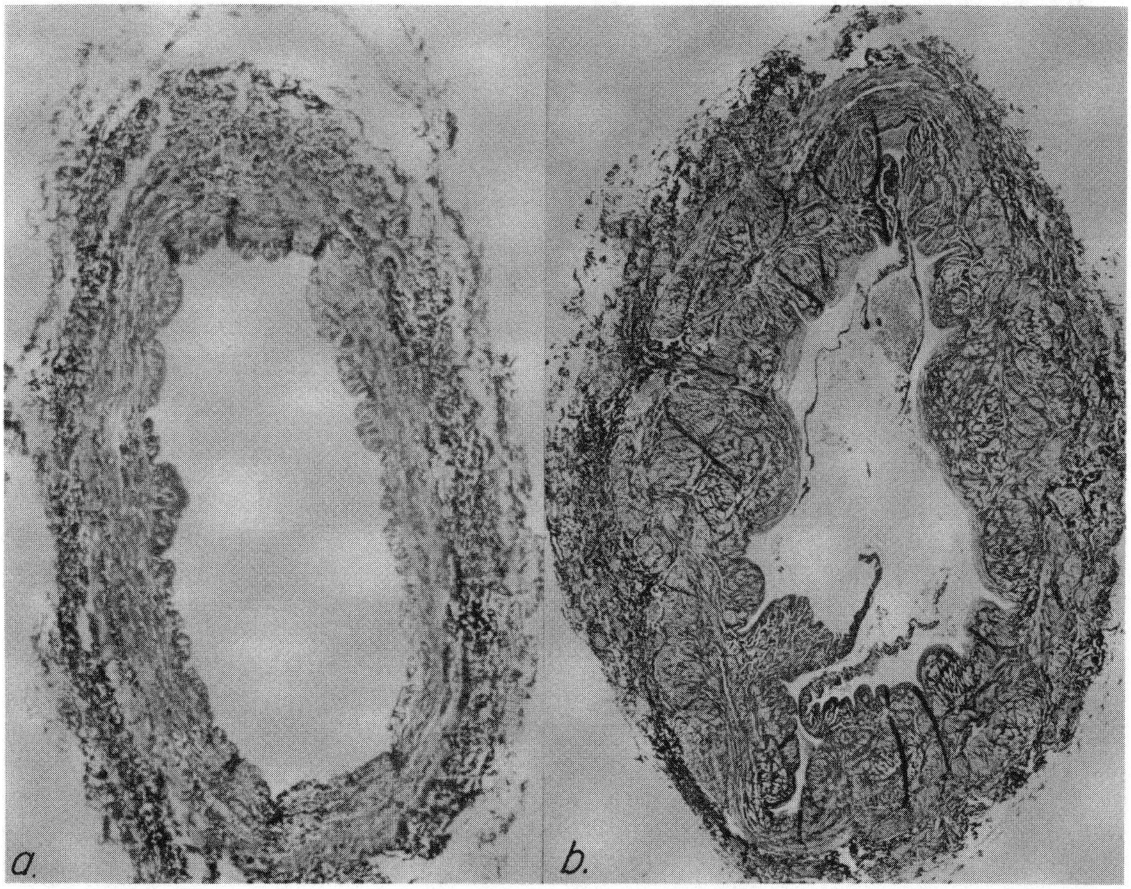

Figure 1

Photomicrographs of normal saphenous veins. (**a.**) *A segment between valves shows a circular medial layer. (Elastic tissue stain, × 25.)* (**b.**) *A segment at the level of a valve shows a thick media in which the fibers are, for the most part, oriented in longitudinal fashion. (Elastic tissue stain, × 20.)*

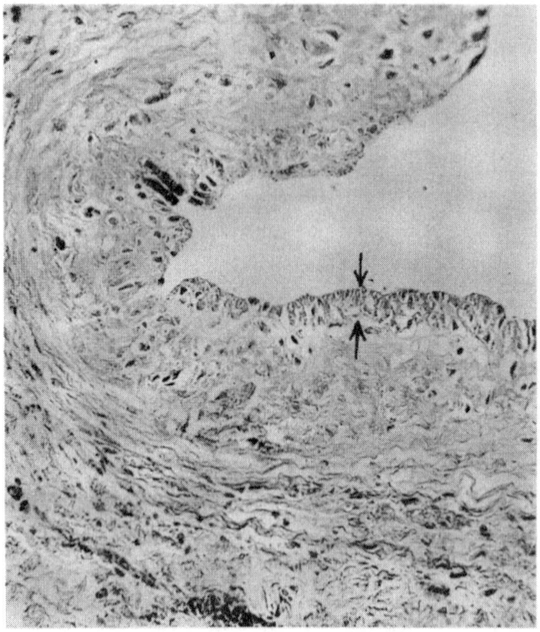

Figure 2

Photomicrograph of saphenous vein graft 1 month after being in place. This shows minimal intimal fibrous proliferation (between arrows) causing little luminal narrowing. (Hematoxylin and eosin, × 50.)

insertion of valves, the circular layer gives way to a longitudinal layer of muscle which blends with the circular layer (fig. 1*b*). The adventitia is composed of bundles of fibrous tissue in which some fascicles of smooth muscle are usually present.

Observations in Vein Grafts

Groups I and II

In the 19 grafts which had been in place for a short time (up to 7 days) no significant differences were noted compared to the normal.

Group III

Each of two grafts had been in place for 1 month. Each showed minimal thickening with avascular mucoid connective tissue (fig. 2). The changes which had caused no significant narrowing of the lumen qualitatively were like the lesions of greater severity observed in group IV. These will be described in greater detail in the next section.

Group IV

Eight grafts which had been in place for periods varying from 3½ to 9 months were obtained from six patients. The findings are summarized in table 1. In four patients (cases 1, 3, 4, and 6) solitary grafts had been

Table 1

Summary of Findings in Group IV

Case	Graft: To	Graft: Time in place (months)	Graft: Lesion*	Graft: Lumen	Atherosclerosis of artery distal to graft (grade)
1	RC	3½	Organized thrombus; (FIP)	Occluded	III
2 a	T-shaped, vertical to RC	3½	FIP	Severe obstruction	III
b	Horizontal to LAD		FIP	Proximal occlusion	II
3	LAD	4½	FIP; (organizing thrombus)	Occlusion	III
4	RC	6½	FIP; (intramural thrombus)	Severe obstruction	Unknown
5 a	RC	7	FIP	Moderate obstruction	II
b	Lt cir		Organized thrombus	Occluded	III
6	RC	9	FIP	Severe obstruction	III

*Lesion listed in parentheses present but of little importance in causing luminal narrowing.

Abbreviations: RC = right coronary artery; LAD = left anterior descending artery; Lt cir = left circumflex coronary artery; FIP = fibrous intimal proliferation.

inserted. In one patient (case 5) two independent grafts had been inserted: (1) one to the right coronary artery and (2) the other to the left circumflex artery.

In case 2, a "T"-shaped graft was used. The "vertical" (main) channel ran from the aorta to the right coronary artery, while a right-angle branch ("horizontal") of this graft had been inserted into the anterior descending coronary artery. In our tabulation, the main part of this graft is considered one graft (case 2a), while the right-angle branch is considered a second graft (case 2b). In each of the eight grafts in group IV, significant lesions were found (table 1).

In each of two grafts (cases 1 and 5b) organized thrombosis caused complete occlusion of the lumen (fig. 3*a*). In one of these cases (case 1) the organized thrombus was superimposed upon minimal intimal fibrous thickening essentially like that observed in group III (fig. 3*b*).

Each of the remaining six grafts showed easily recognizable fibrous intimal proliferation. In one of these (case 5a) moderate narrowing of the lumen was present diffusely (fig. 4). In three grafts (cases 3, 4, and 6), intimal fibrous proliferation caused uniformly severe narrowing of the lumen (fig. 5).

The case with the right-angle graft (case 2) deserves special mention. The vertical segment of the graft (aorta to right coronary artery) showed moderate degrees of luminal narrowing in the proximal half and severe degrees in its distal half. The proximal half of the right-angle graft showed complete obliteration of the lumen while the distal half was moderately narrowed by the intimal change (figs. 6 and 7).

Another case was of special interest (case 3). Three and one-half months after a graft was connected with the anterior descending coronary artery, angiography revealed wide patency of the graft (fig. 8*a*). The patient suffered sudden death 23 days later. At necropsy, the ostium and proximal segment of the graft were occluded by intimal fibrous proliferation (fig. 8*b* and *c*). Distally, including the site of anastomosis to the artery, the lumen of the graft was narrowed severely by

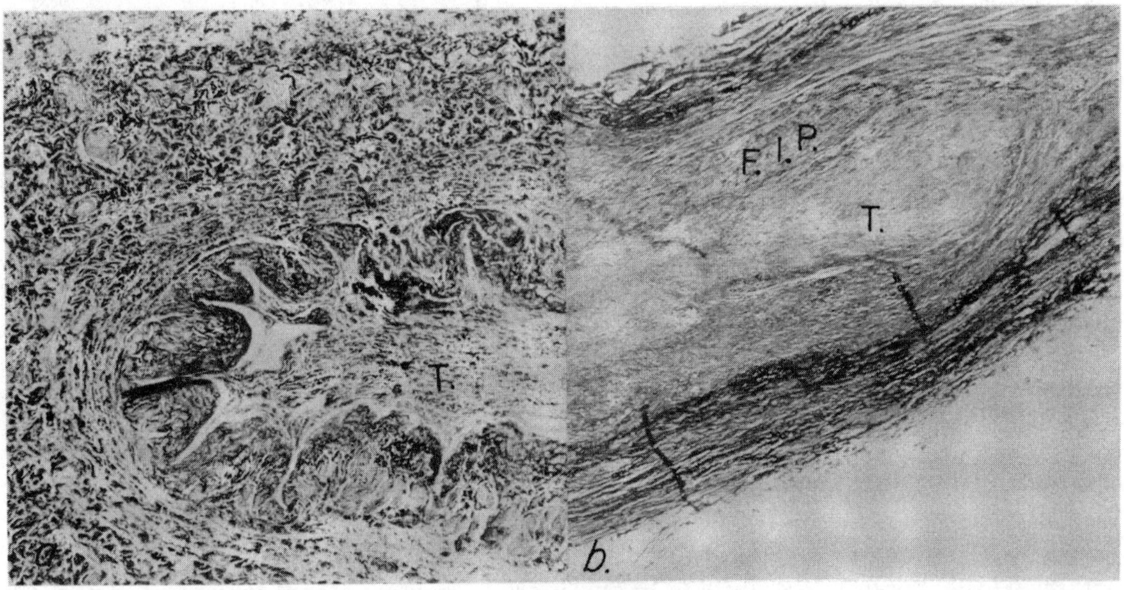

Figure 3

(a.) *Case 5b, with graft in place for 7 months. The lumen is occluded by an organized thrombus* (T.). *(Elastic tissue stain, × 57.)* **(b.)** *Case 1, with graft in place for 3½ months. Longitudinal section of saphenous vein graft. The intima shows fibrous proliferation* (F.I.P.). *In addition, luminal occlusion results from a superimposed organized thrombus* (T.). *(Elastic tissue stain, × 25.)*

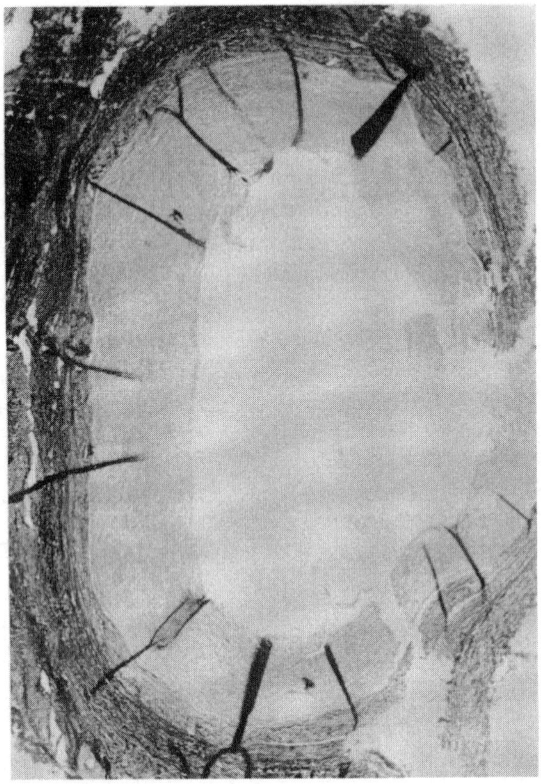

Figure 4

Case 5a, with graft in place for 7 months. Saphenous vein graft shows a zone of distinct intimal fibrous proliferation resulting in only moderate obstruction of the lumen. (Elastic tissue stain, × 22.)

intimal fibrous proliferation. The narrow remaining lumen was entirely compromised by an organizing thrombus (fig. 8*b*). The latter was continuous with a recent thrombus in the coronary artery.

Fibrous intimal proliferation was characterized by thickening of the intima with fibroplastic cells (fig. 9*a* and *b*) lying in a basophilic, mucoid matrix. Foamlike cells surrounded the lumen. With stains for fat, negative reactions were obtained. With stains for acid mucopolysaccharides, the mucoid matrix gave a strongly positive reaction (fig. 9*c*). Blood vessels were either absent or few in number. Blood pigment was absent. The fibrous thickening was usually pure, although in one case the process was complex (case 4). This showed a basal layer of fibrous intimal thickening, an intermediate layer of organized

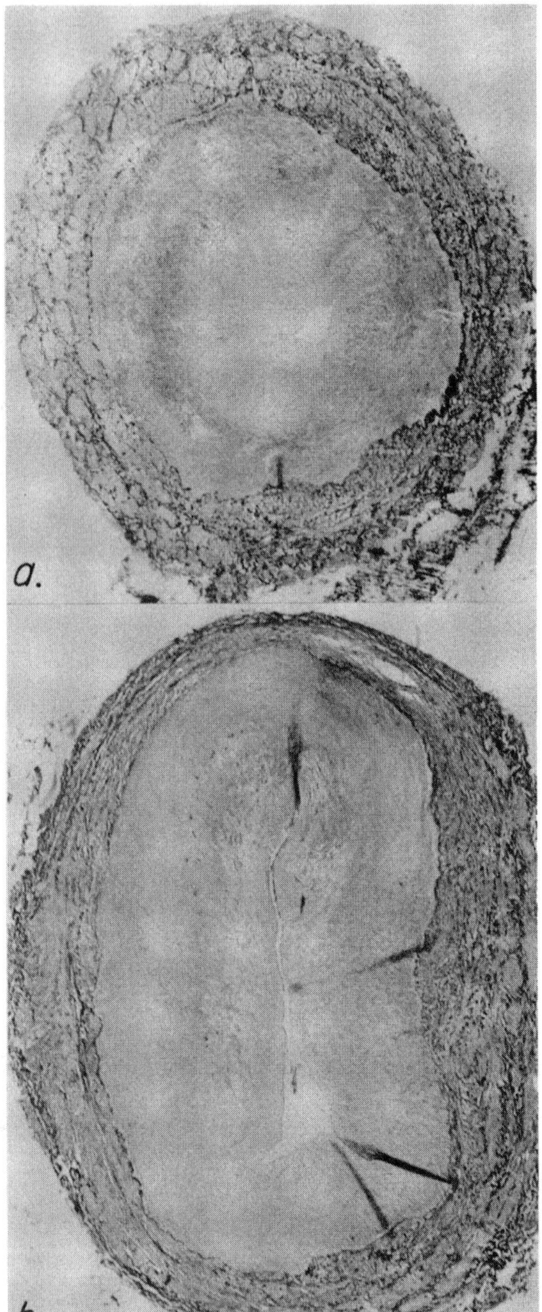

Figure 5

Two cases in which intimal fibrous proliferation of the saphenous vein graft caused severe obstruction of the lumen. **(a.)** *Case 6, with graft in place for 9 months. (Elastic tissue stain, × 14.)* **(b.)** *Case 3, with graft in place for 4½ months. Section through proximal half of graft. The distal half shows the remaining lumen occluded by an organizing thrombus. (Elastic tissue stain, × 15.)*

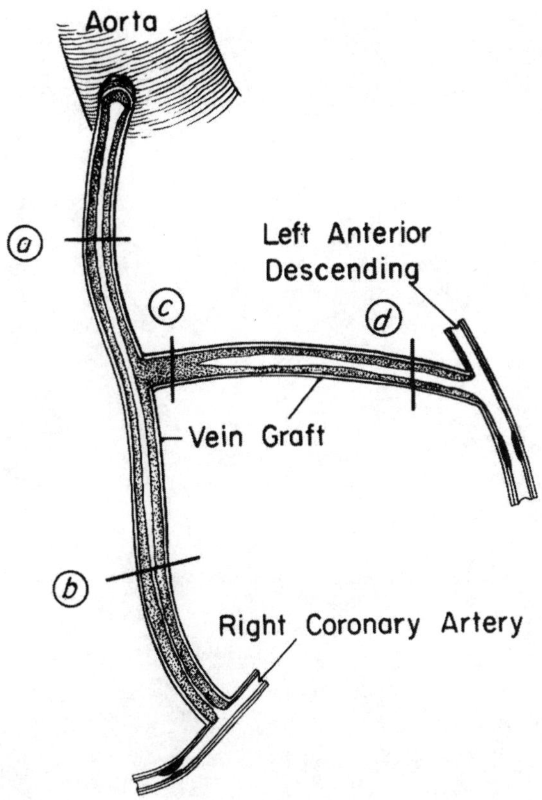

Figure 6

Case 2. Diagrammatic portrayal of the vein grafts employed. That running from the aorta directly to the right coronary artery is designated as case 2a, while that from the graft to the anterior descending artery is 2b. Letters shown on graft correspond to the levels of section shown in figure 7.

thrombosis, and a superficial layer of intimal fibrous thickening. In two cases, superficial thrombosis, either recent or organizing, was present on the surface of the thickened intima (fig. 9*d*). No significant alterations in the media were recognized in any of the grafts.

Since severely obstructive lesions, either thrombotic or proliferative, were common in group IV, it was of interest to determine whether obstructive atherosclerosis was present in the related arteries distal to the insertion of the graft. This opportunity was afforded us in the case of seven grafts. In five of the seven instances, obstructive atherosclerosis of severe degree (grade III) was found in the artery distal to the graft.

Such arterial lesions were found in each of the two cases with organized thrombi and in three cases with obstructive intimal fibrous proliferation. In one of the cases with organized thrombi (case 5b) an additional factor was a narrow aortic ostium of the graft. In one of the two exceptions, in which the artery was devoid to significant obstruction distal to the anastomosis, the graft showed only moderate degrees of intimal fibrous proliferation (case 5a), while in the other (case 2b) occlusion of a right-angled graft by intimal proliferation was observed.

Comment

This study on saphenous veins used as aortocoronary arterial communications revealed significantly obstructive lesion in the grafts to be common among grafts in place 3½ months or longer. It is to be admitted that the material is selected only from patients who failed to survive and, in this way, may not be entirely representative of all patients with such grafts in place. Nevertheless, the lesions observed have reasonable explanations.

It will be recalled that, in two of the eight long-range grafts, the lumen was occluded by organized thrombi. In each of these, significant atherosclerosis was present beyond the site of graft to the coronary artery. The latter phenomenon may explain thrombosis on the basis of restricted flow through the graft. The phenomenon of thrombosis may perhaps not be a natural phenomenon if the anastomosis is made beyond obstructive arterial lesions. An additional factor favoring thrombosis may be a narrow aortic ostium of the graft, as observed in one of our cases. The problem of thrombosis, therefore, appears mainly to be one in identifying unobstructed segments in the coronary arteries.

The second lesion observed was more common, being seen in six of the eight long-range grafts. This lesion is characterized by intimal thickening with avascular highly cellular connective tissue, a lesion which we have chosen to call *intimal fibrous proliferation.* Similar lesions in saphenous vein aortocoronary arterial grafts have been described recently by Johnson and associates[8] and by Grondin and associates.[9]

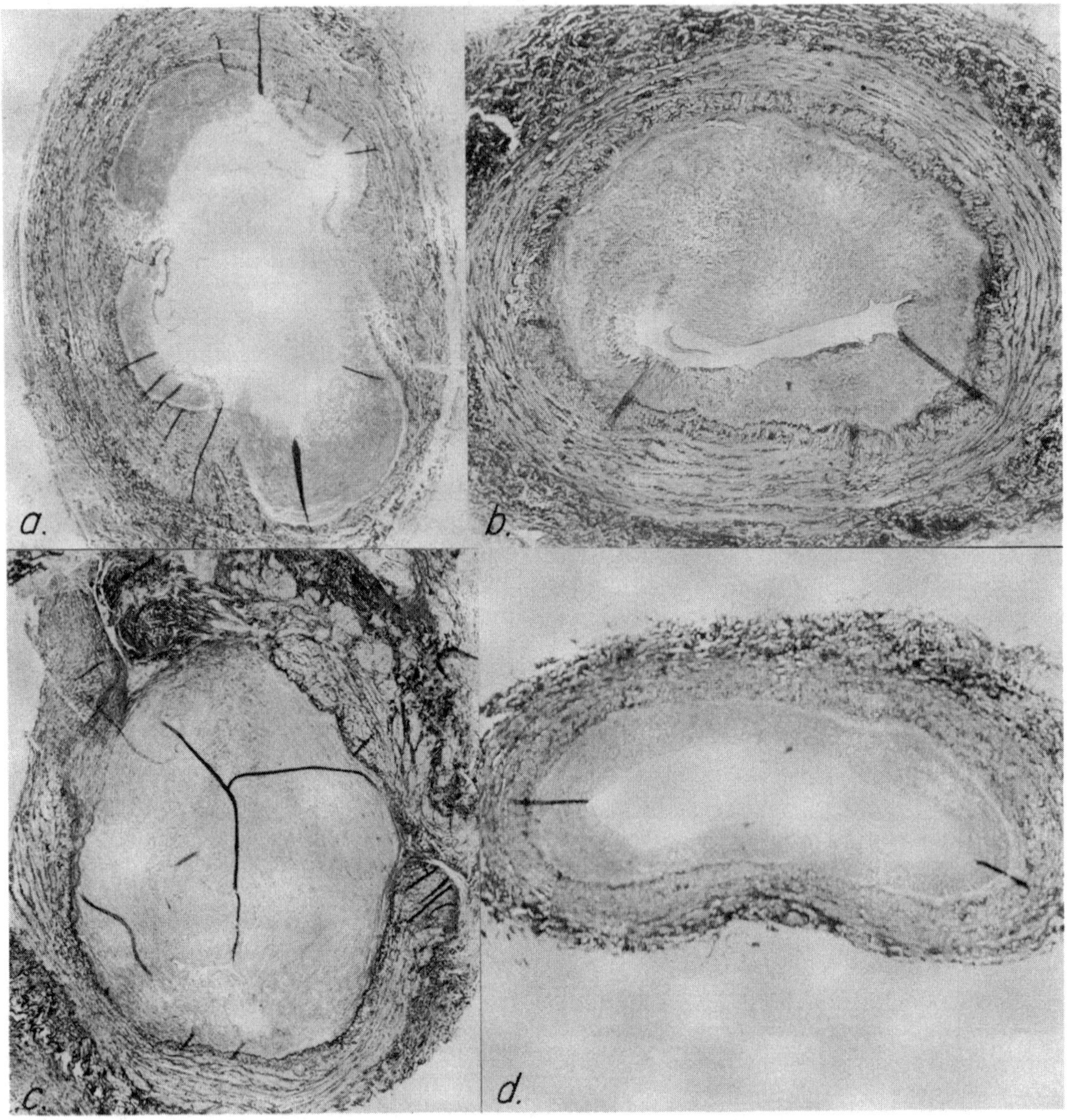

Figure 7

Case 2, with graft in place for 3½ months. Photomicrographs of cross sections of saphenous grafts. Levels of section correspond to letters shown in figure 6. **(a.)** *Vertical segment of "T"-shaped graft. Its proximal segment shows mild to moderate degrees of intimal fibrous proliferation. (Elastic tissue stain, × 13.)* **(b.)** *Distal segment of vertical graft shows severe intimal fibrous proliferation with corresponding severe luminal narrowing. (Elastic tissue stain, × 21.)* **(c.)** *Proximal portion of horizontal segment of "T"-shaped graft showing complete occlusion of lumen. (Elastic tissue stain, × 15.)* **(d.)** *Distal portion of horizontal segment of "T"-shaped graft showing mild to minimal intimal fibrous proliferation. (Elastic tissue stain, × 22.)*

The intimal fibrous proliferative lesion appears to be a natural consequence of subjecting a vein to arterial pressure. Similar lesions are present in veins associated with arteriovenous fistulae. Such lesions have been used to support the concept of "arterializa-

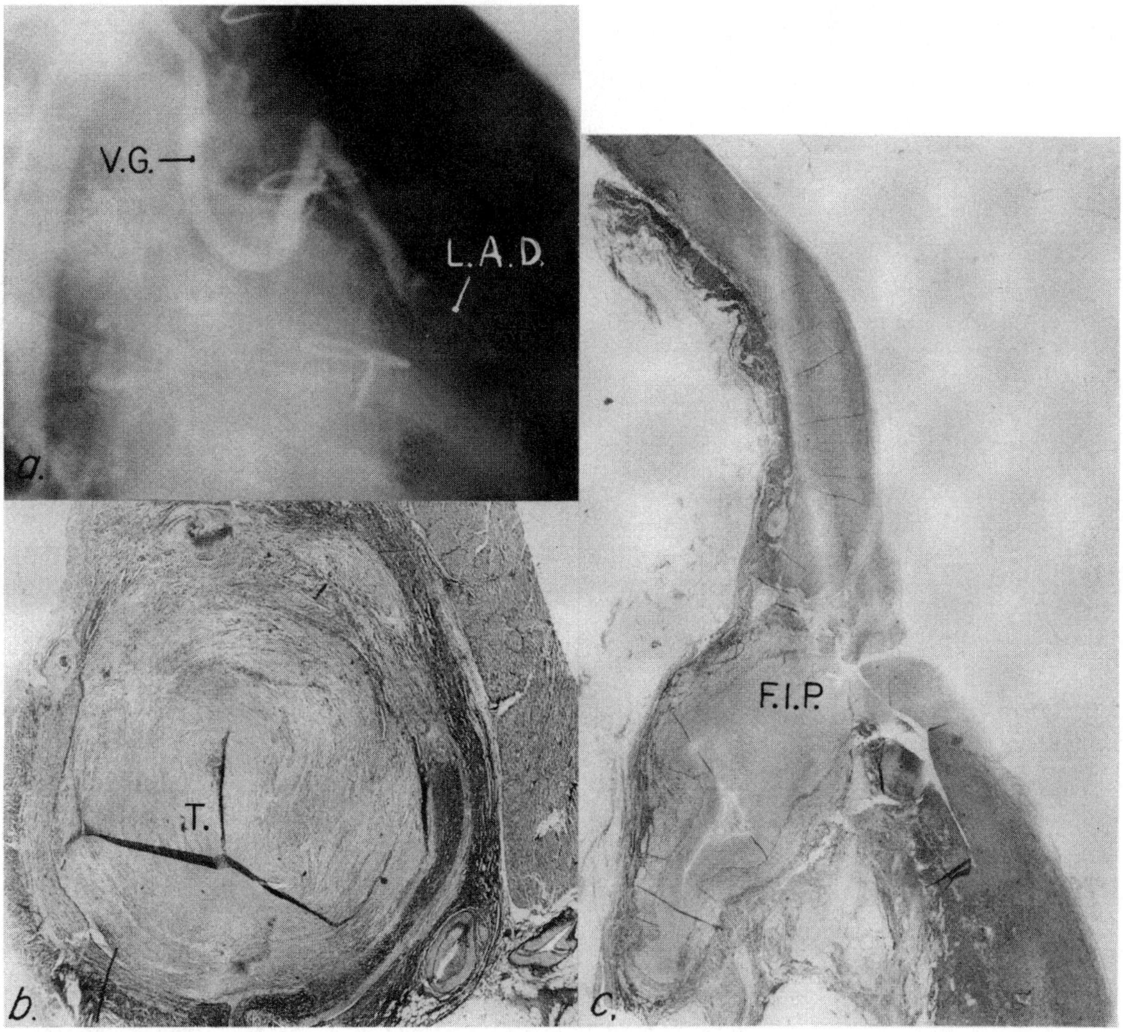

Figure 8

Case 3, with graft in place for 4½ months. **(a.)** *Angiogram made 3½ months after insertion of graft between aorta and anterior descending coronary artery* (L.A.D.) *Patency of the graft* (V.G.) *is indicated.* **(b.** *and* **c.)** *Photomicrographs of graft taken at the time of death about 3 weeks after the angiogram shown in* **a. (b.)** *Segment of the saphenous vein graft showing almost complete occlusion of the lumen by intimal fibrous proliferation. The narrowed lumen shows complete occlusion by a small amount of organizing thrombotic material* (T.). **(c.)** *Longitudinal section through aorta and anastomosis with vein. The latter shows severe intimal proliferation* (F.I.P.) *including involvement of the aortic ostium. (Elastic tissue stain,* × *4.)*

tion" of veins. We prefer not to use this term, since the venous structure of the media remains essentially unchanged and normal arteries do not show an intimal structure comparable to the intimal proliferative changes in veins. Rather, we would consider the intimal fibrous proliferation of veins subjected to arterial pressure as a reparative phenomenon responding to unusual hemodynamic stress. It is appropriate to consider factors which, in addition to the arterial pressure in the graft, may favor the development of the intimal fibrous lesion.

Among the five grafts with intimal fibrous proliferation and in which the nature of the coronary artery beyond the graft was known,

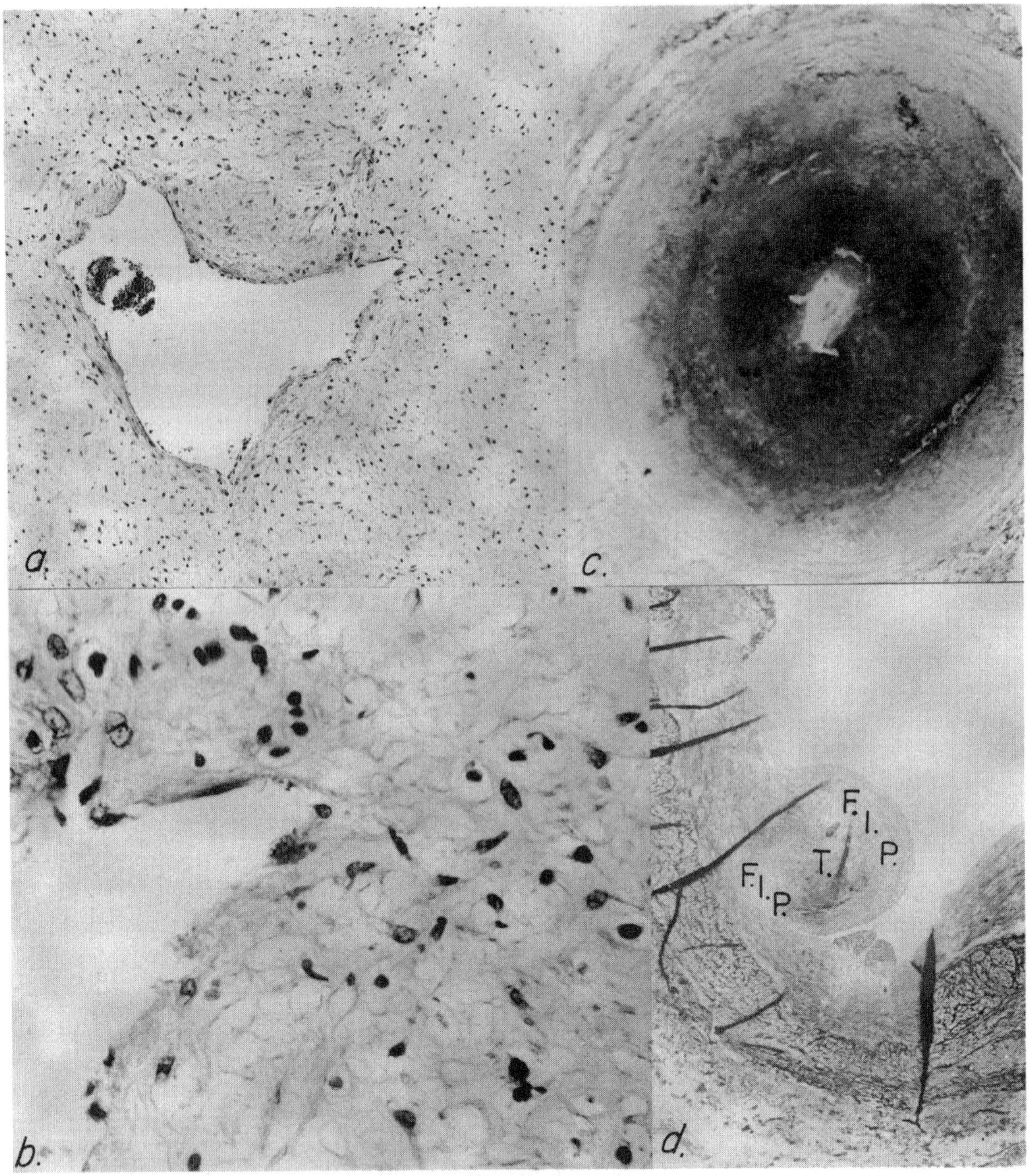

Figure 9

Characteristics of fibrous intimal proliferation. **(a.)** *Surrounding a narrowed lumen, intimal fibrous proliferation is characterized by the presence of fibroblastic cells lying in a basophilic matrix. (Hematoxylin and eosin, × 80.)* **(b.)** *High-power magnification of intimal fibrous proliferation in relation to the lumen. Large cells with clear cytoplasm are present. These stain negatively for fat. (Hematoxylin and eosin, × 400.)* **(c.)** *Severe thickening of the intima by intimal fibrous proliferation showing heavily positive reaction for acid mucopolysaccharides. (Acid mucopolysaccharide stain, × 20.)* **(d.)** *Encasement of organized thrombotic material within intimal fibrous proliferation. In a longitudinal section of the vein the organized thrombotic material* (T.) *lies superimposed on a zone of intimal fibrous proliferation* (F.I.P.) *and secondarily capped by similar tissue. (Elastic tissue stain, × 24.)*

the venous lesion was severe in three cases with distal severely obstructive atherosclerosis. In two grafts, the arterial lesion was only moderate in degree. Obstructive atherosclerosis beyond the level of anastomosis may have represented the basis for additional mechanical stress to the graft in the form of a water-hammer effect.

In the case of two grafts, the artery beyond the site of anastomosis showed only grade II atherosclerosis. In one of these, the graft had been in place for 7 months and the intimal lesion was only moderate in extent. The case may support the water-hammer concept as being in effect when obstructive atherosclerosis is present downstream from the graft.

In the second case without significantly obstructive atherosclerosis beyond the graft (anterior descending artery), complete occlusion of the graft was present near the right-angle anastomosis of the graft to a vertical graft running between the aorta and the right coronary artery. This case may perhaps represent the phenomenon that at right-angled branching there are mechanical stresses peculiar to this phenomenon.

The nature of the intimal fibrous proliferative lesions suggests that it is made up of young connective tissue. The presence of tissue rich in fibroblasts and in acid mucopolysaccharides may support this concept. That the proliferative lesion may progress rapidly is supported by one of our cases (case 3). In this case, it will be recalled, the graft was demonstrated to be widely patent 3½ months after being in place, while 3 weeks later, at the time of death, pathologic examination showed severe restriction in the caliber of the lumen of the graft by the proliferative lesion. In this case, although an organizing thrombus occluded the remaining lumen, the lumen had been severely narrowed by the proliferative lesion.

References

1. FAVALORO RG: Saphenous vein graft in the surgical treatment of coronary artery disease: Operative technique. J Thorac Cardiovasc Surg **58**: 178, 1969
2. JOHNSON WD, LEPLEY D JR: An aggressive surgical approach to coronary disease. J Thorac Cardiovasc Surg **59**: 128, 1970
3. SPENCER FC: Venous bypass grafts for occlusive disease of the coronary arteries. Amer Heart J **79**: 568, 1970
4. MITCHEL BF, ADAM M, LAMBERT CJ, SUNGU U, SHIEKH S: Ascending aorta-to-coronary artery saphenous vein bypass grafts. J Thorac Cardiovasc Surg **60**: 457, 1970
5. FAVALORO RG, EFFLER DB, GROVES LK, SHELDON WC, SHIREY EK, SONES FM JR: Severe segmental obstruction of the left main coronary artery and its divisions. J Thorac Cardiovasc Surg **60**: 469, 1970
6. ROBINSON G, KAPLITT MJ, PHILIPS P, PATEL B: Complete surgical correction of the totally occluded and diffusely diseased right coronary artery. J Thorac Cardiovasc Surg **60**: 504, 1970
7. JOHNSON WD, FLEMMA RJ, LEPLEY D JR: Determinants of blood flow in aortic-coronary saphenous vein bypass grafts. Arch Surg **101**: 806, 1970
8. JOHNSON WD, AUER JE, TECTOR AJ: Late changes in coronary vein grafts. (Abstr) Amer J Cardiol **26**: 640, 1970
9. GRONDIN CM, MEERE C, CASTONGUAY Y, LEPAGE G, GRONDIN P: Progressive and late obstruction of an aorto-coronary venous bypass graft: A case report. Circulation **43**: 698, 1971

Pathologic Changes in Aortic-Coronary Arterial Saphenous Vein Grafts

Zeev Vlodaver, M.D.

In the early 1970s, the popular use of surgical treatment for obstructive coronary artery disease with a bypassing graft stimulated many clinical reports. The mortality at operation, incidence of patency of grafts, flow rates and clinical manifestations after operation were commonly described.

What was missing, and in our minds was of considerable practical importance, were pathologic studies on long-term character of the vein graft, and determination of the nature of the graft system (both in the graft and the artery distal to the graft), the nature of the non-grafted arteries, the state of the myocardium, and the relation of these observations to various postoperative clinical manifestations.

Our findings published in this and subsequent articles demonstrated that the pathology of saphenous vein bypass grafts was related to both early and late complications, and consisted of three main changes: fibrous intimal proliferation, thrombosis and atherosclerosis. Early vein graft occlusion, within one month after operation, is usually caused by thrombosis. The thrombus organizes and causes total graft occlusion. Virtually all vein bypass grafts have some intimal thickening from fibrous proliferation composed of fibroblasts and smooth muscle cells in an extracellular matrix. These changes can be seen as early as one month postoperatively. It may also progress to nearly total graft occlusion.

The pathogenesis of fibrointimal proliferation in vein grafts is unknown, but probably relates to reparative processes after vein ischemia or hemodynamic stresses causing endothelial damage. This may be accelerated by systemic hypertension. More importantly, fibrointimal proliferation promotes the foundation for graft atherosclerosis.

We have observed similar changes following coronary artery cannulation and in segments of coronary arteries in which endoarterectomy had been performed. Because of the occlusion of grafts and changes in coronary arteries in other procedures by proliferative tissue, this has prompted the use of the internal mammary arteries as bypass vessels. An increased patency rate following bypass surgery has resulted.

In the arena of the bypass operation for coronary disease, one factor that is controllable to a certain extent is the manner in which the potential graft is handled. That was emphasized thirty years ago and is still an important consideration.

New "no touch" technique of harvesting the saphenous vein for coronary bypass surgery appears promising in increasing the rate of patency of vein grafts following bypass surgery.

Our studies of fatal cases after coronary bypass surgery in the early days demonstrated that while occlusive disease may develop in long range grafts, the major problem responsible for death of the patients we studied was residual atherosclerotic disease. In some instances the location of the lesion precluded an effective bypass procedure, according to the current practice. Perhaps a more important factor contributing to death was residual obstructed segments which, if identified, might have been bypassed. In all probability, that latter point has been recognized in subsequent years. Surgeons are now more likely to insert multiple grafts than in the earlier years of bypass surgery. A low morbidity and mortality has resulted following this procedure.

In my near decade of working with Jesse, I will always remember the uniquely delicate manner in which he handled and described each specimen. Jesse would always emphasize that "We owe full respect to the deceased patient and his family."

All of us who worked with Jesse became better physicians because of his extraordinary passion for teaching and learning. Furthermore, we also became better individuals because of his extraordinary humanity, compassion and humility.

Ventricular Septal Rupture Complicating Acute Myocardial Infarction: Identification of Simple and Complex Types in 53 Autopsied Hearts

BROOKS S. EDWARDS, MD, WILLIAM D. EDWARDS, MD, and JESSE E. EDWARDS, MD

Fifty-three hearts with rupture of the ventricular septum complicating acute myocardial infarction (AMI) were studied. Thirty-three of the hearts were from men (average age 76 years) and 20 were from women (average age 73 years). The study showed 2 types of rupture of the ventricular septum: *simple* (28 patients) and *complex* (25 patients). Simple ruptures were direct through-and-through defects. Complex ruptures were associated with serpiginous dissection tracts remote from the primary site of tear of the ventricular septum. Specimens were classified as to the location of the underlying AMI and the level of the septum (apex to base) at which the rupture occurred. Twenty-nine hearts had an inferior AMI and 24 an anterior AMI. Complex ruptures occurred in 20 of the inferior AMIs (69%) and in 5 of the anterior AMIs (21%) ($p < 0.001$). Ruptures that involved the inferobasal portion of the septum were much more likely to be complex (94%) than ruptures in all other locations (27%, $p < 0.001$). Significant 3-vessel obstructive coronary arterial atherosclerosis was present in 48 hearts. Rupture of a second structure in addition to the ventricular septum was observed in 11 hearts (left ventricular free wall in 9 cases and papillary muscle in 2). The interval from the onset of the AMI to rupture of the septum could be estimated in 22 patients and averaged 4 days (median 2.5 days). Complete heart block reportedly occurred in 6 patients during hospitalization. **(Am J Cardiol 1984;54:1201–1205)**

Rupture of the ventricular septum is a recognized serious complication of acute myocardial infarction (AMI). Among cases of ruptured ventricular septum, the pathologic state of the ventricular septum varies widely. Consequently, we performed a pilot study from which 2 types of ruptured septum complicating AMI could be identified: *simple* and *complex*. This study was undertaken to determine whether, in cases of AMI with complicating septal rupture, there are features that favor the occurrence of the simple or complex types.

Definitions

A *simple* rupture of the ventricular septum is defined as a direct, through-and-through opening connecting the 2 ventricular chambers (Fig. 1 and 2). Neither gross hemorrhage nor laceration are present in the tissues around the septal defect. The left and right ventricular openings are at about the same horizontal level of the ventricular septum.

A *complex* rupture of the ventricular septum is defined as an interventricular communication that ascribes an undulating or serpiginous course (Fig. 3 to 5). The tract may extend, in part, into regions remote from the site of the primary AMI. Branching zones with disruption of myocardial tissue and hemorrhage occur. Frequently, the openings into the 2 ventricles are at different planes of the ventricular septum.

Methods

Fifty-three autopsy specimens of the heart with rupture of the ventricular septum complicating AMI were obtained from 2 sources: 35 were collected from the Cardiovascular Registry of United Hospitals, and 18 were obtained from the Tissue Registry of the Mayo Clinic. Some cases were included in earlier reports.[1–4] Surgical repair had been performed in 13 of the 53 patients.

Each specimen was examined grossly and histologically. As part of the gross examination, the rupture of the ventricular septum was classified as either simple or complex according to the definitions given herein. In a few cases the nature of the rupture of the ventricular septum tended to be intermediate between the 2 types defined. In such cases, agreement as to definition had to be obtained from at least 2 of the investigators. For each case, in order to categorize the location of the septal rupture, the ventricles were divided into 5 cross-sec-

From the Departments of Pathology, United Hospitals, St. Paul, and the University of Minnesota, Minneapolis, and the Department of Pathology, Mayo Clinic and Foundation, Rochester, Minnesota. This study was supported by Research Grant 5 RO1 HL05694 from the National Heart, Lung, and Blood Institute, Bethesda, Maryland. Manuscript received April 11, 1984; revised manuscript received June 8, 1984, accepted June 11, 1984.

Address for reprints: Jesse E. Edwards, MD, Department of Pathology, United Hospitals, 333 North Smith Avenue, St. Paul, Minnesota 55102.

December 1, 1984 THE AMERICAN JOURNAL OF CARDIOLOGY Volume 54 1203

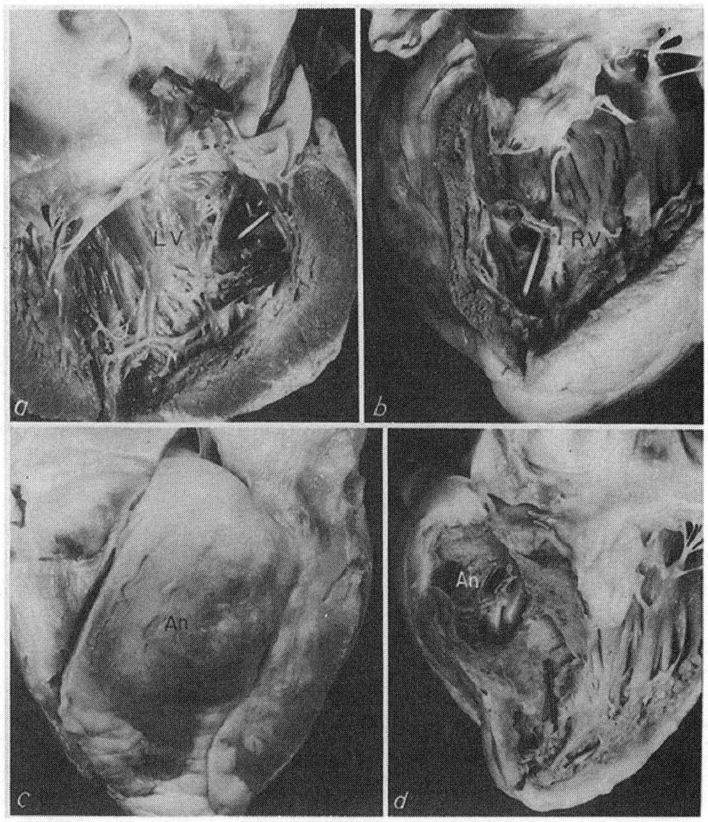

FIGURE 4. A complex type of septal rupture with an associated aneurysm of the ventricular septum from a 66-year-old woman in whom a history of acute myocardial infarction had not been obtained, but in whom the age of the acute myocardial infarction at the time of autopsy was estimated to be 1 month. **a,** interior of left atrium and left ventricle (LV). The posteromedial papillary muscle of the mitral valve has been divided and reflected upward to expose the inferior basal aspect of the left ventricle and a rupture of the ventricular septum (**probe**). **b,** interior of right ventricle (RV). The rupture tract of the ventricular septum contains a probe. The right ventricular opening is in a more apical position than the left ventricular opening. **c,** external view of inferior aspect of heart reveals the left ventricular aneurysm (An). **d,** interior of the right atrium and right ventricle after a sagittal section has been made through the posterior aspect of the ventricular septum to show the aneurysm involving the basal inferior portion of the ventricular septum. The aneurysm had communicated with the left ventricle through the septal rupture and leads by way of a septal tract (containing black probe) into the apical part of the right ventricular cavity.

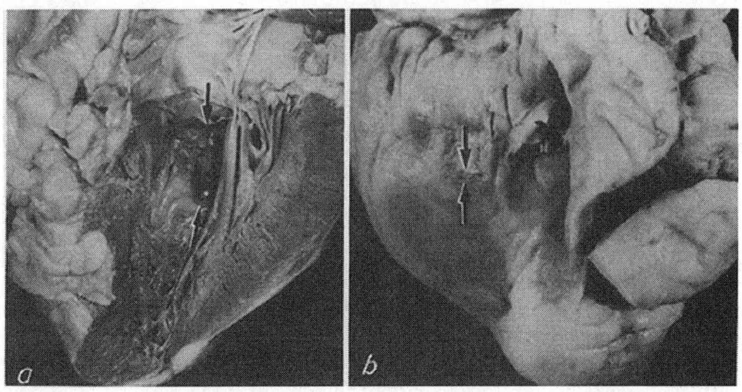

FIGURE 5. A complex septal rupture associated with rupture of the left ventricular free wall from a 68-year-old woman in whom the estimated age of the index acute myocardial infarction was 10 to 12 days. **a,** the interior of the left ventricle. The site of the septal tear (**probe and between arrows**) is in the inferior basal portion of the ventricular septum near the posteromedial papillary muscle. **b,** external view of the inferior aspect of the ventricles. A laceration of the epicardium (**between arrows**) represents the site of associated rupture of the left ventricular free wall.

classified as simple in 28 (53%) and complex in 25 (47%). Of the 29 cases of inferior AMI, the septal rupture was complex in 20 (69% of all inferior AMIs). In the group of 24 patients with anterior AMI, only 5 complex ruptures (21% of anterior AMIs) were identified (Fig. 6). The differences in the frequency of complex ruptures between anterior and inferior AMI was statistically significant ($p < 0.001$).

Among the 28 cases of simple rupture, inferior AMI was observed in 9 (32%) and anterior AMI in 19 (68%). In contrast, within the group of 25 cases of complex rupture, inferior AMI was observed in 20 (80%) and anterior AMI in 5 (20%).

An alternative approach was to categorize septal ruptures according to site of primary tear, dividing the ventricles into apical (slices 1 to 3) and basal (slices 4 to 5) segments. When this was done, septal ruptures could be classified as simple or complex for each region of the septum at which the primary tear occurred. In cases in which the rupture included multiple levels, for this analysis, the most basal level was designated as the 1 in which the primary tear occurred. By this approach, 27% of ruptures occurring in the apical half of the septum were complex, whereas 80% of basal ruptures were complex ($p < 0.001$). Going from apex to base, there is an increasing trend toward complexity of rupture (Fig.

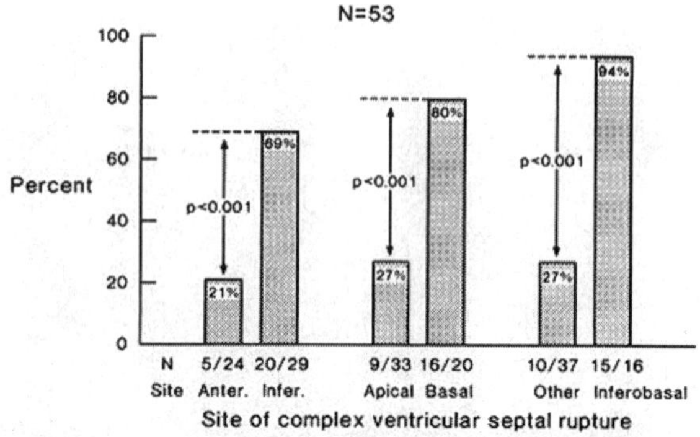

FIGURE 6. The frequencies of complex ventricular septal ruptures among (**left**) anterior (Anter.) and inferior (Infer.) infarctions, (**center**) apical and basal ruptures, and (**right**) inferobasal ruptures compared with all others.

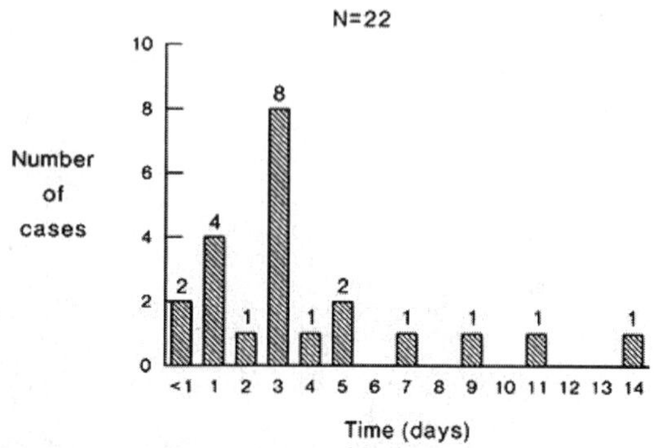

FIGURE 8. Estimation of time interval between onset of acute myocardial infarction and rupture of ventricular septum in 22 patients (mean interval 4 days, median 2.5).

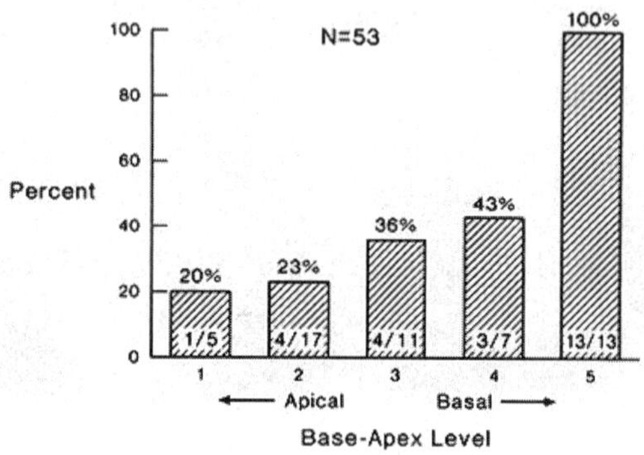

FIGURE 7. Frequency of complex ventricular septal ruptures occurring at each level of the ventricle from apex (slice 1) to base (slice 5).

7). The most basal level (slice 5) showed the greatest incidence of complex ruptures. All of the 13 ruptures identified as occurring at slice 5 were complex.

Although the complex tears varied considerably in appearance and extent (one from the other), certain characteristics were common among them (Fig. 3 to 5). Ruptures that started in the basal aspect of the inferior part of the septum were more extensive than ruptures that originated in the anterior and apical sites. Basal ruptures were accompanied by extensive hemorrhage into the neighboring tissue, the hemorrhage frequently extending to the epicardium at the level of the crux or over the atria and including the atrial walls. In some cases a tract extended into the inferior right ventricular free wall from which a rupture into the right ventricular cavity was observed.

Rupture of a second structure, in addition to that of the ventricular septum, occurred in 11 cases—9 had involvement of the left ventricular free wall and 2, a papillary muscle (1 mitral and 1 tricuspid). Among the 9 patients with rupture of the left ventricular free wall, 7 had inferior AMI (all with complex ventricular septal ruptures) and 2 demonstrated anterior AMI (1 case each of simple and complex rupture).

The average cardiac weight was 514 g for men and 430 g for women. Twenty-four of 33 men (73%) and 10 of 20 women (50%) had a cardiac weight over 450 g and 400 g, respectively. In none of the patients was there significant valvular disease to account for cardiomegaly, and thus, the most likely explanation for the cardiomegaly was chronic hypertension.

The histologic age of AMI correlated well with the available clinical history in all but 8 cases. In 7 of these 8, the AMI was distinctly older histologically than clinically. In the eighth case, the clinical history included an AMI that was older than it appeared to be histologically. Based on available clinical histories and histologic examination, the interval between the onset of AMI and septal rupture could be estimated in 22 of the 53 cases. The average time was 4 days (range 12 hours to 14 days) (Fig. 8). The median time was 2.5 days. Four patients had never sought medical attention and died unexpectedly.

Forty-eight of the 53 cases in this study showed atherosclerosis that caused a reduction in the luminal cross-sectional area of 75% or more in each of the 3 coronary arteries. In 5 specimens, 2-vessel disease of the same degree was found. No cases of 1-vessel disease were found. An acute or organizing thrombus was present in the vessel that supplied the region of infarcted myocardium in 21 of the cases (40%).

In 6 patients, complete heart block had occurred during the hospitalization. Five of these 6 had inferior AMI (4 with complex and 1 with simple ventricular septal rupture) and 1 patient had an anterior AMI and a simple ventricular septal rupture.

Discussion

In this study, 53 specimens with rupture of the ventricular septum after AMI were analyzed pathologically.

In some cases, the septal rupture was of the simple type, whereas in others the rupture was considered to be of the complex type. The simple type of rupture is defined as a direct through-and-through communication between the ventricles without associated major hemorrhagic tracts or laceration of surrounding tissue.

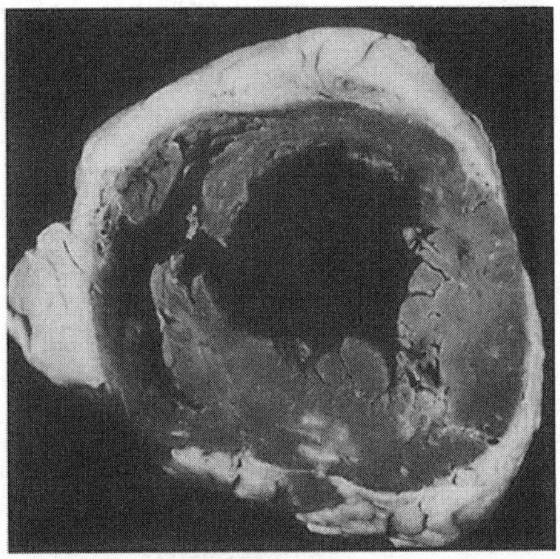

FIGURE 1. Cross section, viewed from the apex, of the ventricular portion of the heart. A simple type rupture of the ventricular septum at the level of slice 3 is apparent. The patient had sustained an acute anteroseptal myocardial infarction 10 days before death. Scars of old inferior acute myocardial infarction are also present.

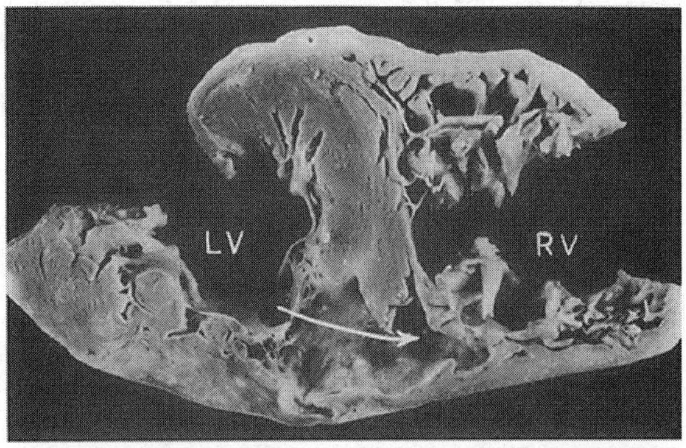

FIGURE 2. The only case of a simple type of ventricular septal rupture involving level 4 of the ventricles. Cross section of ventricular portion of heart after the ventricles have been opened. Specimen viewed from above. In the inferior basal aspect an endothelialized tract (**arrow**) directly connects the 2 ventricles. Histologically, the acute myocardial infarction was approximately 4 weeks old. LV = left ventricle; RV = right ventricle.

tional levels or slices, of which the apex was designated as slice 1 and the base as slice 5. Additionally, the ventricular septum was separated into 3 equal portions for each level of section: anterior, mid and posterior (inferior). The location of the septal rupture was determined from both the left and right ventricular aspects. Additional observations made grossly included determination of the location of the underlying AMI, cardiac weight and degree and distribution of coronary arterial disease.

Tissues from each specimen were examined histologically. The age and location of the underlying AMI were determined, initially without knowledge of the clinical data, and then correlated with the clinical history.

Clinical data were collected when available. Because of the referral nature of the collections from which the specimens were obtained, some cases were accompanied by complete clinical records, whereas in others the clinical history was incomplete.

Results

Among the patients constituting the 53 cases of ventricular septal rupture, there were 33 men and 20 women. The ages were known in all except 1 of the men. The average age among the men was 67 years (range 40 to 84) and among the women, 73 years (range 63 to 88).

In each case the underlying AMI was transmural. The index AMI was inferior in 29 cases (19 men and 10 women) and anterior in 24 (14 men and 10 women). Among the 53 cases in this study, the septal rupture was

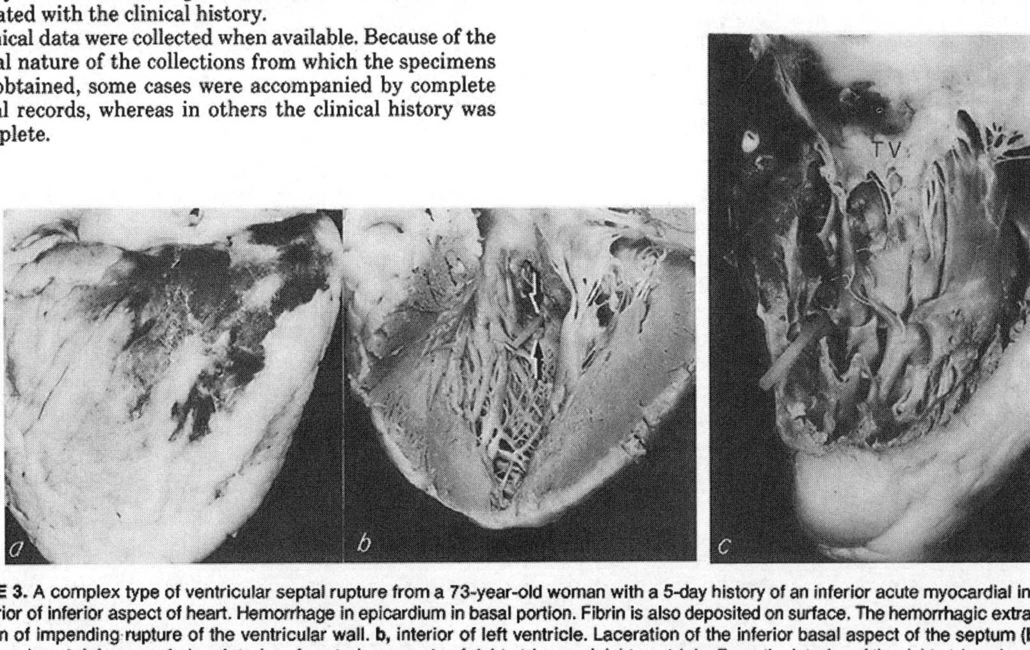

FIGURE 3. A complex type of ventricular septal rupture from a 73-year-old woman with a 5-day history of an inferior acute myocardial infarction. **a,** exterior of inferior aspect of heart. Hemorrhage in epicardium in basal portion. Fibrin is also deposited on surface. The hemorrhagic extravasation is a sign of impending rupture of the ventricular wall. **b,** interior of left ventricle. Laceration of the inferior basal aspect of the septum (**between arrows and containing a probe**). **c,** interior of posterior aspects of right atrium and right ventricle. From the interior of the right atrium, hemorrhage has apparently extended into the lowermost part of the atrial septum. Hemorrhage has also extended to the epicardium over the basal aspect of the right ventricle. An extensive laceration is present in the most posterior part of the ventricular septum and runs from a subtricuspid position approximately two-thirds of the distance to the apex. Lowermost part of laceration contains a probe. TV = tricuspid valve.

December 1, 1984 THE AMERICAN JOURNAL OF CARDIOLOGY Volume 54 1205

The complex type was characterized by the presence of hemorrhagic tracts with myocardial disruption that extended beyond the primary laceration of the ventricular septum, and the communication between the ventricles frequently ascribed an undulating course so that the openings into the 2 ventricles might be at different levels of the ventricular septum.

Simple and complex ruptures were about equally distributed (simple 53% and complex 47%). Predictors for a simple type of rupture were anterior AMI or inferoapical AMI. Complex ruptures most often occurred in the setting of inferior AMI, particularly in the inferobasal position.

Published surgical studies on the treatment of ventricular septal ruptures have reported that when the underlying AMI is inferior the mortality rate is higher than when the underlying AMI is anterior.[5-11] The complex type of rupture, as defined, poses greater challenges to surgical repair than does the simple type of rupture. Ruptures complicating inferior AMI tend to be complex, yielding greater surgicoanatomic challenges, and thus may explain the poorer surgical outcome for ruptures that complicate inferior AMI than those that complicate anterior AMI.

Beyond identification of simple and complex types of rupture, this study revealed other information on rupture of the ventricular septum as a complication of AMI. The interval from the onset of AMI to ventricular septal rupture could be estimated in 22 patients. The period averaged 4.0 days (range 0.5 and 14, median 2.5). This time frame is similar to that observed for rupture of the free wall of the left ventricle[3] and is slightly shorter than that reported for rupture of a papillary muscle.[12] In our study, when there was a discrepancy between the clinical age of the AMI and the histologic age, in most cases the histologic age was older. In this group of patients, tearing of the septum may have caused them to seek medical attention, and the underlying AMI may have been initially "silent," a phenomenon similar to that observed in earlier studies.[3]

Complete heart block was found in the hearts from 6 patients in this study, 5 of which had underlying inferior AMI. The occurrence of atrioventricular conduction disturbance among patients with septal ruptures has been previously noted.[4,13] In our study, among the 5 cases with inferior AMI and complete heart block, 4 had complex septal rupture. The clinical combination of inferior AMI, complete heart block and rupture of the ventricular septum may provide a preoperative indication that the septal rupture is complex.

Based in part on angiographic studies, septal rupture has been reported to occur often in patients with 1-vessel coronary artery disease.[8,9,11,14-17] Among the specimens in our series, this was not the case. Eighty-eight percent of the specimens in this study showed significant 3-vessel obstructive coronary atherosclerosis. One explanation for this discrepancy may be the greater sensitivity for diagnosing obstructive atherosclerotic disease by autopsy than by angiography.[18] Alternatively, because ours is an autopsy series, some inherent bias may be present, because patients with less extensive coronary artery disease may be more likely to survive than those with more extensive disease.

Acknowledgment: We acknowledge with gratitude the assistance of Duane M. Ilstrup, Department of Medical Statistics and Epidemiology, Mayo Clinic, for the statistical analyses for this study.

References

1. **Chesler E, Korns ME, Semba T, Edwards JE.** False aneurysms of the left ventricle following myocardial infarction. Am J Cardiol 1969;23:76–82.
2. **Ersek RA, Chesler E, Korns ME, Edwards JE.** Spontaneous rupture of a false left ventricular aneurysm following myocardial infarction. Am Heart J 1969;77:677–680.
3. **Van Tassel RA, Edwards JE.** Rupture of heart complicating myocardial infarction. Analysis of 40 cases including nine examples of left ventricular false aneurysm. Chest 1972;61:104–116.
4. **Vlodaver Z, Edwards JE.** Rupture of ventricular septum or papillary muscle complicating myocardial infarction. Circulation 1977;55:815–822.
5. **Graham AF, Stinson EB, Daily PO, Harrison DC.** Ventricular septal defects after myocardial infarction. Early operative treatment. JAMA 1973;225: 708–711.
6. **Giuliani ER, Danielson GK, Pluth JR, Odyniec NA, Wallace RB.** Postinfarction ventricular septal rupture. Surgical considerations and results. Circulation 1974;49:455–459.
7. **Gaudiani VA, Miller DC, Stinson EB, Oyer PE, Reitz BA, Moreno-Cabral RJ, Shumway NE.** Postinfarction ventricular septal defect. Argument for early operation. Surgery 1981;89:48–55.
8. **Montoya A, McKeever L, Scanlon P, Sullivan HJ, Gunnar R, Pifarré R.** Early repair of ventricular septal rupture after infarction. Am J Cardiol 1980; 45:345–348.
9. **Killen DA, Reed WA, Wathanacharoen S, McCallister BD, Fell HH.** Postinfarction rupture of the interventricular septum. J Cardiovasc Surg 1981;22:113–126.
10. **Donahoo JS, Brawley RK, Taylor D, Gott VL.** Factors influencing survival following postinfarction ventricular septal defects. Ann Thorac Surg 1975;19:648–653.
11. **Buckley MJ, Mundth ED, Daggett WM, Gold HK, Leinbach RC, Austen WG.** Surgical management of ventricular septal defects and mitral regurgitation complicating acute myocardial infarction. Ann Thorac Surg 1973;16: 598–609.
12. **Nishimura RA, Schaff HV, Shub C, Gersh BJ, Edwards WD, Tajik AJ.** Papillary muscle rupture complicating acute myocardial infarction: analysis of 17 patients. Am J Cardiol 1983;51:373–377.
13. **James TN.** De Subitaneis Mortibus. XXIV. Ruptured interventricular septum and heart block. Circulation 1977;55:934–946.
14. **Radford MJ, Johnson RA, Daggett WM Jr, Fallon JT, Buckley MJ, Gold HK, Leinbach RC.** Ventricular septal rupture: a review of clinical and physiologic features and an analysis of survival. Circulation 1981;64: 545–555.
15. **Wessler S, Zoll PM, Schlesinger MJ.** The pathogenesis of spontaneous cardiac rupture. Circulation 1952;6:334–351.
16. **Roberts WC, Ronan JA Jr, Harvey WP.** Rupture of the left ventricular free wall (LVFW) or ventricular septum (VS) secondary to acute myocardial infarction (AMI): an occurrence virtually limited to the first transmural AMI in a hypertensive individual (abstr). Am J Cardiol 1975;35:166.
17. **Edmondson HA, Hoxie HJ.** Hypertension and cardiac rupture: a clinical and pathologic study of seventy-two cases, in thirteen of which rupture of the interventricular septum occurred. Am Heart J 1942;24:719–733.
18. **Vlodaver Z, Frech R, Van Tassel RA, Edwards JE.** Correlation of the antemortem coronary arteriogram and the postmortem specimen. Circulation 1973;47:162–169.

Reprinted from the December 1 issue of **The American Journal of Cardiology,** A Yorke Medical Journal, Published by Technical Publishing, a Division of Dun-Donnelley Publishing Corporation, a Company of The Dun & Bradstreet Corporation, 875 Third Avenue, New York, N.Y. 10022.
Copyright 1984. All rights reserved. Printed in the U.S.A.

Ventricular Septal Rupture Complicating Acute Myocardial Infarction:

Identification of Simple and Complex Types in 53 Autopsied Hearts

Robert F. Wilson, M.D.

In this paper, Edwards, Edwards and Edwards (!) examined the morphology of ventricular septal rupture complicating acute myocardial infarction. They divided post-infarction septal ruptures into simple and complex morphologies. Complex ruptures created serpiginous tears through the septum and more commonly started near the base of the heart. They found that inferior infarctions, particularly infero-basal infarctions, were associated much more commonly with a complex rupture. Moreover, complex ruptures were more often associated with extension into the right or left ventricular free-wall, and sometimes associated with rupture into the pericardium.

These observations helped shape our understanding of one of the most dreaded and lethal complications of acute myocardial infarction. Since this paper, we have learned that postinfarction septal ruptures are usually associated with complete occlusion of the infarct related artery, often in the setting of poor collateral blood supply to the myocardium supplied by the infarct-related artery. Much about the factors leading to postinfarction septal rupture, however, remains to be understood. For unclear reasons, compared to men, women have a 2.5 fold risk of postinfarction VSD, even when their older age at presentation is taken into account. Conversely, current smokers with an acute infarction have about half the risk of a postinfarction VSD as do non-smokers.[1] This further emphasizes what little we still know about coronary and infarct physiology, and how much we need the "Jesse Edwards type" investigators in the present day.

The incidence of infarct related VSD has fallen significantly in the "reperfusion era" of treating acute myocardial infarction.[1] Rapid reperfusion, especially with PCI, reduces transmural myocyte necrosis and appears to reduce the likelihood of a through-and-through tear that leads to a VSD. VSD's are now seen primarily in patients who present late after ST segment elevation infarction (STEMI)- too late for effective restoration of coronary blood flow to salvage muscle.

Treatment of ischemic VSD's is also changing. Simple VSD's can now be treated with transcatheter closure using an occluder device placed across the VSD (the most used having been developed by a friend of Jesse Edwards, Kurt Amplatz).[2,3] The Amplatzer ventricular septal occluder (intended for congenital muscular VSD's) and others have been used to close septal defects without the need for on-pump surgery that even in the current era has a very high mortality. The importance of identifying the morphology of a VSD outlined by Edwards is even more important in the percutaneous closure era. Placement and retention of occluder devices into complex VSD's is still challenging and the present devices will require modification in order to achieve reliable and durable closure.

Surgical treatment has also progressed with the use of bioglue, infarct exclusion, a variety of patching techniques, and even surgical placement of transcatheter devices though the right atrium or ventricle. Regardless of the repair method, however, the outcomes for patients suffering a postinfarction VSD remain fairly grim, especially for patients with the complex VSD's described and defined by Jesse Edwards. Regenerative therapies (such as stem cell infusion) and ventricular assist devices- only a dream three decades ago, provide hope for better treatment. Twenty six years after the Edwards classification of VSD morphology, we still have a lot of work ahead to invent effective treatment.

References:

1) Crenshaw BS, Granger CB, Birnbaum Y, Pieper KS, Morris DC, Kleiman NS, Vahanian A, Califf RM, Topol EJ: Risk factors, angiographic patterns, and outcomes in paients with ventricular septal defect complicating acute myocardial infarction. Circulation 2000;101:27-32

2) Lock JE, Block PC, McKay RG, Baim DS, Keane JF: Transcatheter closure of ventricular septal defects. Circulation 1988;78:361-368

3) Thiele H, Kaulfersch C, Daehnert I, Schoenuer M, Eitel I, Borger M, Schuler G: Immediate primary transcatheter closure of postinfarction ventricular septal defects. Eur Heart J 2009;30:81-88

Circulation

APRIL 1961
VOL. XXIII NO. 4

AN OFFICIAL JOURNAL of the AMERICAN HEART ASSOCIATION

Editorial

The Congenital Bicuspid Aortic Valve

IT IS commonly taught that the congenital bicuspid aortic valve may function as perfectly as does the normal tricuspid aortic valve. One may wonder, however, about the wisdom of this teaching when certain facts concerning the congenital bicuspid aortic valve are reviewed.

The congenital bicuspid aortic valve in its pure state, without the addition of acquired disease, may be grossly incompetent as proved by clinical and necropsy observations. For example, a congenital bicuspid valve occurs in about 85 per cent of patients who have coarctation of the aorta; Christensen and Hines[1] observed basal diastolic murmurs in 20 per cent of a clinical series of 96 patients with coarctation of the aorta.

Bacterial endocarditis, which tends to involve tissue subjected to trauma, has a distinct predilection for the congenital bicuspid aortic valve. In almost half of the cases of aortic valvular bacterial endocarditis, the underlying disease is a congenital bicuspid aortic valve.

Smith and Matthews[2] re-emphasized the views of Peacock, expressed in the last century, that the congenital bicuspid valve is particularly prone to become calcified and therefore stenotic. It is recognized that a form of congenital aortic stenosis exists but, in this condition, the valve is essentially dome-shaped and not bicuspid. This anomaly is not the subject of this editorial, although the valve may acquire calcific change and in this way, perhaps, the degree of stenosis may become accentuated.

One must assume that the occurrence in a congenital bicuspid aortic valve of intrinsic insufficiency and the traumatic background leading to bacterial endocarditis results from improper closure of the valve. Furthermore, the tendency for congenital bicuspid aortic valves to calcify is perhaps also a manifestation of trauma related to improper closure. With this background suggesting that the congenital bicuspid aortic valve may close improperly, one may present some theoretic considerations on the relationship of function to the structure of the bicuspid aortic valve.

Consideration of the normal tricuspid aortic valve emphasizes how nearly perfect its structure is for its function. The three cusps of the normal aortic valve may be looked on as three independent units, each being connected to its respective segment of the aortic wall. Each cusp has two lateral attachments to the aortic wall and an inferior attachment to the root of the aorta. Between the two lateral attachments of a cusp the tissue is greater than the straight-line distance between the points of attachments. This extra length of tissue of a normal tricuspid aortic valve allows the central part of each cusp to extend to the center of the aortic orifice where it touches the other cusps during closure of the valve (fig. 1*a*). The excess

From the Section of Pathologic Anatomy, Mayo Clinic, Rochester, Minnesota.

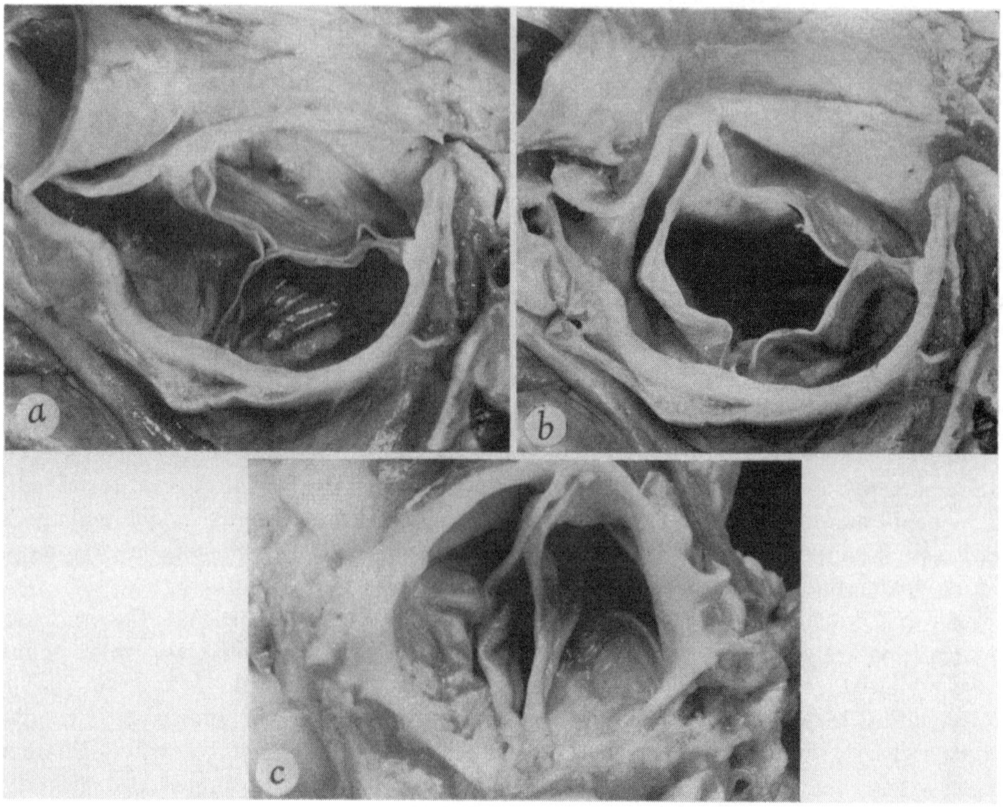

Figure 1

Normal tricuspid aortic valve in closed (a) *and opened* (b) *states.* (c) *Congenital bicuspid aortic valve.*

length also allows the individual cusps to balloon freely from the center of the orifice during systole, thereby allowing unobstructed opening of the valve (fig. 1*b*).

The anatomically perfect bicuspid aortic valve, if it actually ever exists, may now be considered. The length of the two cusps may be equal, or, as is more common, unequal. The length of each cusp is the same as the length of a straight line running between its two lateral attachments to the aortic wall. The individual cusp of the anatomically perfect congenital bicuspid aortic valve differs in this important way from the individual cusp of the normal tricuspid aortic valve. Because of this lack of extra length for free motion, the valve is held essentially fixed in a nearly closed state throughout the cardiac cycle (fig. 1*c*).

Thus, it becomes apparent that the anatomically perfect congenital bicuspid aortic valve would be stenotic because the individual cusps lack the extra length necessary for proper opening of the valve (fig. 2*a*). No evidence exists, however, that a congenital bicuspid aortic valve is intrinsically stenotic. One must therefore presume that two phenomena occur, singly or in combination, to prevent stenosis: (1) during ventricular systole, the aortic orifice becomes smaller, thereby creating a redundancy in the cusps that allows them to move freely away from the center of the orifice or (2) one or both of the cusps are longer than the straight-line length between their two lateral attachments. The extra length of the cusp would allow the mobility necessary for the valve to open during systole (fig. 2*b*, *c*, and *d*).

From the anatomic relationships of the aortic root to the myocardium, it is difficult to envision a mechanism that would cause the aortic orifice to narrow during ventricular systole. Therefore, absence of stenosis of the congenital bicuspid aortic valve is explained more readily by excessive length of one or both cusps. This is actually the usual finding.

While this anatomic fact is readily understood as a preventive of stenosis, it also explains the possibility of imperfect closure and of aortic valvular incompetence. During diastole, the free end of the cusp with excessive length may prolapse (fig. 2*b′* and *d′*). The regurgitant stream may strike the opposite cusp and traumatize it, causing it to be susceptible to bacterial endocarditis or to changes leading to calcification and stenosis. Moreover, the regurgitant stream, once established, may exert a greater force on the ventricular surface of the cusps than is the force on the sinus surface. In this way, the regurgitant stream perhaps may force open the aortic valve during diastole. If this does not happen, one cusp is pressed against its neighbor during diastole, the folding and unfolding of the long cusp may cause intrinsic trauma, and the pressure of the wrinkles of the elongated cusp on its opposite member may be

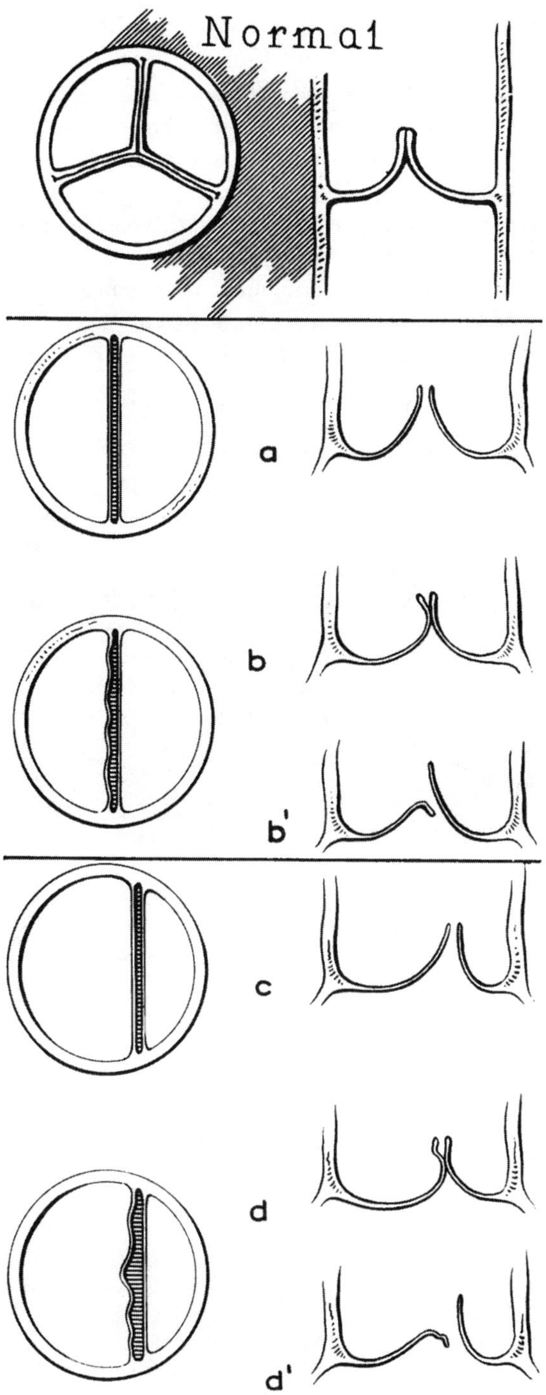

Figure 2

Diagrams of normal tricuspid aortic valve (top) *and congenital bicuspid aortic valve* (middle and bottom, a-d′). *In each instance the valve is viewed from above on the left and in a sagittal section on the right. In* a, b, *and* b′ (middle) *is portrayed a congenital bicuspid aortic valve in which the two leaflets are about the same length. In* a *is shown the hypothetically perfect bicuspid aortic valve in which the distance between the two lateral attachments of each cusp is equivalent to the straight-line distance between these two points. In* b *and* b′ *is portrayed the usual situation in which at least one of the two leaflets is longer than the hypothetically perfect cusp. This allows unobstructed opening of the valve. Closure of such a valve may be accomplished without incompetence* (b), *or with prolapse of the redundant cusp and resultant insufficiency* (b′). *A large regurgitant stream may push the opposite cusp away from the center of the aortic lumen during ventricular diastole and so accentuate the degree of aortic incompetence. In* c, d, *and* d′ (bottom) *is portrayed a congenital bicuspid aortic valve in which one leaflet is larger than the other. If there is no redundant tissue* (c), *the valve would be stenotic. If redundant tissue exists* (d *and* d′), *as is usually the case, the valve, while not stenotic, may be competent, or incompetent if prolapse occurs. The stresses resulting from redundant tissue with or without incompetence may be responsible for traumatic changes in the leaflet.*

traumatic to the latter. Thus, the congenital bicuspid aortic valve, whether competent or incompetent, is potentially subjected to mechanical injury.

One begins to wonder about the validity of the theory that the anatomically perfect bicuspid aortic valve may be stenotic when one considers the state of the venous valves. The latter usually are bicuspid semilunar valves with considerable similarity in structure to the congenital bicuspid aortic valve. Yet the normal peripheral venous system offers no evidence of an obstructive factor. Perhaps this may be the result not of imperfections in the venous valves, as suggested for the congenital bicuspid aortic valve, but rather the result of dilatation of the vein at the site of a valve. Thus, while the venous valve may be so constructed as to be stenotic, the vein is larger at the site of the valve, and the diameter of the "stenotic" valvular orifice may be equal to that of the nondilated parts of the vein both above and below the valve.

The foregoing observations may be summarized as follows: the anatomic basis for the absence of intrinsic stenosis in the congenital bicuspid aortic valve is the very basis for the occurrence in this congenital anomaly of aortic valvular incompetence and also of traumatic influences that represent a tendency to the development of bacterial endocarditis and acquired calcific stenosis.

JESSE E. EDWARDS

References

1. CHRISTENSEN, N. A., AND HINES, E. A., JR.: Clinical features in coarctation of the aorta: A review of 96 cases. Proc. Staff Meet., Mayo Clin. 23: 339, 1948.
2. SMITH, D. E., AND MATTHEWS, M. B.: Aortic valvular stenosis with coarctation of the aorta: With special reference to the development of aortic stenosis upon congenital bicuspid valves. Brit. Heart J. 17: 198, 1955.

The Congenital Bicuspid Aortic Valve

William C. Roberts, M.D.

The editorial "*The Congenital Bicuspid Aortic Valve*" by Dr. Jesse E. Edwards was published 50 years ago (April 1961) and it is a classic. JEE by that time was the world's foremost student of the bicuspid aortic valve. In this piece he asked the simple question, "How does a congenitally bicuspid valve open and close during the 2 phases of the cardiac cycle?" To my knowledge, that question had never been asked previously. JEE preceded his answer to the question by describing how the normal 3-cuspid aortic valve opens and closes. He demonstrated that the latter does so because the distance between any two commissures (lateral attachments of each independent cusp) along their free margins is greater than a straight line. The greater-than-a-straight-line distance allows each cusps to move to the center of the aortic lumen during ventricular diastole, thus closing the orifice, and then move near to the wall of the aorta during ventricular systole, thus opening the orifice maximally or nearly so.

So how does a congenitally bicuspid aortic valve open if theoretically the distance between the two commissures across the aortic orifice is a straight-line? JEE demonstrated that the length of at least one of the two cusps along its free margin is not a straight line but indeed is greater than a straight line. This fact is both its savior and its defeater. It is a "savior" because if at least one of the two cusps was not longer than a straight line, the valve could not open during ventricular systole. That the length of at least one of the two cusps along its free margin is greater than a straight line is also its "defeater" because the elongation allows each cusp to contact each other during ventricular diastole in a traumatic fashion and that trauma over a prolonged period (many years) causes the cusps to thicken and eventually to calcify leading to stenosis. If the cusps do not calcify, pure regurgitation is the usual hemodynamic consequence. Rarely does a congenitally bicuspid valve function normally or nearly normally during an entire lifetime.

JEE additionally pointed out that a congenitally bicuspid aortic valve was rarely, if ever, stenotic from birth. These aortic valves that are stenotic from birth are nearly always unicuspid, mainly unicommissural.

JEE's piece was a great step forward in our understanding of the congenitally bicuspid aortic valve.

News from the American Heart Association

44 East 23rd Street, New York, New York 10010
Telephone: Gramercy 7-9170

PRESIDENTIAL ADDRESS

AHA 41st Scientific Sessions

Atherosclerosis: An Impossible Mission?

IN THE American Heart Association, the Presidental Address comes at the end of the term. Therefore, this either might serve as a review of the accomplishments of the year rapidly closing or it could highlight that which is left undone. The field of cardiovascular disease is so complex that currently the unaccomplished far exceeds that totally solved. It seems proper, therefore, that we concentrate our attention on what needs to be done.

A motto of the U. S. Army Engineers says, "The difficult we do immediately. The impossible takes a little longer." These words are applicable with respect to the cardiovascular field. We recognize that a cornerstone in the history of cardiovascular disease was laid twenty years ago, when two organizations were established.

In 1948 the American Heart Association, which for years had been purely a scientific society, converted itself into a national voluntary health agency. In the same year, the National Heart Institute of the National Institutes of Health was founded. One concept was common to these two organizations.

This concept represented a pivotal point in medicine; it was that the time was right for sustained support of cardiovascular research. The support had two aspects. One was for projects initiated by investigators and the other for the development of people. It was from this newly created program of sustained research support that the difficult was done "immediately." Within a short period of twenty years, an instant in the history of time, problems which for centuries had been insurmountable, were solved. Treatment of hypertension, an impact on prevention of rheumatic fever, treatment and prevention of bacterial endocarditis, cardiac catheterization, angiocardiography, the heart-lung machine, intracardiac surgical procedures, development of artificial valves and blood vessels, control of arrhythmias, assisted circulation, and even cardiac transplantation are to be numbered among the new tools or accomplishments that have peaked to mountainous proportions in the instant of time since 1948.

It would be unrealistic to say that as of today we have achieved perfection in each of these areas. Yet, once the secret is exposed, technical alteration leading to improvement is inevitable. For example, once a heart-lung machine or a pacemaker was developed, improvements through modification were to be expected. We can, therefore, accept that time will take care of the current deficiencies among our accomplishments.

At the present time we find ourselves in the hiatus between the difficult and the "impossible," the "impossible that will take a little longer" to solve.

The "impossible" is the problem of atherosclerosis in its various aspects. It includes a need for an understanding of its pathogenesis and its counterpart in prevention. The "impossible" includes a need for an understanding of the mechanisms which lead to complications of established atherosclerosis.

When we obtain such an understanding we shall have the tools and the concepts with which to accomplish prevention and to apply realistic and predictable methods of treatment.

Quite realistically, before we reach the promised land with regard to atherosclerosis, many investigators will have been put to the trials not only of hard work but of frustration and disappointment. As we look ahead to the solution of the complex problem posed by atherosclerosis, I am reminded of the many trials of Moses in leading his people from bondage in a foreign country to freedom in their native land.

The first step was to obtain permission for release, a release that was not the end but a means to an end. In atherosclerosis our bondage took a certain form, namely the apparent reluctance of large numbers of investigators to tackle the problem in the first place. Here we must pay tribute to the vision of the late Dr. Robert Grant. As a newly installed Director of the National Heart Institute, he immediately recognized the disparity between the incidence of coronary heart disease and the level of research support as contrasted to other cardiovascular diseases and the support they were receiving.

It was through his influence that attention was directed toward this relatively neglected area. Earmarking of money for the study of myocardial infarction represented a release from bondage. The program which he instituted should not be called directed research in the usual sense. It provided a basis for stimulating the interest of investigators and for application for funds on a competitive basis. The latter point was all important in maintaining the vital rule in research; that is, the initiative for formulating a research plan must rest with the investigator who is to do the work. In this way, the energetic and enthusiastic attitude toward the program is maintained. Moreover, an intensive involvement in research exposes unanswered questions and these serve to expand the quest toward the goal of solving the problem.

A review of the subjects of this year's scientific program attests to the fact that Bob Grant did indeed obtain our release from bondage.

To continue the comparison of our task with that of Moses, we recall that his mission, once the movement of his people started was twofold, (1) to obtain a position of freedom and security for the people and (2) to instill a concept of morality as the expressed will of God.

In atherosclerosis we are also faced with two missions (1) to prevent atherosclerosis and (2) to cope with the problem of the millions who currently carry the lesion so fully established that in these the immediate problem is prevention and treatment of complications.

Moses was met with many difficulties both from within his people, and from the outside environment.

From within, he had to cope with the doubters, those who would rather return to slavery than face the uncertainties and hardships leading to freedom. From the external environment he had difficult terrain, trying climatic conditions and hostile tribes or those of uncertain attitude toward him and his people.

The level of support for research in atherosclerosis and in myocardial infarction, although significant, falls far short of the capability of funding all meritorious applications in these areas. In this and in other aspects we are far from having reached our goal as we too have both internal and external problems.

In prevention of the fundamental lesion we are faced with internal genetic and metabolic factors so strong that at the moment we are incapable of manipulating these to the advantage of the individual.

Application of those factors which have promise, in particular maintenance of low levels of serum cholesterol, also meets with internal resistance. This resistance comes from the national habit of building up our arterial linings through the oral route. It will be a herculean task to change the national eating habits (both from the view point of the producer and the consumer) if the dietary factor favoring atherogenesis will ever be controlled.

Internal resistance stops not with prevention of atherosclerosis but is also felt in the area of prevention of complications. Although preventive measures have been adequately publicized, general acceptance of these in practice is still lacking.

Our external hardships are underscored by the half-million Americans who die of coronary arterial disease annually, one quarter of a million in hospital and one quarter acutely outside of the hospital.

Some inroads into the problem seem to be in the making by the establishment of the so-called coronary care units. Perhaps half of the 5,000 hospitals which admit patients with acute coronary attacks are equipped with physical facilities that provide monitoring and resuscitative equipment. Equipment is easy to come by to the point that the number of units outstrips our present capability of providing adequately trained personnel to man these units.

Even more, were we to have an utopian situation, coronary care facilities and adequate personnel for every hospitalized patient, our potential appears to be about 50,000 lives saved annually. This salvage would come from the quarter of a million Americans now dying in hospitals annually from coronary disease.

With coronary care facilities our potential is even greater for the one quarter of a million who die acutely outside the hospital, since these people predominantly die arrhythmic deaths. It is from this group that we are particularly impressed with the pertinence of the statement that the patient died with a "heart too good to die."

Why are we failing with this group in the shadows of facilities that might give life saving help? Several factors come to mind and, for some, appropriate adjustment could be made. Among these factors is sudden death. When, however, one reviews cases of so-called sudden death from coronary disease, one finds that some patients will have had some deviation from normal for a period of time sufficient to have allowed initiation of monitoring. Some have even consulted physicians without being recognized as being in potential danger. Clearly, our clinical interpretation of impending trouble falls short of perfection. Appropriate research may serve to lower the threshold of clinical suspicion by crystalizing criteria so that available facilities will be put at the disposal of the person who, without care is about to "die suddenly."

Physical problems of obvious nature revolve around the person in whom there is no question about the diagnosis. How best to bring the patient into contact with the machinery he obviously needs? Should the machinery move to him or should he move to the machinery? This question can be argued either way and the specific answer is less important than is the awareness of the need and the development of adequate mechanics. I need not detail the various complexities involved in this hoped for accomplishment. These will vary with each community and even with different areas of a given community.

Awareness of the need is the pivotal point upon which such programs will be developed.

In a conference on Program Priorities held last March, the American Heart Association identified Prevention of Atherosclerosis as its number one priority for program. As a result, a number of community projects will inevitably follow.

Here, one must be careful not to worship the golden calf. A project, perhaps involving thousands of people, but without a built-in means of learning what a particular manipulation accomplishes, is a false god. These words of admonition are applicable not only to projects involving health measures in population groups but also to the surgical procedures for coronary disease that are proceeding at an ever-increasing pace.

The effort, money and risk spent in doing something are wasted unless we learn what was or was not accomplished.

The road ahead may be devious, difficult and trying. At the same time, the traveller will

274

encounter the friendly and helpful attitude of the American Heart Association as it continues to take its established place beside other agencies. If we keep faith with the true experimental method, we shall not falter. We shall move forward. However time-consuming and difficult the effort, we shall reach our goal!

Jesse E. Edwards, M.D.

Atherosclerosis: An Impossible Mission?

Brooks S. Edwards, M.D.

This paper represents a transcript of an address my father gave as President of the American Heart Association (AHA) in 1968 and reprinted in 1969. It's the speech in which my father focused on the identification of atherosclerosis and coronary heart disease as the number one priority for the AHA at that time.

The late 1960's were a particularly interesting time for cardiology, and Dad's tenure as President of the AHA in 1968 was a hot bed of activity. As noted in the speech, at that time there were about 500,000 annual deaths attributed to coronary artery disease. Less then half of the hospitals in American had specialized units for monitoring and treating patients with acute myocardial infarction (CCU's), acute intervention was not an option and specialized cardiovascular nursing was in its infancy.

My father often taught by analogy, and in this speech he likened the prevention or treatment of atherosclerosis to the work of Moses leading the Israelites out of Egyptian bondage. The bondage he saw in 1968 was the bondage of progressive atherosclerosis that was becoming the plague of a whole generation. As a pathologist, he often saw the young person suddenly and unexpectedly cut down in the prime of life. While the victim often "never saw it coming," Dad usually found the harbingers of premature death had been present for years. He especially was bothered by the occurrence of so called "fatty streaks" found in the vessels of healthy soldiers who died traumatic deaths. He understood, before many others, that the seeds of coronary atherosclerosis were sowed often decades ahead of the index event. He reasoned that understanding the basic biology of atherosclerosis was critical to arresting its progression and effects. As President of AHA, he lobbied for increased funding for basic research, and while the field has advanced considerably since the 1960s I believe he would continue to make a strong and clear case for the support of basic research in the field. He understood the importance of research, both basic and applied as a prerequisite to clinical advances.

To carry his biblical analogy further, in this speech he likened clinical interventions without rigorous outcomes measures to the worship of a golden calf. He was particularly concerned about high cost, high tech medical and surgical interventions that were proceeding without appropriate study. His words of admonishment (and encouragement) and the works and words of many others, ultimately lead to large clinical trials like CASS and BARI and the evidenced based medicine we now try to practice.

While President of the AHA, Dad traveled the country promoting the development of coronary care units for every community. As a pathologist, he all too frequently saw in the autopsy of the heart "too good to die," and he recognized the importance of monitored beds and CCU teams as a means to identify and treating life-threatening arrhythmias associated with acute infarction. Today, while the monitored bed has become the standard of care for acute infarction, Dad might bemoan the fact that many of the patients who could benefit from implantable cardioverter defibrillators (ICD) are not all receiving this therapy, while others who don't meet guidelines are perhaps receiving inappropriate therapy. Dad would tell us that today's healthcare disparities represent another reason for evidence-based care and translating clinical trials results into practice.

Since my father's service as President of the AHA, great progress has been made. Basic biology and genetics of the atherosclerotic plaque are now better understood, and that has translated into therapeutic gains. Statin therapy for treatment of atherosclerosis has changed the natural history of hyperlipidemia and hence coronary artery disease. Acute intervention for myocardial infarction has saved hundreds of thousands of lives (including my fathers own acute coronary event more then a dozen years ago), and antiarrhythmic device therapies continues to reduce the risk of sudden cardiac death. The death rate for coronary artery disease has fallen more then 50 percent since this lecture was delivered, and for that my father would be pleased. Still, he would remind us, the fatty streak has not disappeared, and the enemy continues to knock at the door. Much work remains to be done but the foundation has been set, and the agenda laid out in 1968 remains relevant today.

The Mechanism of Balloon Angioplasty[1]

Wilfrido R. Castaneda-Zuniga, M.D., Augustin Formanek, M.D., Murthy Tadavarthy, M.D., Zeev Vlodaver, M.D., Jesse E. Edwards, M.D., Christoph Zollikofer, M.D., and Kurt Amplatz, M.D.

A new theory of the mechanism of percutaneous arterial angioplasty is advanced. For this study, abdominal aortas and coronary, renal, superior mesenteric, and iliac arteries were obtained from cadavers. In addition, the iliac arteries of dogs were dilated and studied. No evidence of significant compression or redistribution of plaques could be found, supporting the theory that atheromatous material is incompressible. Cracking of the intima and separation of it from the media were histologically demonstrated following angioplasty. It is proposed that the stretched media distends following dilatation, carrying with it the intima and atheromatous material. Once the media is freed from the encasing effect of the intima, it adapts to the circulatory needs of the body. Beyond a certain point, the arterial widening becomes permanent, due to an overstretching of the muscle fibers, which is demonstrated by a corkscrew deformity of the muscle cell nuclei.

INDEX TERMS: Arteries, stenosis, 9.721 • Arteries, transluminal angioplasty • (Arteries, transluminal dilatation, 9.454)

Radiology 135:565–571, June 1980

PERCUTANEOUS arterial angioplasty is rapidly gaining popularity in the United States. The clinical usefulness of this procedure in certain types of obstructive atheromatous disease is well established. Since the introduction of this technique by Dotter and Judkins (1), the mechanism of angioplasty has been thought to be the compression of atheromatous material. It is our purpose to challenge this classic concept and to advance a new theory based on recent animal and cadaver studies.

MATERIAL AND METHODS

Abdominal aortas and coronary, renal, superior mesenteric, and iliac arteries were obtained from cadavers. Only cadavers of older patients (age range 53–75 years) were used. If significant atheromatous disease was palpable, the arteries were filled with barium sulfate suspension and anteroposterior and lateral radiographs were obtained. If the radiographic examination showed a significant lesion, a guidewire and a Grüntzig balloon catheter of appropriate size were passed across the stenosis. The balloon was inflated to 4 to 6 atmospheres over a period of one minute. Inflation was repeated three times. The catheter was withdrawn, the artery was filled with barium sulfate suspension, and additional radiographs were obtained at right angles. Some of the specimens were injected with India ink. In a cadaver with severe bilateral iliac disease, one iliac artery was placed in a test tube to restrict dilatation (Fig. 1). A balloon was introduced and inflated to the same pressure as a balloon catheter which had been introduced into the contralateral iliac artery. All specimens were fixed in 40% formaldehyde and examined by light microscopy using hematoxylin and eosin as well as stains for elastic tissue.

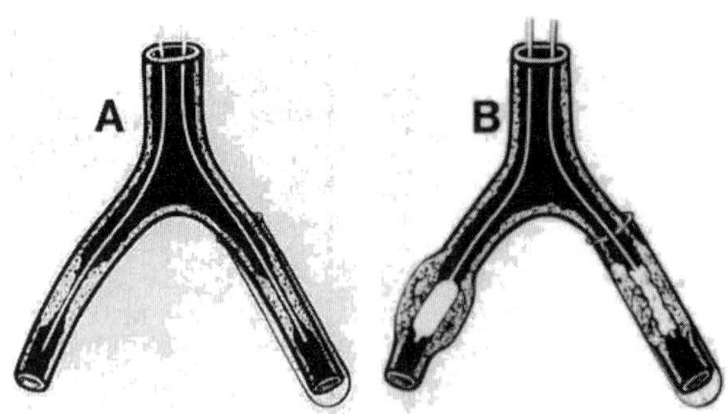

Fig. 1. Cadaver aorto-iliac specimen with severe bilateral iliac atherosclerosis. The left common iliac artery has been placed in a glass test tube. Balloon catheters have been placed across areas of stenosis (*A*). During inflation of the balloon catheters (*B*), the dilated segment of the right common iliac artery expands, while the segment of left common iliac artery being dilated is restrained by the test tube.

Seven mongrel dogs weighing 18 to 20 kg were anesthetized with sodium Pentothal and underwent angiography. The iliac arteries were dilated using a Grüntzig balloon catheter that was 9 mm in diameter. In one animal, 9-mm balloon catheters were introduced into both femoral arteries and advanced into the abdominal aorta. Balloon dilatation of the aorta was accomplished by simultaneous

[1] From the Radiology Department, University of Minnesota Hospitals, Minneapolis (W.R.C-Z., A.F., M.T., C.Z., K.A.), and the Department of Pathology, United Hospitals-Miller Division, St. Paul (Z.V., J.E.E.), MN. Presented at the Sixty-fifth Scientific Assembly and Annual Meeting of the Radiological Society of North America, Georgia World Congress Center, Atlanta, GA, Nov. 25–30, 1979. Received Jan. 16, 1980; accepted Mar. 12.

This work supported by Public Health Service Research Grant #5-R01-HL05694 from the National Heart, Lung and Blood Institute. cd

2,3a,3b

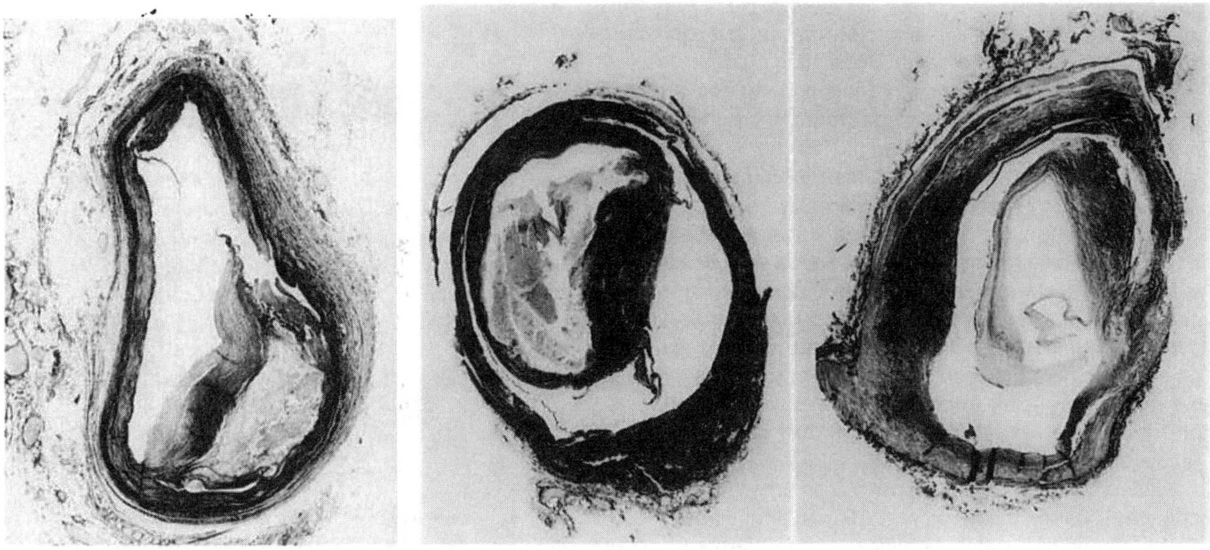

Fig. 2. Superior mesenteric artery. After dilatation with a 9-mm balloon for three minutes, there is a florid lipoid atheroma covered by fibrous tissue, and a tear at the junction of the atheroma with the walls. The tear goes through the intima and into the junction of the media and intima.

Fig. 3a. Left renal artery, after balloon dilatation. On gross examination, before dilatation the renal artery showed major stenosis. The microscopic section shows a highly lipomatous atheroma. There has been fragmentation of the intima from the media in relation to the existing lumen. The fragmentation extends a considerable distance around the circumference of the vessel. In one area the intimal separation extends within the media.

b. Anterior descending coronary artery from a cadaver. Barium angiogram obtained after balloon dilatation. A tear is seen in the intima, extending into a focus of lipoid accumulation. Barium is present in the tract.

inflation of both balloons, as previously described in a patient undergoing abdominal angioplasty (2). In all cases, an inflation pressure of 5 atmospheres was used. Follow-up angiograms were obtained immediately after dilatation and from one week to three months after the procedure in some animals. Some animals were killed immediately after dilatation, and others were killed from one day to four months after the procedure. The arterial specimens were excised and fixed in formalin for histopathologic examination.

RESULTS

On all arterial cadaver specimens that had been dilated with balloon catheters, rupture and fragmentation of the

4a,b

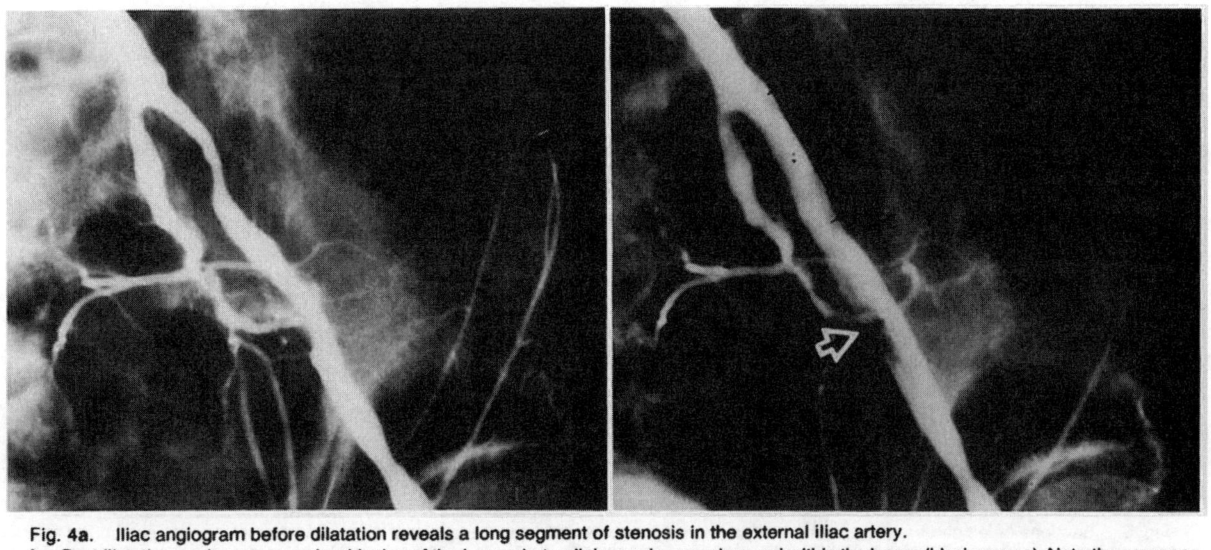

Fig. 4a. Iliac angiogram before dilatation reveals a long segment of stenosis in the external iliac artery.

b. Postdilatation angiogram reveals widening of the lumen, but radiolucencies are observed within the lumen (black arrows). Note the presence of contrast material in the cleft behind the detached atherosclerotic plaque, giving the appearance of subintimal dissection (open arrow).

intima were found (Fig. 2). Large clefts between the intima and denuded media were demonstrated (Fig. 3), which very likely accounted for the angiographic appearance of dissection (Fig. 4). In all cases, the fragmented intima remained attached to the arterial wall. Thinning of all arterial layers was observed in one specimen, which was dilated and fixed with the balloon inflated (Fig. 5).

The iliac artery which was dilated with the restraint of a test tube showed compaction of the media without intimal tears. Clefts were identified in the atheroma, but no compression or remodeling of atheromatous material was seen. In the unrestricted contralateral iliac artery, extensive intimal fragmentation and dehiscence of the intima from the media were found, undoubtedly due to stretching of the arterial media. Again, no remodeling of atheromatous plaques occurred.

In the animal specimens, a correlation among histologic changes, balloon diameter, and inflation time was found. Three stages of histologic changes were observed:

1. No histologic or morphologic alterations.
2. Widening of the artery due to compaction and stretching of elastic fibers, particularly smooth muscle cells. The nuclei of the muscle cells elongated, which resulted in a typical corkscrew appearance. Some of the elastic fibers lost their undulation, apparently due to overstretching (Fig. 6).
3. Disruption of the media, and healing by fibrous tissue. Rupture of the intima and its complete repair by the formation of a neointima was seen. There was no evidence of extravasation or false aneurysm (Fig. 7).

Angiography immediately after balloon dilatation demonstrated a significant widening of the arterial lumen. Angiography at one and four months following balloon dilatation showed persistent arterial widening (Fig. 8).

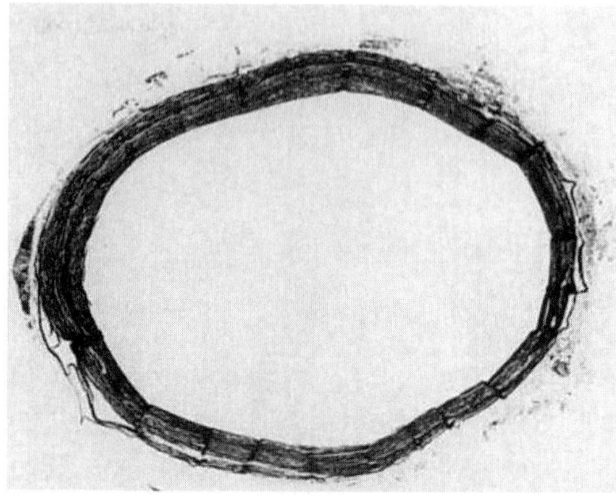

Fig. 5. Iliac artery fixed with balloon in place. The intima is thin. The media is also thin and apparently stretched. Stain for elastic tissue was used.

DISCUSSION

In their original description, Dotter and Judkins attributed the mechanism of transluminal angioplasty to the redistribution and compression of the atheromatous intima (1). Particularly in cases with 100% occlusion, the dilating catheter was supposed to induce a "cold flow" of the

6a,b

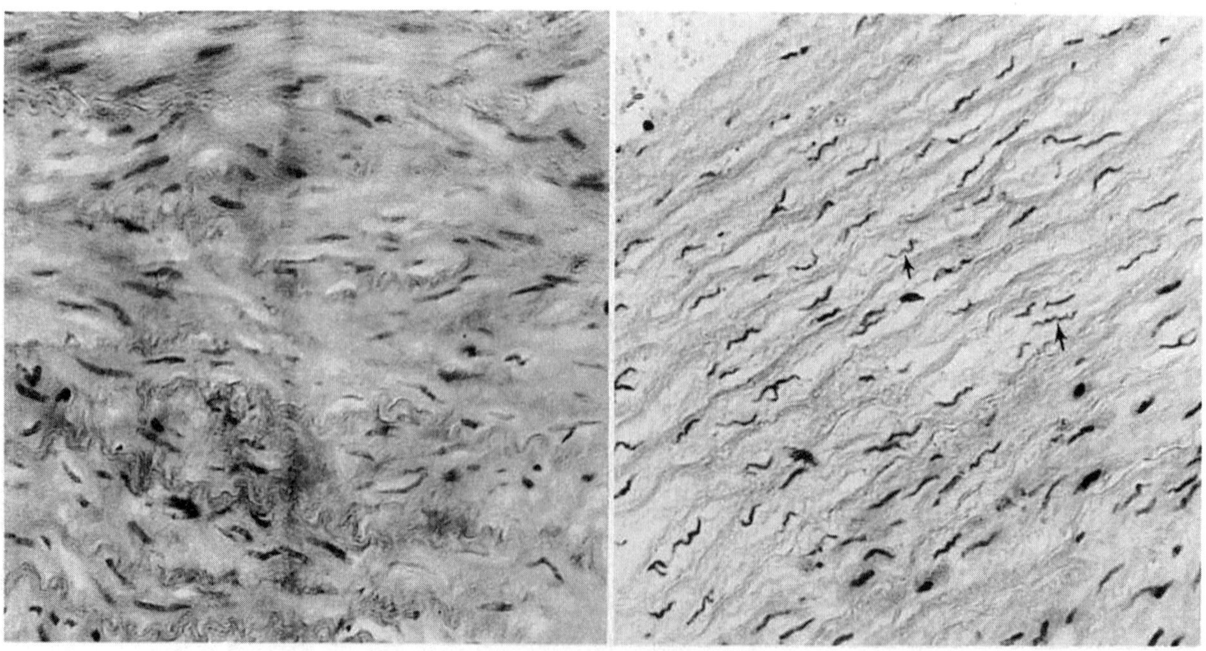

Fig. 6. Sections of left carotid artery. In the control section (a) observe the normal appearance of the different components of the arterial wall. In the dilated area (b) the lumen is wider, and in the inner half of the media the elastic fibers are closely related to each other and there is loss of undulation of the elastic fibers. Note the characteristic corkscrew shape of the nuclei of the smooth muscle fibers of the media (arrows).

7a 7c

7b

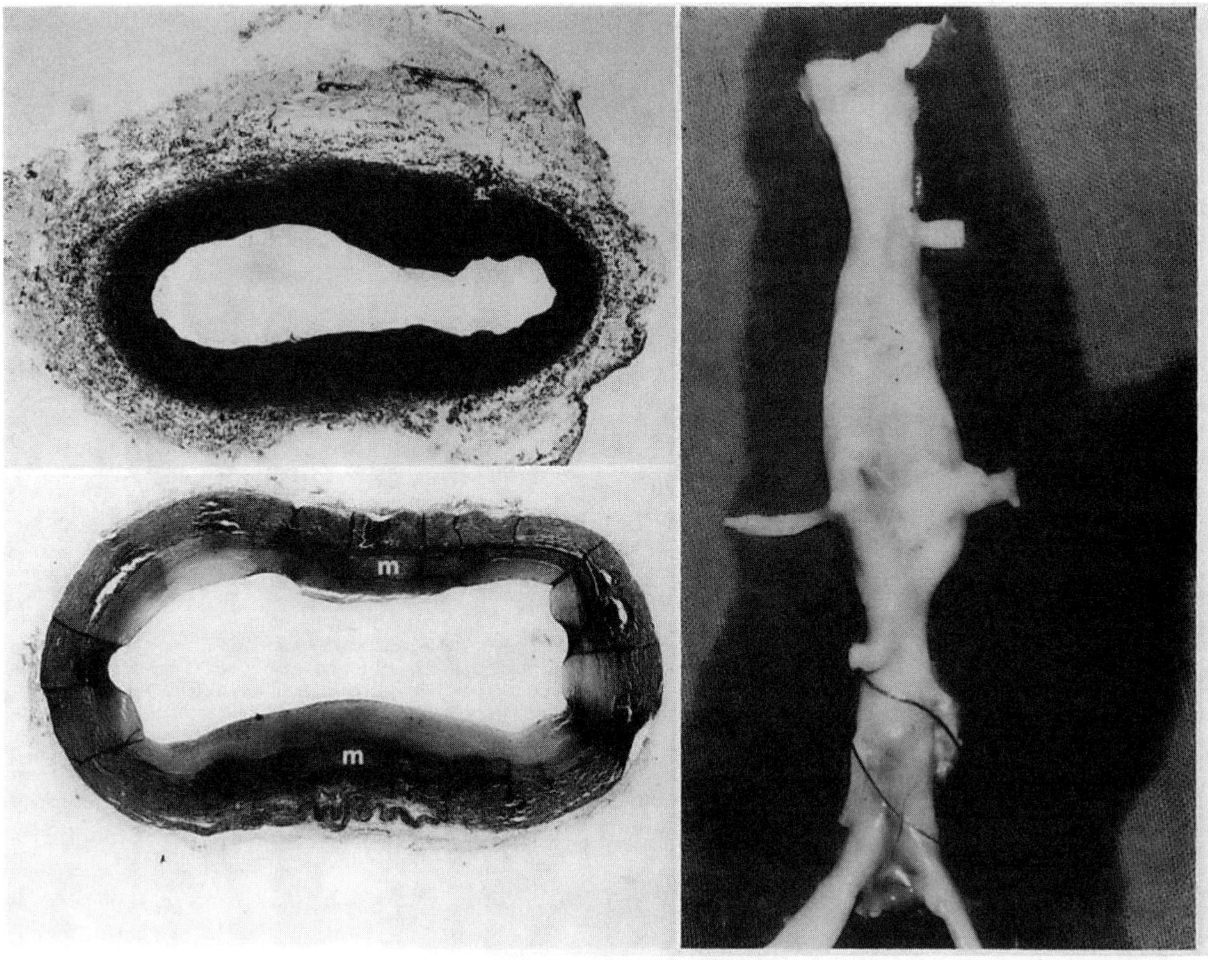

Fig. 7a. Abdominal aorta, section above the area of dilatation. The aortic media appears to be intact. The intima shows focal fibroelastic thickening. The lumen is considerably narrowed compared with levels at which dilatation was done.
b. Section through the site of dilatation. The lumen is considerably wider than it is at the level above dilatation. The media shows focal interruptions (*m*), and related to these there is a neointima composed of laminated fibrous tissue. The neointima over the sites of rupture is continuous with diffuse fibroelastic thickening of the intima at sites where the media is intact.
c. Specimen of abdominal aorta in the same dog shows marked widening of the lumen, without evidence of extravasation or false aneurysm.

puttylike atheromatous material (Fig. 9), (3–5). This theory was universally accepted and supported by Grüntzig and others (6–9). Lue and Grüntzig (10) described a transient increase in the caliber of the artery following balloon dilatation, but basically the intimal compression theory was accepted by all investigators.

Since atheromatous material is a solid, or sometimes a semiliquid, it is basically incompressible unless empty spaces are present within the atheroma, something which is not found histologically. As is true of other solids and liquids, therefore, atheromatous deposits can be considered to be incompressible.

If we assume that soft atheromatous material and thrombi could undergo a cold flow as postulated by Dotter, and could be redistributed, in the absence of dilatation of the artery itself, such a redistribution of soft material would obviously result in an enlongation of the lesion, since no material is removed (Fig. 10). Postdilatation angiograms of such lesions would therefore demonstrate a patent lumen, but an obvious increase in the length of the lesion (9), a phenomenon that has not been observed. In addition, clinical experience shows that arterial dilatation is also effective in old fibrotic, or even calcified, atheromatous plaques in which a cold flow or compressibility can be excluded with certainty.

Balloon dilatation in the arteries of cadavers demonstrated that the arteries stretched, and then assumed their original size as soon as the balloon was deflated. This is very likely due to the lack of blood pressure. Histologic examination clearly demonstrated a cracking of the intima and a pulling away of the intimal layer from the media. In the large clefts between intima and media, barium or India ink was easily demonstrable (Fig. 3). At angiography, contrast medium enters these large spaces between the stretched media and dehisced intima, giving the angiographic appearance of a subintimal dissection (Fig. 4). Very rarely, the intimal tube remains grossly intact, and the appearance of a double lumen can be observed.

If atheromatous plaques are indeed incompressible, as we postulate, such overstretching and dilatation of the media and adventitia occurs also with the original Dotter technique. As soon as the media is freed from the restraint of the atherosclerotic intima, it can stretch and remain stretched by the blood pressure. A similar increased caliber of the artery, due to a stretching of the thin media and adventitia, is observed following endarterectomy.

What we are proposing as a possible mechanism to explain the increase in the lumen size is based on the fact that there are no changes in the atheromatous plaques, and that experimentally in cadavers and laboratory animals there is evidence of intimal disruption and stretching of the media, which beyond a certain point has proven to be irreversible. What probably happens is that a stretched media distends, carrying the intima and atheromatous plaques with it (Fig. 11). Furthermore, as soon as the media is freed from the encasing effect of the intima by balloon dilatation, it can readily adapt to the circulatory needs. It is therefore likely that a vigorous exercise following balloon dilatation may result in progressive, further widening of the arterial lumen due to an increase in blood flow. Further improvement weeks and months after balloon dilatation has been a puzzle to the angiographer, and has been explained by additional removal of atheromatous plaques by phagocytosis. It is our opinion that this later improvement simply represents adaptation of the freed media to the demands of the blood flow.

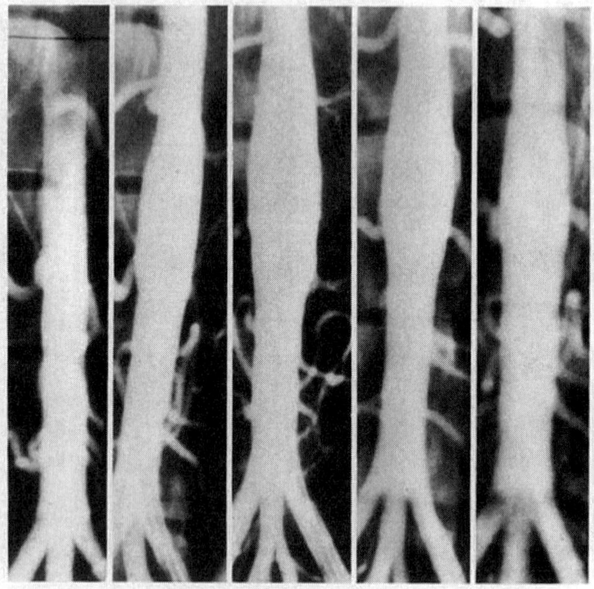

8a–e

Fig. 8a. Predilatation angiogram.
b. Angiogram obtained after dilatation up to 18 mm for three minutes at a pressure of 5 atmospheres. Note widening of the lumen.
c. Angiogram obtained after dilatation for six minutes at 5 atmospheres. Observe further widening of the lumen.
d. Follow-up angiogram at four weeks postdilatation reveals persistent widening of the lumen.
e. Follow-up angiogram at three months postdilatation reveals some decrease of caliber.

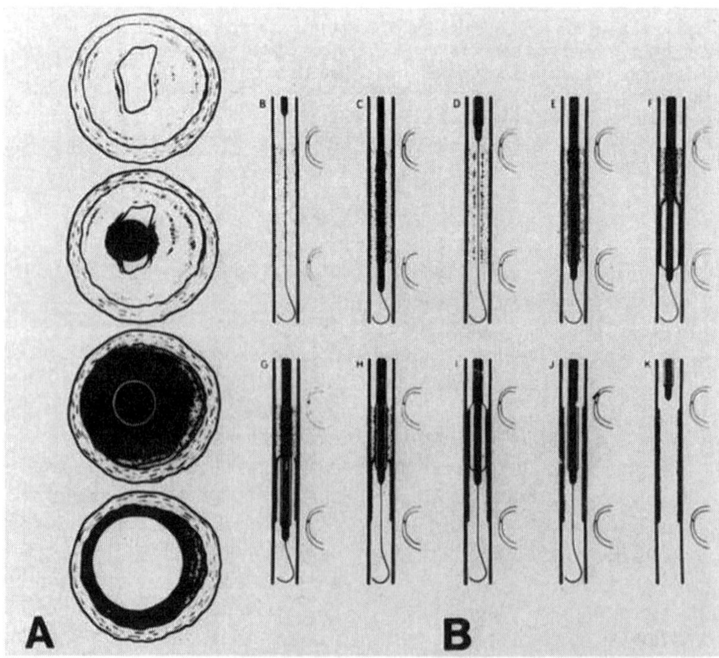

Fig. 9. Schematic representation of events in transluminal dilatation according to Dotter's theory (*A*), showing widening of the lumen without increase in the caliber of the artery itself (5). A diagram of recanalization of atherosclerotic obstruction according to Grüntzig's theory (*B*) shows widening of the lumen, with no evidence of an increase in the caliber of the artery, or of increase in the length of the lesion (6).

10,11

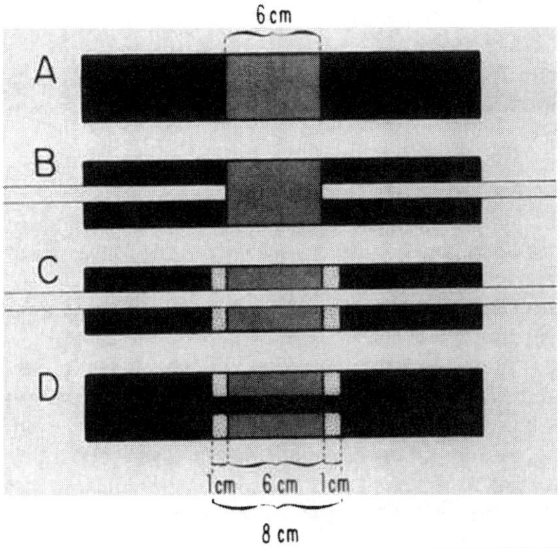

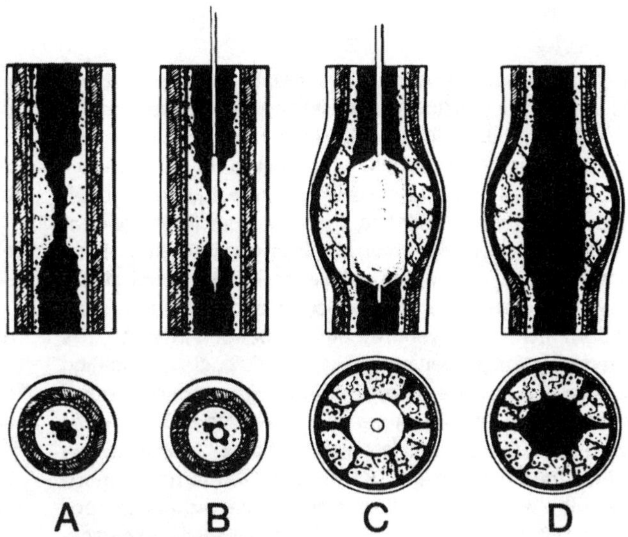

12

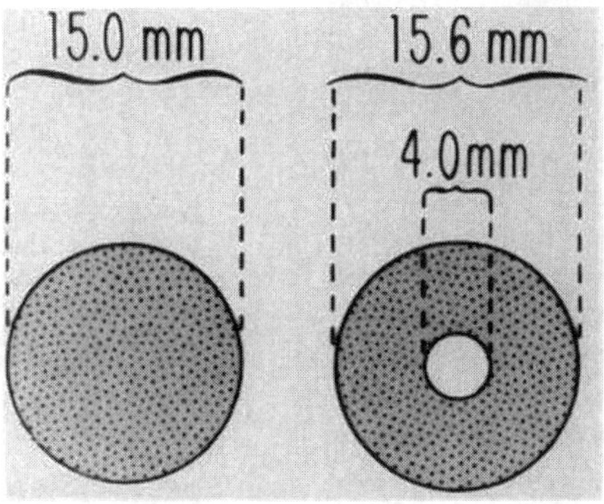

Fig. 10. This diagram illustrates a localized segment of obstruction 6 cm in length (*A*) through which a 12-Fr Dotter dilator is introduced (*B*). If no material is removed, it will have to be redistributed along the adjacent arterial wall (*C*). The calculated volume of the cylinder that has been displaced will occupy an area 2 cm in length (*D*).

Fig. 11. Diagram of proposed theory: *A*. A segment of artery with large atherosclerotic plaques is demonstrated. *B*. Grüntzig's balloon catheter is passed across area of stenosis. *C*. With the inflation of the balloon, the plaques are pushed outwards, and the arterial wall layers are overstretched. *D*. After the balloon is removed, the lumen is widened by the ballooning of the overstretched intima and media, and the plaques remain essentially unchanged.

Fig. 12. Diagram showing a completely occluded arterial segment through which a 12-Fr Dotter dilator has been introduced. The increased area caused by the dilatation causes only a minimal widening of the overall dimension of the artery.

The reason that the overall increase in the outside arterial diameter following angioplasty has not been observed previously is demonstrated by a simple drawing. The increase caused by the use of a 12-Fr Dotter catheter results in only a minimal widening of the overall dimension of the artery (Fig. 12). It is quite conceivable that such a minimal change was overlooked at the time of postmortem examinations.

One of the most intriguing findings of our study is the stretching and widening of the normal canine artery following balloon dilatation. The artery's increased diameter following inflation of the balloon causes an increased wall tension according to the law of LaPlace, which results in arterial widening. This widening may be transient and no histopathologic changes are found.

With an oversized balloon diameter, rupture of the intima and media occurs, resulting in a permanent arterial widening. Such widening was also easily observable at postmortem examination in our animal subjects (Fig. 7c). It is interesting to note that there was no hematoma formation, and complete healing of the dehisced intima and media occurred. The histologic picture was very similar to that of an endarterectomy and it is likely that no permanent sequelae would occur in the smaller arteries, although our longest follow-up was only four months.

Before dehiscence of the media occurs, the elastic fibers, and particularly muscle fibers, undergo an irreversible stretching, which was well demonstrated by the corkscrew appearance of the nuclei of the smooth muscle cells. A similar deformation occurs in elastomers if the modulus of elasticity is exceeded by overstretching. The elastic properties of arteries have been studied extensively. When a small amount of stress is applied, the arteries behave as truly elastic, assuming their original size as soon as the stress disappears. This finding is consistent with our histopathologic observations, which fail to reveal any morphologic changes in arteries which were subjected to dilatation with small balloons. It is therefore likely that angioplasty performed within the true elastic limits of the artery will have no effect unless the intima is ruptured.

With increasing stress, which in our experiment was accomplished by overstretching by balloon inflation, the arteries no longer behave as truly elastic bodies, according to Hooke's law. Permanent deformation occurs and the artery will no longer resume its original size and shape. At what point this plastic deformation occurs is well known for various elastomers, but the problem is much more complex with arteries. This is due to the various components of the arterial wall, since elastic collagen and muscle fibers have different modules of elasticity. The yield point of these various components will therefore be reached at different levels of stress.

Once the muscle fibers are stretched, as demonstrated by the corkscrew deformity of their nuclei (Fig. 6), the artery no longer resumes its original size following deflation of the balloon, and a permanent widening occurs. It is likely that in clinical angioplasty this second stage of overstretching of the arterial wall has to be reached in order to yield beneficial results.

If the yield point of the elastic components of the media is exceeded, disruption of the media occurs, which corresponds to the third stage of the balloon dilatation of the arteries (Fig. 7 a,b). It is likely that the third stage of dilatation is commonly reached in clinical angioplasty, particularly if tight stenotic lesions are dilated.

The fourth stage of dilatation, which also causes rupture of the adventitia, occurs only with massive overstretching. This results in extravasation of blood and has so far not been described in clinical practice.

SUMMARY

1. Significant compression or redistribution of atherosclerotic plaques could not be demonstrated histologically following balloon angioplasty.
2. Atheromatous material is believed to be incompressible.
3. Balloon dilatation of postmortem arteries caused cracking and dehiscence of the intima and media.
4. The increased caliber of arteries following angioplasty is believed to be caused by the permanent overstretching of the media.
5. The angiographic appearance of dissection following angioplasty is believed to be due to a collection of contrast medium between the cracked intima and denuded media.
6. The basic mechanism of arterial angioplasty is believed to be a stretching of intima, media, and adventitia.
7. Stretching can occur without demonstrable histopathologic changes.
8. Increased stretching causes straightening of elastic fibers and a corkscrew deformity of the nuclei of smooth muscle cells.
9. Further stretching results in rupture of the intima and media.
10. Rupture of the intima and media results in permanent widening of arteries in normal dogs (observation time, four months).
11. Healing of the disrupted arterial layers occurs by the formation of a neointima and scar tissue similar to that which is formed following an endarterectomy.

REFERENCES

1. Dotter CT, Judkins MP: Transluminal treatment of arteriosclerotic obstruction. Description of a new technique and a preliminary report of its application. Circulation 30:654–670, Nov 1964
2. Velasquez G, Castaneda-Zuniga W, Formanek A, et al: Nonsurgical aortoplasty in Leriche syndrome. Radiology 134:359–360, Feb 1980
3. Dotter CT, Rösch J, Judkins MP: Transluminal dilatation of arteriosclerotic stenosis. Surg Gynecol Obstet 127:794–804, Oct 1968
4. Dotter CT, Rösch J, Anderson JM, et al: Transluminal iliac artery dilatation. Nonsurgical catheter treatment of atheromatous narrowing. JAMA 230:117–124, 7 Oct 1974
5. Dotter CT: Transluminal angioplasty. Pathologic basis. [In] Zeitler E, Grüntzig A, Schoop W, eds: Percutaneous Vascular Recanalization. New York, Springer-Verlag, 1978, pp 3–12
6. Grüntzig A: Percutaneous transluminal recanalization (PTR) with the double lumen dilatation catheter. [In] Zeitler E. Grüntzig A, Schoop W, eds: Percutaneous Vascular Recanalization. New York, Springer-Verlag, 1978, pp 17–23
7. Wierny L, Plass R, Porstmann W: Long-term results in 100 consecutive patients treated by transluminal angioplasty. Radiology 112:543–548, Sep 1974
8. van Andel GJ: Transluminal dilatation with separate Teflon catheters. [In] Zeitler E, Grüntzig A, Schoop W, eds: Percutaneous Vascular Recanalization. New York, Springer-Verlag, 1978, pp 13–16
9. Zeitler E, Schoop W, Zahnow W: The treatment of occlusive arterial disease by transluminal catheter angioplasty. Radiology 99:19–26, Apr 1971
10. Lue H, Grüntzig A: Histopathologic aspects of transluminal recanalization. [In] Zeitler E, Grüntzig A, Schoop W, eds: Percutaneous Vascular Recanalization. New York, Springer-Verlag, 1978, pp 39–50

Radiology Department
University of Minnesota Hospitals
420 Delaware Street, S.E.
Minneapolis, MN 55455

The Mechanism of Balloon Angioplasty.

John L. Bass, M.D.

Clinical effectiveness of balloon dilation angioplasty (BDA) in relieving vascular stenosis produced by atheromatous plaque in arteries was described in the 1960s and 1970s. The mechanism of relieving stenosis was proposed to be redistribution of atheromatous plaque. In 1980, Dr. Jesse Edwards' group of pathologists in the "Miller basement" in St. Paul, Minnesota, joined Dr. Kurt Amplatz's group of interventional radiologists to examine the mechanism by which BDA relieved atheromatous vascular stenosis. They chose two models to examine the pathology of balloon dilated arteries: cadaver atheromatous arteries, and a canine model of BDA. The studies showed that atheroma were undisturbed in contrast to the prevailing theory of remodeling plaque. Instead, luminal enlargement resulted from rupture of intima partially torn from the media, and damage and stretching of the vascular media. This explained the clinical observation that permanent enlargement and remodeling of the lumen continued after BDA.

The methods Edwards and Amplatz used to investigate the mechanism of intervention -- review of autopsy specimens and in an animal model -- served as guides to further investigations of BDA in congenital heart disease. The stenosis in congenitally narrowed arteries is very different from that of atherosclerosis. Pediatric cardiologists at the University of Minnesota studied the effect of BDA in pathologic material and animal models of coarctation and peripheral pulmonary artery stenosis.

In 1981, Lock and colleagues in freshly excised specimens of human coarctation of the aorta found that high balloon pressures were needed for successful dilatation and resulted in intimal and medial tears. In other studies, similar findings followed BDA for abdominal coarctation and subsequently in an animal model of juxtaductal coarctation. Only after careful evaluation of the anatomy and BDA effects in pathology specimens and animal models was BDA performed in infants.

Following similar studies in an animal model of bilateral pulmonary artery stenosis, BDA was used to treat congenital peripheral pulmonary artery stenosis in children. With the exception of significantly lower balloon pressures required to enlarge pulmonary artery stenosis, the protocol from the animal trial was effective.

Edwards' and Amplatz's groups had uncovered the mechanism of relieving acquired vascular stenosis. Their approaches pointed the direction for progress in evaluating the effectiveness of BDA: 1] examine the anatomy and pathology of the lesion to be treated, 2] develop an animal model to perfect technique and evaluate the effects of treatment, and 3] only then begin human trials. Careful attention to anatomic features of abnormalities before designing preclinical testing is critical. Failure of BDA may result when the animal model does not accurately mimic the human condition. The effectiveness of techniques is best developed in animal trials, not in a patient.

BDA continues to be used to dilate congenital and postoperative vascular narrowing's including coarctation of the aorta, branch pulmonary artery stenosis, systemic and pulmonary venous stenosis, and even aortic, mitral and pulmonary valve stenosis. Resistant lesions may require cutting balloons followed by traditional BDA. Compliant vascular lesions may additionally need stents to maintain the effect of BDA. For each new technique or method to be successful the anatomic features must be linked to the clinical use.

Perspectives

Editorial

The Autopsy: Do We Still Need It?

An index of quality of medical care in an institution has, in the past, been the autopsy rate of that institution. Currently, there is a disturbing decline in autopsy rates. This leads us to the question posed by the title of this editorial. Some would give an unqualified positive answer.

If others for whom the autopsy has peripheral or actual involvement were confronted by the question, the answer from many would be, "Yes" and, after a period of hesitation, "But." Such an answer might come from a clinician, a member of an accrediting agency, a medical administrator, a pathologist, and even a resident in pathology. It is to this group that this communication is directed.

Each has his own reason for the "But," and the process starts with the clinician. In a very short span of time, including that of the career of the undersigned, we have seen astonishing improvement in the quality of clinical diagnosis. This happy state has resulted from expansion and greater sophistication of tests in the broad field of clinical pathology and from development and upgrading of the various types of imaging.

The clinician may therefore explain his reservation primarily on the basis that the autopsy does not usually give him any new essential facts—no surprises. He may expand upon his reserved attitude by relating how reports of autopsies come to him so late that the details of the case, as he recalls them, have blurred with time. Additionally, in support of his attitude, he may indicate that the pathologist does not clearly answer those questions that he, the clinician, has about specific abnormalities in clinical tests and, in particular, about anatomic details as they relate to results of imaging tests or physical examination.

The permissive attitude of the accrediting agencies is hard for me to believe. It may be the case that, inasmuch as input into the policies of these groups is derived mainly from clinicians, the attitude of the agencies simply reflects the attitude of their component parts.

The medical administrator stands ready to support his medical staff while being conscious of costs. The autopsy is expensive to perform and it is non-revenue-producing. Thus, from declining autopsy rates the medical administrator gains satisfaction from savings without any suspicion cast upon him of attempting to manipulate the medical staff.

The reservation of the pathologist is derived from several sources. In the majority of hospitals in this country, both surgical pathology and autopsy pathology are grouped under anatomic pathology. Because autopsies come up at unpredictable times, the autopsy represents an incursion into an otherwise regulated schedule. Time and energy must be devoted to it, and if the clinician fails to attend, the effort of the pathologist is, to a great extent, a hollow exercise. The apparent lack of interest on the part of the clinician and the pressure of other requirements on the pathologist tend to delay the time when the clinician receives a copy of the report of autopsy. The clinician's reaction to the late report has a negative influence on him. It adds a compounding effect on the disinterest of the pathologist, and the vicious cycle continues.

In hospitals with residents, the resident's reservation about the autopsy is, in part, fostered by the disinterest of the staff of pathologists, and the reservation is furthered by the situation that when the resident performs the autopsy his usual companion is only the diener. The absence of a member of the pathology staff, and certainly of the clinician, is a common occurrence.

Without guidance and without sound appreciation of clinical medicine, the resident obediently takes the standard samples of each organ for histologic study, while running the chance of failing to uncover or describe in detail the specific features that may have been unanswered by or perplexing to the clinician.

A very important and practical point is that the resident who is preparing himself or herself for postresidency practice realizes that the talents of correct immediate diagnosis for patients in the operating room must be gained and the many facets of clinical pathology must be mastered. Thus, other areas command the resident's major interests, and the autopsy occupies a secondary position.

There is an appropriate response to each of the groups identified in the foregoing.

To the clinician who has reservations about the autopsy on the basis that the clinical tests performed upon his or her patients serve sufficiently well, it should be pointed out that the reliability of many of those tests is based on a foundation of earlier correlations with autopsies on many patients. To continue to compare findings obtained clinically with autopsy findings forms a firm basis for the identification of conditions as yet unrecognized and undescribed.

The lack of detail given the clinician by the pathologist is, in part, the result of the clinician's deficiency in communicating with the pathologist. Discussing unresolved clinical questions with the pathologist before the autopsy and, better still, the clinician's being present at the autopsy and relating unresolved problems or details are the substrates from which advances in knowledge to the clinical field come.

It should also be recognized that the fruits of the autopsy may, with proper planning, continue to be gathered long after a particular autopsy procedure has been completed. Specific questions as to anatomic details arise anew or change in concert with advances in the field. Verbal description may not with precision give answers that arise at some time after the autopsy, but adequately preserved pathologic material allows for details of observation that are in tune with questions posed by new diagnostic and therapeutic techniques.

The member of an accrediting team who knows the potential advantages of the autopsy will recognize simultaneously that one index of quality of care is the rate of autopsies performed and, inevitably connected with this, the quality of the autopsy.

The medical administrator who relishes the savings from low autopsy rates would be placed in an even better position from increasing occupancy based on the general recognition of high quality of care offered by his institution.

The pathologist is in excellent position not only to teach but to learn continuously on the basis of autopsies. The autopsy is part of clinical medicine. It would be ideal if it could be done by the clinician, but because of present-day routine, one person does the clinical part and another the autopsy. As a bridge to this gap, there should be close association between the clinician and the pathologist—so close that the pathologist is keenly aware of clinical phenomena and specific clinical events of the subject autopsied. Such teamwork or association depends on admixture of the efforts and thinking processes of both the clinician and the pathologist. It is not, in my opinion, an exaggeration to state that, over time, the quality of the autopsy is a measure of the quality of the clinician as a physician.

The resident in training must learn an almost overwhelming number of facts and methods. There is no gainsaying that the resident in pathology must become proficient in immediate diagnosis of surgical pathologic conditions and in the varied intricacies of clinical pathology. Nevertheless, he or she is in training to become a consultant and a close associate of the clinician. To this end, the resident in pathology needs the example and guidance of the pathology staff with whom he or she is in residence. As part of the training, the resident in pathology, to become an effective pathologist, should have some prior clinical training that includes responsibility for patient care. In this way he or she sets the stage for becoming an effective member of a clinician-pathologist team.

For those who have taken the trouble to read the foregoing and whose initial answer to the question posed included "But," it is my hope that at this point, at least for some, the answer will be a simple "Yes."

Jesse E. Edwards, M.D.
United Hospitals of St. Paul
St. Paul, Minnesota

The Autopsy:

Do We Still Need It?

Michael J. Ackerman, M.D., Ph.D.

Nearly 30 years ago, Dr. Edwards opined on the need for the autopsy and on the reasons/excuses why clinicians, administrators, pathologists and pathologists-in-training have said "Yes, but" when pressed on whether we still need them. Like most of Dr. Edwards' works, he was far ahead of his time with his insights on this issue. Like the Greek derivation itself, *autopsia* (*aut* = "self" and *opsis* = "site/ appearance,") Dr. Edwards saw with his own eyes the situation facing the autopsy. Unfortunately, few in the United States, and the Western World for that matter, heeded his admonition to simply say "Yes, the autopsy is still needed." Instead, the rates of autopsy continue to decline substantially. Less than a decade before his editorial, about half of all cases involving hospital deaths and approximately 20 percent of all deaths were subject to an autopsy. Now a decade into the new millennium, the same constituencies that were saying "yes, but" back then are in fact increasingly saying "no, why bother" as the autopsy rates have declined to only about 5 percent of all cases involving hospital deaths and less than 8.5 percent of all deaths. It seems that there is little need for *autopsia* (seeing with one's own eyes) any more.

Unfortunately, this is farthest from the truth. The same case for and benefits of an autopsy exist today as 30 years ago. However, as the "yes, buts" have carried the day, we now have a situation where we have to wonder just how good are the eyes doing the autopsy when it is performed. Nowhere is this more apparent than for the autopsy, the necropsy, the postmortem examination of the sudden unexplained death of a young person. Disturbingly, even in this setting, an autopsy is often not performed. When it is, the primary mandate to be satisfied by the coroner, pathologist, or medical examiner is "ruling out" bad behavior such as homicide or suicide. As long as it is deemed "natural causes," then case closed. Perhaps, because of the dwindling rates of autopsy, the eyes no longer see with precision and accuracy the clues that once emerged before the trained eyes of someone like Dr. Jesse Edwards. Instead, a touch of lymphocytic involvement is now signed out as myocarditis, slight peculiarities in the conduction system prompt a rendering of "fibrosis and apoptosis of the AV node," and a sliver of epicardial fat yields a postmortem rendering of arrhythmogenic right ventricular cardiomyopathy. Then, when one has the autopsy materials examined by another set of eyes, we learn a different story. Because we aren't accustomed to "autopsia" with regularity anymore, perhaps "cataracts" have blurred our pathological vision.

When it comes to the postmortem examination of sudden unexplained deaths, there should be no "Yes, buts." In fact, there should be no "If, Ands, or Buts about it." An autopsy should be performed. The eyes must have a look. But we need to ensure that the right eyes are staring at it, trained eyes, seeing eyes. These eyes must be able to see not only what is there but what lies hidden within the decedent's genetic code. Not only is an autopsy needed, but it is now time to fully usher in the molecular autopsy, i.e. postmortem genetic testing. To do so, the eyes that look for the cause must begin a new standard operating procedure and retain tissue in a DNA friendly fashion (blood in EDTA, blood spot card, or frozen liver, spleen, thymus, or heart) so that this newer way of *autopsia* can be performed.

Epilogue: The Pathologist

JESSE E. EDWARDS, MD

St. Paul, Minnesota

The pathologist writing an epilogue on postoperative pediatric cardiology reflects in an inverse way on the striking progress that has been made in this field. Mary Allen Engle and Joseph Perloff, who invited me to write this piece, suggested that I concentrate on personal experiences. Thus, I review some experiences of the past 35 years as a pathologist whose work involved the field of congenital heart disease. I shall concentrate on my own experiences and, in doing so, I shall not refer to the specific and significant contributions of others to our present knowledge of the pathology of congenital heart disease. Nevertheless, it would be inappropriate to omit the names of others who, during the period involved, have provided numerous additions to our understanding of the pathologic complexities of the area simply called congenital heart disease. Particular recognition should paid to Maurice Lev, whose work in the field antedates my own. Properly added to Lev's name are those of Richard Van Praagh, Robert Van Mierop, William Roberts, Jack Titus and Saroja Bharati.

In 1946, after almost 4 years of active duty as a pathologist in the Army during and after World War II, I was invited to join the Mayo Clinic staff. Here I found adequate material, a willingness of the institution to aid one in his work and, in particular, an accumulation of people from whom a team, without committee planning, naturally developed. I found those people involved in cardiovascular disease to be generous in sharing their special knowledge and skills with those in other subspecialties, recognizing that interchange of ideas is a stimulus for progress—progress to the point where the total effect is greater than the sum of its parts. Also, the time was ripe for progress.

Cardiac Surgery: Historical Background

When my story begins, the only two cardiac operations that had been done at the Mayo Clinic and in many other institutions were decortication for constrictive pericarditis and ligation of patent ductus arteriosus. Although the Blalock-Taussig operation had been introduced in 1944, two years earlier, this procedure had not yet been carried out at the Clinic. Cardiac catheterization as a clinical tool was yet to come, and open heart surgery was far beyond the horizon.

The driving force from which a team ultimately developed came from Howard Burchell, an established cardiologist with personal experience in both physiology and pathology. It was Burchell's capacity to speak the language of the basic scientists and his imagination and drive that served foremost to knit the fabric of a cardiovascular team. It was he who stimulated my interest in various correlations based on a pivot of pathology. Important were the many persons who showed me the relation between their specialty and pathology. Thus, Raymond Pruitt gave me some insight on the electrocardiographic manifestations of what I was seeing as a pathologist. Earl Wood exercised considerable patience in teaching me basic cardiovascular physiology by the technique of case by case review. The relation of symptoms and clinical findings to pathology was highlighted by James DuShane.

By 1955, when the first open heart operation was to be done, John Kirklin had availed himself of existing specimens bearing conditions that were to be subjects of operation. Such studies allowed for a close interpersonal association between us. They also led to a mutual understanding and, later, to fruitful analysis of postoperative cases when similar situations arose. I may add parenthetically for the young cardiovascular surgeon that time after time, as the surgical field was developing, Kirklin would review available pathologic specimens bearing the particular condition that he was to operate on for the first time. The time for such an experience by the young surgeon will, in my opinion, never pass.

Before programs of intracardiac surgery were established, it was thought that the development of a pump oxygenator would solve all difficulties. This proved not to be the case. Among the early problems were obstructive pulmonary vascular disease in ventricular septal defect and inadequate relief of pulmonary stenosis in tetralogy of Fallot. Analysis of these problems led to better selection of patients for closure of ven-

From the Department of Pathology, United Hospitals, St. Paul, Minnesota.

Address for reprints: Jesse E. Edwards, MD, Department of Pathology, United Hospitals, 330 North Smith Avenue, St. Paul, Minnesota 55102.

tricular septal defect and to gradual improvement in surgical techniques for relief of pulmonary stenosis. Surgical induction of complete heart block became infrequent as surgical techniques took applied anatomy into account.

As surgical results improved, a perplexing problem was still present, the "successful operation" with a dead patient. Sometimes, although the patient had undergone the surgical procedure without apparent complication, death occurred in the early days after operation. A striking phenomenon among many such patients was the observation at autopsy that the tracheobronchial system was obstructed by massive accumulations of secretions and death seemed to be of respiratory origin.

It became evident that the pump-oxygenator was not the only requirement; a unique type of complex postoperative care was also needed: The surgical procedure was a continuum from the operating room into the postoperative bed and beyond. Major credit is due John Kirklin for his vision and drive in setting up a special unit for postoperative cardiac surgical patients. Today, cardiac surgery without a postoperative intensive care unit would be unthinkable. In such units today specially trained personnel using appropriate equipment give full expression to the "successful operation."

It was my good fortune to be associated with two pioneer groups in the field of congenital heart disease. The second association occurred in 1960, when I moved to the University of Minnesota. I was cordially received by Richard Varco and C. Walton Lillehei, whose experience in open heart surgery antedated that of Kirklin by 1 year. The new setting provided a stimulating experience both with these surgical pioneers and with their clinical counterparts, Paul Adams and Raymond Anderson. These associations contributed additional ideas and created a vital laboratory to which young people interested in clinical pediatric cardiology came and continue to come in order to gain insight into abnormalities of the heart—both the anatomic states and their various clinical and surgical counterparts.

Present Problems Resulting From Cardiac Surgery

At the present time, over a quarter of a century after the establishment of standard methods for cardiopulmonary bypass, the pathologist has many fewer hearts with postoperative congenital heart disease to examine. But particular problems resulting from the surgical treatment of congenital heart disease remain. These include late death, the unsolved problems in the young infant and secondary changes in artificial conduits.

The late postoperative deaths include cases of sudden death from surgically induced complete heart block. Fortunately, this problem is less common today than in the first half of the period of open heart surgery. The problem of progression of pulmonary vascular disease has not been solved, but the evidence suggests that it may occur in patients with marginal pulmonary vascular disease who survive operation, such as closure of a large ventricular septal defect. This topic is discussed by William Friedman in this Symposium.[1]

The pathologist is often puzzled by the patient who dies suddenly after correction of an intracardiac malformation and many years of apparent health. In such cases one is led to wonder whether cardiac hypertrophy, which had been part of the basic condition, remained and served to underlie a ventricular arrhythmia, perhaps through focal myocardial ischemia. Careful analysis may give us insight into this unfortunate outcome.

A specific problem is the patient with complete transposition of the great arteries who has survived for some years after a Mustard repair or functionally similar operation. Troublesome problems remain in some of these patients. These include pulmonary venous hypertension, not universally established as resulting from postoperative stenosis of the pulmonary veins. The common matter of postoperative superior vena caval obstruction remains an enigma both as to its long-range effects and as to means of preventing this complication of the operation.

Although there has been noticeable improvement in the general management of the young infant, not all the problems have been solved. The respiratory tract still remains crucial, with compounding factors of effects of tracheal intubation, thoracotomy and, in those conditions with pulmonary hypertension, compression of bronchi by pulmonary arterial segments.

A specific challenge remains in the fairly common condition of persistent common atrioventricular canal. Surgical techniques are taxed by the great variations among these cases, variations such as the amount of ventricular septal deficiency, amount of available atrioventricular valve tissue, chordal insertion, size of defects, conduction system and associated pulmonary vascular disease.

The concepts and surgical competence of using conduits of man-made materials fall short of accomplishing the development of a healthy adult from a sick infant or child. Quite apart from the problem of lack of growth of such ducts, there is a more immediate problem, that of the common formation of a lining pannus that leads to obstruction of important lifelines. Dwight McGoon provides information on this topic in the symposium.[2]

Future Challenges

The future poses many challenges to all members of the cardiovascular team. Some of these challenges are identified by the troublesome and still unsolved operative sequelae and residua known to exist at the present time. The pathologist has a part to play in identification of areas for improvement and in making suggestions derived from his observations and concepts. Solutions will be made not only by persons now engaged in the field but also by those who are just entering the arena or have even not yet begun to be involved. These persons will introduce new thoughts and techniques. At the same time, they will need to know why currently successful techniques have developed from the trial and error of the past. They will be dealing with specific abnormalities in given anatomic structures. Therefore, it will behoove these people in their own professional development to learn anatomic facts, as did those who have or will have come before them. To teach these anatomic facts, the pathologist of the future stands as prepared and ready as did the pathologist of the past.

Progress of the past represented a composite result of teamwork. In the future, as established methods in pathology and physiology continue to be applied, and as new fields and techniques develop, the full impact and effect of those involved in the work will be enhanced if they are themselves part of a whole—a whole that one may call a team.

References

1. **Friedman, WF, Heiferman MF.** Clinical problems of postoperative pulmonary vascular disease. Am J Cardiol 1982;50:631–6.
2. **McGoon DC.** Long-term effects of prosthetic materials. Am J Cardiol 1982;50:621–30.

Reprinted from the September issue of **The American Journal of Cardiology.**
A Yorke Medical Journal. Published by Technical Publishing
Company, A Division of Dun-Donnelley Publishing Corporation,
a Dun & Bradstreet Co., 875 Third Avenue, New York, N.Y., 10022.
Copyright 1982. All rights reserved. Printed in the U.S.A.

Epilogue:

The Pathologist

Brooks S. Edwards, M.D.

"Progress of the past represented a composite result of teamwork. In the future, as established methods in pathology and physiology continue to be applied, and as new fields and techniques develop, the full impact and the effect of those involved in the work will be enhanced if they are themselves part of a whole--a whole that one may call a team."

These words, which my father wrote in 1982 as part of an essay entitled "Epilogue: The Pathologist," ring true today perhaps even more strongly than they did when he penned them almost thirty years ago. This short essay provides an interesting window into my father's career and shows a strategy for life and work as relevant today as ever, a strategy that allowed in part for both my father's success and satisfaction in life.

Long before the field of organizational psychology started using terms like "integrated multispecialty approach," my Dad saw the value, and promoted the development of a team approach. His essay articulates the fundamental concept that we are stronger and more effective as a team than as individuals.

When my father arrived at Mayo Clinic in 1946, he was hired as a cancer pathologist and officed among his pathology colleagues, removed from the core of the clinical practice. With the wisdom and blessing of his chief Dr. James Kernahan, a neuropathologist, Dad started to dabble with some old cardiac specimens that had been tucked away in a corner in the pathology department.

The developing field of cardiac surgery was on the horizon, and Dad recognized that those old formalin-fixed specimens might hold one of the necessary keys to help move the fields of cardiology and cardiac surgery forward. He also realized that his contributions would be more valuable if he worked with clinicians to better understand their challenges and needs. Today we might call it a "gap analysis," but back then Dad just looked upon it as an opportunity to help piece together a puzzle.

Dad quickly found an intellectual soul mate in the person of Dr. Howard Burchell, a dedicated clinician and cardiologist (before the term was used) with prior training in classical pathology. Dad reasoned that if he was to provide valuable service as a pathologist, he needed to better understand the clinical issues Dr. Burchell and his colleagues faced everyday. In spite of his appointment as a staff pathologist, Dad arranged to spend several months back on the hospital wards with Dr. Burchell, admitting new patients and carrying on daily rounds. A second internship if you will.

During this time, the other young men (all were under 40 years of age at the time) who would develop the field of cardiac surgery were coming together at Mayo Clinic. Dr. Earl Wood was a physiologist whose lab would focus on cardiac catherization, and Dr. John Kirklin would become the first cardiac surgeon at Mayo Clinic (when no such specialty existed) and a true pioneer in the field.

Without any official appointment or designation, the four of them--Kirklin, Wood, Burchell and my father--would get together to dream, discuss and plan what the fields of cardiology and cardiac surgery could become. Without any fanfare, the team was born. Additional members would later include pediatricians, anesthesiologists, radiologists and dedicated nurses. What made this team special, and what made my father a life-long believer in the team approach, was the shared vision, the mutual respect and the absence of ego. Each member brought special talents and training, and each member believed the words of Will Mayo: "The best interest of the patient is the only interest to be considered, and in order that the sick may have the benefit of advancing knowledge, a union of forces is necessary."

Throughout Dad's long career, the principals of collaboration and "teamwork" served to guide him. Most of his more than 800 multi-authored publications have two or three unique specialties represented in the authorship. This was not just gratuitous authorship on Dad's part, this was the "union of forces" that Dad believed in so strongly. For Dad, the whole was always greater than the sum of the parts, and individuals with unique training and perspective could enhance a study and strengthen a paper. It was never about competition but always about collaboration.

After Dad left Mayo Clinic in 1960, he found new collaborators in the Twin Cities. These individuals--including Jim Moller, Kurt Amplatz, Bob Benassi, Russ Lucas, Walt Lillehei, Demetre Nicoloff and Ken Jue, just to name a few--continued the tradition that began in Rochester now more then sixty years ago. These pioneers not only enhanced the science and made major contributions in their own right, they enhanced my father's life. Dad never constructed barriers between work and play. Fellows became collaborators, and collaborators became friends. All other distinctions were invisible to Dad.

In closing, I would like to recognize the one additional and most important collaborator and teammate in my father's life--my mother Marjorie Edwards. Throughout more than fifty-five years of marriage the two of them approached every day as an opportunity to do good. They were the ultimate team and for that, and so many other gifts, I remain grateful everyday.

Final Thoughts

Brooks S. Edwards, M.D.

"A teacher affects eternity; he can never tell where his influence stops"

That's how my dad began the 1956 Conner Lecture at the Annual Meeting of the American Heart Association. At that time, Dad applied those words to Dr. Lewis Conner, but today even more so, they apply to my father. A teacher affects eternity...and as this collection of reprints and commentaries demonstrate, Dad's influence continues to be felt throughout the world of adult and congenital heart disease. With the occasion of what would have been my father's 100th birthday, this book celebrates and acknowledges his years of wisdom, teaching and sharing.

My father loved to teach, and while he was an invited lecturer around the world, he most enjoyed the "show and tell" sessions, first at Mayo Clinic and later in the Twin Cities. Whether in the Miller basement surrounded by his adoring fellows or on his Thursday "rounds" at the University of Minnesota, Hennepin County or Ramsey County Hospitals and the Minneapolis VA, he gave freely of his time to share his knowledge, to ensure that someone would learn something from every specimen he held in his hand.

My father was a child of the Depression, and as such he didn't believe in wasting anything, especially something as precious as a human heart or, for that matter, a teachable moment that could come from that heart. In a way, this book is intended to carry on that philosophy. Many of the papers reprinted here are decades old, and in our "what have you done for me lately" world they could be easily lost or forgotten. However, their importance and relevance is as fresh today as when they were written. The clarity of his writing, the importance of focused and compelling illustrations and the message that understanding the functional pathology remains as critical today as ever, make this book relevant to a new generation of cardiac specialists. By republishing these papers with the beautiful and thoughtful commentaries, many written by Dad's former students and colleagues, it is our hope that cardiovascular experts will be introduced (or reintroduced) to some of these important manuscripts.

Dr. James H. Moller has been the driving force behind this book. Not only has Jim worked tirelessly to see this project successfully completed, more importantly he has been an ardent supporter of the *Jesse E. Edwards Registry of Cardiovascular Disease* since his fellowship days. Jim's advocacy for study of applied pathology in general, and the Edwards Registry in particular, has been steadfast through his time as Chairman of Pediatrics at the University of Minnesota, during his tenure as president of the American Heart Association and now back as a Senior Clinical Consultant and teacher in the Registry. Above all else, my father would point out, Jim has been a true and loyal friend to all of us.

Steven Korn, our publisher, has been far more than just a publisher providing encouragement, experience and support for this project and previous book projects. Steven's dedication to the importance of high quality publications serves to guide and inspire all of us. His integrity and commitment to quality in the midst of a bottom-line focused world should be a role model for the publishing industry.

Robert Benassi worked alongside Dad for

more than 40 years, making clear and instructive illustrations of many complex lesions, ensuring the reader could both understand and visualize the important functional anatomy. Bob has done many of the illustrations reprinted in this book. He had a special ability to transform my father's rough sketch (sometimes done on the back of an envelope) into a masterpiece telling a complex story in a clear and focused manner. Beyond that, Bob's friendship and support for my father never waived, and his friendship is something we all value greatly.

No epilogue would be complete without recognizing the critically important role my mother Marjorie Edwards played in the creation of all these manuscripts. While not a physician or scientist, her contribution to this body of work is equal to all the specialists who collaborated with Dad. She created the environment that not only allowed my father to be productive, but she encouraged him to remain active well into his 90s. Her drive and his natural abilities created a winning team that resulted in this body of work. Her support of this current project is an extension of a lifetime commitment to my father's passion and talents.

Finally, my father would want me to emphasize the importance of his many students and colleagues whose questioning and inquisitive minds inspired and challenged him over the years. It is our hope that this book will not simply be viewed as a historical account, but rather will serve to inspire the reader that lesions once thought "untreatable" just a generation ago are now often easily and successfully approached with new medical, surgical and percutaneous strategies. While great progress has been made, far more is needed, and we hope the lessons of the past will serve to stimulate the advancements of the future.

Permissions Granted By

This article was published in Medical Clinics of North America, July 1948, Edwards JE: Anomalies of the derivatives of the aortic arch system, pp 925-949, © Elsevier, 1948.

Edwards JE, Clagett OT, Drake RL, Christensen NA: The collateral circulation in coarctation of the aorta. Proc Mayo Clin 23: 333-339 (July 21) 1948.
Reproduced with permission
© July 21, 1948 Mayo Clinic Proceedings

This article was published in Surgical Clinics of North America, August 1949, Collett RW, Edwards JE: Persistent truncus: A classification according to anatomic types, pp 1245-1270, © Elsevier, 1949.

Edwards JE, Helmholz HF Jr: A classification of total anomalous pulmonary venous connection based on developmental considerations. Proc Mayo Clin 31: 151-160 (Mar 21) 1956.
Reproduced with permission
© March 21, 1956, Mayo Clinic Proceedings

Edwards JE: The Lewis A. Conner Memorial Lecture. Functional pathology of the pulmonary vascular tree in congenital cardiac disease.
Reproduced with permission:
Circulation 1957;15:164-196
© 1957 American Heart Association, Inc.

Edwards JE, Burchell HB: Pathologic anatomy of mitral insufficiency. Proc Mayo Clin 33: 497-509 (Oct 15) 1958 (330)
Reproduced with permission
© October 15, 1958, Mayo Clinic Proceedings

Heath D, Edwards JE: The pathology of hypertensive pulmonary vascular disease. A description of six grades of structural changes in the pulmonary arteries with special reference to congenital cardiac septal defect.
Reproduced with permission
Circulation 1958;18:533-547
© 1958 American Heart Association, Inc.

Neufeld HN, DuShane JW, Wood EH, Kirklin JW, Edwards JE: Origin of both great vessels from the right ventricle. I. Without pulmonary stenosis.
Reproduced with permission
Circulation 1961;23:399-412
© 1961 American Heart Association

Edwards JE: The congenital bicuspid aortic valve.
Reproduced with permission
Circulation 1961;23:485-488
© 1961 American Heart Association, Inc.

Neufeld HN, DuShane JW, Edwards JE: Origin of both great vessels from the right ventricle. II. With pulmonary stenosis.
Reproduced with permission
Circulation 1961;23:603-612
© 1961 American Heart Association, Inc.

This article was published in American Journal of Cardiology, Volume 11, Shone JD, Sellers RD, Anderson RC, Adams P Jr, Lillehei CW, Edwards JE: The developmental complex of "parachute mitral valve", supravalvular ring of left atrium, subaortic stenosis, and coarctation of aorta, pp 714-725. © Elsevier 1963.

Titus JL, Daugherty GW, Kirklin JW, Edwards JE: Lesions of the atrioventricular conduction system after repair of ventricular septal defect. Relation to heart block.

Reproduced with permission
Circulation 1963;36:28:82-88
© 1963 American Heart Association, Inc.

Titus JL, Daugherty GW, Edwards JE: Anatomy of the atrioventricular conduction system in ventricular septal defect.

Reproduced with permission
Circulation 1963;36:28:82-88
© 1963 American Heart Association, Inc.

Raghib G, Ruttenberg HD, Anderson RC, Amplatz K, Adams P Jr, Edwards JE: Termination of left superior vena cava in left atrium, atrial septal defect, and absence of coronary sinus. A developmental complex.

Reproduced with permission
Circulation 1965;31:906-918
©1965 American Heart Association, Inc.

This article was published in American Journal of Cardiology, Volume 17, Elliott LP, Amplatz K, Edwards JE: Coronary arterial patterns in transposition complexes. Anatomic and angiocardiographic studies, pp 362-378, © Elsevier, 1966.

Moller JH, Nakib A, Anderson RC, Edwards JE: Congenital cardiac disease associated with polysplenia. A developmental complex of bilateral "left-sidedness".

Reproduced with permission
Circulation 1967;36:789-799
© 1967 American Heart Association, Inc.

Stanger P, Benassi RC, Korns ME, Jue KL, Edwards JE: Diagrammatic portrayal of variations in cardiac structure. Reference to transposition, dextrocardia and the concept of four normal hearts.

Reproduced with permission
Circulation 1968;37 and 38(Suppl IV):1-16
© 1968 American Heart Association, Inc.

Edwards JE: Atherosclerosis: An impossible mission?

Reproduced with permission
Circulation 1969;39:271-274
© 1969 American Heart Association, Inc.

This article was published in American Heart Journal, Volume 77, Grondin CM, Steinberg CL, Edwards JE: Dissecting aneurysm complicating Marfan's syndrome (arachnodactyly) in a mother and son, pp 301-306, © Elsevier, 1969.

Becker AE, Becker MJ, Edwards JE: Pathologic spectrum of dysplasia of the tricuspid valve. Features in common with Ebstein's malformation. Arch Path 91: 167-178 (Feb), 1971.

Reproduced with permission
© 1971 American Medical Association. All rights reserved.

Vlodaver Z, Edwards JE: Pathologic changes in aortic-coronary arterial saphenous vein grafts.

Reproduced with permission
Circulation 1971;44:719-728.
© 1971 American Heart Association, Inc.

This article was published in American Journal of Cardiology, Volume 41, Maron BJ, Roberts WC, Edwards JE, McAllister HA Jr, Foley DD, Epstein SE: Sudden death in patients with hypertrophic cardiomyopathy: Characterization of 26 patients without functional limitation, pp 803-810, © Elsevier 1978.

Castaneda-Zuniga WR, Formanek A, Tadavarthy M, Vlodaver Z, Edwards JE, Zollikofer C, Amplatz K: The mechanism of balloon angioplasty. Radiology 135: 565-571 (June) 1980.

Reproduced with permission
© The Radiological Society of North America (RNSA®).

Edwards JE: The autopsy: Do we still need it? Mayo Clin Proc 56: 457-458 (July), 1981.

Reproduced with permission
© July 1981 Mayo Clinic Proceedings.

This article was published in American Journal of Cardiology, Volume 50, Edwards, JE: Epilogue: The Pathologist, pp 652-654, © Elsevier 1982.

Chesler E, King RA, Edwards JE: The myxomatous mitral valve and sudden death.
Reproduced with permission
Circulation 1983;67:632-639.
© 1983 American Heart Association, Inc.

This article was published in American Journal of Cardiology, Volume 54, Edwards BS, Edwards WD, Edwards JE: Ventricular septal rupture complicating acute myocardial infarction: Identification of simple and complex types in 53 autopsied hearts, pp 1201-1205, © Elsevier 1985.